Fundamentals of Family Medicine

Springer
New York
Berlin
Heidelberg
Barcelona
Budapest
Hong Kong
London
Milan
Paris
Tokyo

ROBERT B. TAYLOR

Editor

Fundamentals of Family Medicine

Associate Editors

ALAN K. DAVID   THOMAS A. JOHNSON, JR.
D. MELESSA PHILLIPS   JOSEPH E. SCHERGER

With 30 Illustrations

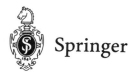 Springer

Robert B. Taylor, M.D.
Professor and Chairman
Department of Family Medicine
Oregon Health Sciences University
School of Medicine
Portland, OR 97201 USA

Alan K. David, M.D.
The Fred Lazarus Jr. Professor and Director
Department of Family Medicine
University of Cincinnati College of Medicine
Cincinnati, OH 45267 USA

Thomas A. Johnson, Jr., M.D.
Chairman
Department of Family Medicine
St. John's Mercy Medical Center
St. Louis, MO 63141 USA

D. Melessa Philips, M.D.
Professor and Chairman
Department of Family Medicine
University of Mississippi School of Medicine
Jackson, MS 39216 USA

Joseph E. Scherger, M.D., M.P.H.
Vice President
Family Practice and Primary Care Education
Sharp HealthCare
San Diego, CA 92123 USA

Library of Congress Cataloging in Publication Data

Fundamentals of family medicine / [edited by] Robert B. Taylor
     p.   cm.
    Includes selected chapters from the 4th ed. of Family medicine: principles and practice.
    Includes bibliographical references and index.
    ISBN 0-387-94448-6 (softcover: alk. paper)
    1. Family medicine. II. Taylor, Robert B. II. Family medicine.
    [DNLM: 1. Family Practice. 2. Primary Health Care. 3. Education, Medical. WB 110 F981]
    RC46.F945   1995
    616—dc20
    DNLM/DLC
    for Library of Congress   95-1788

Printed on acid-free paper.

Production managed by Princeton Editorial Associates and supervised by Theresa Kornak; manufacturing supervised by Jeffrey Taub.
Typeset by Princeton Editorial Associates, Princeton, NJ.
Printed and bound by Hamilton Printing Co., Rensselaer, NY.
Printed in the United States of America.

9 8 7 6 5 4 3 2 1

ISBN 0-387-94448-6 Springer-Verlag New York Berlin Heidelberg

To medical students choosing Family Practice and other generalist careers

Who value continuity in the care of patients

Who seek diversity of experience and can be comfortable with ambiguity

Who believe that service is still the reason for being a physician

This book is dedicated.

Preface

Fundamentals of Family Medicine has a focused purpose: to be the course text for family medicine/primary care clerkships in medical schools. The book is intended to present common problems in generalist practice, to explain the process by which family physicians provide high-quality comprehensive and continuing care to patients, and to serve as the basis for small group discussions by faculty and students.

The factual content in the book consists of selected chapters from the fourth edition of *Family Medicine: Principles and Practice;* all chapters have been updated by the authors. I selected chapters based on the philosophy of the generalist curriculum: "patient-, not discipline-centered and community-, not hospital based."[1] The principal diagnoses recorded on office visits in the National Ambulatory Medical Care Survey are covered as they apply to generalist practice (see Chapter 1, Table 1.1). I also looked ahead to the generalist physician's residency training, including the broad competencies necessary for primary care practice.[2] The book covers five types of topics: *common acute problems* such as otitis media, *common chronic problems* including diabetes mellitus and hypertension, *"must-never-miss" problems* such as myocardial infarction, *changing problems* that represent current areas of investigation such as human immunodeficiency virus disease, and *emerging areas of emphasis in family medicine* such as geriatric care, sports medicine, and domestic violence. Selection has also been influenced by problems recorded in the Oregon Health Sciences University Family Health Centers in Portland and by the patients seen by students in the family medicine clerkship over the past seven years.

The key to understanding family practice is the *process*—how the family physician can define, prioritize, and manage the diverse problems of many patients in time-limited visits. The *how* is the generalist approach, described in Chapter 1. This approach, which emphasizes patient-centered concepts and high-payoff inquiries, is reinforced through the case presentations and related discussion questions that follow each chapter. The patients in the 26 cases are all members of one extended family, allowing the reader a sense of continuity of care and awareness of the effects of illness ⌐

various family members. The Nelson family and the case presentations are explained in Notes for the Reader.

I appreciate the contributions of the authors and the four associate editors: Alan David, Lessa Phillips, Tom Johnson, and Joe Scherger. All the editors and all the primary authors of chapters are family physicians. Special recognition is due Anita D. Taylor, M.A. Ed., for sharing her expertise in medical student education. I also thank Coelleda O'Neil and Laurie Charron of Oregon Health Sciences University for their assistance in manuscript preparation.

In preparing this book, I have spoken with many medical students and family medicine educators, and some of their ideas are reflected in the pages that follow. I continue to encourage suggestions from readers in North America and around the world.

Robert B. Taylor, M.D.
Portland, Oregon, USA

References

1. Noble J, Bithoney W, MacDonald P, et al. The core content of a generalist curriculum for general internal medicine, family practice, and pediatrics. J Gen Intern Med 1994;9(Suppl1):S31–S42.
2. Rivo ML, Saultz JW, Wartman SA, DeWitt TG. Defining the generalist physician's training. JAMA 1994;271:1499–504.

Contents

Notes for the Reader

To the Student

Your time on the family medicine/primary care clerkship may be the most important of all in medical school.[1] Here you will encounter concepts that will shape your future patient care—whether or not you choose a generalist speciality as a career: concepts such as personal care, longitudinal care, the meaning of illness, and the investment of self in the therapeutic relationship. This book presents these and other principles of generalist health care plus factual data regarding selected clinical problems, supplemented by case presentations that involve members of a single family.

The discussion questions are not intended to be post-tests of the factual content of each chapter and the answers to some questions may not actually be in the chapter, but in your own reasoning abilities and personal experiences. The questions are designed to stimulate thought about the issues, encourage discussion, and even inspire a quest for more information.

To the Faculty

This book, intended to be a single source text for your clerkship, has been prepared to meet the General Guidelines for a Third-Year Family Medicine Clerkship as developed by the Society of Teachers of Family Medicine (Table 1).[1] The 26 clinical chapters present a broad spectrum of family practice problems. The case presentations and questions that follow each chapter are intended to be the basis of small group discussions, including both traditional questions about medical history, physical examination, diagnosis, and management, as well as psychosocial issues such as the reason for the visit, the impact of illness on the family, the patient's adaptation to illness, and the resources used in management. The case discussions have been "field-tested" with third-year medical students, and they work. Try them.

TABLE 1. General guidelines for a third-year family medicine clerkship

By the completion of a third-year family medicine clerkship, the medical student is expected to possess, at a level appropriate for a third-year student, the knowledge, attitudes, and skills needed to:

1. Provide personal care for individuals and families as the physician of first contact and continuing care in health as well as in illness
2. Assess and manage acute and chronic medical problems frequently encountered in the community
3. Provide anticipatory health care using education, risk reduction, and health enhancement strategies
4. Provide continuous as well as episodic health care, not limited by a specific disease, patient characteristics, or setting of the patient encounter
5. Provide and coordinate comprehensive care of complex and severe problems using biomedical, social, personal, economic, and community resources, including consultation and referral
6. Establish effective physician–patient relationships by using appropriate interpersonal communication skills to provide quality health care

Source: Working Committee to Develop Curricular Guidelines for a Third-Year Family Medicine Clerkship. Curricular Guidelines for a Third-Year Family Medicine Clerkship. Kansas City, MO: The Society of Teachers of Family Medicine. With permission.

About the Case Discussions in this Book: The Nelson Family

Each chapter is followed by a case presentation with discussion questions, all involving members of a single extended family: the Nelsons. The Nelson family genogram is shown in Figure 1. During a period of 12 months, various members of the Nelson family come to the office for care, some making two or three visits during the year. The reader will find that the problems of various family members are interconnected and that they evolve over time.

The following introduces the four-generation Nelson family, some of whom have been your patients for more than a decade and who look to you as their personal physician. You and your patients live in a community of 40,000 people.

Harold and Mary Nelson

The senior family members are Harold and Mary Nelson, both in their 70s. Harold Nelson retired from his job as a welder at age 61. He now leads a quiet life and seldom leaves the house. He has had type 2 diabetes mellitus for 24 years and osteoarthritis of the hands for 20 years, both of which were considerations in his early retirement.

Mary Nelson, aged 71, is a retired nursery school teacher. She has been hypertensive, taking medication, for 10 years. Also, she has episodes of

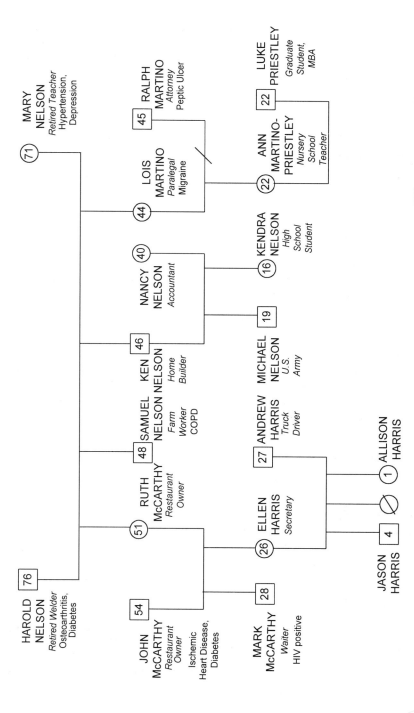

Nelson family genogram: family members, occupations, chronic health problems. Symbols used: ⬚76⬚, male, age 76; Ⓐ71, female, age 71; ⬚, marriage; ⟋, divorce; ⊘, deceased.

depression that require treatment. She wishes that she and Harold were "doing more" in their retirement and worries about what will happen to their son Samuel when they die.

Harold and Mary Nelson have four children: Ruth, Samuel, Ken, and Lois—all in their 40s and 50s.

John and Ruth McCarthy

Ruth, the oldest Nelson daughter, is married to John McCarthy. Together they own and operate a small delicatessen-style restaurant. Their restaurant business struggles financially, and Ruth and John sometimes seek "loans" from her parents during lean times. Both work long hours in the restaurant. Ruth enjoys good health, but John has coronary artery disease with angina pectoris for which he had been treated by an internist who retired recently, and John has decided to transfer his care to you.

John and Ruth McCarthy have two children. Their oldest son is Mark, aged 28, who dropped out of college to organize a rock group that disbanded about 2 years ago. Mark now works as a waiter in his parents' restaurant. John and Ruth openly disapprove of Mark's life style, which includes cigarette smoking, marijuana use, and many sexual contacts. Recently, Mark was found to be human immunodeficiency virus (HIV)-positive.

The McCarthys' second child is Ellen, aged 26, who works as a secretary in a business office. Ellen is married to Andrew Harris, a truck driver who is on the road a good deal of the time. Ellen and Andrew Harris have two children: Jason, aged 4, and Allison, aged 1. A third child, who would have been 3 years old this year, died in infancy of meningitis.

Samuel Nelson

Samuel Nelson, aged 48, is the second child of Harold and Mary Nelson. Samuel was a high school dropout at age 16 when he began work at a nearby orchard. Today, he lives with his parents and has no close friends. He has kept the same job as a farm worker for 32 years and spends his spare time watching television. Samuel has been a heavy smoker since his teens and now has chronic obstructive pulmonary disease.

Ken and Nancy Nelson

The third son is Kenneth Nelson, aged 46, who works as a contractor, building new homes in middle-class neighborhoods. Ken is married to Nancy, who has an accounting degree and works part-time for a public accounting firm. Nancy has always described herself as "nervous," which has limited her ability to take a full-time job.

Ken and Nancy Nelson have two children. The oldest is Michael Nelson, aged 19, a U.S. Army paratrooper stationed at Fort Bragg, North Carolina. Still living at home is their 16-year-old daughter, Kendra, a high school sophomore. Kendra is an above-average student and a varsity athlete. She has had her first serious relationship with a boyfriend for the past year.

Lois and Ralph Martino

The fourth child is Lois, aged 44, who has training as a paralegal and works in a large law firm. Ten years ago, Lois separated from her husband, Ralph Martino, an attorney previously employed in the same law firm as Lois and now in solo practice. Although Ralph's relationship with Lois and the Nelson family is strained, he has continued to consider you his personal physician.

Lois and Ralph have one child, Ann, aged 22, who works mornings as a nursery school teacher. A year ago, Ann married Luke Priestley, a graduate student now working on his Masters of Business Administration degree. Ann's parents secretly worry about Ann's marriage because Luke seems very distant and moody.

Reference

1. Senf JH, Campos-Outcalt D. The effect of a required third-year family medicine clerkship on medical students' attitudes: value indoctrination and value clarification. Acad Med 1995;70:142–8.

Contributors

Alan M. Adelman, M.D., M.S., Associate Professor of Family and Community Medicine, The Milton S. Hershey Medical Center, Pennsylvania State University, Hershey, PA 17033.

Bruce Ambuel, Ph.D., Assistant Professor of Family Medicine, Medical College of Wisconsin, Milwaukee, WI 53226.

Elizabeth E. Brownell, M.D., Private Practice, Waukesha, WI 53188.

Stephen A. Brunton, M.D., Clinical Professor of Family Medicine, University of California-Irvine, Orange, CA, and Director of Family Residency Program, Long Beach Memorial Medical Center, Long Beach, CA 90806.

Walter L. Calmbach, M.D., Assistant Professor of Family Practice, University of Texas Health Science Center, San Antonio, TX 78284-7795.

Elise M. Coletta, M.D., Assistant Professor of Family Medicine, Brown University School of Medicine, Providence, RI 02912, and Family Practice Residency, Memorial Hospital of Rhode Island, Pawtucket, RI 02860.

Rita K. Edwards, Pharm.D., Assistant Clinical Professor of Family Medicine, University of California-Irvine, School of Medicine, Orange, CA, and Family Practice Residency, Long Beach Memorial Medical Center, Long Beach, CA 90806.

M. Patrice Eiff, M.D., Assistant Professor of Family Medicine, Oregon Health Sciences University, School of Medicine, Portland, OR 97201.

Scott A. Fields, M.D., Assistant Professor of Family Medicine, Oregon Health Sciences University, School of Medicine, Portland, OR 97201.

Valerie J. Gilchrist, M.D., Professor of Family Medicine, Northeastern Ohio Universities College of Medicine, Rootstown, OH, and Associate Program Director, Aultman Hospital Family Practice Program, Canton, OH 44710.

Rupert R. Goetz, M.D., Assistant Professor of Family Medicine and Psychiatry, Oregon Health Sciences University, School of Medicine, Portland, OR 97201.

Ronald H. Goldschmidt, M.D., Professor and Vice Chair of Family and Community Medicine, University of California-San Francisco School of Medicine, San Francisco, CA, and Director, Family Practice Inpatient Service, San Francisco General Hospital, San Francisco, CA 94110.

Geoffrey Goldsmith, M.D., M.P.H., Professor and Chairman, Department of Family and Community Medicine, University of Arkansas College of Medicine, Little Rock, AR 72205-7199.

Melinda Strouse Graham, M.Ed., Aultman Hospital, Canton, OH 44710.

Frank A. Hale, Ph.D., Professor of Clinical Family and Community Medicine, University of Arizona College of Medicine, Tucson, AZ 85724.

Daniel E. Halm, M.D., Assistant Professor of Family Medicine, Department of Family Practice, University of Nebraska Medical Center, Omaha, NE 68198-3075.

Larry W. Johnson, M.D., Associate Professor of Family Medicine, Medical College of Ohio, Toledo, OH 43699.

David A. Katerndahl, M.D., Associate Professor of Family Practice, University of Texas Health Science Center, San Antonio, TX 78284-7795.

George L. Kirkpatrick, M.D., Associate Professor of Family Practice, University of South Alabama, Mobile, AL 36604.

Evan W. Kligman, M.D., Associate Professor and Head, Department of Family and Community Medicine, University of Arizona College of Medicine, Tucson, AZ 85724.

Richard B. Lewan, M.D., Associate Professor of Family Medicine, Medical College of Wisconsin, Milwaukee, WI 53226.

Timothy R. Malloy, M.D., Assistant Professor of Family Medicine, Department of Family Practice, University of Nebraska Medical Center, Omaha, NE 68198-3075.

John B. Murphy, M.D., Associate Professor of Family Medicine, Brown University School of Medicine, Providence, RI 02912, and Residency Director, Brown University, Department of Family Medicine, Pawtucket, RI 02860.

Sandra B. Nichols, M.D., Director, Arkansas Department of Health, Little Rock, AR 72205-7199.

Jim Nuovo, M.D., Assistant Professor of Family Medicine, University of California School of Medicine, Davis, CA, and Director, Family Practice Residency, University of California-Davis Medical Center, Sacramento, CA 95817.

Judith A. Pauwels, M.D., Private Practice, Saint Croix Falls, WI 54024.

Barbara D. Reed, M.D., M.S.P.H., Associate Professor of Family Practice, University of Michigan School of Medicine, Ann Arbor, MI 48109-0708.

James P. Richardson, M.D., Associate Professor of Family Medicine, Division of Geriatric Medicine, University of Maryland, School of Medicine, Baltimore, MD 21201-1509.

Jo Ann Rosenfeld, M.D., Associate Professor of Family Medicine, East Tennessee State University School of Medicine, Bristol, TN 37620.

Joseph E. Scherger, M.D., M.P.H., Vice President, Family Practice and Primary Care Education, Sharp HealthCare, San Diego, CA 92123.

John P. Sheehan, M.D., Assistant Professor of Medicine, Case Western Reserve University School of Medicine, Cleveland, OH 44106-4901.

Henry F. Simmons, M.D., Ph.D., Associate Professor of Emergency Medicine, University of Arkansas College of Medicine, Little Rock, AR 72205-7199.

Charles Kent Smith, M.D., Professor and Chairman, Department of Family Medicine, Case Western Reserve University School of Medicine, Cleveland, OH 44106-4901.

George F. Snell, M.D., formerly Associate Professor of Family and Preventive Medicine, University of Utah College of Medicine, Salt Lake City, UT 84102, and Director, Family Practice Residency Program, McKay Dee Hospital, Ogden, UT 84403; currently Philippines Bacolod Mission, Bacolod City, Philippines.

Jeffrey L. Susman, M.D., Associate Professor of Family Practice, University of Nebraska Medical Center, Omaha, NE 68198-3075.

Robert B. Taylor, M.D., Professor and Chairman, Department of Family Medicine, Oregon Health Sciences University, School of Medicine, Portland, OR 97201.

William L. Toffler, M.D., Associate Professor of Family Medicine, Oregon Health Sciences University, School of Medicine, Portland, OR 97201.

Joseph L. Torres, M.D., Private Practice, Kissimmee, FL 34743.

Margaret M. Ulchaker, M.S.N., R.N., C.D.E., Clinical Instructor, Manager-Diabetes Program, Department of Medicine, Case Western Reserve University School of Medicine, Cleveland, OH 44106-4901.

Daniel J. Van Durme, M.D., Clinical Assistant Professor of Family Medicine, University of South Florida, College of Medicine, Tampa, FL 33612.

Anne D. Walling, M.D., Professor and Vice Chairman, Department of Family and Community Medicine, University of Kansas-Wichita, School of Medicine, Wichita, KS 67214.

Howard Weinberg, M.D., Staff Physician, Sentara Norfolk and Leigh Hospitals, Norfolk, VA 23452.

Mary A. Willard, M.D., Director, Family Practice Residency, West Jersey Health System, West Jersey Family Practice Residency, Voorhees, NJ 08043.

1
Principles of Generalist Health Care

ROBERT B. TAYLOR

This first chapter in the book is about caring for *patients*—as distinct from diseases or organs—and the generalists who provide personal health care. It is about the baby with a fever, the teenager with concerns about sexually transmitted disease, the laborer with back pain, and the manager with heartburn. It is about home visits to the young man with the flu and nursing home care of the elderly woman with a stroke—and about how these illnesses affect their lives and the lives of those close to them. Because such care is, to a great degree, a characteristic of the individual physician, I have written this chapter in the first person.

I was a general practitioner before family practice existed. In 1969, when general practice became family practice, I began to think of myself as a family physician (FP), and then I became a board-certified FP in 1971. In the 1980s, the term *primary care physician* became popular, although I never really embraced it. Now I—along with my colleagues in general internal medicine and general pediatrics—are called generalists. I have practiced in the U.S. Public Health Service and in small town group practice. I spent 10 years in rural solo practice before entering academic medicine. Although I am currently chairman of a family medicine department in an academic medical center, I still think of myself as a rural FP and what follows reflects that practice-oriented viewpoint.

In this book, I have decided to use the term *generalist,* which, seems to be the favored designation for the foreseeable future.

What Is Generalist Health Care and Who Provides It?

Generalist health care is continuing, comprehensive, and coordinated medical care provided to a population undifferentiated by gender, disease, or organ system.[1] This type of care is also called primary care, and the terms are often used interchangeably. Generalists offer first-contact and longitudinal care for persons with diverse problems such as earache, chest pain, fracture, or cancer. They provide care that is not problem- or technology-specific. They coordinate the patient's health care, whether provided in the generalist's own office or in the emergency department, consultant's office, or hospital. The spectrum of generalist care varies with the setting—suburban, rural, inner city, community health clinic, or academic medical center—and melds into a continuum in which some generalists, in fact, include tertiary care activities as part of their practice.[2] My current practice is in an academic medical center, and hence my patients tend to have much more complicated problems than did my patients when I was in private practice.

The U.S. Department of Health and Human Services describes four primary care/generalist competencies[3]:

Health promotion and disease prevention
Assessment and diagnosis of common symptoms and physical signs
Management of common acute and chronic medical conditions
Identification of and appropriate referral for other needed health services

Persons who choose careers in the generalist specialties are those who—like me—want to do it all. We worked hard to learn the full spectrum of medicine and do not want to give anything up. By offering a broad range of services, I can offer truly comprehensive care to my patients. If Mrs. Jones, for example, has migraine headaches, a skin rash, and irregular menstrual periods, I can provide care for all these complaints, often in a single office visit and without referrals. What is more, with each encounter the patient and I add to a cumulative fund of medical and personal knowledge—what Balint called the "mutual investment company"—that allows increasingly effective health care.[4] As I learn more and more about Mrs. Jones and her stress at work, her problems with her teenage son, and her concern about her husband's alcohol use, she and I can better manage her various problems, but these data are never fully elucidated in one visit or two.

Exactly what does the generalist do? Most generalist practice is office practice and the variety of problems is reflected in the top 20 principal diagnoses in office visits as recorded in the National Ambulatory Medical Care Survey (Table 1.1).[5] Of course, this list covers all ambulatory care, not just generalist practice, and thus contains some other data, such as the many repeat visits to subspecialists for glaucoma, cataracts, and chronic sinusitis. Also, prenatal care includes visits to both family physicians and obstetricians. With these qualifications, however, the list approximates the daily problem list of the generalist physician.

Generalists provide a wide spectrum of care, which includes *anticipatory care,* counseling the teenager on avoidance of injury or unplanned pregnancy, and *symptomatic care* to relieve the pain of a back strain. There is *therapeutic care* of acute asthma or chronic ulcerative colitis and the *palliative*

TABLE 1.1. U.S. National Ambulatory Medical Care Survey:
Office visits by principal diagnosis, 1991

Principal diagnosis	All visits (%)
Hypertension	3.5
Normal pregnancy	3.1
Adult examination	2.7
Infant/child examination	2.6
Acute upper respiratory infection	2.5
Otitis media	2.4
Diabetes mellitus	1.9
Chronic sinusitis	1.7
Glaucoma	1.6
Acute pharyngitis	1.6
Bronchitis	1.5
Diseases of sebaceous glands	1.4
Allergic rhinitis	1.4
Asthma	1.3
Cataract	1.1
Contact dermatitis and other eczema	1.1
Back strain	1.0
Laboratory investigations	0.9
Neurotic disorders	0.9
General symptoms	0.9
All visits	100.0%

Source: Schappert SM.[5]

care of the person with terminal cancer or late-stage acquired immuno-deficiency syndrome.

Generalist care occurs in many sites in addition to the physician's office. Most generalists provide hospital and nursing home services for their patients. Home care is an important part of care in many communities, allowing the physician to visit the patient in his or her own "habitat." Other generalists work in schools, community health centers, the military, or government service.

Some generalists develop special areas of expertise such as care of the elderly, adolescent medicine, sports medicine, occupational medicine, or administrative medicine. At times, the focus may be on the community—community-oriented primary care—an expression of generalism in which the target is a community and the health problems that affect it (e.g., preventing cervical cancer by increasing the number of women screened with Pap smears) rather than concentrating exclusively on health problems at the level of the individual patient.

We are in the midst of profound changes in the U.S. medical workforce. "As a policy, the Association of American Medical Colleges (AAMC) advocates an overall national goal that a majority of graduating medical students be committed to generalist careers (family medicine, general internal medicine, or general pediatrics) and that appropriate efforts be made by all schools so that this goal can be reached within the shortest possible time."[6] In its Fourth Report to Congress and the Department of Health and Human Services Secretary, the Council on Graduate Medical Education (COGME) recommended in 1994 that "at least 50 percent of residency graduates should enter practice as generalist physicians (FPs, general internists, and general pediatricians)."[7] U.S. health care reform discussions emphasize the importance of primary care physicians.[8] But most significant is the tremendous need of managed care organizations for generalists. We are entering a "managed care era," which calls for some 50% generalists and 50% limited specialists. The medical workforce is now only about 30% generalists, and the current imbalance only emphasizes the value of the primary care physician and underscores the need to balance the ratio of generalists to specialists in the United States.

Of course, the AAMC, COGME, and managed care organizations are important considerations, but the key to the future is the people who receive health care. Family practice arose in the 1960s as a social movement to combat the fragmentation in medicine, to put medicine back together again, and to deliver it to the people. This same spirit is present today. Generalism is about the public need for personal health care, for a physician about whom one can say, "That's my doctor." It is about the physician who will make the commitment inherent in saying, "I am your personal physician. I will be there when you need me."

How to Provide Generalist Health Care: Asking the High-Payoff Questions

How do we do it? How do I as a generalist physician stay current with all of medicine and see 25 patients per day? First of all, I do not know all of medicine any more than a cardiologist knows *everything* about heart disease. As a specialist in family practice, I maintain broad-based knowledge of common health problems and the generalist competencies previously described. I believe that this fund of information is about the same "quantity" of information as that of, for example, the cardiologist; it is just that mine is about people's general health problems and the heart specialist's is about heart problems.

I manage to apply this generalist fund of knowledge and competencies to help a relatively large number of patients daily by efficient application of the most commonly performed generalist procedure: *the focused clinical encounter.* Typically compressed into a 15-minute time slot, the focused clinical encounter flows seamlessly through five phases: offering of the problem, elucidation of key issues, a targeted physical examination, explanation of the diagnosis, and negotiation of plans for management and follow-up. In less than a quarter hour, I can elicit a history of epigastric distress and what makes it better and worse, explore life stresses, examine the abdomen, explain my findings, and work with the patient to plan for dietary change, stress management, and appropriate use of antacids or an H_2-receptor blocker.

Of necessity, the time-limited visit targets the high-probability diagnosis (e.g., gastritis, duodenitis) while considering the possibility of the "must-never-miss" diagnoses (e.g., gastric cancer). The focused clinical encounter will include exploration of psychosocial topics such as the patient's need to take a second job to cover credit card debt or concerns about a child in trouble at school. The experienced physician knows how often these nonphysical issues hold the key to understanding the patient's illness.

High-payoff questions are how the skilled generalist focuses the time-limited clinical encounter. These questions are open-ended and can often begin with, "Tell me about. . . ." They can be phrased in ways that are most comfortable to each physician and in complexity appropriate to the patient's understanding. The high-payoff questions are used along with standard queries about, "How long have you had chest pain?" "Does the pain radiate anywhere?" and "Have you taken any medicine for the chest pain?" Among all the clarifying but closed-ended queries, the full scope of the problem may become clear with the response to, "Tell me about what's been going on lately" or "Let's talk about what's most stressful in your life right now."

The following are five areas of high-payoff questions. For each, I have described a rationale, with some examples. Specific questions are listed—in varying levels of specificity—for both the patient and for you or me, the physician.

What Is the Reason for the Visit?

Patients visit physicians for many reasons, which are not always self-evident.[9] A 65-year-old man came on a first visit, requesting a "complete examination." In response to a question, "Why?" I learned that the patient was planning a second marriage, that there had been a question of a prostate nodule in the past, and that he needed to know more about his health outlook to make some financial decisions. If I had not dug deeper, I would have failed to meet the patient's needs for the encounter.

The reasons for a visit may be classified under five headings (Table 1.2). Most new-problem visits are for the diagnosis and treatment of physical problems, such as earache. The next most common category—concern about the meaning of a sign or symptom—includes many instances in which the patient with a problem is less bothered by the discomfort than

TABLE 1.2. Why patients visit physicians: problems and
needs that prompt patients to initiate medical encounters

Reason	Example
Physical problem	Ankle sprain
Worry or concern	Coughed up bloody sputum
Administrative purpose	Insurance medical examination
Emotional problem	Anxiety
Social problem	Loneliness

by what the discomfort might *mean*. For example, in Chapter 17, Andrew Harris comes to the physician with back pain that began while lifting boxes at work; there is some radiation of pain to the right leg and foot. Is Mr. Harris in the office for relief of his pain so that he can sleep at night or return to work soon? Is he here because he is concerned about the possibility of a herniated disc necessitating back surgery, as happened to his brother? Or is the visit for an administrative purpose—to establish a workers' compensation claim?

Patients sometimes identify their problems as social or emotional, but more often such problems are offered as physical complaints—sometimes referred to as a "ticket of admission" (to health care). One young married woman visited my office repeatedly with lower abdominal pains. She and her husband had three small children, and their income was limited. The chief problem seemed to be that he spent most evenings playing softball and drinking with his friends, leaving her alone at home with the children. Although the patient continued to offer a physical complaint, her "reason for the visit" was, in my opinion, a social problem.

Questions for the Patient

• What do we need to accomplish on this visit?
• Is there anything you are concerned (or worried) about?
• Tell me why you are here with this problem *at this time*.
• How can I help you at this visit?

Questions for the Physician to Consider

• Does the patient's stated problem seem "not quite right"?
• Might the patient, for some reason, have misled the receptionist or nurse (or me) about the complaint?
• Have I possibly made an incorrect assumption about the patient's objectives?
• Is the patient here today for someone else's reason (i.e., to satisfy the wishes of a spouse or parent)?

What Is the Meaning of the Illness to the Patient?

Think back to the last time you had the flu, with high fever, achiness, and fatigue. Along with the need to stay in bed for a few days to get well, what did the flu mean to you? Did it mean that you would miss class or a sports event? Might it have meant that you would be absent for an important examination or that you might perform poorly on the test? Could it be that you were not prepared for the examination and were, in fact, happy for a delay? Perhaps the chief concern was the economic impact of the flu—the cost of care or the loss of a weekend job. Did the chills and fever remind you of the first stages of pneumonia that ended with the death of a grandparent? Or did the flu symptoms have some other special meaning for you?

Disease and illness are not synonymous. Disease refers to a biomechanical, physiologic, or psychologic dysfunction. Illness includes the patient's disease—with all its pain, worry, inconvenience, or loss—and places it in the context of the life, family, community, and society of the affected individual. Ellen Harris (Chapter 16) visits your office with a complaint of vaginal discharge. She is married and works as a secretary. A straightforward problem? Probably, but not necessarily. Could the symptom mean loss of sexual relations with her husband for a week or more? Does this mean he will be angry? Could she have passed an infection to him? Could the infection have been caught from him? Could that mean that he acquired it somewhere?

The physician must never neglect the patient's unspoken concerns: Will I be able to return to work after my heart attack? Will my husband still love me after my mastectomy? Might I pass my chest cold (or infectious mononucleosis, or skin rash, or chlamydia infection) to my partner?

Another example: In Chapter 5, Harold Nelson, aged 76, develops urinary incontinence. What might this mean to him? "Will I have to go to the hospital?" "Will I need an operation?" "Will I need to go to a nursing home?" Although Mr. Nelson may be hesitant to ask these questions, it is likely that they have occurred to him.

It is important to understand the meaning of the sick role and the legitimization of illness. When you or I are sick, we are excused from our usual duties, and others offer medicine, food, and support. That is, we are allowed to assume *the sick role.* Part of the contract, however, is that we will make every effort to get well—and no longer assume the sick role. Of course, the sick role has definite advantages, not the least of which are reduced responsibility and increased service by others. Not surprisingly, some persons would prefer to prolong the sick role, and the physician may become involved. Many office visits are concerned with legitimization of the sick role, whether explicitly by signing an excuse for work or implicitly by writing a prescription for a cough or renewing a physical therapy order for a painful neck.

If you overlook the contextual meaning of the illness to patients such as Mrs. Harris or Mr. Nelson, has your clinical encounter—your "procedure"—been successful?

Questions for the Patient

• What do you believe is the cause of the illness?
• Tell me how you feel about this illness.
• How does this illness affect your activities at home or at work?
• What would getting well mean to you?

Questions for the Physician to Consider

• How might this illness be affecting the patient's self-image?
• What are the implications of the patient assuming the sick role?
• Might this illness remind the patient of something that happened to a family member or friend?
• Might you—the physician—have personal experience or feelings that are affecting your judgment about this patient's illness?

What Is the Impact of the Illness on the Family?

If you have any doubt that illness is a family affair, ask any child, sibling, or parent of a person with a chronic problem such as asthma, diabetes mellitus, or cerebral palsy. Resources and attention that should be equally shared are diverted to the identified "patient." The patient's sick role eventually becomes a family burden, and other family members come to think of themselves as caretakers. Anger begets guilt, and the illness permeates all family relationships. Eventually, the illness becomes part of the family lore.

Describing the legacy of migraine in her own family, Anne Walling, MD (author of Chapter 7) writes, "My father's severe attacks were part of our family's normal pattern of life. Like spells of bad weather, they were unpredictable, significant events that appeared to take a perverse delight in disrupting the most intricately planned and eagerly anticipated events." And then, "My mother abhorred migraine and grimly warned us against developing even remotely migrainous symptoms."[10]

The effect of illness on a family is not predictable. Chronic, recurrent childhood illness such as renal failure or hyperactivity can be the stress that results in disruption of a young family, and many parents of leukemic children see their marriages end in divorce. However, I have cared for a family with a child whose asthma attacks seemed to occur at just the times needed to divert parental attention to the child and away from their own arguments.

In Chapter 3, you will meet Ann Martino-Priestley, aged 22, and her husband, Luke. Ann is pregnant with their first child. Of course, pregnancy is not an illness, but it will have an impact on the couple/family. How does each feel about the pregnancy? How will a child affect their relationship? Can they afford to have a baby at this time? Will Ann be able to continue to work? What about Luke's studies for his MBA degree? How might all these issues affect health care decisions?

Questions for the Patient

- How is your spouse (or children, parents, partner, etc.) affected by this illness?
- What are you hearing from others about your illness?
- Tell me what has changed in your relationships since the illness began.
- How would things be different at home if you were well?

Questions for the Physician to Consider

- Who, besides the patient, is affected by this illness?
- What emotions might the patient's family be experiencing: sorrow, anger, abandonment, frustration, guilt?
- Have I, as physician, spoken with key people in my patient's life?
- By engaging in the care of this patient's illness, what might be the effect on me and my family?

What Is the Appropriate Locus of Care for This Person's Illness?

The seminal work on the locus of care was the 1961 paper by White et al[11] showing that of 1000 adults "at risk" each month

750 reported one or more illnesses or injuries
250 of these persons consulted a physician one or more times
    9 of these patients were admitted to hospital
    5 patients were referred to another physician
    1 patient was referred to a university medical center

Some thoughts about this study and what it means today: Note that although 75% of adults reported an illness or injury during a month, only one illness/injury in three resulted in a medical encounter; fully two-thirds of care was home care in which the physician was not directly involved. The consultation rate was 2%, less than the 7% to 10% generalist consultation rates of today, but, of course, the White study recorded contact with any physician, which necessarily recorded many self-referrals to specialists. Finally, there was only one academic medical center admission among the 1000 at-risk adults, a key finding considering that research data and therapeutic guidelines tend to come from academic medical centers and thus are based on 0.1% of the population.

A current issue in managed care centers around appropriate use of consultation and referral. The family practice approach to locus of care is presented in the first edition of *Family Medicine: Principles and Practice.*[12]

Definitive Care: The physician provides independent care, perhaps with the participation of ancillary personnel but without subspecialist consultation or referral. Examples include depression, type 2 diabetes mellitus, and an undisplaced fracture of the fibular malleolus. The residency-trained FP generalist should be competent to manage 85% to 90% of definitive care problems without need for consultation or referral.

Shared Care: These problems generally necessitate consultation for some aspect of diagnosis or therapy. Care is thus shared by the generalist and subspecialist for problems such as thyroid mass or active pulmonary tuberculosis. Some 7% to 10% of problems will be best managed by shared care.

Supportive Care: These are clearly subspecialty problems such as extensive third-degree burns or retinal detachment. The generalist has the responsibility to direct the patient to appropriate care and to maintain educational and emotional support for the patient and family.

The physician's decisions in locus of care options will be guided by individual choices in interest, competence, and comfort levels. In our Family Practice Center, some physicians perform colposcopy (as a definitive care procedure); others refer patients needing colposcopy (for them, it is thereby a shared care procedure). Of course, physicians are only part of the decision making. Patient preferences play a role, as do practice guidelines of the health care organization or hospital.

In Chapter 21, we encounter an increasingly common locus-of-care decision: Mark McCarthy, age 28, is human-immunodeficiency-virus-positive and for 3 weeks has had a fever and cough productive of yellow-gray sputum. His parents ask, "Is it safe for him to stay at home, or should he be in the hospital? Should he have a consultation with a specialist? Should a specialist be in charge of his care? By having him living at home, are we—his parents—at risk?" Answers to these and related questions are often complex and may be clouded by misinformation, fear, protection of turf, and concerns about maintaining practice volume.

Questions for the Patient

- Have you had this problem before and how was it managed?
- Tell me your view of the treatment needed today.
- What concerns do you have about our plans for management and follow-up?
- Tell me your understanding of the reason we might seek consultation and the questions we are hoping to answer.

Questions for the Physician to Consider

- Is the problem within my area of competence and comfort?
- Does the patient expect a consultation and, if so, is it medically appropriate?
- Is there an administrative need that would call for a consultation or referral: insurance, litigation, disability determination, or other?
- Am I making my consultation/referral recommendation for the right reasons?

What Resources Are Available to Help in Managing the Illness?

The rise in managed care in the United States is a reflection of what families have known all along: Health care resources are not limitless. Individuals and families have always had to face limits on care that can be given in the home, cost of medication purchased, and nursing home care provided. Recognition of resources that are available—and what are not available—is important in assuring optimal care for patients.

The categories of resources are listed in Table 1.3. Financial resources include the direct ability to pay and also medical insurance, emergency assistance in times of disaster, and loans or gifts from family. Care by family members, visiting nurses, community health workers, nurses, physicians, and other providers all constitute medical care resources. The time and energy resources may come from the patient, the family, medical personnel, and volunteers such as neighbors or church members. Patient and family knowledge of medicine, community contacts, and funding sources can affect the quality of care ultimately received as can the availability of medical equipment and supplies.

In Chapter 4, Allison Harris is brought to your office by her mother "for her 1-year-old checkup and shots." There are resource implications even in this routine visit: Mrs. Harris missed several hours of work to bring Allison to the appointment. There is a cost to the Harris family for the checkup

TABLE 1.3. Resources used to manage patients' health care problems

Resource	Example
Financial	Health insurance
Medical care	Office visit to physician
Time and energy	Middle-aged person stays at home caring for elderly parent
Knowledge	Information from medical reference book
Equipment and supplies	Wheelchair from community loan program

that is not covered by their health insurance. There is a vaccine cost that, although covered by a state subsidized program, is inflated by the hidden cost of vaccine-related litigation.

Generalists work together with patients, families, community agencies, hospitals, and others to help ensure the appropriate and cost-effective deployment of resources. The higher-priced prescription is not necessarily better, and not every patient with pneumonia needs hospitalization. The Medical Outcomes Study demonstrated that, even when data are controlled for patient mix, generalists use less health care resources than subspecialists. Among the generalist specialties, FPs use resources most cost-effectively of all.[13]

Questions for the Patient

- Who is your most important support person, and how is he or she involved in caring for this illness?
- Are you now a client of any community agencies that could help today?
- Tell me about family or friends that could help us at this time.
- Is there some special way you deal with problems—reading about them, meditation, pastoral counseling—and how can we put this to work now?

Questions for the Physician to Consider

- What are the patient's personal and family resources that can be used?
- What community resources might be useful in management?
- Does the illness have public health or community implications?
- Have I fully used all my office staff to help coordinate resource access and use?

Why Is Generalist Care Important?

Writing on his own decision to become a general practitioner, British physician Robin Hull recalls, "I began to look at patients not as a means of locomotion of interesting pathology, but as people who were quite fascinating in their own right."[14] Dr. Hull's comment provides insight into why technological medicine is unsatisfying to many. Patients are people, not machines with broken parts, and their illnesses have diverse origins, which include the family, the community, the workplace, and the tangled relationships of a lifetime.

Generalist health care is not a substitute for scientifically oriented and research-based clinical activity; actually, generalist care expands the dimensions of disease-oriented clinical practice by adding the contextual basis through which both physician and patient come to understand the *illness*. Is there a clinical payoff to such patient-centered behavior? Certainly, the diagnosis of acute myocardial infarction—documented on the electrocardiogram (ECG)—is enhanced by understanding the patient's high-fat diet that began in childhood at the family diningroom table, the cigarette smoking started with friends in high school, the long hours at work, and the recent concern about the company takeover that may cost him his job at age 56. Is all this reflected on the ECG tracing? No. Is the context important? Definitely!

Generalist health care calls for a committed investment of self. As an FP, I become, in a sense, a member of the family; on home visits, I see my name and telephone number posted on the refrigerator door along with those of other family members and the clergy. The generalist physician is a member of the community; he or she is active in clubs, civic groups, and church— and enjoys dealing with patients in these settings.

Most of all, generalist health care means *being there* for the patient and family. This has been called accessibility, but it is more. It is making the follow-up telephone call. It is asking the patient about the disabled parent at home. It is showing the patient that you care. Almost 30 years ago, I cared for an elderly man dying at home of the multiple complications of a hard life and a poor genetic endowment. He and his wife lived in a trailer in the woods about 40 minutes from my office, and I visited him every Wednesday afternoon—my day for house calls for my practice group. One Monday morning, the patient died at home, somewhat unexpectedly. My schedule was overbooked and the waiting room was full of patients. I did the logical thing. I sent my partner to pronounce the patient dead, sign the death certificate, and comfort the widow. After all, it was my partner's day to do the house calls. I next saw the widow at the viewing (yes, many generalists make a final visit to their patients). Here, she quietly let me know that she had expected *me* to come when he died. I had failed to *be there* when she needed me. She taught me a lesson about being a physician that I still remember.

Family practice and today's generalist physicians are the current expression of the "horse and buggy" doctors of early America. We have assumed the role of maintaining patient-centered values while providing state-of-the-art health care in an increasingly technical age. Changing health care economics predict that the health care systems of the next few decades will be based on a primary care-centered model. The secret of keeping our commitment to patients and yet achieving the universally accessible, affordable new care model will be to remain true to our first principles— offering our patients competent medical care that includes consideration of how their acute or chronic illness is part of the fabric of their lives.

References

1. Kimball HR, Young PR. A statement on the generalist physician from the American Boards of Family Practice and Internal Medicine. JAMA 1994; 271:315–6.
2. Wartman SA, Wilson M, Kahn N. The generalist health work force: issues and goals. J Gen Intern Med 1994;9(Suppl1):S7–S13.

3. Rivo ML. Division of Medicine Update. Washington, DC: USPHS Health Resources and Services Administration, Bureau of Health Professions. Summer, 1992.
4. Balint M. The doctor, his patient and the illness. New York: International Universities Press, 1957.
5. Schappert SM. National Ambulatory Medical Care Survey: 1991 summary. Hyattsville, MD: National Center for Health Statistics, 1992.
6. AAMC policy on the generalist physician. Acad Med 1993;68(1):1–6.
7. Council on Graduate Medical Education. Fourth report to Congress and the Department of Health and Human Services Secretary. Washington, DC: U.S. Public Health Services, Health Resources and Services Administration, 1994.
8. Starfield B, Simpson L. Primary care as part of US health services reform. JAMA 1993;269:3136–9.
9. Taylor RB, Burdette JA, Camp L, Edwards J. Purpose of the medical encounter: identification and influence on process and outcome in 200 encounters in a model family practice center. J Fam Pract 1980;10:495–500.
10. Walling AD. The legacy of migraine. J Fam Pract 1994;38:629–30.
11. White KL, Williams F, Greenberg B. Ecology of medical care. N Engl J Med 1961:265:885–91.
12. Taylor RB. Family medicine: principles and practice, 1st edition. New York: Springer-Verlag, 1978.
13. Tarlov AR, Ware JE, Greenfield S. The medical outcomes study: an application of methods for monitoring the results of medical care. JAMA 1989;262: 925–30.
14. Hull R. Just a GP. Oxford, England: Radcliff, 1994.

2
Clinical Prevention

EVAN W. KLIGMAN AND FRANK A. HALE

Clinical prevention is the connecting link between public health and primary care. Health education and health promotion counseling skills are among the most important tools in the family physician's medical bag. A major challenge facing the family physician is how to bridge the gap between clinical prevention knowledge and practice, recognizing the impact of personal behaviors on health. The traditional biomedical approach to the diagnosis and treatment of disease is only a partial response to addressing the health care needs of patients. Patient care must encompass a prospective preventive approach toward helping individuals and families assume major responsibility for their own health-related behaviors.[1,2]

Background

Family Physician's Office

Many factors affecting preventive care can be modified by the physician: office hours, convenience, location, private dressing rooms to prepare for procedures and screening tests, flow charts and check lists, colored chart stickers to flag certain risk factors, and follow-up protocols for behavior change counseling or screening tests initiated.[3] Modifications in the reception area, examination rooms, and patient flow alterations are environmental strategies that can enhance the delivery of preventive services.[4] The office should have a system of continuous improvement and monitoring, inclusive of self-audits, to promote a high level of patient satisfaction and acceptance of clinical preventive services.[5]

Physician–Patient Encounter

Family physicians must incorporate a preventive attitude in the context of each patient encounter. The *Guide to Clinical Preventive Services*[6] of the U.S.

Preventive Services Task Force places great emphasis on integrating clinical prevention into patient care, noting that counseling and patient education may be the most valuable clinical prevention activities, that preventive services are an appropriate part of all visits, and that all patients should be counseled. Every acute and chronic problem cared for in the family physician's office should have a prevention component. However, a recent study suggests that physicians offer more preventive services during routine physical examination visits rather than when patients are seen for illnesses. Further, those physicians who seem to order the most appropriate preventive services based on U.S. Preventive Services Task Force recommendations are those who are younger, residency-trained, in a group practice, and who have greater experience with these recommendations.[7]

The concept of offering clinical prevention to all patients based on their age, sex, and risk level is important for the family physician. Clinical preventive services identified by the U.S. Preventive Services Task Force[6] encompass four categories: counseling, screening, immunizations, and chemoprophylactic agents. The Task Force's report, when combined with the preventive recommendations for asymptomatic adults generated by other groups,[8,9] the American Cancer Society,[10] and the work of individual clinicians,[11] provides a database to justify the selection of appropriate preventive clinical services for individuals and families.

Preventable Factors Contributing to Premature Death

Although the role of the family physician is critical to the management of disease and acute care, the overwhelming threat to health for most people is related to nonmedical factors,[12] including health-related life-style behaviors, the environment, and genetic background. Family physicians must base clinical prevention strategies on a spectrum of influences.

About 10% of premature deaths result from inadequate access to health care services. Shorter life expectancy is associated with lower educational and income levels. Common life-style risk factors, such as smoking, obesity, stress, poor nutrition, and alcohol and drug use, contribute to more than 50% of premature deaths. Environmental factors, such as sanitation, food safety, pollution, toxic exposures, and occupational risks and hazards, contribute to about 20% of premature deaths. Family history, genetic influence, and inherited susceptibility to certain diseases is believed to be responsible for another 20% of premature deaths.[13] For instance, the relative risk related to genetic susceptibility for many adult-onset disorders may range from 2 to 180.

Selection of Clinical Preventive Services for Individuals and Families

General Guidelines for Developing Protocols

Clinical preventive services are an integral part of the patient care process. The traditional concept of the annual physical examination has been replaced by the practice of conducting selective health maintenance procedures at periodic intervals based on rational guidelines. Practice guidelines have been developed to reduce inappropriate services, control geographic variations in practice patterns, and encourage more efficient and effective use of resources.[13] Efficient delivery of clinical preventive services means that not all patients need every clinical intervention. Identification of high-risk patients (see Tables 2.1, 2.3–2.6, and 2.8–2.10), whether based on personal or family medical history (or both), a particular life-style behavior, or "physiologic" rather than "chronologic" age, is important when customizing clinical prevention.

Periodic Health Examination

Periodic health examination is the centerpiece of prevention in the office setting.[14] These examinations should be streamlined, allowing sufficient time for discussion with the patient on how to promote and prolong healthy living. No longer are annual checkups encompassing complete histories and comprehensive physical examinations with a spectrum of appropriate laboratory tests.[9] Such visits should be targeted to the patient's risk profile and include a review of screening needs, health promotion counseling, and identification of immunization and chemoprophylaxis needs. It is now customary to include clinical prevention as a component of any acute or chronic care visit. For most patients and most family physicians caring for patients in managed care plans, these visits provide the only opportunity for receiving preventive services. These visits may, in fact, provide both appropriate and timely opportunities for physicians to counsel patients. Thus, one or two preventive interventions should be delivered at all patient encounters. The discovery of a pregnancy may become a "teachable moment" to counsel the mother-to-be on the hazards of smoking, or knowledge of a family history of breast cancer may be the basis for recommending that a patient obtain a mammogram.

Revising and Updating Protocols

Because guidelines and recommendations may change as new data become available, it is important for family physicians to stay abreast of current information. The field of clinical prevention is rapidly advancing. Several large group practices and health maintenance organizations (HMOs) have standing committees to update their prevention protocols, taking into consideration such factors as cost, effectiveness, efficacy, and the unique profile and needs of their enrollees.

Delivery of Preventive Services to Special or High-Risk Populations

Populations at risk pose important health challenges to our society owing to higher rates of death and disability based on environmental, cultural, or economic risk factors and life-style practices. Special populations include low-income groups, minorities, and people with disabilities.[15] For each of these subgroups, special clinical prevention efforts may be indicated. They must frequently compensate for economic, racial, or linguistic barriers. Many underserved populations are cared for on an acute need basis, and the clinical preventive needs ordinarily available to the mainstream population are not as readily available.

Special training in understanding other cultural perspectives is necessary to be effective at prevention with special populations. The physician needs to develop sensitivity toward individual perspectives on health and well-being as well as familiarity with particular health beliefs of culturally or ethnically defined populations. Ethnosensitivity can enhance communication, patient satisfaction, and willingness to modify behaviors.[16]

Family practice training is increasingly recognized as providing physicians with the necessary skill to practice population-based medicine. Indeed, several governmental strategic plans and directives indicate that family physicians will be expected to play an increasing role in improving the well-being of underserved Americans and take the lead in designing preventive health care strategies and personal health promotion activities.[15] One of these efforts comprises linkages between family medicine education programs and Public Health Service clinics established to provide community-based, comprehensive, prevention-oriented primary care services. The delivery of preventive services in these settings is based on a team approach involving health educators, midlevel health providers, and often volunteer lay health promoters from the community.

Clinical Preventive Services Guidelines

The most effective way to develop and maintain a preventive-oriented attitude is to care for patients using a framework of specific guidelines and strategies for implementing preventive services. When focusing the preventive interventions, physicians should take into consideration the leading causes of death and disability for the patient's age group. The life cycle presented in this chapter is divided into nine stages. Providers should develop a stage system that most clearly reflects the age distribution of patients in their practice.

The system that follows is oriented toward a balanced family practice population. The age-specific Tables 2.1, 2.3, 2.4, 2.5, 2.6, 2.8, 2.9, and 2.10 are based on *The Guide to Clinical Preventive Services* by the U.S. Preventive Services Task Force[6] and recommendations of the AAFP Subcommittee on Periodic Health Intervention.[17] General recommendations made by the Subcommittee include the following.

1. All new patients should undergo a comprehensive history and physical examination, have a database/health risk appraisal completed, and be exposed to various preventive services based on the recommended guidelines (outlined below).
2. Previous health records should be obtained to avoid duplication of services (e.g., pneumonia vaccine).
3. Additional services may be added routinely based on (1) protocols developed by each physician or practice or (2) the individual patient's risk profile.
4. Physicians must update their protocols as new scientific findings become available.

Birth to Eighteen Months

After preconception care and the prenatal period, the first 18 months of life remain the most formidable for establishing health patterns for years to come. During the first week, several screening interventions are recommended. Counseling topics during the first year and a half include nutritional intake and injury prevention. Other preventive services include immunizations[18] and chemoprophylaxis to prevent infectious diseases. Flow sheets and tracking forms are most useful during infancy and early childhood given the number of recommended interventions at each visit (Tables 2.1 and 2.2).

Nineteen Months to Six Years

Universal immunization over the past 40 years has eliminated the threat of major infectious diseases to many children, a significant cause of mortality and morbidity in this age group. Yet, with decreases in immunization rates among some groups of young children in the United States, there are regions with sporadic outbreaks of pertussis, measles, and other preventable communicable infectious diseases. Thus a second measles/mumps/rubella immunization is now recommended at 4 to 6 years.

Unintentional injuries are the major health problem for children in this age group. Periodic preventive interventions during this life period should

TABLE 2.1. Periodic health examination: Birth to 18 months[a]
Schedule: 2, 4, 6, (12), 15, 18 months[b]

First week
Ophthalmic antibiotics (at birth)
Hemoglobin electrophoresis (HR1) (at birth)
T_4/TSH (days 3–6 preferred for testing)

Screening
History: interval medical and family history (an updating of the previously obtained
   medical and family medical history)
Physical examination: height and weight
Laboratory/diagnostic procedures
   Hemoglobin and/or hematocrit (once during infancy; either test is acceptable)
   High-risk groups
      Hearing (HR2) (by age 18 months, if not tested earlier)
      Serum lead level or erythrocyte protoporphyrin (HR3)

Parent counseling

Diet and exercise	Injury prevention (*continued*)
Breast-feeding	Hot water heater temperature (≤120°F)
Nutrient intake, especially	Stairway gates, window guards, pool fence
iron-rich foods	Storage of drugs and toxic chemicals
Substance use	Syrup of ipecac, poison control telephone number
Sexual practices	Dental health: baby bottle tooth decay
Injury prevention	Other primary preventive measures: effects of passive
Child safety seats	smoking
Smoke detector	

Immunizations and chemoprophylaxis
Diphtheria/tetanus/pertussis (DTP) vaccine (at ages 2, 4, 6, and 15 or 18 months)
Oral poliovirus vaccine (OPV) (at ages 2, 4, and 6 months)
Measles/mumps/rubella (MMR) vaccine (at age 12 or 15 months)
Hemophilus influenzae type b (Hib) conjugate vaccine (if using HbOC, at ages 2, 4, 6,
   and 15 months; if using PRP-OMP, at ages 2, 4, and 12 months; if using PRP-D, one
   dose at 18 months)
Hepatitis B vaccine (at birth, ages 1–2, and 16–18 months)
High-risk groups: Fluoride supplements (HR4)

Additional notes

Leading causes of death	Remain alert for
Conditions originating in perinatal period	Ocular misalignment
Congenital anomalies	Tooth decay
Heart disease	Signs of child abuse or neglect
Injuries (nonmotor vehicle)	
Pneumonia/influenza	

High-risk categories
HR1: Newborns of Caribbean, Latin American, Asian, Mediterranean, or African descent.
HR2: Infants with a family history of childhood hearing impairment or a personal
   history of congenital perinatal infection with herpes, syphilis, rubella, cytomegalovirus, or toxoplasmosis; malformations involving the head or neck (e.g.,
   dysmorphic and syndromal abnormalities, cleft palate, abnormal pinna); birth
   weight less than 1500 g; bacterial meningitis; hyperbilirubinemia requiring
   exchange transfusion; or severe perinatal asphyxia (Apgar scores 0–3, absence of
   spontaneous respirations for 10 minutes, or hypotonia at 2 hours of age).

TABLE 2.1. *(continued)*

HR3: Infants who live in or frequently visit housing built before 1950 that is dilapidated or undergoing renovation; who come in contact with other children with known lead toxicity; who live near lead processing plants or whose parents or household members work in a lead-related occupation; or who live near busy highways or hazardous waste sites. Some communities are currently providing universal screening.

HR4: Infants living in areas with inadequate water fluoridation (<0.7 ppm).

*a*This list of preventive services is not exhaustive. It is adapted from the U.S. Preventive Services Task Force and the *AAFP Commission on Public Health and Scientific Affairs.* Clinicians may wish to add other preventive services on a routine basis and after considering the patient's medical history and other individual circumstances. Examples of target conditions not specifically examined by the task force include developmental disorders, musculoskeletal malformations, cardiac anomalies, genitourinary disorders, metabolic disorders, speech problems, behavioral disorders, parent/family dysfunction.

*b*Five visits are required for immunizations. Because of lack of data and differing patient risk profiles, the scheduling of additional visits and the frequency of the individual preventive services listed in this table are left to clinical discretion (except as indicated in other footnotes).

focus on injury prevention. Environmental and socioeconomic factors are also significant determinants of health and illness in this age group. Poor children have a higher prevalence of learning disorders, mental retardation, vision and speech impairments, and emotional and behavioral problems. One serious cause of such developmental problems is lead exposure. More than 3 million children between age 6 months and 5 years showed high levels of serum lead in 1984.[15] Respiratory problems such as influenza and asthma are the chief illness-related reasons young children miss school. The role of parental smoking and passive smoking exposure, a major trigger of these illnesses, should be addressed periodically during this age period (Tables 2.2 and 2.3).

Seven to Twelve Years

Healthy child development depends on establishing healthy behaviors during this age period to avoid smoking and alcohol abuse and develop good nutrition and physical activity. Three-fourths of children have smoked their first cigarette by grade 9, and the average age of first use of alcohol and marijuana is age 13.[15] Important screening and counseling topics include fat in diet, cholesterol/lipoprotein analysis as indicated, selection of an exercise program, sex education, maintenance of dental health, and injury prevention.

Screening for hypercholesterolemia in all children older than age 2 years is controversial. Without data on the costs, risk, and benefits of intervention strategies for children with high cholesterol concentrations, general screening of all children for total cholesterol values must be considered

TABLE 2.2. Childhood immunization schedule

Age	Hepatitis B vaccine[a]	DTP	TOPV	HbCV	MMR	Td
Birth (first visit)	Hepatitis B vaccine 1					
1–2 Months	Hepatitis B vaccine 2 (or vaccine 1)					
2 Months (earliest age)		DTP1 (6 weeks)	TOPV1 (6 weeks)	HbCV1 (6 weeks)		
4 Months (minimum interval)	Or vaccine 2	DTP2 (4 weeks after first dose)	TOPV2 (6 weeks after first dose)	HbCV2 (4 weeks after first dose)		
6 Months (minimum interval)		DTP3 (4 weeks after second dose)		HbCV3 (only if HbOC is used; 4 weeks after second dose)		
6–18 Months (minimum interval)	Hepatitis B vaccine 3[b] (2 months)					
12 Months (minimum interval)				HbCV3 (only if PRP-OMP is used; 2 months after second dose and 12 months old[e]		
15 Months (earliest age or minimum interval)		DTP4 (do not give earlier than 15 months and 6 months after third dose)	TOPV3 (do not give earlier than 15 months 6 weeks after second dose)	HbCV4 (if HbOC is used, 2 months after third dose and 15 months old[e])	MMR1 (12 months in high-risk areas only)	

	DTP5[c]	TOPV4[d]	HbCV	MMR	HB
4–6+ Years (minimum interval)			Four (three if PRP-OMP is used)	MMR2 (1 month after first dose and 4–14 years old)	
14–16 Years	Td1				N/A
Usual number of doses in series	Five	Four		2	
Dose	IM / 0.5 ml IM	0.5 mL oral	0.5 ml IM	0.5 mL SQ	0.5 mL IM

Source: Based on recommendations from the Immunization Practices Advisory Committee, American Academy of Pediatrics and American Academy of Family Physicians. Adapted from Zimmerman and Giebink.[18] With permission.

Note: Use Td, not DTP, for series at age 7 years or later. Do not give split doses of DTP. Except in special circumstances, HbCV is not given at age 5 years or later; IM doses should be given in the anterolateral thigh for infants. For children, hepatitis B vaccine is given in the deltoid muscle.

[a] Children younger than 7 years of age should receive 2.5-μg (0.25-ml) doses of Recombivax HB or 10-μg doses of Engerix-B as part of universal childhood immunization. Offspring of hepatitis B carriers should receive hepatitis B immunoglobulin at birth and the hepatitis B vaccine series with Recombivax HB at the 5.0-μg (0.5-ml) dose or Engerix-B at the 10-μg dose.

[b] If hepatitis B vaccine 2 is late, give hepatitis B vaccine 3 at 3–5 months after hepatitis B vaccine 2.

[c] This dose is not needed if the fourth dose is given after the fourth birthday.

[d] This dose is not needed if the third dose is given after the fourth birthday.

[e] See Table 2.3 for HbCV vaccine schedules when starting series late.

DTP = diphtheria/tetanus/pertussis; TOPV = trivalent oral poliovirus vaccine; HbCV = *Haemophilus* b conjugate vaccine; MMR = measles/mumps/rubella; HbOC = diphtheria CRM 197 protein conjugate; PRP-OMP = meningococcal protein conjugate; IM = intramuscularly; SQ = subcutaneously.

TABLE 2.3. Periodic health examination: Ages 19 months to 6 years
Schedule: See footnote[a]

Screening
  History
    Interval medical and family history
    Developmental/behavioral assessment
  Physical examination[a]
    Height and weight
    Blood pressure
    Eye examination for amblyopia and strabismus (ages 3–4 years)
  Laboratory/diagnostic procedures
    Urinalysis for bacteriuria (The optimal frequency for urine testing has not been
      determined and is left to clinical discretion. In general, dipsticks combining the
      leukocyte esterase and nitrite tests should be used to detect asymptomatic
      bacteriuria.)
  High-risk groups
    Serum lead or erythrocyte protoporphyrin (HR1)
    Tuberculin skin test (PPD) (HR2)
    Hearing (before age 3 years, if not tested earlier) (HR3)

Patient and parent counseling

  Diet and exercise
    Sweets and between-meal snacks,
      iron-enriched foods, sodium
    Nutritional assessment
    Selection of exercise program
  Substance use
  Sexual practices: initiate sex education
  Injury prevention
    Safety belts
    Smoke detector
    Hot water heater temperature (≤120°F)
    Burn protection
    Electrical cords and outlets
    Warning about strangers

  Injury prevention (*continued*)
    Window guards and pool
      fence
    Bicycle safety helmets
    Storage of drugs, toxic chemicals,
      matches, and firearms
    Syrup of ipecac, poison control
      telephone number
  Dental health
    Tooth brushing
    Dental visits starting at age 3 years
  Other primary preventive measures
    Effects of passive smoking
  High-risk groups
    Skin protection from ultraviolet light (HR4)

Immunizations and chemoprophylaxis
  Diphtheria/tetanus/pertussis (DTP) vaccine (once before ages 4 and 6 years)
  Oral poliovirus vaccine (OPV) (once between ages 4 and 6 years)
  Measles/mumps/rubella (MMR) vaccine (before school entry) between ages 4 and
    6 years
  Review *Haemophilus influenzae* type b (Hib) conjugate vaccine immunization status
  High-risk groups
    Fluoride supplements (HR5)

Additional notes

  Leading causes of death
    Injuries (nonmotor vehicle)
    Motor vehicle crashes
    Congenital anomalies
    Homicide
    Heart disease

  Remain alert for
    Vision disorders
    Dental decay, malalignment, premature loss of teeth,
      mouth breathing
    Signs of child abuse or neglect
    Abnormal bereavement

TABLE 2.3. (continued)

High-risk categories

HR1: Children who live in or frequently visit housing built before 1950 that is dilapidated or undergoing renovation; who come in contact with other children with known lead toxicity; who live near lead processing plants or whose parents or household members work in a lead-related occupation; or who live near busy highways or hazardous waste sites.

HR2: Household members of persons with tuberculosis or others at risk for close contact with the disease; recent immigrants or refugees from countries in which tuberculosis is common (e.g., Asia, Africa, Central and South America, Pacific islands); family members of migrant workers; residents of homeless shelters; or persons with certain underlying medical disorders.

HR3: Children with a family history of childhood hearing impairment or a personal history of congenital perinatal infection with herpes, syphilis, rubella, cytomegalovirus, or toxoplasmosis; malformations involving the head or neck (e.g., dysmorphic and syndromal abnormalities, cleft palate, abnormal pinna); birth weight less than 1500 g; bacterial meningitis; hyperbilirubinemia requiring exchange transfusion; or severe perinatal asphyxia (Apgar scores of 0–3, absence of spontaneous respirations for 10 minutes, or hypotonia at 2 hours of age).

HR4: Children with increased exposure to sunlight.

HR5: Children living in areas with inadequate water fluoridation (<0.7 ppm).

This list of preventive services is not exhaustive. It is adapted from the U.S. Preventive Services Task Force and the *AAFP Commission on Public Health and Scientific Affairs*. Clinicians may wish to add other preventive services on a routine basis and after considering the patient's medical history and other individual circumstances. Examples of target conditions not specifically examined by the task force include developmental disorders, speech problems, behavioral and learning disorders, parent/family dysfunction.

[a]One visit is required for immunizations. Because of lack of data and differing patient risk profiles, the scheduling of additional visits and the frequency of the individual preventive services listed in this table are left to clinical discretion (except as indicated in other footnotes).

carefully.[19] Many children with high cholesterol levels have normal levels during young adulthood in the absence of prescribed individual interventions.

The controversy regarding universal cholesterol screening in children is addressed in the National Cholesterol Education Program's "Report of the Expert Panel on Blood Cholesterol Levels in Children and Adolescents." It calls for a dietary approach aimed at lowering the average cholesterol levels of all Americans older than the age of 2 years[20] by consuming less than 30% of total calories from fat (with no more than 10% from saturated fatty acids) and less than 300 mg of dietary cholesterol intake per day. Selective screening is also recommended for children and adolescents at greatest risk of having high cholesterol as adults: (1) those whose parents or grandparents had coronary atherosclerosis or angiography before age 56; (2) those whose parents or grandparents had a myocardial infarction, angina, peripheral vascular disease, or sudden cardiac death before age 56; and (3) those whose parents' blood cholesterol level is greater than 240 mg/dl.

Other important interventions to promote cardiovascular health in children include counseling about obesity and smoking. Also routine updating of the family history of cardiovascular disease during well-child visits is important. Physicians should practice targeted screening to be effective in this area[21] (Table 2.4).

Thirteen to Eighteen Years

Adolescence through early adulthood represents a time of changing health hazards. Major health impediments to screen for and counsel about include injuries, violence, tobacco use and substance abuse, school failure, delinquency, suicide, unwanted pregnancy, and sexually transmitted diseases (Table 2.5).

Nineteen to Thirty-nine Years

Young adults have an opportunity to assume personal responsibility for their health and life expectancy; most of the leading causes of mortality during this age period are preventable through adoption of healthy behaviors. Important screening recommendations cover identification of infectious and sexually transmitted diseases; clinical and personal examinations for the early detection of breast, testicular, and skin cancer; and tests to identify coronary heart disease risk factors, as heart disease is the leading cause of mortality beyond age 40. Topics of concern for counseling include diet and exercise, substance use, sexual practices, and injury prevention. It is important to remember to offer immunizations (e.g., diphtheria toxoid boosters) and initiate preconception care routinely to women before pregnancy (Table 2.6).

Forty to Sixty-four Years

Heart disease, cancer, stroke, and chronic lung disease are the leading causes of mortality from age 40 to 64 years. Each has precursor health behaviors that are totally preventable or modifiable through effective physician intervention.

Coronary Heart Disease

More than 20% of persons who die from heart disease fall into this age group. The following interventions are recommended for primary prevention of myocardial infarction[22]: smoking cessation, lower cholesterol level, treatment of hypertension, maintenance of a physically active life style, avoidance of obesity, maintenance of normal glucose tolerance, postmenopausal estrogen-replacement therapy, mild-to-moderate consump-

TABLE 2.4. Periodic health examination: Ages 7–12 years
Schedule: See footnote[a]

Screening
History: interval medical and family history
Physical examination[a]
　Height and weight
　Blood pressure
　Tanner staging (A physical examination including Tanner stage is recommended at
　　least once in this age group.)
Laboratory/diagnostic procedures
　High-risk groups
　　Total cholesterol (Child of a parent with blood cholesterol 240 mg/dl or higher)
　　　(Exact frequency is not determined. It should be performed at least once.)
　　Lipoprotein analysis (Child of a parent or grandparent with a documented history
　　　of premature [age <55 years] cardiovascular disease. Exact frequency is not
　　　determined. It should be performed at least once.)
　　Tuberculin skin test (PPD) (HR1)

Patient and parent counseling
Diet and exercise
　Fat (especially saturated fat), cholesterol, sweets,
　　and between-meal snacks, sodium
Nutritional assessment
Selection of exercise program
Substance use: tobacco, alcohol, and other drugs:
　primary prevention
Sexual practices: sex education
Injury prevention
　Safety belts
　Smoke detector

Injury prevention (*continued*)
　Storage of drugs, toxic chemicals,
　　matches, and firearms
　Bicycle safety helmets
Dental health: regular tooth brushing
　and dental visits
Other primary preventive measures
　High-risk groups: skin protection
　　from ultraviolet light (HR2)

Immunizations and chemoprophylaxis
Update of immunization status, including measles/mumps/rubella (MMR) at ages 11–
　12 (if second dose)
High-risk groups: fluoride supplements (HR3)

Additional notes
Leading causes of death
　Motor vehicle crashes
　Injuries (nonmotor vehicle)
　Congenital anomalies
　Leukemia
　Homicide
　Heart disease

Remain alert for
　Vision disorders
　Diminished hearing
　Dental decay, malalignment, mouth
　　breathing
　Signs of child abuse or neglect
　Abnormal bereavement

High-risk categories
HR1: Household members of persons with tuberculosis or others at risk for close
　　contact with the disease; recent immigrants or refugees from countries in which
　　tuberculosis is common (e.g., Asia, Africa, Central and South America, Pacific
　　islands); family members of migrant workers; residents of homeless shelters; or
　　persons with certain underlying medical disorders.
HR2: Children with increased exposure to sunlight.
HR3: Children living in areas with inadequate water fluoridation (<0.7 ppm).

This list of preventive services is not exhaustive. It is adapted from the U.S. Preventive
Services Task Force and the *AAFP Commission on Public Health and Scientific Affairs*. Clinicians
may wish to add other preventive services on a routine basis and after considering the
patient's medical history and other individual circumstances. Examples of target conditions
not specifically examined by the task force include developmental disorders, scoliosis,
behavioral and learning disorders, parent/family dysfunction.
[a]Because of lack of data and differing patient risk profiles, the scheduling of visits and the
frequency of the individual preventive services listed in this table are left to clinical
discretion (except as indicated in other footnotes). Additional visits should occur as risk
factors are determined. Achievement of developmental or social milestones, such as entry
to junior high school, may also warrant a visit. Each visit by patients in this age group
should be considered an opportunity to assess and address risks.

TABLE 2.5. Periodic health examination: Ages 13–18
Schedule: At least one visit for preventive services[a]

Screening

History
  Interval medical and family history
  Dietary intake
  Physical activity
  Tobacco/alcohol/drug use
  Sexual practices
Physical examination
  Height and weight
  Blood pressure
  Tanner staging (A physical examination
    including Tanner stage is recommended at
    least once in this age group.)
  High-risk groups
    Complete skin examination (HR1)
    Clinical testicular examination (HR2)

Laboratory/diagnostic procedures
  High-risk groups
    Rubella antibodies (HR3)
    VDRL/RPR (HR4)
    Chlamydial testing (HR5)
    Gonorrhea culture (HR6)
    Counseling and testing for HIV (HR7)
    Tuberculin skin test (PPD) (HR8)
    Hearing (HR9)
    Papanicolaou smear (every 1–
      3 years) (HR10)
    Total cholesterol (Child of a parent
      with a blood cholesterol of
      240 mg/dl or higher)
    Lipoprotein analysis (Child of a
      parent or grandparent
      with a documented history of
      premature (age <55 years) cardio-
      vascular disease)

Counseling

Diet and exercise
  Fat (especially saturated fat), cholesterol,
    sodium, iron (girls), calcium (girls)
  Nutritional assessment
  Selection of exercise program
Substance use
  Tobacco: cessation/primary
    prevention
  Alcohol and other drugs: cessation/
    primary prevention
  Driving/other dangerous activities while
    under the influence
  Treatment for abuse
  High-risk groups
    Sharing/using unsterilized needles and
      syringes (HR11)
Sexual practices
  Sexual development and behavior (often best
    performed early in adolescence and with
    the involvement of parents)
  Sexually transmitted diseases: partner selection,
    condoms
  Unintended pregnancy and contraceptive
    options

Injury prevention
  Safety belts
  Safety helmets
  Violent behavior (especially boys)
  Firearms (especially boys)
  Smoke detector
  Noise-induced hearing loss (Education
    regarding hearing loss from
    recreational and personal
    listening devices is recommended.)
Dental health: regular tooth brushing,
  flossing, and dental visits
Other primary preventive measures
  Breast self-examination (Teaching
    of breast self-examination is
    recommended at the time of
    initiation of pelvic examinations.)
  Testicular self-examination
    (Teaching of testicular self-
    examination is recommended for boys.)
  High-risk groups
    Discussion of hemoglobin testing (HR12)
    Skin protection from ultraviolet
      light (HR13)

Immunizations and chemoprophylaxis
  Tetanus/diphtheria (Td) booster (once between ages 14 and 16)
  High-risk groups
    Measles/mumps/rubella (MMR) vaccine (A second measles immunization, preferably
      as MMR (measles/mumps/rubella vaccine, live) is recommended for all patients
      unable to show proof of immunity who are entering postsecondary education
      and for those becoming employed in medical occupations with direct patient care.)
    Hepatitis B vaccine (homosexually and bisexually active men, intravenous drug users,
      recipients of some blood products, persons in health-related jobs with frequent
      exposure to blood or blood products, household and sexual contacts of HBV

TABLE 2.5 *(continued)*

carriers, sexually active heterosexual persons with multiple sexual partners diagnosed as having recently acquired sexually transmitted disease, prostitutes, and persons who have a history of sexual activity with multiple partners in the previous 6 months)

Additional notes

Leading causes of death	Remain alert for
Motor vehicle crashes	Depressive symptoms
Homicide	Suicide risk factors (HR14)
Suicide	Abnormal bereavement
Injuries (nonmotor vehicle)	Tooth decay, malalignment, gingivitis
Heart disease	Signs of child abuse or neglect

High-risk categories

HR1: Persons with increased recreational or occupational exposure to sunlight, a family or personal history of skin cancer, or clinical evidence of precursor lesions (e.g., dysplastic nevi, certain congenital nevi).

HR2: Men with a history of cryptorchidism, orchiopexy, or testicular atrophy.

HR3: Women of childbearing age lacking evidence of immunity.

HR4: Persons who engage in sex with multiple partners in areas in which syphilis is prevalent, prostitutes, or contacts of persons with active syphilis.

HR5: Persons who attend clinics for sexually transmitted diseases; attend other high-risk health care facilities (e.g., adolescent and family planning clinics); or have other risk factors for chlamydial infection (e.g., multiple sexual partners or a sexual partner with multiple sexual contacts).

HR6: Persons with multiple sexual partners or a sexual partner with multiple contacts, sexual contacts of persons with culture-proved gonorrhea or persons with a history of repeated episodes of gonorrhea.

HR7: Persons seeking treatment for sexually transmitted diseases; homosexual and bisexual men; past or present intravenous (IV) drug users; persons with a history of prostitution or multiple sexual partners; women whose past or present sexual partners were infected bisexual or IV drug users; persons with long-term residence or birth in an area with high prevalence of HIV infection; or persons with a history of transfusion between 1978 and 1985.

HR8: Household members of persons with tuberculosis or others at risk for close contact with the disease; recent immigrants or refugees from countries in which tuberculosis is common (e.g., Asia, Africa, Central and South America, Pacific islands); family members of migrant workers; residents of homeless shelters; or persons with certain underlying medical disorders.

HR9: Persons exposed regularly to excessive noise in recreational or other settings.

HR10: Women who are sexually active or (if the sexual history is thought to be unreliable) aged 18 or older.

HR11: Intravenous drug users.

HR12: Persons of Caribbean, Latin American, Asian, Mediterranean, or African descent.

HR13: Persons with increased exposure to sunlight.

HR14: Recent divorce, separation, unemployment, depression, alcohol or other drug abuse, serious medical illnesses, living alone, or recent bereavement.

This list of preventive services is not exhaustive. It is adapted from the U.S. Preventive Services Task Force and the *AAFP Commission on Public Health and Scientific Affairs.* Clinicians may wish to add other preventive services on a routine basis and after considering the patient's medical history and other individual circumstances. Examples of target conditions not specifically examined by the task force include developmental disorders, scoliosis, behavioral and learning disorders, parent/family dysfunction.

*a*Additional visits should occur as other risk factors are determined, such as initiation of sexual activity, experimentation with alcohol or other drugs, or licensure for operating a motor vehicle. Achievement of developmental milestones, such as entry to high school, may also warrant a visit. Each visit by patients in this age group should be considered an opportunity to assess and address risks.

Screening

History
  Interval medical and family history
  Dietary intake
  Physical activity
  Tobacco/alcohol/drug use
  Sexual practices
Physical examination
  Height and weight
  Blood pressure (at every physician visit, with a minimum of every 2 years)
  Pelvic examination (women)
  Clinical breast examination (women) (HR1)
  Clinical testicular examination (men) (HR2)
  High-risk groups
    Complete oral cavity examination (HR3)
    Palpation for thyroid nodules (HR4)
    Complete skin examination (HR5)
Laboratory/diagnostic procedures
  Nonfasting or fasting total blood cholesterol (at least every 5 years)
  Papanicolaou smear (All women who are or who have been sexually active should
    have an annual Papanicolaou test and pelvic examination. After a woman has had
    three or more consecutive satisfactory normal annual examinations, the
    Papanicolaou test may be performed at the discretion of the physician and the
    patient, but not less frequently than every 3 years.)
  High-risk groups
    Fasting plasma glucose (HR6)
    Rubella antibodies (HR7)
    VDRL/RPR (HR8)
    Urinalysis for bacteriuria (Optimal frequency for urine testing has not been
      determined. In general, dipsticks combining the leukocyte esterase and nitrite
      tests should be used to detect asymptomatic bacteriuria.) (HR9)
    Chlamydia testing (HR10)
    Gonorrhea culture (HR11)
    Counseling and testing for HIV (HR12)
    Hearing (HR13)
    Tuberculin skin test (PPD) (HR14)
    Electrocardiogram (HR15)
    Mammogram (HR1)
    Colonoscopy (HR16)

Counseling

Diet and exercise
  Fat (especially saturated fat), cholesterol,
    complex carbohydrates, fiber, sodium, iron
    (women), calcium (women)
  Nutritional assessment
  Selection of exercise program
Substance use
  Tobacco: cessation/primary prevention
  Alcohol and other drugs: limiting alcohol
    consumption
  Driving/other dangerous activities while
    under the influence

Sexual practices
  Sexually transmitted diseases:
    partner selection, condoms,
    anal intercourse
  Unintended pregnancy and
    contraceptive options for men
    and women
Injury prevention
  Safety belts
  Safety helmets
  Violent behavior (especially young men)
  Firearms (especially young men)

TABLE 2.6. *(continued)*

Counseling *(continued)*

Substance use *(continued)*
  Treatment for abuse
  High-risk groups
    Sharing/using unsterilized needles and syringes (HR17)
  High-risk groups
    Back-conditioning exercises (HR18)
    Prevention of childhood injuries (HR19)
    Falls by the elderly (HR20)
Dental health: regular tooth brushing, flossing, dental visits
Other primary preventive measures
  Breast self-examination (Teaching breast self-examination is recommended at the time of initiation of pelvic examination.)
  Testicular self-examination (Teaching testicular self-examination is recommended for male patients.)
  High-risk groups
    Discussion of hemoglobin testing (HR21)
    Skin protection from ultraviolet light (HR22)

Injury prevention *(continued)*
  Smoke detector
  Smoking near bedding or upholstery

Immunizations and chemoprophylaxis

Tetanus/diphtheria (Td) booster (every 10 years)
High-risk groups
  Hepatitis B vaccine (HR23)
  Pneumococcal vaccine (HR24)
  Influenza vaccine (annually) (HR25)
  Measles/mumps/rubella vaccine (HR26)

Additional notes

Leading causes of death	Remain alert for
Motor vehicle crashes	Depressive symptoms
Homicide	Suicide risk factors (HR27)
Suicide	Abnormal bereavement
Injuries (nonmotor vehicle)	Malignant skin lesions
Heart disease	Tooth decay, gingivitis
AIDS	Signs of physical abuse

High-risk categories

HR1: Women aged 35 and older with a family history of premenopausally diagnosed breast cancer in a first-degree relative.

HR2: Men with a history of cryptorchidism, orchiopexy, or testicular atrophy.

HR3: Persons with exposure to tobacco or excessive amounts of alcohol or those with suspicious symptoms or lesions detected through self-examination.

HR4: Persons with a history of upper-body irradiation.

HR5: Persons with a family or personal history of skin cancer, increased recreational or occupational exposure to sunlight, or clinical evidence of precursor lesions (e.g., dysplastic nevi, certain congenital nevi).

HR6: Markedly obese, persons with a family history of diabetes, or women with a history of gestational diabetes.

HR7: Women lacking evidence of immunity.

HR8: Persons who engage in sex with multiple partners in areas in which syphilis is prevalent, prostitutes, or contacts of persons with active syphilis.

HR9: Persons with diabetes.

HR10: Persons who attend clinics for sexually transmitted diseases; attend other high-risk health care facilities (e.g., adolescent and family planning clinics); or have other risk factors for chlamydial infection (e.g., multiple sexual partners or a sexual partner with multiple sexual contacts, age <20).

(continued)

TABLE 2.6. (*continued*)

HR11: Persons with multiple sexual partners or a sexual partner with multiple contacts, sexual contacts of persons with culture-proved gonorrhea or persons with a history of repeated episodes of gonorrhea.

HR12: Persons seeking treatment for sexually transmitted diseases; homosexual and bisexual men; past or present intravenous (IV) drug users; persons with a history of prostitution or multiple sexual partners; women whose past or present sexual partners were infected bisexual or IV drug users; persons with long-term residence or birth in an area with high prevalence of HIV infection; or persons with a history of transfusion between 1978 and 1985.

HR13: Persons exposed regularly to excessive noise.

HR14: Household members of persons with tuberculosis or others at risk for close contact with the disease; recent immigrants or refugees from countries in which tuberculosis is common (e.g., Asia, Africa, Central and South America, Pacific islands); family members of migrant workers; residents of homeless shelters; or persons with certain underlying medical disorders.

HR15: Men who would endanger public safety were they to experience sudden cardiac events (e.g., commercial airline pilot).

HR16: Persons with a family history of familial polyposis coli or cancer family syndrome.

HR17: Intravenous drug users.

HR18: Persons at increased risk for low back injury because of past history, body configuration, or type of activities.

HR19: Persons with children in the home or automobile.

HR20: Persons with older adults in the home.

HR21: Young adults of Caribbean, Latin American, Asian, Mediterranean, or African descent.

HR22: Persons with increased exposure to sunlight.

HR23: Homosexually and bisexually active men, intravenous drug users, recipients of some blood products, persons in health-related jobs with frequent exposure to blood or blood products, household and sexual contacts of HBV carriers, sexually active heterosexual persons with multiple sexual partners diagnosed as having recently acquired sexually transmitted disease, prostitutes, and persons who have a history of sexual activity with multiple partners in the previous 6 months.

HR24: Persons with medical conditions that increase the risk of pneumococcal infection (e.g., chronic cardiac or pulmonary disease, sickle cell disease, nephrotic syndrome, Hodgkin's disease, asplenia, diabetes mellitus, alcoholism, cirrhosis, multiple myeloma, renal disease, or conditions associated with immunosuppression).

HR25: Residents of chronic care facilities or persons suffering from chronic cardiopulmonary disorders, metabolic diseases (including diabetes mellitus), hemoglobinopathies, immunosuppression, or renal dysfunction.

HR26: Persons born after 1956 who lack evidence of immunity to measles (receipt of live vaccine on or after first birthday, laboratory evidence of immunity, or a history of physician-diagnosed measles).

HR27: Recent divorce, separation, unemployment, depression, alcohol or other drug abuse, serious medical illnesses, living alone, or recent bereavement.

This list of preventive services is not exhaustive. It is adapted from the U.S. Preventive Services Task Force and the *AAFP Commission on Public Health and Scientific Affairs*. Clinicians may wish to add other preventive services on a routine basis and after considering the patient's medical history and other individual circumstances. Examples of target conditions not specifically examined by the task force include chronic obstructive pulmonary disease, hepatobiliary disease, bladder cancer, endometrial disease, travel-related illness, prescription drug abuse, occupational illness and injuries.

*a*The recommended schedule applies only to the periodic visit itself. The frequency of the individual preventive services listed in this table is left to clinical discretion, except as indicated in other footnotes.

TABLE 2.7. Primary prevention of myocardial infarction

Intervention	Estimated mean risk reduction[a]	Efficacy of strategies to modify risk
Smoking cessation	50–70% ↓ if stop within 5 years	Fair
↓Serum cholesterol	2–3% ↓ per 1% ↓ in level	Fair to good
Hypertension treatment	2–3% ↓ per 1 mm ↓ in DBP	Good
Exercise	45% ↓ if maintain active life style	Fair
Ideal body weight	35–55% ↓ if within 20% of IBW	Poor
Normoglycemia in diabetics	Insufficient data	Fair to poor
Postmenopausal ERT	44% ↓ with estrogen alone	NA
Mild-to-moderate ETOH use	25–45% ↓ compared with nondrinkers	NA
Aspirin	35% ↓ compared with nonusers	NA

Source: Adapted from Manson et al.[22] With permission.
[a]Estimated reductions in risk refer to independent contribution of each risk factor to myocardial infarction.
DBP = diastolic blood pressure; IBW = ideal body weight; ERT = estrogen replacement therapy; NA = not applicable; ETOH = alcohol.

tion of alcohol, and prophylactic low-dose aspirin (Table 2.7). Individual lifetime excess risks of heart disease death due to environmental tobacco smoke is 1 to 3 per 100.[23] Exercise stress testing is available to screen for ischemic heart disease in asymptomatic men at risk, to determine functional capacity, and to generate an exercise prescription.[24]

Cancer

More than 30% of cancer deaths are linked to smoking, and about 35% may be associated with diet. Many primary and secondary prevention interventions are recommended by the National Cancer Institute and Healthy People 2000. Counseling regarding tobacco use with an integrated office-based program best supports physician activities[25]: organized identification, progress records, brief physician messages, follow-up assistance, and a focus on those most interested in quitting. Passive smoking exposure is responsible for 3000 lung cancer cases each year in the United States among never-smokers.

Breast Cancer

Breast cancer is the most commonly diagnosed cancer and the second leading cause of mortality due to cancer.[26] Although there has been an increased incidence in recent years, perhaps because of improved screening, the death rate remains stable. Unalterable risk factors include family history and age at menarche and menopause. Other factors, such as parity and age at first pregnancy, are not easily modifiable. Thus, primary prevention interventions such as maintaining a low-fat diet and secondary prevention screening by mammography are essential. In 1990, only 58% of women aged 40 or older had had a mammogram within the preceding 2 years.[27]

Colon Cancer

Screening for colon cancer is controversial. The U.S. Preventive Services Task Force did not recommend any tests,[6] as they thought there was insufficient evidence to recommend screening for asymptomatic persons. However, the most common recommendation for persons 50 years or older is an annual fecal occult blood test (FOBT).[28] If the test is positive, follow-up examination with either colonoscopy or flexible sigmoidoscopy plus air-contrast barium enema (ACBE) should be undertaken. Persons between 50 and 75 may also benefit from screening with flexible sigmoidoscopy every 3 to 5 years.[29] There were 150,000 new cases of colon cancer diagnosed in 1991, with more than 60,000 related deaths. The percentage of lesions detected by each method and the relative cost of the tests are estimated to be as follows.[28]

FOBT	20–50%	$5
Flexible sigmoidoscopy	40%	$100–$200
ACBE	66–92%	$200
Colonoscopy	95%	$300–$500

One study found that screening with rigid sigmoidoscopy can lead to a 60% to 70% reduction in risk of death due to rectal or distal colon cancer.[29] In patients with a history of colon or rectal cancer in one or more first-degree relatives, screening colonoscopy should be performed at age 40 to 50 years, especially if the cancer was diagnosed when the relative was younger than age 40.[28]

Prostate Cancer

Diagnosed in more than 122,000 men each year, prostate cancer kills more than 32,000 annually, making it the second leading cause of cancer death of men older than age 55. One in 11 men develop this cancer in their lifetime, 1 in 9 if they are African-American. The median age at diagnosis is 72. An annual digital rectal examination (DRE) is recommended by age 40.[10] Both the U.S. and Canadian task forces, as of 1991, concluded that there is insufficient evidence to recommend prostate-specific antigen (PSA) serum levels routinely beginning at age 40 for men with a positive family history and age 50 for all other men. Nevertheless, PSA at present is the most accurate diagnostic marker available for prostate cancer, although it lacks adequate sensitivity and specificity to recommend generalized screen-

ing. Following the rate of change in serum PSA over tim'
to detect a greater percentage of curable prostate ca'
probably has no clinically important effect on the PS.
urinary tract infection, urinary tract manipulations, and ᵖ.
can cause spurious elevations in PSA levels. Thus, serum PSA lev.
be obtained before DRE or at a minimum of 6 weeks after any uᵣ.
infection or manipulation.

Osteoporosis

Osteoporosis is another major public health problem, affecting 24 million
Americans including 50% of women older than age 45 and 90% of women
older than age 75. Three groups of women are most likely to benefit from
increased risk-reduction strategies: premenopausal women; perimenopausal or postmenopausal women without previous estrogen supplementation; and women with multiple risk factors[31] (Table 2.8).

Chemoprophylaxis

Aspirin administration should be considered for the prevention of coronary heart disease and possibly colon cancer.[32] Adults who take aspirin
16 times a month for at least 1 year reduce their risk of dying from
colon cancer by 40% compared with nonaspirin users. Regular use of
nonsteroidal antiinflammatory drugs is associated with a 50% reduction
in combined risk of colon and rectal cancer. Estrogen, calcium, vitamin
D, and exercise for osteoporosis prevention and estrogen for heart disease prevention in postmenopausal women have been recommended.
Other recommendations include sunscreen with sun protection factor
16 or higher and active against both ultraviolet A and B rays and
specific antioxidant vitamins to inhibit cancer promotion and atherosclerosis. Low plasma levels of selenium, vitamins A, C, and E, and
β-carotene may be associated with an increased risk of cancer mortality
late in life.[15] The evidence is particularly strong for men older than
age 60. Low vitamin C intake is associated with increased gastrointestinal and stomach cancer. Vitamins A and E may inhibit cancer promotion. Also, vitamins C and E and β-carotene may protect older persons
against cataract formation (Table 2.8).

Sixty-five to Eighty-four Years

People who reach age 65 can expect to live into their eighties. Many seniors
have successfully "postponed" chronic conditions to later periods of their
life through previous successful risk reduction behaviors. The quality and
the quantity of life remaining are important considerations for the family

Screening

History
  Interval medical and family history
  Dietary intake
  Physical activity
  Tobacco/alcohol/drug use
  Sexual practices
Physical examination
  Height and weight
  Blood pressure (at every physician visit with a minimum of once every 2 years)
  Clinical breast examination (annually) (women)
  Pelvic examination
  Digital rectal examination
  High-risk groups
    Complete skin examination (HR1)
    Complete oral cavity examination (HR2)
    Palpation for thyroid nodules (HR3)
    Auscultation for carotid bruits (HR4)
Laboratory/diagnostic procedures
  Nonfasting or fasting total blood cholesterol (at least every 5 years)
  Papanicolaou smear (All women who are, or who have been, sexually active should have an annual Papanicolaou test and pelvic examination. After a woman has had three or more consecutive satisfactory normal annual examinations, the Papanicolaou test may be performed at the discretion of the physician and the patient but not less frequently than every 3 years.)
  Mammogram (It is recommended that mammography be performed annually for all women beginning at age 50. It may be clinically prudent to perform mammography every 1–2 years in women between the ages of 40 and 49.)
  High-risk groups
    Fasting plasma glucose (HR5)
    VDRL/RPR (HR6)
    Urinalysis for bacteriuria (HR7)
    Chlamydial testing (HR8)
    Gonorrhea culture (HR8)
    Counseling and testing for HIV (HR8)
    Tuberculin skin test (PPD) (HR9)
    Hearing (HR10)
    Electrocardiogram (HR11)
    Fecal occult blood/sigmoidoscopy (HR12)
    Fecal occult blood/colonoscopy (HR13)
    Bone mineral content (HR14)

Counseling

Diet and exercise
  Fat (especially saturated fat), cholesterol, complex carbohydrates, fiber, sodium, calcium (women)
  Nutritional assessment
  Selection of exercise program
Substance use
  Tobacco cessation
  Alcohol and other drugs: limiting alcohol consumption

Substance use (*continued*)
  Driving/other dangerous activities while under the influence
  Treatment for abuse
  High-risk groups
    Sharing/using unsterilized needles and syringes (HR15)
Sexual practices
  Sexually transmitted diseases; partner selection, condoms, anal intercourse

TABLE 2.8. *(continued)*

Sexual practices *(continued)*
  Unintended pregnancy and contraceptive options
Injury prevention
  Safety belts
  Safety helmets
  Snoke detector
  Smoking near bedding or upholstery
  High-risk groups
    Back-conditioning exercises (HR16)
    Prevention of childhood injuries (HR17)
    Falls by the elderly (HR18)
  Dental health: regular tooth brushing, flossing, dental visits
  Other primary preventive measures
    High-risk groups
    Skin protection from ultraviolet light (HR19)
    Discussion of aspirin therapy (HR20)
    Discussion of estrogen replacement therapy (HR21)

Immunizations and chemoprophylaxis
  Tetanus/diphtheria (Td) booster (every 10 years)
  High-risk groups
    Hepatitis B vaccine (HR22)
    Pneumococcal vaccine (HR23)
    Influenza vaccine (annually) (HR24)

Additional notes

Leading causes of death	Remain alert for
Heart disease	Depressive symptoms
Lung cancer	Suicide risk factors (HR25)
Cerebrovascular disease	Abnormal bereavement
Breast cancer	Signs of physical abuse or neglect
Colorectal cancer	Malignant skin lesions
Obstructive lung disease	Peripheral arterial disease (HR26)
	Tooth decay, gingivitis, loose teeth

High-risk categories

HR1: Persons with a family or personal history of skin cancer, increased recreational or occupational exposure to sunlight, or clinical evidence of precursor lesions (e.g., dysplastic nevi, certain congenital nevi).

HR2: Persons with exposure to tobacco or excessive amounts of alcohol, or those with suspicious symptoms or lesions detected through self-examination.

HR3: Persons with a history of upper-body irradiation.

HR4: Persons with risk factors for cerebrovascular or cardiovascular disease (e.g., hypertension, smoking, CAD, atrial fibrillation, diabetes) or those with neurologic symptoms (e.g., transient ischemic attacks) or a history of cerebrovascular disease.

HR5: Markedly obese, persons with a family history of diabetes, or women with a history of gestational diabetes.

HR6: Prostitutes, persons who engage in sex with multiple partners in areas in which syphilis is prevalent, or contacts of persons with active syphilis.

HR7: Persons with diabetes.

HR8: Persons seeking treatment for sexually transmitted diseases; homosexual and bisexual men; past or present intravenous (IV) drug users; persons with a history of prostitution or multiple sexual partners; women whose past or present sexual partners were infected bisexual or IV drug users; persons with long-term residence or birth in an area with high prevalence of HIV infection; or persons with a history of transfusion between 1978 and 1985.

TABLE 2.8. *(continued)*

HR9: Household members of persons with tuberculosis or others at risk for close contact with the disease; recent immigrants or refugees from countries in which tuberculosis is common (e.g., Asia, Africa, Central and South America, Pacific islands); family members of migrant workers; residents of homeless shelters; or persons with certain underlying medical disorders.

HR10: Persons exposed regularly to excessive noise.

HR11: Men with two or more cardiac risk factors (high blood cholesterol, hypertension, cigarette smoking, diabetes mellitus, family history of CAD); men who would endanger public safety were they to experience sudden cardiac events (e.g., commercial airline pilots); or sedentary or high-risk men planning to begin a vigorous exercise program.

HR12: Persons aged 50 and older who have first-degree relatives with colorectal cancer; a personal history of endometrial, ovarian, or breast cancer; or a previous diagnosis of inflammatory bowel disease, adenomatous polyps, or colorectal cancer.

HR13: Persons with a family history of familial polyposis coli or cancer family syndrome.

HR14: Perimenopausal women at increased risk for osteoporosis (e.g., Caucasian, bilateral oophorectomy before menopause, slender build) and for whom estrogen replacement therapy would otherwise not be recommended.

HR15: Intravenous drug users.

HR16: Persons at increased risk for low back injury because of past history, body configuration, or type of activities.

HR17: Persons with children in the home or automobile.

HR18: Persons with older adults in the home.

HR19: Persons with increased exposure to sunlight.

HR20: Men who have risk factors for myocardial infarction (e.g., high blood cholesterol, smoking, diabetes mellitus, family history of early-onset CAD) and who lack a history of gastrointestinal or other bleeding problems, and other risk factors for bleeding or cerebral hemorrhage.

HR21: Perimenopausal women at increased risk for osteoporosis (e.g., Caucasian, low bone mineral content, bilateral oophorectomy before menopause or early menopause, slender build) and who are without known contraindications (e.g., history of undiagnosed vaginal bleeding, active liver disease, thromboembolic disorders, hormone-dependent cancer).

HR22: Homosexually and bisexually active men, intravenous drug users, recipients of some blood products, persons in health-related jobs with frequent exposure to blood or blood product, household and sexual contacts of HBV carriers, sexually active heterosexual persons with multiple sexual partners diagnosed as having recently acquired sexually transmitted disease, prostitutes, and persons who have a history of sexual activity with multiple partners in the previous 6 months.

HR23: Persons with medical conditions that increase the risk of pneumococcal infection (e.g., chronic cardiac or pulmonary disease, sickle cell disease, nephrotic syndrome, Hodgkin's disease, asplenia, diabetes mellitus, alcoholism, cirrhosis, multiple myeloma, renal disease or conditions associated with immunosuppression).

HR24: Residents of chronic care facilities and persons suffering from chronic cardiopulmonary disorders, metabolic diseases (including diabetes mellitus), hemoglobinopathies, immunosuppression, or renal dysfunction.

TABLE 2.8. *(continued)*

HR25: Recent divorce, separation, unemployment, depression, alcohol or other drug abuse, serious medical illnesses, living alone, or recent bereavement.

HR26: Persons older than age 50, smokers, or persons with diabetes mellitus.

This list of preventive services is not exhaustive. It is adapted from the U.S. Preventive Services Task Force and the *AAFP Commission on Public Health and Scientific Affairs.* Clinicians may wish to add other preventive services on a routine basis and after considering the patient's medical history and other individual circumstances. Examples of target conditions not specifically examined by the task force include chronic obstructive pulmonary disease; hepatobiliary disease; bladder cancer; endometrial disease; travel-related illness; prescription drug abuse; occupational illness and injuries.

*a*The recommended schedule applies only to the periodic visit itself. The frequency of the individual preventive services listed in this table is left to clinical discretion, except as indicated in other footnotes.

physician when selecting preventive interventions for this age group. The elderly are not a homogeneous population, a point that must be taken into consideration when customizing a package of prevention services for each patient. Older individuals may be more vulnerable to adverse effects of preventive services so the relative value for certain interventions may be questionable. Cognitive function is impaired in many elderly, which represents a significant health problem in that it may place the individual or others in physical danger. One of the most important considerations for the healthy older adult is sustaining a physically active life style to reduce the incidence of coronary disease, hypertension, diabetes, colon cancer, depression, and anxiety; increase bone mineral content; maintain appropriate body weight; and improve balance, coordination, and strength to reduce falls.

Other counseling topics include review of medication use and the importance of social support networks. Valuable clinical preventive services that are clearly effective in the elderly include identification and control of hypertension; screening for cancers, early signs or symptoms of dementia, depression, reversible sensory deficits, and urinary incontinence; and immunization against pneumonia and influenza.[33] Chemoprophylaxis with aspirin, estrogen, calcium, vitamins, and sunscreen is also recommended.

Indicators of poor nutritional status include physical signs and specific symptoms or sets of symptoms: significant weight loss over time, significant low or high weight for height, significant reduction in serum albumin to less than 3.5 mg/dl, significant reduction in midarm circumference, significant increase or decrease in skinfold measurement, significant obesity, inappropriate food intake, and selected nutrition-related disorders[34] (Table 2.9).

TABLE 2.9. Periodic health examination: Ages 65–84 years
Schedule: Every year[a]

Screening

History
  Interval medical and family history
  Medication use (prescription and
    nonprescription)
  Prior symptoms of transient ischemic
    attack
  Dietary intake
  Physical activity
  Tobacco/alcohol/drug use
  Functional status at home
Physical examination
  Height and weight
  Blood pressure (at every physician visit
    with a minimum of every 2 years)
  Visual acuity
  Hearing and hearing aids
  Clinical breast examination (annually)
  Pelvic examination
  Cardiac auscultation
  Digital rectal examination

Physical examination (continued)
  High-risk groups
    Auscultation for carotid bruits (HR1)
    Complete skin examination (HR2)
    Complete oral cavity examination (HR3)
    Palpation of thyroid nodules (HR4)
Laboratory/diagnostic procedures
  Nonfasting or fasting (at least
    every 5 years) total blood
    cholesterol
  Dipstick urinalysis
  Mammogram (It is recommended
    that mammography be performed
    annually for all women beginning
    at age 50.)
  Thyroid function tests (women)
  High-risk groups
    Fasting plasma glucose (HR5)
    Tuberculin skin test (PPD) (HR6)
    Electrocardiogram (HR7)
    Papanicolaou smear (every
      1–3 years) (HR8)
    Fecal occult blood/sigmoidoscopy (HR9)
    Fecal occult blood/colonoscopy (HR10)

Counseling

Diet and exercise
  Fat (especially saturated fat), cholesterol,
    complex carbohydrates, fiber, sodium,
    calcium (women)
  Nutritional assessment
  Selection of exercise program
Substance use
  Tobacco cessation
  Alcohol and other drugs: limiting alcohol
    consumption
  Driving/other dangerous activities while
    under the influence
  Treatment for abuse
Sexual practices: sexuality
Injury prevention
  Prevention of falls
  Safety belts
  Smoke detector
  Smoking near bedding or upholstery
  Hot water heater temperature (≤120°F)

Injury prevention (continued)
  Safety helmets
  High-risk groups
    Prevention of childhood injuries (HR11)
    Education regarding hearing loss from
      recreational and personal listening
      devices is recommended
Dental health: regular tooth brushing,
  flossing, and dental visits
Other primary preventive measures
  Glaucoma test
  Advance directives/living will/durable
    power of attorney
  High-risk groups
    Discussion of estrogen
      replacement therapy (HR12)
    Discussion of aspirin therapy (HR13)
    Skin protection from ultraviolet
      light (HR14)

TABLE 2.9. (continued)

Immunizations and chemoprophylaxis

Tetanus/diphtheria (Td) booster (every 10 years)
Influenza vaccine (annually)
Pneumococcal vaccine

High-risk groups
Hepatitis B vaccine (HR15)

Additional notes

Leading causes of death
  Heart disease
  Cerebrovascular disease
  Obstructive lung disease
  Pneumonia/influenza
  Lung cancer
  Colorectal cancer

Remain alert for
  Depression symptoms
    Suicide risk factors (HR16)
    Abnormal bereavement
  Changes in cognitive function
  Medications that increase risk of falls
  Signs of physical abuse or neglect
  Malignant skin lesions
  Peripheral arterial disease
  Tooth decay, gingivitis, loose teeth
  Abnormal bereavement

High-risk categories

HR1: Persons with risk factors for cerebrovascular or cardiovascular disease (e.g., hypertension, smoking, CAD, atrial fibrillation, diabetes) or those with neurologic symptoms (e.g., transient attacks) or a history of cerebrovascular disease.

HR2: Persons with increased recreational or occupational exposure to sunlight, a family or personal history of skin cancer, or clinical evidence of precursor lesions (e.g., dysplastic nevi, certain congenital nevi).

HR3: Persons with exposure to tobacco or excessive amounts of alcohol, or those with suspicious symptoms or lesions detected through self-examination.

HR4: Persons with a history of upper-body irradiation.

HR5: Markedly obese, persons with a family history of diabetes, or women with a history of gestational diabetes.

HR6: Household members of persons with tuberculosis or others at risk for close contact with the disease; recent immigrants or refugees from countries in which tuberculosis is common (e.g., Asia, Africa, Central and South America, Pacific islands); family members of migrant workers; residents of homeless shelters; or persons with certain underlying medical disorders.

HR7: Men with two or more cardiac risk factors (high blood cholesterol, hypertension, cigarette smoking, diabetes mellitus, family history of CAD); men who would endanger public safety were they to experience sudden cardiac events (e.g., commercial airline pilots); or sedentary or high-risk men planning to begin a vigorous exercise program.

HR8: Women who have not had previous documented screening in which smears have been consistently negative.

HR9: Persons who have first-degree relatives with colorectal cancer; a personal history of endometrial, ovarian, or breast cancer; or a previous diagnosis of inflammatory bowel disease, adenomatous polyps, or colorectal cancer.

HR10: Persons with a family history of familial polyposis coli or cancer family syndrome.

HR11: Persons with children in the home or automobile.

HR12: Perimenopausal women at increased risk for osteoporosis (e.g., Caucasian, low bone mineral content, bilateral oophorectomy before menopause or early menopause, slender build) and who are without known contraindications (e.g., history of undiagnosed vaginal bleeding, active liver disease, thromboembolic disorders, hormone-dependent cancer).

(continued)

TABLE 2.9. (*continued*)

HR13: Men who have risk factors for myocardial infarction (e.g., high blood cholesterol, smoking, diabetes mellitus, family history of early-onset CAD) and who lack a history of gastrointestinal or other bleeding problems, and other risk factors for bleeding or cerebral hemorrhage.

HR14: Persons with increased exposure to sunlight.

HR15: Homosexually and bisexually active men, intravenous drug users, recipients of some blood products, persons in health-related jobs with frequent exposure to blood or blood products, household and sexual contacts of HBV carriers, sexually active heterosexual persons with multiple sexual partners diagnosed as having recently acquired sexually transmitted disease, prostitutes, and persons who have a history of sexual activity with multiple partners in the previous 6 months.

HR16: Recent divorce, separation, unemployment, depression, alcohol or other drug abuse, serious medical illnesses, living alone, or recent bereavement.

This list of preventive services is not exhaustive. It is adapted from the U.S. Preventive Services Task Force and the *AAFP Commission on Public Health and Scientific Affairs.* Clinicians may wish to add other preventive services on a routine basis and after considering the patient's medical history and other individual circumstances. Examples of target conditions not specifically examined by the task force include chronic obstructive pulmonary disease; travel-related illness; hepatobiliary disease; prescription drug abuse; bladder cancer; occupational illness and injuries; endometrial disease.

*a*The recommended schedule applies only to the periodic visit itself. The frequency of the individual preventive services listed in this table is left to clinical discretion except as indicated in other footnotes.

Age 85 and Older

The most rapid population increase during the 1990s is occurring among those older than age 85.[35] This age group is composed of a substantial number of persons not independent in terms of physical functioning. Thus, the focus for clinical preventive services in this age group should be on maintaining function physically, socially, and emotionally. See Table 2.10 for specific preventive services that have improved or diminished effectiveness in the elderly (>age 85).[33] In this age group, the family physician should change orientation from the prevention of conditions to monitoring and decreasing the impact of chronic conditions on quality of life.

Health Maintenance Strategies for Integrating Clinical Preventive Services into the Family Practice Office

Clinical prevention is best delivered by following protocols and guidelines, and it is enhanced by practice aids such as flow sheets and reminder systems. The health maintenance strategies that follow are tools and competencies that may enhance the ability of physicians to change patient

TABLE 2.10. Periodic health examination ages 85 and older
(preventive services that have improved or diminished
effectiveness in the old old)
Schedule: Every year

Preventive service	Improved effectiveness	Diminished effectiveness
History		
Accidents		
Fall prevention; particularly with a history of previous falls	X	
Motor vehicle		X
Mobility: ADL/IADL assessment	X	
Nutrition (undernutrition) screening or counseling	X	
Podiatry care	X	
Polypharmacy identification	X	
Dementia screening	X	
Urinary incontinence screening	X	
Physical examination		
Blood pressure		X
Cancer screening		
Breast		X
Cervix		X
Hearing screening	X	
Visual acuity screening	X	
Laboratory evaluation		
Cholesterol		X
Interventions		
Advance directives counseling	X	
Vaccinations		
Influenza immunization	X	

Source: Adapted from Zazove et al.[33] With permission of Appleton & Lange, Inc.

behaviors to reduce health risks. They are central to the physician–patient
relationship and parallel the strategies traditionally used in the care of
individuals with acute and chronic problems. Effective physician counseling skills lead to empowering and motivating patients to make changes in
health behavior.

It is helpful to audit charts to determine baseline rates when performing
various preventive interventions, such as immunizations, counseling, identifying smokers, and recommending mammograms. Physicians should
establish reasonable goals for an office-based, age-specific prevention program given existing resources and patient population needs. The goals
include profiling patients based on risk factors and membership in high-
risk groups.

Development and use of a "prevention-friendly" patient record and charting system can improve adherence to preventive service guidelines and recommendations. This system should permit effective organization and management of prevention information longitudinally at both patient and practice population levels. It may include problem lists with risk factors identified, flow sheets, patient-held minirecords, tracking forms, manual and computerized reminders, and health risk appraisals.

Flow sheets for health maintenance are the most commonly used tracking tool.[36] Studies have shown that they improve physician record-keeping, yet physicians do not always record all interventions done on such sheets. Flow sheets should be in examination rooms as posters and on patient charts. They are especially useful in group practices to maintain continuity in the delivery of preventive services when different providers may be involved. Qualities of a good flow sheet include all information on one page per age group to facilitate ease of seeing dates of procedures done; limited writing and codes or initials; prominent location in the chart near the front cover; adequate staff and physician training to use the sheets; and a system of periodic prompts or reminders.[36] Prompts or reminders appear to increase health risk behavior counseling and the efficacy of behavioral prescriptions.[37]

Improved physician cooperation over a 5-year period (from 71% to 85%) has been shown to occur with a "package" of major, noncontroversial, screening interventions (blood pressure, smoking history, alcohol use history, fecal occult blood test, Papanicolaou smear, and clinical breast examination), with systematic placement of a health maintenance flow sheet (age appropriate) on all adult charts.[38]

Patient-held minirecords have been successfully used to promote preventive care.[39] In one study, their use was well accepted by providers and led to improvements in compliance with guidelines. They can help build cooperation between patient, providers, and nursing staff. The pocket-sized booklets allow patients to keep track of their health histories and preventive services they need or have received.

Tracking forms, such as those often mandated for Medicaid populations to deliver Early Periodic Screening and Developmental Testing services, are also useful for prompting and "memory-jogging." Use of these tracking forms at the University of Arizona Family Practice Office led to completion of 91% of all possible clinical prevention interventions (e.g., nutritional assessment of 95% of children seen for well-child care, 89% with developmental assessments, 76% with age-appropriate completed physical examinations, 96% with immunizations up to date, and 88% receiving counseling on anticipatory guidance topics identified on the forms).

Reminder/prompting systems involve the generation of compliance reminders, either manually or by computer, as a systematic approach to tracking patients in need of routine preventive care. Generating an updated report on health care maintenance needs for each visit and distributing the report to the patient is also helpful. Manual prompts include routine charting, a tickler file, or stickers on the charts of patients with life-style risks. Messages can be stamped onto progress notes periodically to remind physicians to update problem lists or flow sheets, ask patients about their physical activity level, whether they use seat belts, and so on. Postcard reminder systems may prompt patients who do not have appointments for acute problems to return for health care maintenance.[36] Mailed influenza vaccine reminders have increased the percentage of patients obtaining immunizations in 1 year from 11.1% to 45.5%.[40] The main weaknesses of manual reminder systems are their dependence on physician motivation and inadequate outreach to inactive patients.

Computer-generated systems range from offering a status report for the physician at each visit (e.g., listing the preventive services that should be delivered to the patient) to programs for recalling inactive patients. Cost-effective programs are linked to the practice's billing system to eliminate duplicate demographic data gathering. Such prompting reports often identify office educational/counseling resources or list appropriate community referrals to streamline physician actions. Often programs generate letters to patients on their birthdays reminding them of recommended annual preventive services. Computer-generated physician and patient reminders have been shown to improve adherence to preventive services. A recent study by Frame et al.[41] concluded that computer-based health maintenance tracking improved the physicians' health maintenance compliance as compared with the manual system. This improvement by using a computer-based system occurred without a significant increase in patient visits or billings. The best results occur when the reminders are given to both groups.[42] In one study,[42] use of reminders increased the percentage of patients with cholesterol screening, an annual fecal occult blood test, a mammogram, and current tetanus vaccination. However, computer reminders to obtain an influenza vaccine may promote independent action among younger patients but engender dependency on the reminder among older patients who have more frequent visits.[43]

The "Put Prevention into Practice" program of the U.S. Public Health Service is an excellent example of a bundled information management system, with kits for physicians that include an updated clinician's handbook on selecting and administering preventive services, flow sheets for patient charts, a set of colored chart stickers to alert physicians to patients who need periodic services (e.g., tobacco use counseling, or influenza vaccines), postcards to notify patients when preventive services are needed, and pocket-sized patient-held minirecords in Spanish and English. Kits, with patient minirecords, are available by contacting AAFP Order Department (1-800-944-0000). Request kit number E-1999 at $60 each.[44]

Health risk appraisals (HRAs) can add impact to initial risk evaluation using flow sheets.[45] These instruments determine an individual's risk of preventable death or chronic illness on the basis of health history, life style, physiologic test findings, age, and gender. The patient's profile is compared with a database of epidemiologic and mortality statistics. They can be used by physicians to motivate and educate patients, encourage them to take greater responsibility for their health, make healthy life-style decisions, and make appropriate use of medical services. They are intended to be used with persons who are free from chronic illnesses, and their use has been mostly with middle-class, middle-aged, white populations. Health risk appraisals should be used only in conjunction with risk reduction counseling or programs. For more information, contact the Society of Prospective Medicine at 402-291-3297. A directory has been prepared by the society to assist providers in selecting the instrument most appropriate for their practice population. Conversational microcomputer-based HRAs seem to be cost-effective with older users.[43] There have been few controlled trials of HRAs in primary care practice.

Availability of Quality Patient Education Materials

Patient education can be streamlined by providing easy-to-read handouts with large print (especially important for the elderly and those with visual impairment) at the literacy level appropriate to a given patient population. Literacy levels usually range from fourth to eighth grade in diverse urban practice settings. Simple tests (e.g., Fog test) are available to determine literacy level. Often comic book formats are effective. If a significant portion of a practice is Spanish-speaking, materials should be available in Spanish.

The patient education newsletter can be an effective tool in family practice, allowing the physician to communicate information about preventive services and health promotion recommendations.[46] Staff should participate in their preparation. Information from a variety of sources can be assimilated. Monthly practice themes with attractive posters and buttons for patients and staff can be rotated periodically. Educational videotapes to view in the waiting room can save time and serve to supplement physician advice. Magazines should exclude tobacco advertising. Explicit and implicit prevention messages should be delivered in the simplest format possible.

Special kits are available for specific types of intervention. For example, the American Academy of Family Physicians (AAFP) Stop Smoking Kit includes a variety of clinical tools, patient materials, chart forms, and staff/physician manuals. The AAFP also has immunization record cards and chart stickers available.

Linkages with the Community

Linkages are recommended in *Healthy People 2000:* it is suggested that physicians become involved with local groups to develop countywide or statewide prevention plans and incorporate the objectives of Healthy Older Adults 2000 or Healthy Youth 2000 into practice plans. Physicians can serve as catalysts within their communities to encourage establishment of local objectives and priorities and implementation of innovative methods to achieve them.[1] Family physicians often provide clinical prevention information to community groups and local media. Family physician involvement with schools can also effectively lead to important preventive health changes. For example, in one study, family physicians volunteering time at six public schools doubled helmet ownership among bicycle riders. During a 1-week educational intervention, family physicians provided 15-minute talks at each school.[47]

Building an Office Team Approach to Manage Time Efficiently

All available office personnel can be included in a team effort to promote and reinforce a healthy environment and life style for patients and staff alike. Office personnel have a vital role in implementing practice prevention policies. Staff and the office setting should reinforce prevention messages.[37] Assigning an office staff member the responsibility of coordinating specific prevention activities can be effective.

Offering group classes as an alternative to well-child care visits can be a time-efficient method of discussing such health issues as feeding, immunizations, and home safety. Such group parent education classes can be successful with as many as 40 parents at once. They drastically reduce the number of times the physician or other providers must give the same preventive advice.

The nursing staff can be effective at tracking preventive care delivered and prompting physicians to recommend interventions. After nurses clipped reminder slips to the front of patient charts, the administration of fecal occult blood tests was increased from 32% to 47%, physician clinical breast examination from 29% to 46%, and influenza vaccination from 18% to 40%.[48] It is also important to involve patients in screening and preventive activities. For example, distributing self-administered fecal occult blood test slide kits to patients at clinic registration increased screening to 57% and was more successful than reminder cards on patient charts and training programs.[49]

Developing "Minicounseling" Topics

Physicians can develop 5 to 10 minicounseling topics, each about 3 to 10 minutes in duration. Selection of topics should be based on the risks and needs of the physician's practice population. A sample list for a practice might be productive activity, nutrition, stress reduction, cancer prevention, tobacco use, injury prevention, discipline and parenting skills, preventing heart disease, midlife challenges, and family health promotion.

Reimbursement Issues and the Economics of Prevention

Thousands of years ago Chinese physicians were reimbursed for their services only when their patients maintained their health. Today prepaid capitated HMO plans offer less health promotion than expected. Fewer than 50% of HMOs allocate funds for clinical preventive services.[50] Access to and payment for preventive services are major issues facing the American health care system during the 1990s. Most proposed health reform plans inadequately address this issue. Despite a growing body of research demonstrating the health benefits and cost-effectiveness of preventive services, physicians remain appropriately frustrated by the current reimbursement system, which for the most part denies payment for preventive screening, counseling, and immunizations.[51]

Use of preventive strategies has been strongly linked with insurance.[52] For instance, poor women with Medicaid are less likely to be referred for mammography.[53] Even enrollees in health insurance plans who are required to share costs made significantly less use of preventive services than did those who received free care.[54] In HMOs and in settings where care is not billed to the patient, there is greater use of preventive services.[55]

It is important for physicians to charge appropriately for the time and resources used when delivering preventive care, based on the length of visit. Fortunately, efforts among private insurers and Medicare suggest that improvements in coverage are occurring rapidly during the 1990s. Medicare's resource-based relative value scale codes allow physicians to include their counseling services as "contributory components" in both inpatient and outpatient settings. Typical areas related to preventive services include discussion with patient, family, or both (the very young and the very old) concerning diagnostic results from screening tests and recommended diagnostic studies, the importance of compliance with management options, risk factor reduction, and patient and family education.

Nationally, Blue Cross and Blue Shield, covering more than 73 million Americans, encourages certain screening tests in policies issued by member employer-based plans based on recommendations by the American College of Physicians. If adopted nationally, it is estimated that the recommended interventions would improve the quality of life for many patients, but it would boost the nation's net health care bill by an estimated $1 billion to $3 billion annually. Nevertheless, the average cost of preventive services benefits would be only about $7.50/month for family coverage. Other estimates for total lifetime preventive costs incurred by age 85 years range from $2900 to $4300 for men and from $4700 to $6600 for women.[56] The Office of Disease Prevention and Health Promotion estimates a cost of $46 per adult per year for preventive services, or around 1% of the nation's annual health spending.

Prevention may not save money; it usually adds to medical expenditures. Thus when assessing preventive interventions, a cost-effective analysis (how much health is obtained by spending money on medical care) is more appropriate than cost-benefit analysis (how much money is saved by spending some). The cost of success is often the price of longer life. Two potential "costs" to society are the cost of diseases that the aged live to develop and the added cost of old-age pensions, including Social Security payments.

During the 1990s, many innovative state and national health plans were drafted in efforts at health care reform. Most ranked high prenatal care and adult and children's preventive services. The AAFP's "Rx for Health" health care reform proposal would require all insurance plans to include a federally mandated basic benefits package that stresses general medical and preventive services. Plans would cover preventive services with no cost-sharing by the patient.

Future Trends in Clinical Prevention Affecting Family Physicians

Family physicians will increasingly practice in settings driven by large-scale computerized database systems to control costs and analyze the quality of clinical care and types of clinical prevention activities being delivered. Group practice environments with sophisticated database systems require that tomorrow's family physicians be recognized for their health promotion expertise. Thus, the professional education of family physicians will be more oriented toward health promotion, disease prevention, and patient counseling activities. These clinical preventive foci will, in turn, reflect the rapidly advancing knowledge base regarding clinical prevention. Thus, a critical competence for the family physician is the ability to absorb new information regarding clinical prevention in a rapid manner and to translate that information into preventive-oriented patient care.

Published reports such as *Healthy People 2000*[15] set standards and goals for family physicians. These goals will be revised and the strategies modified as research in the area of clinical prevention yields new information on which to improve practice guidelines.

The challenge of the 1990s to the family physician is to implement practical, simple, reproducible clinical prevention strategies in the office setting to address the existing barriers to clinical prevention that arise from the health system, patient behaviors, and traditional physician practice styles. Guidelines, outcomes research, randomized controlled studies, and model practices are needed to increase our understanding about how clinical prevention can become more effective. Physicians and health care organizations will inevitably be offering preventive services as a strategy to increase market share.

Based on current state-of-the-art programs, it appears that clinical prevention efforts in the primary care settings of the future can be characterized in the following ways.

1. They will become more widespread as more physicians, especially during their years of training, are exposed to concepts of preventive medicine.
2. As evidence supporting the cost-effectiveness of comprehensive health promotion and disease prevention packages mounts, such services will be mandated by employers, insurance companies, and federal and state regulatory agencies, who will also pay for the delivery of such services.
3. They will be delivered by "teams" creatively using midlevel practitioners to decrease the physicians' time and operating costs.
4. Group practices will identify one physician as their clinical preventive medicine specialist or an interdisciplinary committee of staff members to develop and periodically review their comprehensive health promotion package (assessment instruments, screening procedures, resources for counseling and education, data collection to describe their population) and to help initiate targeted campaigns based on their practice population needs.
5. The quality of care delivered and reimbursement received by physicians will be determined in part by their ability to provide health promotion services and to affect the morbidity and mortality of their defined practice populations.
6. National standards with respect to the quality of clinical prevention activities in primary care will be developed and monitored by regulatory agencies.
7. Health assessment technologic advances will allow physicians to individualize health risk trends more accurately and produce risk profiles for much earlier identification of cancer and cardiovascular disease. Most importantly, impetus for the continued delivery of clinical prevention activities should be documented proof of their impact on improving quality of life and compressing morbidity,[57] rather than on reducing health care dollar expenditures alone.

References

1. Kligman EW, Kamerow DB, Artz LM. Year 2000 health objectives and the family physician. Am Fam Physician 1990;42:851–4.
2. Pew Health Professions Commission. Healthy America: practitioners for 2005, an agenda for action for US health professional schools. In: Shugars DA, O'Neil EH, Baden JD, editors. Durham, NC: The Pew Health Profession, 1991.

3. Pommerenke FA, Dietrich A. Improving and maintaining preventive services. Part 1. Applying the patient model. J Fam Pract 1992;34:86–91.
4. Richards JW, Blum A. Health promotion. In: Taylor R, editor. Family Medicine: Principles and Practice. 2nd ed. New York: Springer-Verlag, 1988.
5. Pommerenke FA, Dietrich AD. Improving and maintaining preventive services. Part 2. Practical principles for primary care. J Fam Pract 1992;34:92–97.
6. US Preventive Services Task Force. Guide to clinical preventive services: an assessment of the effectiveness of 169 interventions. Baltimore: Williams & Wilkins, 1989.
7. Stang KC, Fedirko T, Zyzanski SJ, et al. How do family physicians prioritize delivery of multiple preventive services? J Fam Pract 1994;38:231–7.
8. Canadian Task Force on the Periodic Health Examination. The periodic health examination. Can Med Assoc J 1979;121:1194–254.
9. Sox HC. Preventive health services in adults. N Engl J Med 1994;330(22): 1589–95.
10. American Cancer Society. Report on the cancer-related health checkup. CA 1980;30:194–240.
11. Frame PS. A critical review of adult health maintenance. Part 4. Prevention of metabolic, behavioral, and miscellaneous conditions. J Fam Pract 1986;23: 29–39 (erratum: J Fam Pract 1986;23:537).
12. Healthy people: the Surgeon General's report on health promotion and disease prevention. Washington, DC: Government Printing Office, 1979; DHEW publication No. (PHS) 79-55071.
13. Woolf SH. Practice guidelines: a new reality to medicine. Arch Intern Med 1990;150:1811–8.
14. Kamerow DB, Mickalide AD, Woolf SH. Preventive services in the office. HELP newsletter 1989;3:1–4 (American Academy of Family Physicians, Kansas City, MO).
15. Department of Health and Human Services. Public Health Service. Healthy people 2000: national health promotion and disease prevention objectives. Conference edition. Washington, DC: Department of Health and Human Services, 1990.
16. Borkan JM, Neher JO. A developmental model of ethnosensitivity in family practice training. Fam Med 1991;23:212–7.
17. AAFP Subcommittee on Periodic Health Intervention. Age charts for periodic health examination. Reprint No. 510. Kansas City, MO: American Academy of Family Physicians.
18. Zimmerman RK, Giebink GS. Childhood immunizations: a practical approach for clinicans. Am Fam Physician 1992;45:1759–72.
19. Clarke WR, Lauer RM. The predictive value of childhood cholesterol screening. JAMA 1992;267:101–2.
20. National Cholesterol Education Program. Highlights of the report of the expert panel on blood cholesterol levels in children and adolescents. Am Fam Physician 1992;45:2127–36.
21. Kluger CZ, Morrison JA, Daniels SR. Preventive practices for adult cardiovascular disease in children. J Fam Pract 1991;33:65–72.
22. Manson JE, Tosteson H, Satterfield S, et al. The primary prevention of myocardial infarction. N Engl J Med 1992;326:1406–16.

23. Steenland K. Passive smoking and the risk of heart disease. JAMA 1992;267: 94–99.
24. Evans CH, Karunaratne HB. Exercise stress testing for the family physician. Part I. Performing the test. Am Fam Physician 1991;45: 121–32.
25. Solberg LI, Maxwell PL, Kottke TE, et al. A systematic primary care office-based smoking cessation program. J Fam Pract 1990;30:647–54.
26. National Cancer Institute. Cases diagnosed between 1973 and 1987 and intercensal population estimates by race, sex, and age. Bethesda, MD: US Department of Health and Human Services, Public Health Service, National Institutes of Health, 1990.
27. Public Health Focus: Mammography. MMWR 1992;41:454–9.
28. Levine R, Tenner S, Fromm H. Prevention and early detection of colorectal cancer. Am Fam Physician 1992;45:663–8.
29. Selby JV, Friedman GD, Quesenberry CD, et al. A case-control study of screening sigmoidoscopy and mortality for colorectal cancer. N Engl J Med 1992;326:653–7.
30. Crawford ED, Schutz MJ, Clejan S, et al. The effect of a digital rectal examination on prostate specific antigen levels. JAMA 1992;267:2227–8.
31. Bourguet CC, Hamrick GA, Gilchrist VJ. The prevalence of osteoporosis risk factors and physician intervention. J Fam Pract 1991; 32:265–71.
32. Thun MJ, Namboodiri MM, Health CW. Aspirin use and reduced risk of fatal colon cancer. N Engl J Med 1991;325:1593–6.
33. Zazove P, Mehr DR, Riffin MT, et al. A criterion-based review of preventive health care in the elderly. Part 2. A geriatric health maintenance program. J Fam Pract 1992;34:320–47.
34. Ham RJ. Indicators of poor nutritional status in older Americans. Am Fam Physician 1992;45:219–28.
35. National Research Council. Panel on statistics for an aging population: the aging population in the twenty-first century. Washington, DC: NRC, 1988: 54.
36. Frame PS. Health maintenance in clinical practice: strategies and barriers. Am Fam Physician 1992;45:1192–200.
37. Johns MB, Howell MF, Drastal CA, et al. Promoting preventive services in primary care: a controlled trial. Am J Prev Med 1992;8:135–40.
38. Shank JC, Powell T, Llewelyn J. A five-year demonstration project associated with improvement in physician health maintenance behavior. Fam Med 1989;21:273–8.
39. Dickey LL, Petitti D. A patient-held minirecord to promote preventive care. J Fam Pract 1992;34:457–63.
40. McDowell I, Newell C, Rosser W. A follow-up study of patients advised to obtain influenza immunizations. Fam Med 1990;22: 303–6.
41. Frame PS, Zimmer JC, Werth PL, et al. Computer-based vs. manual health maintenance tracking: a controlled trial. Arch Fam Med 1994;3:581–8.
42. Ornstein SM, Garr DR, Jenkins RG, et al. Computer-generated physician and patient reminders: tools to improve population adherence to selected preventive services. J Fam Pract 1991; 32:82–90.
43. Ellis LBM, Joo H, Gross CR. Use of a computer-based health risk appraisal by older adults. J Fam Pract 1991;33:390–4.

44. American Academy of Family Physicians Directors' Newsletter. Kansas City, MO: AAFP, July 22, 1994.

45. Peterson KW, Hilles SB, editors. Handbook of health risk appraisals. Charlottesville, VA: Society of Prospective Medicine, 1994.

46. Aukerman GF. Developing a patient education newsletter. J Fam Pract 1991; 33:304–5.

47. Towner P, Marvel MK. A school-based intervention to increase the use of bicycle helmets. Fam Med 1992;24:156–8.

48. McDonald CJ, Hui SL, Smith DM, et al. Reminders to physicians from an interactive computer medical record. Ann Intern Med 1984;100:130–8.

49. Struewing JP, Pape DM, Snow DA. Improving colorectal cancer screening in a medical resident's primary care clinic. Am J Prev Med 1991;7:75–81.

50. Nutting PA. Health promotion in primary medical care: problems as potential. Prev Med 1986;15:537–48.

51. Parkinson MD. Paying for prevention: recent developments and future strategies. J Fam Pract 1991;33:529–30.

52. Woolhandler S, Himmelstein DU. Reverse targeting of preventive care due to lack of health insurance. JAMA 1988;259:2872–4.

53. Hamblin JE. Physician recommendations for screening mammography: results of a survey using clinical vignettes. J Fam Pract 1991;32:472–7.

54. Lurie L, Manning WG, Peterson C. Preventive care: do we practice what we preach? Am J Public Health 1987;77:801–4.

55. Warner KE, Murt HA. Economic incentives for health. Annu Rev Public Health 1984;5:107–33.

56. Davis K, Bialek R, Parkinson M, et al. Paying for preventive care: moving the debate forward. Am J Prev Med 1990;6:32.

57. Fries JF. Aging, natural death, and a compression of morbidity. N Engl J Med 1980;303:130–6.

CASE PRESENTATION

Subjective

PATIENT PROFILE

Ruth Nelson McCarthy is a 51-year-old married white female restaurant owner.

PRESENTING PROBLEM

"Here for my pap smear."

PRESENT ILLNESS

Mrs. McCarthy has a periodic examination every 2 years. Her menses ceased 3 years ago, and she has not used estrogen replacement. She has no other medical complaints.

PAST MEDICAL HISTORY

Asthma in childhood.

SOCIAL HISTORY

She and her husband have owned and operated a small restaurant for 11 years. She works long hours 6 days per week.

HABITS

She uses no tobacco, alcohol, or drugs.

FAMILY HISTORY

Her father, aged 76, has diabetes mellitus and "arthritis." Her mother is 71 years old and has high blood pressure. She and her husband have two children. Her daughter is living and well at age 26. Their son, aged 28, has recently been diagnosed as HIV-positive.

REVIEW OF SYSTEMS

She reports an occasional mild rash on her hands that becomes red and itching but is not present at this time.

- What other historical information would be useful for this periodic health maintenance examination?
- What are common areas of concern for patients of this age group, and how would you approach these possibilities?
- What else would you like to know regarding her menopausal symptoms?
- What might be the meaning of her health status to the patient, and what unspoken reasons might be bringing her to the physician today?

Objective

VITAL SIGNS

Height, 5 ft 4 in; weight, 182 lb; blood pressure, 138/90; pulse, 72; temperature, 37.2°C.

EXAMINATION

The patient is overweight for height. The eyes, ears, nose, and throat are normal. The neck and thyroid glands are unremarkable. Examination of the chest, heart, and breasts is normal. There is no mass, tenderness, or organ enlargement in the abdomen. The vaginal introitus is mildly atrophic; the cervix, fundus, adnexa, and rectal examination are normal. The neurologic examination and peripheral pulses are normal. Examination of the skin, including the hands, reveals no abnormalities.

LABORATORY

A pap smear is performed today.

- What more—if anything—should be included in this health maintenance examination? Why?
- What might point to a physical cause for obesity?
- What—if any—laboratory tests would you order today, and why?
- What—if any—diagnostic imaging would you order today, and why?

Assessment

- What is your diagnosis regarding Mrs. McCarthy's menopausal status, and how would you describe this to the patient?
- What is the patient's ideal weight, and how would you initiate a discussion regarding weight control?
- How might decreased estrogen and increased weight influence the patient's relationship with her husband? How might you address this issue?
- What are likely to be key stressors in the patient's life, and how might these affect her future health status?

Plan

- What are the disease prevention and health promotion opportunities for this visit?
- Describe your recommendation regarding weight control.
- Describe your recommendation regarding estrogen use.
- What continuing care would you advise for Mrs. McCarthy?

3
Normal Pregnancy, Labor, and Delivery

JOSEPH E. SCHERGER

Pregnancy and birth are normal physiologic processes for most women. The current cesarean delivery rate of 25% in the United States is a reflection of a higher than expected rate of medical intervention in the birth process. Unfortunately, modern medicine has been guilty of using a disease model for the management of pregnancy and birth, resulting in higher than expected rates of complications. At least 90% of women should have a normal birth outcome without medical intervention.[1]

The disease model for pregnancy and birth took hold during the 1920s, led by Chicago obstetrician Joseph DeLee, who questioned, "What is normal?" and pioneered efforts to improve medically on the "cruelty of nature."[2] During this period, childbirth in America went from the home to the hospital, and the legacy of hospital interventions in the birth process began. Much good has come from modern hospital obstetric care, with maternal mortality having decreased to small levels; moreover, infant mortality has steadily declined for populations having access to perinatal care. Modern prenatal care developed during the first half of the twentieth century, and with a focus on good nutrition and screening for problems in pregnancy, it has improved the birth outcome.[3]

A renewed respect for normal childbirth came about as a reaction to hospital interventions, led by Grantly Dick-Read during the 1930s and 1940s,[4] Ferdinand LaMaze during the 1950s,[5] Sheila Kitzinger during the 1960s,[6] and eventually a social movement in America during the 1970s with the widespread development of childbirth education. Odent's *Birth Reborn* represents a culmination of the effort to rediscover normal pregnancy and birth.[1]

Technologic obstetrics, with its steady focus on improving the uncertainty of nature and sparing women the pain of childbirth, continues to march onward. Prenatal care has become preoccupied with serial ultrasonographic evaluations, screening for α-fetoprotein (AFP) abnormalities, gestational diabetes, genetic disorders, and every potentially infectious agent. Continuous electronic fetal monitoring, developed during the early 1970s, quickly became the standard of care in most American hospitals, despite little evidence of benefit and cumulative evidence that it causes unnecessary cesarean interventions.[7,8] The epidural anesthetic has become so commonplace in some hospitals that labor units are quiet and nurses have little experience in helping women through natural labor.

The family physician active in maternity care has become the exception rather than the norm and is even a rarity in some areas. The current lack of access to prenatal care for many women in both rural and urban areas is a compelling reason for more family physicians to deliver these services. Knowledgeable about scientific medicine, yet with a humanistic approach to pregnancy and birth similar to that of midwives, the family physician is well suited to provide a balance between nature and technology and may be a guiding force to appropriate maternity care.[9]

This chapter focuses on normal pregnancy and delivery from a perspective of family-centered care. *Family-centered maternity care* has been defined by the International Childbirth Education Association as care that focuses on how the birth of a child affects the entire family. A woman who gives birth forms new relationships with those close to her, and all family members take on new responsibilities to each other, the baby, and the community. Family-centered maternity care recognizes the importance of these new relationships and responsibilities and has as its goal the best possible outcome for all family members. Family-centered maternity care is an attitude rather than a specific program. It respects the woman's individuality and need for autonomy; it requires that a woman be guided, not directed, and that she be allowed to make her own decisions in accordance with her goals.[10] The family physician, as physician for the woman, the father, and the children, is well suited to provide family-centered maternity care.

This chapter reviews the principles and practice of normal pregnancy, labor, and delivery. Some of this material has been published in a paper by members of The Working Group on Teaching Family-Centered Perinatal Care of the Society of Teachers of Family Medicine (reprinted with permission).[11]

Prenatal Care

Current prenatal care begins before conception. This important early phase of prevention of complications is referred to as preconception care. Prenatal care after conception should begin as early as possible, as health screening and intervention early during pregnancy may improve birth outcome. For example, taking folic acid in doses present in multivitamins during the first 6 weeks of pregnancy provides a three- to fourfold reduction in the chance of neural tube defects in the offspring.[12] Early screening and intervention may also help in glucose control of diabetes, genetic screening, changing teratogenic drugs such as phenytoin (Dilantin), treating infections, and life-style modifications such as smoking, alcohol use, recreational drugs, and maternal nutrition.

The traditional approach to prenatal care developed early during the twentieth century has been modified by an expert panel convened by the U.S. Public Health Service.[13] Rather than a single comprehensive initial visit followed by monthly visits until the third trimester, this panel recommends more intensive intervention early in pregnancy if risk factors exist that can be modified. For example, women who smoke, have poor nutrition, or have a high-risk home environment may benefit from frequent visits and a multidisciplinary team approach early in the pregnancy. Low-risk women may require fewer visits than are scheduled with the traditional protocol.

Prenatal care in the normal or healthy woman is part of preventive medicine. A biopsychosocial approach with a family perspective should be used, with an emphasis on advocacy for the pregnant woman.[14] Prenatal care encompasses both primary prevention such as proper nutrition to enhance birth outcome and secondary prevention through screening for conditions that can be modified or that will alter patient management.

Health Promotion

All those who care for childbearing women should approach pregnancy as an opportunity to promote the health and well-being of the family. Counseling to reinforce healthful behaviors and education about pregnancy, childbirth, and parenting are crucial parts of perinatal care—not "extras."

In a family practice, education about pregnancy, birth, and parenting begins before the first conception and continues throughout the parenting years. Pregnancy is an opportunity for more intensive involvement. Table 3.1 is an outline of topics to be covered in the education of all pregnant women and their support persons.[15] Experienced parents need only an abbreviated program, focusing on selected areas of interest to them. Preparation for natural childbirth (birth without regional or systemic analgesic drugs) and for vaginal birth after a previous cesarean section can reduce maternal anxiety and the rates of operative delivery and associated complications.[16] Childbirth preparation classes, often run by hospitals, clinics, or private childbirth educators, fulfill this function well. Also, during pregnancy care it is important that the practitioner spend time discussing with the woman recommendations specific to her care, such as the purpose of tests and procedures and the steps to follow when labor begins. The benefits of breast-feeding for baby and mother should be discussed with women and their family members before or early during pregnancy and then modeled at delivery.

TABLE 3.1. Sample topics for birth and parenting classes

Early pregnancy

Nutrition; optimum weight gain; iron, calcium, vitamin supplements

Exercise and sex during pregnancy

Common symptoms and remedies: fatigue, nausea/vomiting, backache, round ligament pain, syncope, constipation

Danger signs: bleeding, contractions, dysuria, vaginitis, weight loss

Psychology of pregnancy: body image, libido; need for security: education for self-help; changing family roles; acceptance of pregnancy

Fevers, hot tubs, saunas

Environmental and occupational hazards and how to mitigate them; stress management

Exposure to infectious agents (e.g., toxoplasmosis, rubella, HIV, varicella)

Avoidance of tobacco, alcohol, x-rays, other drugs

Resources available for pregnant and parenting families

Late pregnancy

Common symptoms and remedies: heartburn, backache, "loose joints," hemorrhoids, edema, insomnia

Nutrition/fetal growth

Avoidance of tobacco and other drugs

Potentially serious symptoms: edema, bleeding, headache, meconium-stained fluid, decreased fetal movements

Exercise (e.g., Kegel's, pelvic tilt), sex, travel (avoid prolonged sitting because of risk of deep vein thrombosis)

Occupational adjustments (avoid excessive exertion, prolonged standing, stress) and postpartum plans

Breast-feeding

Signs of labor

Stages of labor

Techniques for pain control (and practice relaxation, visualization)

Cesarean section, vaginal birth after cesarean, other potential interventions

Birth plan; importance of labor companion and early parent–infant contact

Positions for labor and birth

Seat belt use; infant car seats

Circumcision

Sibling preparation

Postpartum/parenting

Care of the perineum, Kegel's exercises

Practical support for breast-feeding

Reasons to contact provider (e.g., maternal hemorrhage, fever, increased pain; infant jaundice, respiratory distress)

Postpartum exercises

Nutrition, especially calcium and iron

Rest and sleep

Return to work

Sex, contraception

Sibling adjustment

Infant immunizations and preventive care schedule

Infant growth and development: normal expectations and parenting issues at each age

The effectiveness of education on preventing low birth weight has not been proved. However, information about smoking, alcohol and drug use, prevention of sexually transmitted infection, and mobilizing family supports and social services in the community are likely to be beneficial. Health education may have a profound effect on the problem of low birth weight if it is undertaken during preconception, pregnancy, and postpartum, even though the gains may not be noticed until subsequent pregnancies.

Motivation to adopt more healthy behaviors is probably stronger during pregnancy than at most other times. However, pregnancy may intensify the pressure on close relationships, increasing the pregnant women's dependence on them. Many women are motivated to stop smoking during pregnancy but may resume after delivery. During pregnancy, the couple may be involved, and the benefits of a nonsmoking household for children should be emphasized.

Abstention from alcohol and recreational drugs is also important. Alcohol exposure during gestation is now a more common cause of mental retardation than Down syndrome.[17] The prevalence of cocaine use during pregnancy is as high as 17% in some populations but often is not admitted to the physician.[18] With a paucity of research on substance use by women and few treatment programs accepting pregnant women, this area is a challenge to professionals caring for them.

Physicians are often in a position to counsel women about work during perinatal care. The physician should review the effects of physical exertion and prolonged standing during pregnancy, occupational and environmental hazards (e.g., heat, heavy metals, anesthetic gases, x-rays, possibly cathode ray tubes), legal rights of pregnant workers, child care, and breastfeeding.

Physical fitness may improve pregnancy and childbirth. Prescription and occasionally proscription of exercise during pregnancy and discussion of sexuality during perinatal care are appropriate.

Nutrition and weight should be closely monitored during prenatal care. Physicians must be knowledgeable about nutritional requirements and concerning practical suggestions regarding management of nausea and vomiting, reflux esophagitis, constipation, obesity, anticipatory guidance about body image changes, and ways of modifying the diet within various constraints (e.g., vegetarianism, lactose intolerance). Optimal weight gain during pregnancy varies depending on the prepregnancy weight. A thin woman may benefit from gaining 40 pounds, whereas an obese woman might do well gaining 10 pounds. The normal weight gain of 25 to 30 pounds is often exceeded without harm to the fetus. Nutritional advice to pregnant women should focus on a high-quality, high-protein diet with a steady, gradual weight gain profiled to the woman's size and eating habits. Pregnant women should be instructed to avoid cat feces and eating raw meat (toxoplasmosis).

Pregnancy is an opportunity to assess family supports and liabilities and to intervene with the potential of an improved perinatal outcome. If a history of maternal deprivation, postpartum depression, physical abuse, or substance use by significant others is obtained, interventions can be begun during pregnancy and continued during care of the parent(s) and child. The physician must ask explicitly about these issues, which often are not spontaneously mentioned by women. Finally, physicians should be knowledgeable and able to recommend the public social service programs available to aid and support the pregnant patient and family.

Prenatal Screening

The purpose of prenatal screening is to identify problems that could affect the outcome of pregnancy and for which effective interventions are available. The number of conditions for which screening is available seems limitless. Therefore, the choice of items should be based on a rational assessment of the current literature, legislation, the medicolegal climate, cost-effectiveness, and treatment effectiveness. Screening means that the search for the presence of a specific condition is not based on signs or symptoms but is carried out for the prenatal population as a whole or for those with historic or demographic risk factors. Each screening test should be evaluated to ensure that the benefits of the test and the planned intervention outweigh the risks and complications. Unfortunately, not all currently recommended screening techniques have been so rigorously evaluated.

Screening may include identification of conditions of the mother or fetus that require monitoring during the pregnancy or that may be treatable during the pregnancy or after delivery. Prenatal screening should be discussed with each patient at the first prenatal visit. Elective screening items should be recommended and pursued based on a joint decision between physician and patient. It may be helpful to provide written materials for patients to review at home. Screening tests should be scheduled so as to minimize blood drawing and number of visits.

Traditional medical teaching focuses on screening for medical conditions using blood tests, ultrasonography, amniocentesis, and physical examination. A comprehensive approach would also include screening through questioning about family and social dysfunction, such as single parent status, a history of child abuse, economic hardship, and work-related stresses. The relation between psychosocial stress and outcome of pregnancy is now well established.[19,20]

Medical conditions appropriate for prenatal screening can be divided into three groups: universal, selective, and elective. Universal screening tests include Papanicolaou smear, urinalysis, urine culture, complete blood count, blood type and Rh factor, indirect Coombs' test, and tests for syphilis, rubella immunity, *Chlamydia,* gonorrhea, antibody for hepatitis B surface antigen, and blood glucose (diabetes). All these tests are appropriately performed at preconception or at the first prenatal visit, except that for diabetes, which should be performed at 24 to 28 weeks' gestation in low-risk patients. A hemoglobin or hematocrit should be rechecked during the third trimester. The physical examination routinely screens for weight gain or loss, blood pressure, edema, fungal growth, fetal heart sounds, and fetal position.

Screening for gestational diabetes is still controversial, and screening based on risk factors is advocated by some. The current recommended test is the use of an oral 50-g glucose solution with a 1-hour blood glucose, regardless of earlier food intake. This test has a high false-positive rate.[21] One- or two-hour postprandial blood glucose assays may also be used for screening. Positive screening tests are followed by a standard glucose tolerance test before a diagnosis of gestational diabetes is established.

Selective screening tests are chosen for patients who fit a particular risk category. If indicated, tests for sickle cell disease, toxoplasmosis, and human immunodeficiency virus (HIV) should be carried out at the first prenatal visit. All pregnant women at risk should be offered HIV testing and counseled about risk factors and safer sex practices. If indicated by history, tests for HIV, *Chlamydia,* and gonorrhea should be performed again at 36 weeks. Herpes screening remains controversial, and screening by cultures those women with a history of herpes fails to prevent most cases of neonatal herpes. Screening is best done by questioning and by examination early during labor for possible herpes lesions. Rh-negative patients should be screened for Rh antibodies at 28 weeks and should receive antenatal Rho-GAM if these tests are negative. Amniocentesis or chorionic villous sampling, if indicated by maternal age or a previous chromosomal abnormality, is performed during the first trimester or early second trimester.

Elective screening tests include maternal AFP assay and ultrasonography. Some states require that maternal AFP assays be offered to all pregnant women. Maternal serum AFP can be used as a screening test to detect fetal abnormalities, particularly neural tube defects. In some states, screening for AFP in the maternal serum is offered to all pregnant women, despite its low positive predictive value (1.9% for spina bifida) and relatively low sensitivity (90% for spina bifida).[22] An elevated level may be found in patients with inaccurate dates, multiple gestation, neural tube defects, abdominal well defects, congenital nephrotic syndrome, and fetal demise, as well as in normal pregnancy. A low level may be found with inaccurate dates, chromosomal trisomy (e.g., Down syndrome), fetal demise, molar pregnancy, and normal pregnancy. If the initial AFP level is abnormal, it may be necessary to repeat the test or to order diagnostic ultrasonography to confirm the gestational age and to evaluate for fetal abnormalities. Amniocentesis may be indicated to measure amniotic fluid AFP and acetylcholine esterase and for chromosome evaluation. Because the maternal AFP assay is widely available and is considered a standard test by some, the test should be discussed with all patients, with a mutual agreement of patient and practitioner regarding its use.

Routine ultrasonography currently falls into a gray area. In the United States, a National Institutes of Health Consensus Conference recognized 27 indications for prenatal ultrasonography that result in examinations in most pregnancies.[23] The American College of Obstetrics and Gynecology recommends adherence to these guidelines.[24] In most of western Europe, ultrasonography is performed routinely at 16 to 18 weeks. The benefits and cost-effectiveness of universal screening are still controversial and are the subject of ongoing study.[25,26]

Conditions for which routine screening has been considered but not found to be warranted at this time include cytomegalovirus infection and toxoplasmosis. Group B streptococcal infection of the newborn is an important cause of sepsis, and selective prenatal screening may be recommended once the risk factors become clarified and treatment is clearly shown to be effective.[27]

A screening checklist is a valuable memory jogger and should be part of the prenatal record. A useful screening instrument is one that includes the items to be screened and the appropriate patients and timing for screening. Tables 3.2 and 3.3 demonstrate a possible screening instrument for medical problems that requires only a single page, front and back. Table 3.2 is the front of the obstetric screening checklist. Dates and results of testing are noted here. Also noted are conditions that require rescreening at delivery. Table 3.3 is the reverse side of the checklist, which describes indications for selective and elective screening. As psychosocial, substance use, and nutritional screening methods are adopted, they may be added to the checklist.

Risk Assessment

The outcome of screening is the identification of patients at risk for complications during pregnancy. Conventional risk assessment divides patients into low-, medium-, or high-risk categories. Because most family physicians are trained to care for low- and medium-risk patients and to refer or share the care of high-risk patients with perinatal specialists, proper risk assessment is crucial. Complex risk scoring mechanisms have been developed but have failed to cause any improvement over simpler clinical identification of known risk factors.[28] Table 3.4 indicates well-established risk factors recognized by the American Board of Family Practice and the American College of Obstetricians and Gynecologists.[29] Family physicians in some areas and with appropriate training may provide high-risk obstetric care, but the classification of

Table 3.2. Obstetric screening checklist

Test	Pts. to screen at first visit[a]	Additional screening[a]	Pts. subjected
Papanicolaou	All		
Uric acid	All		
Urine culture	All		
CBC	All	Third trimester	All
Blood type	All	Delivery	All
Rh factor	All	28 Weeks	If Rh–
		Delivery	All
Indirect Coombs'	All	28 Weeks	If Rh–
		Delivery	All
Sickle cell	Black pts.		
Syphilis	All	Delivery	
Rubella	All	Delivery	
Gonococcus	All	Second prenatal visit	Risk 1
Hepatitis B	All	36 Weeks	Consider on all
Chlamydia	Risk 2[b]	36 Weeks	Risk 2
Herpes	Risk 3	36 Weeks	Risk 4
HIV	Risk 5		
Diabetes		12 Weeks	Risk 6
		24–28 Weeks	All
		32 Weeks	Risk 7
Serum AFP		15–18 Weeks	Risk 8
Amniocentesis		16–18 Weeks	>35, Risk 9
Ultrasonography		16–18 Weeks	Risk 10

Source: Scherger et al.[11] With permission.
[a]The date performed and result of the test should always be noted on the checklist.
[b]For risk indicators, see Table 3.3.
CBC = complete blood count; HIV = human immunodeficiency virus; AFP = α-fetoprotein.

risk status remains important for guiding clinical care. The prenatal record should conveniently assist in the evaluation and indication of risk status.

High-risk categories should not be absolute contraindications to care by family physicians. For example, family physicians may be the best qualified to handle high-risk social situations and substance abuse. Because of broad medical training, family physicians may have more experience than some obstetricians in an area dealing with medical problems such as thyroid or pulmonary disease. Consultation does not preclude "shared care." Many high-risk problems may resolve during the pregnancy, and the birth may be a low-risk event. The family physician should be encouraged to stay in contact with the patient after consultation or referral is made. The high-risk pregnant woman and her family will continue to benefit from a comprehensive, biopsychosocial approach.

TABLE 3.3. Indicators for selective and elective screening

1. Women with previous gonococcal infection or other sexually transmitted disease (STD) if first screen is negative.
2. Adolescents, women with multiple sexual partners, women with a history of other STD.
3. Women with suspicious lesions, history of previous herpes infection, history of other STD.
4. Same as item 3; but if any positive herpes cultures are found during pregnancy, special considerations apply.
5. Women at risk for HIV infections: IV drug abusers, born in countries with a high risk of heterosexual transmission, prostitutes, women with sexual partners meeting the previous criteria, patients with bisexual or hemophiliac partners. Should offer to all pregnant women; may become mandatory.
6. Previous gestational diabetic family history of diabetes, history of "diabetic tendency," or glucose intolerance outside of pregnancy (known diabetes should not be screened), obesity (more than 120% of ideal body weight), patient's own birth weight >9 pounds, poor obstetric history (recurrent abortions, large infants, current suspected large infant, unexplained stillbirths, congenital anomalies, history of preeclampsia, and polyhydramnios).
7. Women with positive diabetes screen but negative glucose tolerance test at 24 to 28 weeks' gestation, older than age 33, and obesity.
8. Women whose relatives (other than parents or siblings—see item 9) have neural tube defects. Women with diabetes. In many communities, standard of care is to offer to all pregnant women.
9. Women having previously delivered a child with or either parent with neural tube defect, Ashkenazi Jews for Tay-Sachs disease, prior delivery of a child affected by or parent with other chromosomal or metabolic abnormality. Determination of fetal sex if high risk for X-linked recessive heritable disorder.
10. Scan at 16–18 weeks for routine screening. Value of routine scan in all pregnancies not proved at this time. Selective indications include the following:

Maternal factors
  Evaluation of pelvic mass
  Exclusion of hydatidiform mole
  Evaluation of ectopic pregnancy
  Evaluation for uterine anomaly
  Pregnancy after tuboplasty
Prenatal diagnosis and procedures
  Evaluation of suspected fetal anomaly
  Evaluation of abnormal α-fetoprotein
  Localization of intrauterine device
  Adjunct to procedures
    Genetic amniocentesis
    Fetoscopy
    Fetal transfusion
    Chorionic villous sampling
    Cerclage placement
    External version
    Shunt placement
Estimation of gestational age
  Uncertain dates
  Before repeat cesarean section
  Preterm labor
  Premature rupture of membranes
  Before induction
  Adjunct to amniocentesis for fetal maturity

Growth abnormalities
  Evaluation of growth in patients with
    Pregnancy-induced hypertension
    Chronic hypertension
    Diabetes
    Chronic renal disease
    Other chronic maternal disease
  Evaluation of macrosomia
  Evaluation of size or dates discrepancy
  Diagnosis and follow-up of multiple gestation
  Suspected intrauterine growth retardation
  Oligo- or polyhydramnios
Fetal assessment
  Late prenatal care
  Biophysical evaluation
  Suspected fetal death
Antenatal hemorrhage
  Confirmation of intrauterine pregnancy
  Evaluation for placenta previa
  Evaluation for abruption
Delivery
  Confirmation of presentation
  Observation of intrapartum events

Source: Scherger et al.[11] With permission.

Table 3.4. Obstetric risk criteria

Category I: high-risk factors	Category II: medium-risk factors
Initial prenatal factors	*Initial prenatal factors*
Age ≥40 or <16	Ages 35–39, 16–17
Multiple pregnancy	Drug dependency
Insulin-dependent diabetes	High-risk family—lack of family/social support
Chronic hypertension	Uterine or cervical malformation or incompetence
Renal failure	Contracted pelvis
Heart disease, class 2 or greater	Previous cesarean section
Hyperthyroidism	Multiple spontaneous abortions (>3)
Rh isoimmunization	Grand multiparity (>8)
Chronic active hepatitis	History of gestational diabetes
Convulsive disorder	Previous fetal or neonatal demise
Isoimmune thrombocytopenia	Hypothyroidism
Subsequent prenatal and intrapartum factors	Heart disease, class I
Vaginal bleeding, second or third trimester	Severe anemia (unresponsive to iron)
Pregnancy-induced hypertension (or toxemia), moderate or severe	Pelvic mass or neoplasia
Fetal malformation, by α-fetoprotein (AFP) screening, ultrasonography, or amniocentesis	*Subsequent prenatal and intrapartum factors*
Abnormal presentation: breech, face, brow, transverse	Gestational diabetes
Intrauterine growth retardation	Pregnancy-induced hypertension (toxemia), mild
Polyhydramnios	Pregnancy at 42 weeks, obtain appropriate fetal/placental tests
Pregnancy >43 weeks or <35 weeks	Active genital herpes
Abnormal fetal/placental tests	Positive high or low AFP screen
Persistent severe variable or late decelerations	Estimated fetal weight >10 pounds (5.5 kg) or <6 pounds (2.7 kg)
Macrosomia	Abnormal nonstress test
Cord prolapse	Arrest of normal labor curve
Midforceps delivery	Persistent moderate variable decelerations or poor base-line variability
	Ruptured membranes beyond 24 hours
	Second stage beyond 2 hours
	Induction of labor

Prenatal Visits

The schedule of prenatal visits has traditionally been every 4 weeks through week 28 of pregnancy, then every 2 weeks until week 36 of pregnancy, and weekly until delivery. The U.S. Public Health Service Report suggested that low-risk patients may require fewer visits, whereas patients with risk factors may need modified or intensive care.[13] For example, risk factors identified early in pregnancy, such as smoking, alcohol or drug use, family dysfunction, and lack of social support, should be aggressively managed with frequent visits during early pregnancy. Subsequent risk factors, such as elevated blood pressure or preterm labor, require more frequent visits beginning as soon as the condition develops. Accurate dating of the pregnancy is critically important for prenatal care, for the proper performance and interpretation of screening tests and for avoiding unnecessary testing due to misdiagnosis of prematurity or postdates. If the dates are not clear from the initial visit, an ultrasound scan should be obtained during the first or second trimester.

The initial prenatal visit consists of a detailed history, physical examination, and laboratory assessment. A complete physical examination should be performed as early as possible. The pelvic assessment, which includes a bimanual examination, is helpful for dating the pregnancy and evaluating the pelvic structure. Screening laboratory investigations are undertaken as stated in Tables 3.2 and 3.3.

First-trimester prenatal care (up to 14 weeks) includes a determination of the patient's well-being during pregnancy, a review of family and life-style issues, and reevaluation of the risk status. A clinical assessment would include measuring uterine growth and maternal weight gain, detection of fetal heart tones by Doppler ultrasonography, and counseling patients toward a healthy pregnancy. Genetic prenatal diagnostic tests that may be performed during the first trimester include chorionic villous sampling and early amniocentesis.

Second-trimester prenatal care (14–28 weeks) includes confirmation of the estimated date of delivery by quickening at 18 to 20 weeks or earlier and the uterus being at the umbilicus at 20 weeks, with fetal heart tones being heard using a stethoscope. Ultrasonographic evaluation of the fetus may be performed if fetal age is in doubt. Health education during the second trimester includes planning for labor and delivery through childbirth education classes, and initial discussion of infant feeding preferences when planning for parenting by recommending readings or classes. Mothers should be instructed to report symptoms that would indicate a pregnancy risk, such as vaginal bleeding, swelling of the face and/or fingers, continuous headache, blurring of vision, abdominal pain, persistent vomiting, chills, fever, dysuria, escape of fluids per vagina, or a change in the frequency or intensity of fetal movements.

Third-trimester prenatal care (28 weeks–delivery) includes screening for anemia, gestational diabetes, and sexually transmitted diseases if risk is present. More frequent visits are generally made during the third trimester to evaluate for elevated blood pressure or other signs of preeclampsia. Labor signs are taught to the patient with careful attention to the possibility of preterm labor. Labor and delivery preferences of the mother and father should be clarified, and the completed prenatal record including documentation of the parents' birth request should be given to the patient or sent to the hospital.

Fetal Assessment

Several methods have been developed to assess the well-being of the fetus during pregnancy. Noninvasive methods of fetal assessment include fetal movement counting, nonstress test (NST), nipple stimulation contraction stress test (CST), and ultrasonography for amniotic fluid evaluation. A more invasive test is the oxytocin contraction stress test. The Biophysical Profile is a quantitative score that combines fetal heart rate testing with ultrasound evaluation of the fetus and amniotic fluid.[30] This test is time-consuming and requires special training of the sonographer. A combination of fetal heart rate testing (NST or CST) and amniotic fluid evaluation is an alternative to the biophysical profile. These methods are used according to accepted protocols when risk factors occur that may jeopardize the fetus. They are routinely applied when a pregnancy becomes postdated (42 weeks from the last menstrual period) or earlier for such conditions as intrauterine growth retardation, diabetes during pregnancy, chronic hypertension or renal disease, pregnancy-induced hypertension, previous unexplained stillbirth, Rh sensitization, oligohydramnios, multiple gestation, or maternal perception of decreased fetal movement. Family physicians should understand these methods and be aware of their relative usefulness, including their sensitivity, specificity, and predictive values.[31]

Duration of Pregnancy

The normal duration of human pregnancy has considerable variation. The "bell-shaped curve" of human pregnancy is illustrated by Figure 3.1. The median is just past 280 days, or 40 weeks, from the last menstrual period. Two standard deviations from the mean would be 37 to 43 weeks. About 10% of pregnancies reach 42 weeks, confirming the normalcy of postdates pregnancy for many women.

Labor

Labor in the first stage is defined as progressive dilation of the cervix with uterine contractions. The early (latent) phase of labor occurs up to 4 cm of dilation and is variable in duration. Progress during this phase is often slow because of the time needed for effacement of the cervix.

The active phase of labor is more rapid and predictable; yet there is still considerable individual variation. With frequent regular contractions, the average is 1.2 cm dilation per hour in primigravidas and 1.5 cm per hour in multigravidas, but flexibility is important. Friedman attempted to describe labor, not to define parameters women must follow.[32] Arrest of

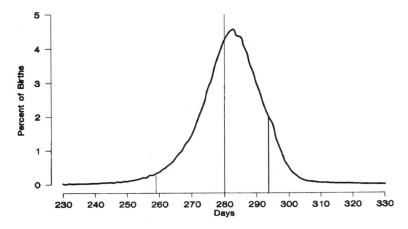

FIGURE 3.1. Distribution of duration of pregnancy (in days from the last menstrual period to birth) for 383,484 singleton, noncesarean births with certain menstrual dates in Sweden, 1976–1980. Vertical lines are drawn at 259, 280, and 294 completed days. The line has been drawn between day-to-day percentages, without any smoothing of the curve ("raw data"). From Bergsjo P, Denman DW III, Hoffman HY, et al. Duration of human singleton pregnancy. Acta Obstet Gynaecol Scand 69:197–207, 1990. With permission.)

labor is present where there has been no cervical dilation for 2 hours during this active phase.

Support and observation are the hallmarks of managing normal labor. Women in labor should be given as much freedom of movement as possible. The dorsal supine (lithotomy) position should be avoided, as the gravid uterus may compress the inferior vena cava and cause maternal hypotension and fetal distress. Upright women in labor report less pain and have greater intrauterine pressure through the cervix.[33] Fatigued women may want to rest on their sides.

During the first stage of labor, the blood pressure and frequency and duration of contractions are measured every 15 to 30 minutes. The fetal heart rate should be monitored during and immediately after a contraction every 30 minutes during the first stage by whatever method is most convenient (electronically, Doppler ultrasonography, or fetoscopic auscultation). Intermittent fetal heart rate monitoring is preferable over continuous monitoring in normal or low-risk patients, as continuous monitoring interferes with freedom of movement and is associated with a high false-positive rate.[7,8] Continuous electronic fetal monitoring in low-risk patients has resulted in three times the diagnosis of fetal distress and twice the frequency of cesarean section without improving birth outcome.[34]

Women succeed best during the second stage of labor (expulsion of the fetus) when they are allowed and encouraged to use their instincts for pushing. Prolonged breath-holding and Valsalva maneuvers should be avoided, as they may result in decreased oxygenation of the placenta and fetal hypoxia. Women push more effectively and with less pain when upright: sitting, squatting, kneeling, or standing.[35] Fatigued or hypotensive women may push while lying on their sides. Again, the lithotomy position should be avoided to prevent inferior vena cava compression and fetal distress. Fetal heart rate should be monitored every 15 minutes during the second stage in low-risk patients.[36]

Support During Labor

Continuous emotional support of the woman in labor enhances the birth process. It may be provided by a "labor support team" consisting of the nurse, the delivering physician or midwife, the father, and any other person close to the mother. A "doula" is a lay person trained to provide continuous support to the woman in labor and may be employed by the hospital to ensure that all women in labor receive optimal emotional support for labor and birth. Support during labor may reduce the need for intrapartum medication and technologic intervention.[37]

Intrapartum Analgesia and Anesthesia

Because all medications given during labor produce side effects in both mother and fetus, none should be given routinely. Pain during labor may be managed by nonpharmacologic methods primarily, such as support from labor attendants, change of position, rest, physical contact, ambulation, and a warm shower or bath. Labor and birth without medication may be satisfying for the woman and her partner.

Some women benefit from pain medication during labor. A short-acting narcotic given parenterally during the first stage of labor may help the woman cope and even facilitate dilation of the cervix.

Lumbar epidural anesthesia has become increasingly common and provides effective pain relief. It has a place in the management of dystocia and is of benefit during cesarean section. Its use during labor should be carefully considered, not be elective. Studies in Europe and North America have shown that elective use of epidural anesthesia for labor increases the need for oxytocin augmentation and may increase the cesarean section rate.[38,39] Documented effects of epidural anesthesia on labor include decreased uterine activity, prolongation of the first stage of labor, relaxation of the pelvic diaphragm predisposing to minor malpresentation, decreased maternal urge and ability to push, prolonged second stage of labor, and increased use of instrumental vaginal delivery.[38]

Despite these effects, epidural anesthesia has become almost routine in many hospitals, including hospitals with residency programs, and is requested by many women. If women and their birth attendants hope to avoid epidural anesthesia, prenatal education, support during labor, and management of the birthing environment must receive high priority. Low-dose epidural anesthesia, perhaps self-administered, may decrease some of the problems associated with its use.[40]

Delivery

Normal delivery of the infant should occur in whatever position is comfortable for the woman, and the physician should be as flexible as possible with birth positions. The infant's head should remain flexed during delivery to lessen the diameter presenting to the perineum. An episiotomy should be avoided unless the infant is large or delivery must occur quickly. Sometimes delivery of the head can be more controlled if accomplished by gentle pushing between contractions. After delivery of the head, the physician should not rush to deliver the shoulders. He or she should assess for shoulder dystocia (Is the infant's head tightly retracted to the perineum?), check for a nuchal cord and reduce or clamp and cut it if necessary, dry off the baby's head, and allow for spontaneous delivery of the shoulders. The anterior and posterior shoulders should be delivered during a contraction with limited traction. Patience and gentleness result in fewer perineal lacerations.

The delivered infant should be assessed immediately for color, tone, and respiratory effort. If no resuscitation efforts are necessary, the infant should be placed against the mother for bonding, warming, and drying. Clamping and cutting the cord and assigning Apgar scores may follow these initial steps.

Delivery of the placenta (third stage of labor) should not be attempted until separation from the uterus has occurred (up to 20 minutes). Placental separation is likely when there is a sudden gush of blood, the uterus becomes globular or firmer and rises in the abdomen, and the cord protrudes farther out of the vagina. Gentle traction on the cord and suprapubic pressure to avoid uterine inversion spontaneously delivers the placenta. The placenta should be examined for completeness, number of vessels, and abnormalities. The mother should be examined for cervical, vaginal, or perineal lacerations. Most first-degree lacerations (skin or mucosal tears) do not require suturing.

Summary

The family physician may be skillful in the management of normal pregnancy, labor, and delivery. Inclusion of this joyous part of the family life cycle into the physician's practice has many benefits to the diversity of the practice and bonds the family with the physician. The family physician may play an important role in advocating for the proper support and management of normal pregnancy, labor, and delivery in an environment filled with technology.

References

1. Odent M. Birth reborn. New York: Pantheon Books, 1984.
2. Wertz RW, Wertz DC. Lying-in: a history of childbirth in America. New Haven: Yale University Press, 1989.
3. Gortmaker SL. The effects of prenatal care on the health of the newborn. Am J Public Health 1979;69:653–60.
4. Dick-Read G. Childbirth without fear. 2nd ed. New York: Harper & Row, 1959.
5. Karmel M. Thank you, Dr. Lamaze. Philadelphia: Lippincott, 1959.
6. Kitzinger S. The experience of childbirth. New York: Pelican Books, 1967.
7. Freeman R. Intrapartum fetal monitoring—a disappointing story. N Engl J Med 1990;322:624–6.
8. Banta HD, Thacker SB. The case for reassessment of health care technology. JAMA 1990;264:235–40.
9. Rosenblatt RA. The future of obstetrics in family practice: time for a new direction. J Fam Pract 1988;26:127–9.
10. International Childbirth Education Association. Definition of family-centered maternity care. Int J Childbirth Educ 1987;2(1): 4.
11. Scherger JE, Levitt C, Acheson LS, et al. Teaching family centered perinatal care in family medicine. Parts 1 and 2. Fam Med 1992;24: 288–98, 368–74.
12. Willett WC. Folic acid and neural tube defect: can't we come to closure? Am J Public Health 1992;82:666–8.
13. Expert Panel on the Content of Prenatal Care. The content of prenatal care. Washington, DC: U.S. Public Health Service, 1989.
14. Midmer OK. Does family-centered maternity care empower women? The development of woman-centered childbirth model. Fam Med 1992;24:216–21.
15. Nichols FH, Humenick SS. Childbirth education: practice, research and theory. Philadelphia: Saunders, 1988.
16. Scott JR, Rose NB. Effect of psychoprophylaxis (Lamaze preparation) on labor and delivery in primiparas. N Engl J Med 1976;294:1205–7.
17. U.S. Preventive Services Task Force. Guide to clinical preventive services. Baltimore: Williams & Wilkins, 1989:289–95.
18. Frank DA, Zuckerman BS, Amaro H, et al. Cocaine use during pregnancy: prevalence and correlates. Pediatrics 1988;82:888–95.
19. Ramsey CN, Abell TD, Baker LC. The relationship between family functioning, life events, family structure, and the outcome of pregnancy. J Fam Pract 1986;22:521–7.
20. Williamson HA, LeFevre M, Hector M. Association between life stress and serious perinatal complications. J Fam Pract 1989;29:489–96.
21. Sacks DA, Abu-Fadil S, Greenspoon JS, et al. How reliable is the fifty-gram, one-hour glucose screening test? Am J Obstet Gynecol 1989;161:642–5.

22. Campbell TL. Maternal serum alpha-fetoprotein screening: benefits, risks, and costs. J Fam Pract 1987;25:461–7.
23. U.S. Department of Health and Human Services, Public Health Service, National Institute of Health. Diagnostic ultrasound imaging in pregnancy. NIH publication no. 84-667. Washington, DC: U.S. Government Printing Office, 1984.
24. American College of Obstetricians and Gynecologists. Ultrasound in pregnancy. ACOG technical bulletin no. 116. Washington, DC: American College of Obstetricians and Gynecologists, 1988.
25. Belfrage P, Fernstrom I, Hallenberg G. Routine or selective ultrasound examinations in early pregnancy. Obstet Gynecol 1987;69: 747–50.
26. Youngblood JP. An affirmative view. Ewigman BG. An opposing view. Should ultrasound be used routinely during pregnancy? J Fam Pract 1989; 29:657–64.
27. Hueston WJ. Preventing group B streptococcal infection in newborns. Am Fam Physician 1991;43:487–92.
28. Alexander S, Keirse JNC. Formal risk scoring during pregnancy. In: Chalmers I, Enkins M, Kierse JNC, editors. Effective care in pregnancy and childbirth. New York: Oxford University Press, 1989:345–64.
29. American Board of Family Practice. Normal pregnancy. Reference guide 17. Lexington, KY: American Board of Family Practice, 1983.
30. Norman LA, Karp LE. Biophysical profile for antepartum fetal assessment. Am Fam Physician 1986;34(4):83–89.
31. American College of Obstetricians and Gynecologists. Antepartum fetal surveillance. ACOG technical bulletin no. 107. Washington, DC: American College of Obstetricians and Gynecologists, 1987.
32. Friedman EA. Disordered labor: objective evaluation and management. J Fam Pract 1975;2:167–72.
33. McKay S, Mahan CS. Laboring patients need more freedom to move. Contemp Ob-Gyn 1984;24(1):90–119.
34. Leveno KJ, Cunningham FG, Nelson S, et al. A prospective comparison of selective and universal electronic fetal monitoring in 34,995 pregnancies. N Engl J Med 1986;315:615–19.
35. Olsen R, Olsen C, Cox NS. Maternal birthing positions and perineal injury. J Fam Pract 1990;30:553–7.
36. American College of Obstetricians and Gynecologists. Intrapartum fetal heart rate monitoring. ACOG technical bulletin no. 132. Washington, DC: American College of Obstetricians and Gynecologists, 1989.
37. Kennell J, Klaus M, McGrath S, et al. Continuous emotional support during labor in a U.S. hospital. JAMA 1991;265:2197–201.
38. Thorp JA, McNitt JO, Leppont PC. Effects of epidural analgesia: some questions and answers. Birth 1990;17:157–62.
39. Niehaus LS, Chaska BW, Nesse RE. The effects of epidural anesthesia on type of delivery. J Am Board Fam Pract 1988;1:238–44.
40. Viscome C, Eisenach JC. Patient-controlled epidural analgesia during labor. Obstet Gynecol 1991;77:348–51.

Case Presentation

Subjective

Patient Profile

Ann Martino-Priestley is a 22-year-old married white female nursery school teacher.

Presenting Problem

"Possible pregnancy."

Present Illness

Mrs. Martino-Priestley, who has never been pregnant in the past, reports that her last normal period was 7 weeks ago. She has had morning nausea and urinary frequency, and an over-the-counter pregnancy test was positive. She has had a few episodes of spotting over the past week.

Past Medical History

No serious illnesses or hospitalization.

Social History

Mrs. Martino-Priestley graduated from college a few months ago and is working part-time as a nursery school teacher. She has been married for 1 year to Luke, who is a graduate student in an MBA program.

Habits

She does not smoke, she takes alcohol occasionally on weekends, and she uses no drugs.

Family History

Her parents are divorced. Her biological father, aged 45, has peptic ulcer disease. Her mother has migraine headaches. She has no siblings.

REVIEW OF SYSTEMS

Her only other symptom is occasional heartburn if she is under stress and drinks too much coffee.

- What other information about her current health status would you like to know? Why?
- What more would you like to know about her social history? Explain.
- What might be the meaning of pregnancy to Ann and Luke at this time, and how would you approach this issue?
- Is there anything in the patient's history that might especially concern you at this time? Why?

Objective

VITAL SIGNS

Height, 5 ft 5 in; weight, 130 lb; blood pressure, 130/88; pulse, 70; temperature, 37.3°C.

EXAMINATION

The head, eyes, ears, nose, and throat are normal. The neck and thyroid glands are normal. The chest and heart are unremarkable. There are no breast masses. The abdomen has no tenderness or mass palpable. On pelvic examination, there is a thin vaginal discharge. The cervical isthmus is soft. The fundus is enlarged to a 6- to 8-week pregnancy size and is nontender. The adnexa and the rectal examination are normal.

LABORATORY

An office pregnancy test is positive.

- What more—if anything—would you include in the physical examination, and why?
- What—if anything—would you do today to evaluate the blood pressure reading of 130/88?
- What are your concerns regarding the vaginal discharge, and what would you do to further evaluate this finding?
- What laboratory studies would you order on this first prenatal visit?

Assessment

- How would you describe your conclusions and prognosis to Mrs. Martino-Priestley?
- What are your concerns regarding this pregnancy?
- What might be the impact of this pregnancy on the patient as an individual? How might you address this topic?
- What changes are this pregnancy likely to cause in Ann and Luke's life as a couple, and how should these issues be addressed?

Plan

- What advice would you offer the patient at this time regarding diet, vitamins, medications, and activity?
- If the patient is found to have a trichomonas vaginitis, how would you explain this to the patient, and what therapy would you recommend?
- What community agencies might be helpful to Ann and Luke, and how might these agencies be contacted?
- Describe your plans for continuing care of this patient and her pregnancy.

4

Problems of the Newborn and Infant

RICHARD B. LEWAN, BRUCE AMBUEL,
ELIZABETH E. BROWNELL, AND JUDITH A. PAUWELS

Family physicians are ideal providers for reducing risk and improving health of newborns and infants. Premarital, preconception, and prenatal visits provide opportunities to assess genetic disorders, ensure healthy life-style changes (e.g., nutrition), provide preconception vitamins, manage chronic diseases such as diabetes, and intervene when prenatal disorders such as toxemia threaten. Optimal care requires preparation for emergencies (e.g., neonatal resuscitation, sepsis), management of common problems, timely referral for complicated conditions, and prevention through early identification of feeding, growth, developmental, and family problems. Full family involvement prepares each member for new roles, recruits participation in healthy habits, and maintains cohesiveness when problems arise.

Newborn Care

Newborn Resuscitation

Skillful resuscitation can prevent lifelong complications of common neonatal emergencies. Proper preparation for the distressed newborn begins with a search for risk factors with every delivery. Participation in a resuscitation course or in hospital-based practice sessions promotes teamwork and leadership and allows team members to develop and maintain skills using an organized plan of assessment and intervention. Figure 4.1 simplifies the approach compared with Apgar scoring by basing interventions on meconium, respiratory effort, heart rate, and color. Figure 4.1 can be posted with a list of tested equipment in a visible location in the resuscitation area. Ready access must be provided to equipment and medications listed. Before intravenous access, note that epinephrine and naloxone can be given by endotracheal tube followed by 1 to 2 ml of saline.

Basic resuscitation skills for a depressed newborn include (1) controlling the *thermal environment* with proper use of a radiant warmer and rapid, thorough drying; (2) *positioning, suctioning,* and gentle *tactile stimulation;* (3) catheter *suctioning of meconium* from the airway when the infant's head is on the perineum followed by gentle bulb syringe suctioning after delivery; tracheal suctioning of thick or particulate meconium through an endotracheal tube (repeat until clear unless the neonate is overly distressed); and (4) providing immediate *bag-and-mask ventilation* for newborns with apnea or poor respiratory effort (short delays greatly prolong recovery time). Effective positioning and skillful assisted ventilation revive most distressed neonates.

Advanced skills for those without immediate consultation include (1) *endotracheal tube placement* with ventilation for those not responding or who require more prolonged bag-and-mask ventilation; (2) *chest compressions* at 120/min for a sustained heart rate less than 80 beats/min; (3) *central circulation* access through the umbilical venous catheter, as peripheral intravenous access is often unsuccessful; and (4) *chest puncture* at the second intercostal space in the midclavicular line with a 20-gauge angiocatheter for tension pneumothorax.

Stabilization for Transport or Transfer to the Nursery

After resuscitation and brief assessment for emergent anomalies, hypothermia, hypoxia, hypoglycemia, hypovolemia, and hypotension should be corrected. The needs for oxygen and assisted ventilation are assessed using a cardiorespiratory monitor and pulse oximeter. Oxygen saturations of 88% to 92% in preterm and 92% to 95% in term infants should be maintained. If ventilatory support continues, feedings are avoided and a nasogastric tube is placed. If intravenous fluids are needed, 10% dextrose in water ($D_{10}W$) at 80 ml/kg/day can be started. After 24 hours, 5% dextrose in 0.2 N saline (add 10 mEq KCl/L once the infant voids) at 100 ml/kg/day should be used. Assess the chest roentgenogram, complete blood count (CBC), venous or capillary glucose level, and blood gases (ABGs; arterial if possible, otherwise capillary). A sepsis workup and other laboratory tests may be indicated.

Common Problems in the Nursery

Neonatal Sepsis

Sepsis is often suspected because of its nonspecific signs and symptoms. Bacterial sepsis occurs in 2 of 1000 neonates. Risk increases with preterm labor, premature rupture of membranes, or intrapartum fever. Group B streptococcus (GBS) and *Escherichia coli* account for 70% of cases and *Listeria,* enterococci, staphylococci, and *Haemophilus influenzae* the rest. Early manifestations include temperature instability, lethargy, and poor feeding. Prompt evaluation and careful observation every few hours can clarify the situation and indicate when a thorough workup is needed.

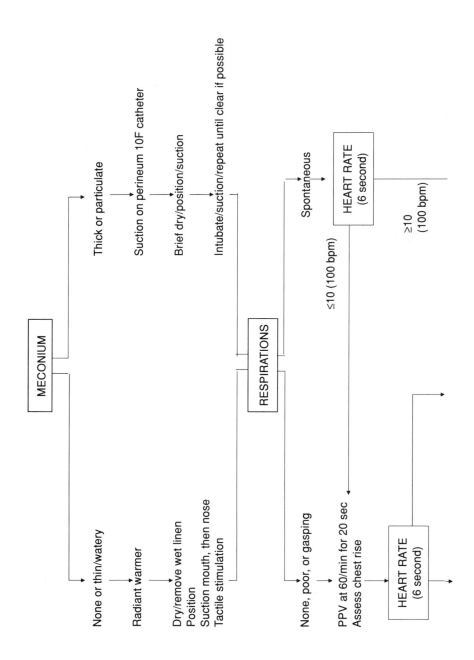

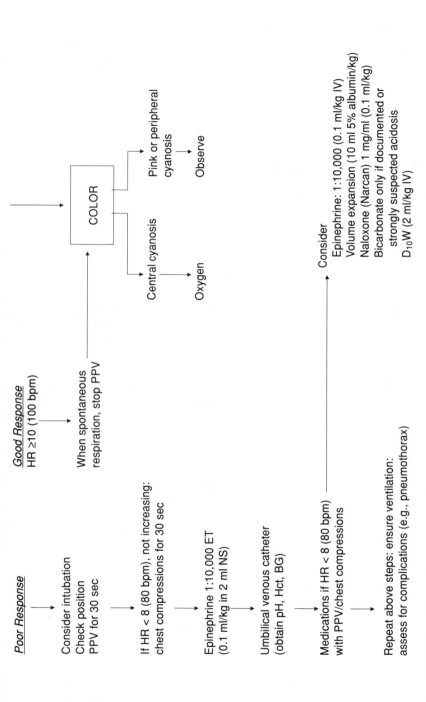

FIGURE 4.1. Neonatal resuscitation. bpm = breaths per minute; HR = heart rate; PPV = positive-pressure ventilation; ET = endotracheal; NS = normal saline; Hct = hematocrit; BG = blood glucose. (From Waukesha Family Practice Residency, Waukesha Memorial Hospital, 1992. With permission.)

Hepatosplenomegaly, jaundice, petechiae, seizures, stiff neck, and bulging fontanel occur late and denote a poor prognosis.

The GBS-induced sepsis is associated with 20% mortality and can present early; it is often symptomatic at birth, with rapid deterioration, unexplained apnea, tachypnea, respiratory distress, or shock. It can also present late (mean onset of 24 days), usually as meningitis.

Diagnosis

Helpful studies include CBC, chest film, and cultures of blood, cerebrospinal fluid (CSF), and urine. Suprapubic aspiration is preferable for culture and rapid antigen test of urine. CSF normally contains up to 32 white blood cells (WBC)/mm^3 during the first few days, so the Gram stain and protein and glucose levels should be checked. Surface cultures are no longer recommended.

Treatment

Antibiotics should be started as soon as sepsis is suspected. A combination of ampicillin (100–200 mg/kg/day *divided* bid for infants during the first week of life, tid thereafter) plus gentamicin (2.5 mg/kg *per dose* bid for the first week, tid thereafter) is frequently used. Dosages are increased for meningitis and decreased for prematurity. Antibiotics can be stopped at 48 hours with sterile cultures unless the suspicion for infection is high, then treat intravenously for at least 7 days and monitor gentamicin levels.[1] If such levels are not available, cefotaxime can be used in place of gentamicin. With onset after 3 days of life, methicillin should be used in place of ampicillin. Bacteremia should be treated for 7 to 10 days depending on response.

Cyanosis

Cyanosis occurs when more than 3 to 5 g of hemoglobin per deciliter are oxygen-desaturated. Central cyanosis involving the trunk and mucous membranes after the first 20 minutes of life implies serious abnormalities. Causes include hypothermia, congenital heart disease, respiratory distress with hypoxia, central nervous system (CNS) disease, polycythemia, sepsis, and metabolic problems such as acidosis or hypoglycemia. Cardiac causes are strongly suggested by an absence of any respiratory abnormalities and a failure to achieve a PO$_2$ of 100 to 150 mm Hg when the infant is placed in 100% oxygen. To reverse cyanosis, oxygen and assisted ventilation may be needed. If serious causes are likely, transfer to a high-risk nursery is suggested.[2]

Jaundice

Jaundice is noted in 50% of newborns, with 6% having bilirubin levels of more than 12.9 mg/dl. Kernicterus leading to death or severe neurologic handicap is preventable if bilirubin levels do not exceed 20 mg/dl (lower in sick premature neonates).

Diagnosis

Icterus, best detected by blanching blood from the skin, is first noted in the face and progresses to the feet as bilirubin levels rise. Transcutaneous bilirubinometry can be used to estimate bilirubin levels but is inaccurate with rapid progression, after phototherapy, or in dark-skinned individuals. Bilirubin levels are necessary in those with severe or rapid-onset jaundice. They may be inaccurate by 1 mg/dl.

Physiologic jaundice is common with a typical pattern of unconjugated hyperbilirubinemia, reaching an average peak of 6 mg/dl by day 3, with resolution within 1 week in term and 2 weeks in preterm infants. Pathologic jaundice is suspected with (1) icterus during the first 24 hours (assess *quickly* for hemolysis); (2) total bilirubin rise of more than 5 mg/dl/day; (3) total bilirubin exceeding 12.9 mg/dl in term bottle-fed infants or 15 mg/dl in preterm or breast-fed infants; (4) direct bilirubin exceeding 1.5 mg/dl; and (5) icterus lasting longer than the pattern of physiologic jaundice noted above. Review the maternal and perinatal history. Search for a family history of hemolysis. If the above criteria are met in a healthy term neonate, obtain blood type and Rh, and direct Coombs' test. In preterm or sick neonates, CBC, smear, and reticulocyte count should be added. A sepsis workup is needed only if other signs of sepsis exist. A direct bilirubin is indicated if jaundice is prolonged or cholestasis is suspected (light stool, dark urine, or jaundice with a green tinge). Normal studies suggest an exaggerated physiologic pattern.[3]

Treatment

Delayed recognition of hemolysis can be life-threatening. Exchange transfusion for hemolysis may be indicated if (1) accompanied by anemia, (2) bilirubin rise exceeds 0.5 mg/dl/hr, or (3) total bilirubin exceeds 20 mg/dl. Phototherapy is *not* a substitute for exchange transfusion.

In healthy term infants, phototherapy is started if the total bilirubin exceeds 17 to 22 mg/dl. Sick or preterm infants should be started earlier. Precautions include increasing fluids to 15 ml/kg/day, patching the eyes, and monitoring for temperature instability. A transient rash, green stools, lethargy, irritability, and abdominal distension may occur. Phototherapy can be stopped after 24 hours when the bilirubin falls below 12 mg/dl on two consecutive tests. A small rebound may occur. Home phototherapy (using a fiberoptic panel) with uncomplicated jaundice and a reliable family allows breast-feeding and bonding to proceed with minimal interruption.

Breast-feeding is associated with elevated bilirubin levels beginning on the third day. Breast-feeding every 2 to 3 hours (not supplementation) can reduce bilirubin levels. "Breast milk jaundice" is a delayed, sometimes alarming, less common (1–2%) form of jaundice. It begins after the third day, peaks by the end of the second week, and gradually resolves over 1 to 4 months. If the evaluation described above is normal but levels reach 20 to 22 mg/dl, breast-feeding can be stopped for 48 hours. A significant decline within 3 days confirms the diagnosis. Alternating breast- and bottle-feeding is also acceptable but may not result in a rapid fall in bilirubin levels. Parental preferences must be considered.

Respiratory Distress

Symptoms of respiratory distress include tachypnea, grunting, nasal flaring, intercostal and subcostal retractions, central cyanosis, apnea, and stridor. Common causes soon after birth are *transient tachypnea of the newborn* (TTN, or "wet lung"), *meconium aspiration,* and *hyaline membrane disease* (HMD). In utero acquired pneumonia or congenital defects compromising the respiratory tract are less common. Several hours after birth sepsis, metabolic abnormalities, cardiac failure, and intraventricular hemorrhage become more likely.

HMD occurs in preterm infants with decreased levels of lung surfactant. After stabilization, tertiary care is needed. Meconium aspiration causes airway obstruction and edema with subsequent peripheral air trapping. After resuscitation, the infant is aggressively supported with ventilation and oxygen to maintain arterial PO_2 at more than 80 mm Hg. These infants have a high incidence of infection, requiring a full sepsis workup and antibiotic coverage.

TTN results from delayed resorption of normal fetal lung fluid; it resolves spontaneously within 24 hours and requires only supportive therapy with oxygen.

Other causes of distress should be considered. *Neonatal pneumonia* may present like TTN or mild HMD. Findings or risks of sepsis require a full sepsis workup and antibiotic coverage.[4]

Apnea

A respiratory pause for 20 seconds (shorter if associated with cyanosis or bradycardia) has many causes. Complete details about the event, including respiratory effort, color, tone, relation to feeding, and unusual movement, should be obtained; and a careful cardiorespiratory and neurologic examination should be performed. Initial workup includes assays for calcium and electrolytes and urinalysis. Based on suspicion, an electrocardiogram (ECG), echocardiogram, ABGs, electroencephalogram (EEG), computed tomographic (CT) scan of the head, or reflux studies must be considered. A 24-hour breathing study (pneumogram) may support the need for home monitoring in preterm infants. All underlying problems should be corrected or managed.

Hypotension

Hypotension, or shock, is categorized as hypovolemic, septic, cardiogenic, neurogenic, or medication-related. Hypovolemic shock results from a 25% loss of blood volume, antepartum bleeding, fluid or electrolyte loss, or congenital anemia. Treat most forms of shock with volume expanders (e.g., 5% albumin 10 ml/kg). Ongoing management depends on the underlying condition. Cardiogenic hypotension or a poor response to volume expanders may indicate the need for a trial of vasopressors.[5]

Cardiac Murmurs

Soft murmurs are common during the first 24 hours of life. Loud early murmurs suggest stenosis or regurgitation through a valve. Murmurs of cardiac shunts usually begin after the second or third day. Loud murmurs or any signs or symptoms suggesting cardiac disease, including cyanosis, poor color, respiratory distress, tachycardia, bradycardia, abnormal blood pressure, or hepatomegaly, should be quickly evaluated by ECG and chest roentgenography. An early office visit or cardiologist consultation may be needed for suspected pathology.

Upper Gastrointestinal Anomalies

High intestinal obstructions often cause hydramnios before delivery but may not be diagnosed until problems with feeding or regurgitation appear. Lack of intestinal air (after 3 hours of age) below the blockage requires emergent surgical referral.

Anal Atresia

Suspect anal atresia with failure to pass meconium after 48 hours of life. Inability to pass a catheter 3 cm into the rectum requires emergent surgical referral.

Other Selected Problems of the Neonate

Table 4.1 outlines the initial approach to common anomalies. Other common serious problems are discussed below.

Small for Gestational Age

Small-for-gestational age (SGA) infants (weight <10th percentile) appear "symmetric" (small head and body size, earlier onset during pregnancy, caused by genetic or TORCH syndromes) or "asymmetric" (normal head size and small body, later onset during pregnancy, caused by uteroplacental insufficiency, and at risk for asphyxia or meconium aspiration at delivery). Both types can have temperature instability, hypoglycemia, or polycythemia.

TABLE 4.1. Approaches to common neonatal anomalies

Abnormality	Causes	Evaluation/treatment
Head		
Macrocephaly (head size >97%)	May be normal; hydrocephalus; metabolic disorders	Check for neurologic impairment; consider ultrasonography, head computed tomogram (CT)
Microcephaly (head size <3%)	Cerebral dysgenesis; prenatal insults	Ultrasonography, head CT
Large fontanels	Skeletal disorders; chromosomal anomalies; hypothyroidism; high intracranial pressure	Check for neurologic impairments
Small fontanels	Hyperthyroidism; microcephaly; craniosynostosis	Check for neurologic impairments
Cephalohematoma (scalp swelling over a skull bone, not crossing a suture line)	Subperiosteal hematoma; rarely skull fracture	Spontaneous resolution over 1–2 months; borders swell and center sinks, creating a "crater"; watch for jaundice, anemia
Craniotabes (softening of cranial bones, giving a "ping-pong ball" sensation)	If local, benign demineralization of bone If generalized, syphilis or osteogenesis imperfecta	Recalcifies and hardens over 3 months VDRL
Eyes		
Abnormal red reflex ("white pupil")	50% of patients have cataracts	Ophthalmologic evaluation
Ears		
Any significant ear anomaly		Investigate for renal abnormalities
Mouth/palate		
Long philtrum, thin upper lip, small jaw, large tongue		Check for genetic abnormalities
Bohn's or Epstein's pearls (2- to 3-mm white papules on the gums or palate)	Keratogenous cysts	Spontaneous resolution in weeks
Short lingual frenulum ("tongue-tie")	Normal	Clip if tip of tongue notches when extruded or tongue cannot touch upper gums

Cleft lip or palate	Isolated variant; some genetic anomalies	Feeding assessment; lip repair usually at 3 months, palate at 1 year

Neck

Fistulas, sinuses, or cysts midline or anterior to the sternocleidomastoid (SCM); may retract with swallowing	Branchial cleft anomalies; thyroglossal duct cysts	Nonemergent surgical referral
Cystic hygroma (soft mass of variable size in the neck or axilla)	Dilated lymphatic spaces	Semiurgent surgical referral as lesion can expand rapidly
Congenital torticollis (tilting of the infant's head due to SCM spasm)	Isolated abnormality	Physical therapy

Skin

Cafe au lait spots (flat, light brown macules usually <2 cm)	Neurofibromatosis if more than six spots or large lesions	No treatment
Hemangiomas (often raised, red, vascular nodules, but deeper lesions appear blue; usually <4 cm; onset during first 3–4 weeks, increases over 6–12 months)	Multiple lesions suggest possible dissemination involving internal organs	Most involute and disappear by 7–9 years of age; observe without treatment unless involving vital structures; evaluate further if multiple
Mongolian spots (gray-blue plaques, up to several centimeters, often lumbosacral, may appear elsewhere)	Hyperpigmentation, seen in up to 70% of nonwhite infants	Benign; most fade over first year; document location
Nevi (variably sized light to dark brown macules; some congenital; others appear later during infancy)	Congenital giant (>20 cm) nevi may undergo malignant degeneration	No treatment needed, although some advise removal of congenital nevi at puberty; refer giant nevi for evaluation
Petechiae (normal on head or upper body after vaginal births, abnormal elsewhere)	Infection or hematologic problem if abnormal	If abnormal, look for signs of TORCH syndrome
Port-wine stains (permanent vascular macules)	Possible associated ocular or CNS abnormalities	Cosmetic problem only, unless other abnormalities
Subcutaneous fat necrosis (hard, purplish, defined areas on cheeks, back, buttocks, arms, or thighs, appearing during the first week)	Necrosis of fat from trauma or asphyxia	Spontaneous resolution over several weeks; rare complication of fluctuance or ulceration

(continued)

TABLE 4.1. (*continued*)

Abnormality	Causes	Evaluation/treatment
Abdomen		
Mass	Genitourinary (GU) in 50% (either kidney or bladder)	Emergent ultrasonography of urinary tract
Single umbilical artery	Other congenital defects in 4–7% of infants	Careful examination for other defects
Genitourinary tract		
Hypospadias (urethral opening proximal to tip of glans; may be associated chordee: abnormal penile curvature)	Isolated defect unless other GU anomalies	Avoid circumcision; surgical referral, with repair at 6–9 months of age
Cryptorchidism (failure of testicular descent)	May be normal: seen in 33% of preterm, 3% of term; if bilateral, consider ambiguous genitalia; if hypospadias and bilateral, urologic or endocrine problems	Observe for descent by 3 months; if not, treatment by age 2 years; if bilateral, perform chromosomal analysis; if also hypospadias, do full urologic and endocrine evaluation
Hydrocele (scrotal swelling that transilluminates)	Communication of testicular tunic with abdominal cavity	If no hernia, observe for spontaneous resolution in 3–12 months; surgical referral if hernia, increasing size, or persistence
Nervous system		
Spina bifida occulta (spinal defect with cutaneous signs: patch of abnormal hair, dimple, lipoma, hemangioma)	Nonfusion of posterior arches of spine; may be tethering of cord or sinus connecting to intraspinal space	Examine for neurologic deficits; nonemergent referral to neurosurgeon if dermal sinus or tethering suspected, or if deficits present

Prematurity

Preterm infants cared for in a level I nursery are ready for discharge when they are (1) medically stable; (2) feeding well (100 kcal/kg/day); (3) weigh more than 2 kg with consistent weight gain; (4) maintain stable body temperature in an open crib; (5) apnea-free (or home monitoring and parental instruction is complete); and (6) born to parents who are able to cope with the infant at home.[6]

Hypoglycemia

Hypoglycemia, a blood glucose level of less than 35 mg/dl during the first 24 hours or 40 mg/dl after 24 hours, may occur with no risk factors and be asymptomatic. Signs range from lethargy and hypotonia to irritability, seizures, or coma. There may be respiratory or circulatory instability, diaphoresis, weak cry, hypothermia, or difficulty feeding. For high-risk or symptomatic infants, check a capillary glucose strip early. Confirm any value of less than 45 mg/dl by venipuncture. Begin treatment for symptomatic infants immediately. Give a bolus of $D_{10}W$, 3 to 4 ml/kg, over 5 minutes and recheck the glucose strip in 15 minutes while continuing maintenance fluids. Optimal management begins with prevention. Keep infants warm and feed high-risk infants early and often. Repeat the glucose 1 hour after feedings to monitor the response until three consecutive normal values are noted.

Metabolic Disorders

Inborn errors of metabolism often present during the first few days of life. Common symptoms are persistent vomiting and failure to thrive. Initial tests include blood glucose, electrolyte and ammonia levels, and urine for reducing substances. Early consultation and treatment avoids severe metabolic disturbances.

Polycythemia

A hematocrit value of more than 65% (venous blood) or 70% (capillary blood) can result in plethora with subsequent jaundice from red blood cell (RBC) breakdown. Lethargy, apnea, irritability, seizures, feeding difficulties, respiratory distress, cyanosis, or hypoglycemia requires a partial exchange transfusion with albumin. Phlebotomy alone can cause acute hypoxic injury and should be avoided.

Anemia

A venous hematocrit value of less than 45% is often caused by blood loss or hemolysis and rarely by congenital anemias. Determine the RBC indices, perform a reticulocyte count and Coombs' test, and examine a peripheral smear. Consider a Kleihauer-Betke stain of maternal blood to look for fetomaternal transfusion. Treatment of shock includes crossmatched blood or, if time is not available, O-negative whole blood crossmatched with maternal blood. For a hematocrit value below 30% without shock, give packed RBCs 10 ml/kg over 1 to 2 hours. Rh or severe ABO incompatibility requires exchange transfusion.

Seizures

Signs of seizure are usually focal and include subtle, rhythmic movements (staring, blinking, sucking), rigidity, limpness, apnea, or repetitive movements of the extremities; or autonomic (salivation, unstable vital signs). Causes of seizures include intrapartum anoxia (symptoms manifest during the first 24 hours), infection, metabolic problems, CNS abnormalities, intracranial hemorrhage, and drug withdrawal. After a prenatal history and examination, evaluation includes a sepsis workup, ABGs, glucose, calcium, and electrolyte levels, and urinalysis with reducing substances. Head ultrasonography or CT, EEG, and other tests may also be needed. Status epilepticus is treated with phenobarbital (15 mg/kg IV load, then 5 mg/kg/day *divided* bid PO or IV).[7]

Brachial Plexus Injuries

Erb's palsy (neuritis of C5–C7 roots due to delivery trauma) causes arm adduction and internal rotation, elbow extension, forearm pronation, and wrist flexion ("waiter's tip" posture). Diaphragm paralysis occurs in 5% to 9%. Recovery begins within 2 weeks and ends by 5 months. If there are no fractures of the shoulder, arm, or clavicle, arm immobilization for 7 to 10 days in a functional position is followed by physical therapy.

Guidelines for Early Hospital Discharge of the Newborn

With discharge frequently occurring before 24 hours of life, ongoing medical supervision must be secured. Each hospital must implement guidelines to assess medical risk and stability, educate parents on proper care and warning signs, and provide early follow-up. Discharge should be delayed if there is no prior prenatal care, prolonged rupture of membranes, maternal diabetes, low Apgar score (<7 at 1 minute, <8 at 5 minutes), weight below 2500 g or SGA, heart murmur, hypoglycemia, poor feeding, fever, unstable vital signs or medical condition, inappropriate parent–newborn interaction, or inability for parents to verbalize instructions and complete education. A home visit by a physician or nurse within 2 to 3 days greatly improves infant assessment and educational efforts.

Infant Care

Well-Child Care and Normal Development

Well-infant visits help build the doctor–family relationship, educate parents about child development, promote health through immunization and anticipatory guidance, and identify medical, developmental, and family problems early. An efficient, thorough approach to examination, education, prevention, and early identification uses standard, developmentally appropriate chart forms for each well-child visit, including assessment of (1) basic sensory function (sight and hearing); (2) gross and fine motor development; (3) language expression and comprehension; (4) social behavior; and (5) family function. Early identification and treatment of infant and family problems can make a dramatic difference in infant outcome.

Nutrition, Feeding, and Associated Problems

Because breast or formula feedings are the primary source of nutrition during the first 4 to 6 months, an unbiased discussion of options well before delivery supports the mother's personal and well-informed choice. There are many advantages to breast-feeding for the normal healthy infant. Contraindications include (1) maternal contagious disease (hepatitis B if immune globulin has not been given to the infant and positive tests for human immunodeficiency virus (HIV) and cytomegalovirus); (2) inborn errors of metabolism requiring special formula; and (3) cytotoxic or illicit drugs.

Frequent breast-feedings started soon after delivery enhance milk flow and supply. As breast milk is well digested, the infant's stomach empties rapidly, necessitating more frequent feedings than bottle-fed infants (8–12 feedings in 24 hours). Feedings should be guided by infant demand. Current recommendations suggest 8 to 15 minutes per breast per feeding. Prolonged suction, more than 15 minutes at one breast, can cause nipple damage. Other complications of breast feeding include mastitis (not a contraindication) and breast abscess. Regurgitation is a benign, self-limiting condition. Availability of hospital support or consultants (i.e., La Leche League) can be helpful for additional instruction and encouragement.

Most formulas are preparations of modified cow's milk simulating human breast milk. Other formulas are available for specific problems, such as prematurity, lactose intolerance, and malabsorption. A demand schedule for bottle-feeding is encouraged and is every 3 to 4 hours initially with 2 to 4 ounces.[8]

Feeding Supplements

Exclusively breast-fed infants should receive 0.25 mg fluoride daily. Vitamin D should be given (400 IU daily) if the maternal diet is lacking or if sunlight exposure is limited. Iron should be added after the first 6 months in term infants and 2 months in preterm infants to avoid depleted iron stores (elemental iron; 2 mg/kg/day).[9] Bottle-fed infants should receive iron-fortified formulas. Add fluoride (0.25 mg daily) if water sources do not contain adequate amounts. Local public health departments can measure fluoride levels.

Weaning and Solids

Weaning from breast-feeding is based on individual preference and usually occurs over 1 to 4 weeks at 6 to 15 months of age. Formula may be substituted for the midday feeding and may gradually replace breast-feedings, or whole milk may replace breast-feeding by 9 to 12 months of age. Solids are usually introduced at 4 to 6 months (iron-fortified cereals, fruits, and vegetables). Meats can be added at 6 to 7 months, finger foods at 7 to 8 months, and table food at 8 to 12 months. Frequently aspirated foods such as chunks of hot dogs, popcorn, and nuts must be avoided.

Colic

Episodic fussiness and crying that lasts minutes to hours, "colic" is common in healthy well-fed infants; it usually starts at 2 to 3 weeks of age with resolution by 3 months. Episodes are often worse at night. Infants become stiff with clenched fists and legs drawn up rigidly. Suggested causes are food intolerance (specifically, lactose intolerance or allergy to cow's milk protein), immature gastrointestinal tract, CNS hypersensitivity, and tension transferred from caregiver to infant. Careful history, physical examination, and baseline laboratory tests can rule out pathology such as intestinal obstruction or infection. Although all causes must be considered, colic most often seems to be a variant of normal. It is important not to minimize the concerns of tired and distressed parents, who should be reassured that they are not at fault. The following specific suggestions can be offered in a stepwise fashion:

1. *Behavioral factors:* Calm, gentle interactions (e.g., rock in a quiet, dim room; rub the back while lying prone; use wind-up swings or strollers); help avoid overstimulation.
2. *Feeding:* Air swallowing can be minimized by ensuring that the nipple opening is not too large and using a semiupright feeding position with frequent burping. A change of formula to avoid possible cow's milk intolerance can be tried. If breast-feeding, discontinuation of dairy products in the mother's diet can be tried for 1 week, then gradually restarted if tolerated.

3. *Caregiver:* Parents should be encouraged to take time away, leaving their infant with a supportive experienced sitter.
4. *Pharmacologic factors:* In general, medications are not encouraged nor are they curative. Antispasmodics, phenobarbital, simethicone, or a combination of these agents may help, although side effects are possible.

Obesity

Ten percent of children younger than 1 year of age are obese owing to caloric intake exceeding expenditure, with excess calories being stored as fat. Specific disease processes and endocrinopathies are rare causes in the absence of delayed height and bone growth. Infants at risk are those with a high birth weight, rapid weight gain during the early months, or an obese parent (40% incidence with one obese parent; 80% incidence with two). Obesity should not be diagnosed based on appearance. Age, sex, and length-matched growth charts should be carefully monitored and plotted at each well-child visit to detect weight greater than 120% of normal or weight for height greater than the 95th percentile.

Treatment is directed at stabilizing weight but avoiding low-calorie diets, which may decrease linear growth. Parent education addressing nutrition counseling at each well-child examination is the primary means of preventing obesity. By encouraging breast-feeding and introducing solids after 4 to 5 months, caloric intake can be appropriate. Help parents avoid excess feedings to meet the infant's needs, especially for attention. Encourage activity at all ages.

Failure to Thrive

Failure to grow at an appropriate rate is weight crossing two major channels on the National Center for Health Statistics growth curve or less than the 5th percentile for age and sex after correcting for parents' stature, prematurity, or growth retardation at birth.[10] Because of a 10% to 20% prevalence in urban and rural areas[11] and significant morbidity (developmental delay, permanent cognitive deficits, behavioral disorders, short stature, chronic physical problems, and medical illness), it is advisable to follow carefully any child whose weight declines across one channel on the growth curve or if the parent suspects a growth problem.[12] Assume that multiple infant, social, and environmental factors contribute. Malnutrition is the common denominator that can trigger organic, behavioral, and family problems that obscure the original cause.

Diagnosis

A thorough history and examination detects most contributing organic factors. Prior records, including growth charts and prenatal history (prematurity, growth retardation), are essential. Nutrition (diet, behavior), development (cognitive, motor, behavioral, emotional), social context (parental knowledge, family dysfunction, drug abuse, social support, isolation), and environment (poverty, adequate shelter, toxic exposures to lead or pesticides) should be assessed. Initial laboratory tests include CBC, fasting chemistry panel, electrolytes, thyroid tests, urinalysis, stool tests (culture, ova and parasite, fat), and a sweat chloride test. Other studies, based on risk, may include those for tuberculosis, HIV, skeletal survey, and renal studies.

Treatment

The parents, physician, social worker, nutritionist, and psychologist may need to collaborate on the following specific strategies: (1) treating organic factors first; (2) implementing a written nutrition plan for meals and snacks with caloric intake 1.5 to 2.0 times normal; (3) beginning a vitamin supplement; (4) supporting parents with mealtime observation and coaching; (5) treating specific family problems that interfere with the family's ability to care for the infant (misunderstanding, depression, drug abuse); (6) enlisting social support (family, friends, church); (7) mobilizing community and economic resources for the family; (8) establishing continuity of care and accessibility to the treatment team; and (9) promoting parental competence and the child's nutrition and weight gain.

Outpatient treatment is appropriate with moderate failure to thrive (not <60% weight for age, 80% weight for height). Weekly follow-up may be lengthened after *sustained* weight gain. Inpatient treatment is indicated when there is (1) severe malnutrition or suspected abuse or neglect; (2) an extreme problem with parent–child interaction; (3) family dysfunction (e.g., barriers to follow-up, disorganization, depression, chemical dependency); or (4) a failure of outpatient treatment.

Iron Deficiency Anemia

Prevention or early treatment can prevent developmental delays such as impaired learning, poor academic achievement, and low psychomotor test scores. Most infants are asymptomatic, but others display easy fatigability, irritability, decreased attention span, generalized weakness, headaches, poor feeding, anorexia, pica, or poor weight gain. Skin and mucous membrane pallor may be noted on physical examination. Uncommon findings include glossitis, stomatitis, koilonychia, lymphadenopathy, and hepatosplenomegaly.

Preterm infants have reduced iron stores at birth and increased growth requirements, which may lead to depletion of iron stores by 3 months of age. Healthy term infants have adequate iron stores for 6 months even without adequate iron intake. After 6 months, dietary deficiency is the most common cause. Other etiologies are blood loss, both perinatal and postnatal (primarily gastrointestinal), and impaired absorption. Parents should be educated regarding proper diet and encouraged to breast-feed during the first 6 months, as breast milk contains an adequate amount of bioavailable iron. Infant formulas with iron are an acceptable alternative during this time. After 6 months, cow's milk should be limited to 1 quart/day due to low iron concentration and bioavailability and intestinal loss of blood. Solids are delayed until 4 months, as they may impair iron absorption. Solids (e.g., cereals) should be iron-fortified.

"At risk" term infants should be tested at 6 months. A hemoglobin level lower than 11 g/dl or hematocrit value less than 33% can be treated with elemental iron (ferrous sulfate drops) 3 to 6 mg/kd/day *divided* tid. The hemoglobin level should be rechecked in 3 months.

Selected Problems of Infancy

Table 4.2 provides a quick reference for addressing many important problems encountered by family physicians. Sepsis and sudden infant death syndrome are discussed in more detail below.

Sepsis

Except for the neonatal period, 3 months to 2 years is the highest risk period for sepsis. Bacteremia (multiplication of bacteria in the blood) and septicemia (systemic disease due to bacteremia) may result from unrecognized or untreated infections. Early recognition and treatment are essential. Risk factors include fever greater than 39.0°C, elevated WBC count greater than 15,000/mm^3, and age.[13] Common organisms are pneumococcus (65%) and *Haemophilus influenzae* B (20–25%). Others are *Neisseria meningiditis, Escherichia coli, Salmonella, Klebsiella, Enterobacter,* and *Streptococcus pyogenes.* A careful search for foci of infection is required. There may be a history of upper respiratory infection, otitis media, urinary tract infection, or pneumonia. The examination may reveal a "toxic" child with poor color, dehydration, lethargy, and inconsolability. Meningeal signs should be sought but are not always found in this age group.

All febrile (≥39.0°C) toxic infants should be hospitalized and undergo a septic workup: CBC with differential, chest roentgenogram, and cultures of urine, blood, and CSF. Infants older than 3 months without an identified focus should receive ceftriaxone (Rocephin) 100 mg/kg/day *divided* bid. Antibiotics can be discontinued if cultures remain negative after 48 hours without an identified focus. If cultures are positive, change antibiotics based on sensitivities and continue intravenous treatment until the infant is afebrile for 48 to 72 hours. A comparable oral antibiotic can then be used to complete a 10-day course.[14]

Febrile (38.0°C) newborns younger than 28 days of age should also be cultured and hospitalized for parenteral antibiotic therapy. Febrile infants 28 to 90 days of age who are nontoxic and low risk (previously healthy, no

TABLE 4.2. Approaches to common problems of the infant

Problem	Causes	Evaluation/treatment
HEENT		
Thrush (white, curdlike, adherent to oropharyngeal mucosa)	Candida albicans	Self-limited Nystatin suspension: continue 48 hours after plaques disappear
Nasolacrimal duct obstruction (excessive tearing and mucous discharge, no conjunctival injection)	Congenital; first few days to weeks of life	Nasolacrimal duct massage Topical antibiotics for secondary conjunctivitis
Strabismus (deviation of eyes on distant gaze)	Muscular imbalance of extraocular muscles	Ophthalmology consult by 3 months if fixed or by 5 months if intermittent
Hearing loss (often see delay in speech and comprehension; associated with birth weight <1.5 kg, bilirubin >20 mg/dl, hereditary hearing loss)	Asphyxia (5-min Apgar ≤5) TORCH infections Congenital head and neck deformities Recurrent ear infections	Auditory testing ENT referral
Teething (gingival swelling and inflammation)	Deciduous teeth erupt by 6 months of life	Cold teething ring Topical anesthetic gel Acetaminophen
Skin problems		
Circumcision (within 48 hours after birth, not medically indicated unless paraphimosis)	Complications: bleeding, infection Excess foreskin removal	Contraindications: hypospadias, ambiguous genitalia, bleeding disorders Silver nitrate q3–6 days until dry
Umbilical granuloma (pink, soft, vascular tissue at base of umbilicus)	Excess granulation after cord separation	
Diaper rash		
Primary irritant contact dermatitis (erythematous papules, pustules, or erosions with intertriginous folds spared)	Excessive moisture, maceration, erosion of skin	Maintain dry area: frequent diaper change and topical zinc oxide Treat secondary bacterial infection
Candida diaper rash (intensely erythematous, well demarcated; intertriginous folds involved; satellite papules and pustules)	C. albicans from GI tract seeding or recent antibiotic use	Treat as for primary contact dermatitis Topical antifungal ointment Treat thrush if present

Miliaria (prickly heat) (pinpoint blisters on an erythematous base)	Inspissated sweat glands	Spontaneous resolution with cooling
Cradle cap (dry, white to greasy yellow-brown scales over scalp; focal or diffuse)	Form of seborrheic dermatitis Appears at 2–10 weeks	Self-limited; apply mineral oil directly to scales and comb out after 10 minutes
Atopic dermatitis		
Acute (erythema, vesicles, crusts, oozing, and pruritus of scalp, face, and extremities)	Inflammatory reaction of unknown cause Family history in 60–70% Asthma and allergic rhinitis develop later in 30–50%	Relieve pruritus and inflammation Wet, tepid compresses Antihistamines Topical steroids
Chronic (scaling, lichenified skin and altered pigmentation)		Environmental changes Lubricate affected areas Avoid irritants (smoke, soaps, perspiration) Topical steroids Tar, keratolytic preparations, if resistant

Cardiac murmurs

Innocent

Peripheral pulmonary murmur (systolic ejection murmur, left intercostal space)	Turbulent blood flow at branching of left, right, and main pulmonary arteries	Reassurance
Pulmonary souffle (midsystolic murmur, left intercostal space)	High cardiac output states (fever, infection, anemia, anxiety)	Increases supine, decreases sitting, radiates to axilla and back
Venous hum (holosystolic and diastolic murmur)	Turbulent blood flow in jugular venous system Present in up to 50% of healthy children	Increases with inspiration, disappears supine Increases with fever, exercise
Still's: (grade I–III/IV midsystolic ejection, vibratory, at left lower sternal border)		
Pathologic murmurs (suspected: features not typical of innocent murmurs)	VSD, ADS, pulmonic or aortic stenosis, coarctation	ECG, chest film, cardiology consult if symptomatic or not consistent with above murmurs

Respiratory problems

Apnea (cessation of spontaneous respiratory effort)	Associated with prematurity, metabolic disorders, sepsis, hypoxemia, anemia, child abuse	Hospitalize for observation, laboratory evaluation, and apnea monitor

(continued)

TABLE 4.2. (*continued*)

Problem	Causes	Evaluation/treatment
Gastrointestinal problems		
Constipation (hard, firm stools; may be difficult to expel)	Anal fissures	Rule out underlying organic cause
	Perianal dermatitis	Treat perianal rashes or fissures
	Dietary	Dietary measures: increase osmotic load in formula and increase fruits and vegetables
	Medications (codeine)	If >3 months old, use oral laxative for resistant cases
	Aganglionic megacolon (1/25,000)	
	Systemic disorders (hypothyroidism, lead intoxication)	
	Neuromuscular diseases	
Pyloric stenosis (gastric outflow obstruction with projectile vomiting; onset at 2–8 weeks; often seen in first-born boy)	Narrowed pyloric lumen secondary to hyperplasia and hypertrophy of smooth muscle	Palpate "olive"; if not palpable, do ultrasonography (97% accurate) or barium study ("string sign")
		Surgery curative

VSD, ASD = ventral or atrial septal defect.

focal infection, WBC count 5 to 15,000/mm³, normal urinalysis) may be managed as outpatients if close follow-up is assured. Blood, urine, and CSF cultures are encouraged, followed by ceftriaxone 50 mg/kg IM (up to 1 g) daily until culture results are complete.

Sudden Infant Death Syndrome

Unexplained death in healthy infants—sudden infant death syndrome (SIDS)—is the leading cause of infant death after the neonatal period. The incidence is 2 to 3 per 1000 live births in the United States, with the peak incidence at age 2 to 3 months. Rates are higher among African and Native American infants, probably because of an increased incidence of risk factors. Maternal risk factors include high-risk pregnancy, substance abuse, smoking, and illness during pregnancy. Infant risk factors include prematurity, SGA, multiple births, male gender, and prior SIDS in a sibling. Despite many theories, autopsy studies have failed to clarify the etiology. Unless contraindicated by a medical condition, advise all parents to use firm bedding, keep soft pillows out of the crib, and place infants on their side or back. Studies for apneic or near-miss infants are noted in the section Apnea. If apneic episodes are documented, consider training parents in home monitoring and cardiopulmonary resuscitation. Reevaluate monitoring at 6 months of age and set a discontinuation date.

Family and Community Issues

Child Care

More than 50% of infants younger than 1 year of age have working mothers. Although child care is not intrinsically harmful, many settings do not protect health and safety or provide adequate developmental stimulation. Therefore, parents benefit from guidance and information. Encourage parents to use paid and unpaid leave to maximize time spent with their child during the first year of life. When selecting child care, quality is more important than location in the home or a care center; however, nonprofit centers generally provide higher quality care than for-profit centers.[15] Encourage parents to compare several programs by making scheduled and unscheduled visits to judge the emotional atmosphere and sanitation. The adult/child ratio should not exceed 1:4 before 1 year of age; 1:3 is optimal. Staff should (1) be trained in child development and paid sufficiently to minimize turnover; (2) enjoy their interactions with children, respond positively to the children's accomplishments, and attend quickly when a child is upset; and (3) wash their hands after diapering and before food preparation, use disposable tissue for wiping runny noses, and routinely wash changing tables. After enrollment, encourage parents to continue making occasional unscheduled visits and investigate sudden changes in their child's behavior such as withdrawal, anxiety, or agitation.

Families and Infants at Risk

Normal infant development is threatened by many risk factors. *Individual factors* include chronic illness, physical handicap, low birth weight, growth failure, or developmental delay. *Family factors* include physical or sexual abuse, family violence, neglect, and parents' chemical dependency. *Environmental factors* include poverty and environmental toxins such as lead. By engaging the family in early intervention programs, developmental delay can be prevented or minimized even in families facing serious medical, psychological, social, and environmental obstacles. Effective early intervention has five elements.

1. *Crisis intervention.* Take quick action to treat immediate threats to safety (e.g., family violence, physical or sexual abuse, severe neglect).
2. *Family-centered care.* Collaborate with parents and avoid labeling a child or parent. Describe the challenge the family faces and the strengths and resources they have to assist them. Teach parents about the unique needs and abilities of their infant. Be optimistic and adapt your interventions to the family's culture.
3. *Social support.* Help families identify *mutual-help groups* and supportive family or friends.
4. *Community resources.* Help the parents mobilize community resources to treat specific needs of the infant and family (e.g., specialized day care, treatment for parent problems).
5. *Ecologic model of intervention.* Assess the individual infant, family, and physical environment; customize your intervention to use the specific strengths of the family. Continue to coordinate the involvement of multiple professionals and ensure that the overall plan remains suitable for the family. Serve as an advocate and catalyst to ensure the treatment team addresses unanswered questions.

Chaotic families disrupted by family violence, sexual abuse, or chemical dependency may be difficult to work with, as these same problems tend to disrupt the physician–patient relationship. It is important that family-centered care be respectful, culturally sensitive, and nonstigmatizing. The physician can take a leadership role by helping the team and family focus on the developmental potential of the infant.

Infants of Substance-Abusing Mothers

Drug abuse during pregnancy significantly increases the risk for many anomalies, low birth weight, growth retardation, and microcephaly. Suspected substance abuse by a mother requires careful infant assessment for medical and neuropsychological complications.

Fetal alcohol syndrome is well described and includes the triad of growth retardation before or after birth, nervous system abnormalities, and midfacial hypoplasia. Cardiac and renal systems may also be affected. Infants are typically irritable with difficulty feeding and disorganized sleep patterns. The full syndrome occurs with heavy drinking throughout pregnancy, although lower levels of exposure may produce some effects.

Specific effects of prenatal exposure to cocaine and other drugs of abuse are less well described because of the difficulty linking dose to response.[16] Studies of infant outcome have been confounded by social and environmental factors (e.g., diet and prenatal care) correlated with chemical dependency and known to affect infant outcome and by a high rate of abuse of multiple substances. When maternal drug abuse is suspected, infants should be evaluated and treated for acute withdrawal symptoms and referred for early intervention. Parents should be encouraged to seek treatment for chemical dependency at any point during pregnancy or after birth.

Adolescent Parents

Adolescent parents are often *perceived* as high risk when, in fact, adolescent girls who have access to appropriate resources, including pre- and postnatal care, give birth to healthy infants and raise children who are well adjusted. True risk factors are poverty, lack of access to health care, family violence, and substance abuse. Adolescents who grow up in a family with violence, sexual abuse, or chemical dependency initiate sexual intercourse at an earlier age than the general population and experience a higher rate of pregnancy.

When working with adolescent parents, (1) expect a positive outcome while offering respect and dignity; (2) encourage family support, if appropriate, including support of the father and his family; (3) encourage use of community resources (child care, parenting classes, education, early intervention programs); (4) initiate family planning early in the pregnancy; and (5) encourage continued education and delay in the birth of another child (delay by as little as 6 months and completion of high school improves long-term economic outcome).

Public Policy

Federal law (PL99-457) encourages states to develop programs that identify and provide services to children at risk from birth to age 3 years. By statute, these early intervention programs are to be individualized, family-centered, and *involve the primary care physician.* Implementation varies from state to state, making it important for physicians to familiarize themselves with local programs and resources.

References

1. Cole FS. Bacterial infections of the newborn. In: Taeusch HW, Ballard RA, Avery MA, editors. Schaeffer and Avery's diseases of the newborn. 6th ed. Philadelphia: Saunders, 1991.
2. Driscoll DJ. Evaluation of the cyanotic newborn. Pediatr Clin North Am 1990;37:1–23.
3. Newman TB, Maisels MJ. Evaluation and treatment of jaundice in the term newborn: a kinder, gentler approach. Pediatrics 1992;89:809–18.
4. Schreiner RL, Bradburn NC. Newborns with acute respiratory distress: diagnosis and management. Pediatr Rev 1988;9:279–85.
5. Lees MH, King DH. Cardiogenic shock in the neonate. Pediatr Rev 1988;9: 258–66.
6. Bernbaum JC, Friedman S, Hoffman-Williamson M, et al. Preterm infant care after hospital discharge. Pediatr Rev 1989;10:195–206.
7. Mizrahi EM. Consensus and controversy in the clinical management of neonatal seizures. Clin Perinatol 1989;16:485–93.
8. Hoekelman RA, Friedman SB, Nelson NM, Seidel HM. Primary pediatric care. 2nd ed. St. Louis: Mosby, 1992.
9. Lawrence R. Breast feeding. 3rd ed. St. Louis: Mosby, 1989.
10. Casey PH. Failure to thrive. In: Levine MD, Carey WB, Crocker AC, editors. Developmental-behavioral pediatrics. Philadelphia: Saunders, 1992:375–83.
11. Drotar D. Failure to thrive. In: Routh DK, editor. Handbook of pediatric psychology. New York: Guilford Press, 1988:71–107.
12. Ambuel JP, Harris B. Failure to thrive: a study of failure to grow in height or weight. Ohio State Med J 1963;59:997–1001.
13. Behrman R. Nelson textbook of pediatrics. 14th ed. Philadelphia: Saunders, 1992:503–4.
14. Baroff LJ. Practice guidelines for the management of infants and children 0 to 36 months of age with fever without a source. Pediatrics 1993;92:1–2.
15. Phillips DA, Howes C, Whitebook M. The social policy context of child care: effects on quality. Am J Community Psychol 1992; 20(1):25–52.
16. Singer L, Farkos K, Kliegman R. Childhood medical and behavioral consequences of maternal cocaine use. J Pediatr Psychol 1992;17:389–406.

Case Presentation

Subjective

Patient Profile

Allison Harris is a 1-year-old white female child, here today with her mother.

Presenting Problem

"For checkup and shots."

Present Illness

Over the first year of life, you have treated Allison for three episodes of otitis media. She has otherwise been well. She knows three words, walks alone, eats some table food, and drinks almost 2 quarts of milk daily.

Past Medical History

No serious illnesses or hospitalization during her first year of life.

Social History

She is the second child of her father who is a truck driver and her mother who works as a secretary in a business office.

Family History

Her parents are living and well. Her grandfather has diabetes and coronary artery disease with angina, and her uncle is HIV-positive.

- What other information regarding Allison's health status would you like to know? Why?
- What are the possible implications of both parents working, and how might you address this issue?
- What more would you like to know about Allison's ear infections and her ability to hear?
- What is the possible significance of her milk consumption, and what else would you ask about her current diet?

Objective

VITAL SIGNS

Height 28 in; weight 32 lb; pulse, 82; respirations, 22; temperature, 37.2°C.

EXAMINATION

The 1-year-old child is alert and cheerful and makes good eye contact. Her left tympanic membrane is slightly dull but moves freely. Her eyes, throat, and neck are normal. The chest, heart, abdomen, and genitalia are unremarkable. Her musculoskeletal examination, including gait, is normal for her age.

- What other information derived from the physical examination might be important, and why?
- Are the patient's weight and height appropriate for her age, and how is this calculation made?
- How might you further evaluate Allison's ability to hear?
- What—if any—laboratory tests would you perform today?

Assessment

- How would you describe Allison's health status to her parents?
- What is the developmental status of this patient?
- What are your concerns regarding Allison's diet, and how would you further assess the potential problem?
- Would you do anything special in view of the family history of diabetes mellitus and coronary artery disease? Explain.

Plan

- Describe your recommendation regarding vitamins, medication, and follow-up on her ear infections.
- What immunizations would generally be appropriate at this visit?
- What diet recommendations would be appropriate? How might a problem have developed?
- Describe your recommendations for follow-up care of Allison.

5

Common Problems of the Elderly

TIMOTHY R. MALLOY, DANIEL E. HALM,
JOSEPH L. TORRES, AND JEFFREY L. SUSMAN

As the baby boom generation comes of age, the geriatric imperative becomes increasingly clear. By the year 2030, the current geriatric population will have almost doubled and represent close to one-fourth the population.[1] Moreover, the fastest growing population in the United States is the old-old, age 85 and older.[2] The elder population is dominated by women, and this predominance increases with age. Older men are more likely than women to be married and to live with their families.[3] This increasing population of older adults has profound social and economic implications. Despite changes in mandatory retirement, only 12% of elders work after age 65. Social Security is the prime income source for most elders, and although their median net worth is almost twice that of younger adults[4] the burden of health care becomes overwhelming.

More than 40% of hospital days and 20% of physician expenses are accounted for by the elderly, some 36% of total national health expenditures. Medicare or private insurance accounts for most physician and hospital payments. Unfortunately, nursing home, home health care, and preventive and mental health services are paid for largely by the elderly themselves. In today's world of incomplete coverage and complex rules, the family physician is in a prime position to act as coordinator of care.

Prevention

Although few data exist to support or refute the need for most preventive health services for the elderly, care for the older adult should aim to forestall morbidity and increase active life expectancy. The following recommendations, which encompass expert opinion,[5-7] must be modified to reflect patient and family preferences, expected benefits to a given individual, and estimated risks and costs of the intervention.

Primary Prevention

Primary preventive services, aimed at preventing a condition from occurring, should include counseling, exercise, immunization, and chemoprophylaxis (see Table 2.9).

Counseling

Counseling concerning smoking, nutrition, alcohol and substance use, and injury prevention (including the use of seatbelts and prevention of falls) are of relatively low cost and without significant side effects (see Table 2.10).

Exercise

Despite steady declines in strength, flexibility, and maximum oxygen uptake with age, exercise helps maintain agility, independence, and a sense of well-being.[8] Before recommending an exercise program, the physician must take into account the individual person's level of fitness, preexisting conditions, and medical treatments. For example, are there problems with ambulation, cardiopulmonary disorders, or deficits in balance or vision that limit activity? Is the patient on a medication, such as a β-blocker, that might limit the heart rate response to exercise, or does the patient need an adjustment in a medication dosage, such as insulin? To set a goal for aerobic exercise, a target heart rate should be calculated.[9] There is a simple equation for calculating a target heart rate:

$$\text{Target heart rate} = 0.7 \text{ (max. heart rate} - \text{resting heart rate)} + \text{resting heart rate}$$

where maximum heart rate is estimated by 200 − age. The family physician should recommend an exercise treadmill test when prescribing a vigorous exercise program to most elders to assess baseline fitness, ascertain maximum heart rate, and rule out coronary disease.

Exercise not only helps preserve health and function, but several studies have shown that moderate regular activity lowers the incidence of new-onset cardiovascular disease and decreases all causes of mortality when compared with individuals who do not exercise.[10] Moderate exercise is also helpful for overweight patients suffering from significant complications of their obesity. It is important when prescribing an exercise program to tailor recommendations to the individual's needs and limitations and then begin gradually. An exercise program not only helps people age gracefully but lets them age vigorously.

Immunizations

By missing opportunities to immunize older patients, physicians are overlooking the chance to positively affect the care of older Americans.[5,6] Tetanus immunization is efficacious, and reports indicate that 20% to 50%

of patients older than age 60 may lack adequate protection.[7] If a patient has had a primary series of immunizations, booster immunizations should be administered every 10 years. If a patient has not had a primary series, two doses of tetanus-diphtheria toxoid 1 month apart are recommended. Tetanus immune globulin should be reserved for patients with major trauma in whom the status of tetanus immunity is uncertain.

Influenza vaccine should be routinely administered during the fall season to all patients older than age 65. The vaccine differs from year to year, and so annual recommendations for use should be consulted.

Pneumococcal vaccine provides substantial protection against common strains of streptococcal pneumonia. The vaccine, administered once, is more effective when given to younger patients. Some authorities recommend pneumococcal vaccination before age 65 to improve the immunogenic response. Vaccination to prevent other diseases should be based on risk factors and performed according to current guidelines for the adult population[5] (see Chapter 2).

Chemoprophylaxis

Chemoprophylaxis with low-dose aspirin is currently recommended by the U.S. Preventive Services Task Force for male elders with two or more cardiac risk factors who lack a history of gastrointestinal or other bleeding problems or of other risk factors for bleeding or cerebral hemorrhage. Estrogen prophylaxis is also recommended for women without contraindications because of its effect on preservation of bone mass and its cardioprotective effects[5-7] (see Chapter 2).

Secondary Prevention

Elements of the physical examination, laboratory workup, and other testing aim at detecting disease in an early asymptomatic state. Few elements of the physical examination have been proved effective for screening in the elderly. Screening for hypertension is perhaps the most clear. Nonetheless, most other recommendations may be implemented easily with low risk for side effects.

Vision

These are several anatomic and physiologic changes of the eye that occur during the life-span that are considered part of normal aging. These changes, such as increased lens rigidity and impaired accommodation for light and distance, do not significantly impair functional vision. Cataracts, macular degeneration, diabetic retinopathy, and glaucoma increase in prevalence with age and are responsible for most visual impairment in the elderly.

Serious visual impairment may lead to isolation, apathy, and both functional and cognitive decline in elders. The 5-year survival rate for the visually impaired is lower than for the normally sighted elderly.[11] As vision declines, there is a significant increase in the risk of falling and hip fractures. This is increasingly true as visual impairment becomes severe (20/100 or worse after best correction) and as vision is lost altogether in one eye. Monocular vision, even if vision is good in the remaining eye, presents significant problems for safe ambulation.

Primary care physicians are key to the early detection of visual problems. Whereas a detailed ophthalmologic examination is neither practical nor necessary in the family physician's office, a screening visual acuity examination should be performed during a routine physical examination. An ophthalmologist should examine all elders on a yearly basis. When visual impairment is significant, the physician should counsel concerning adequate lighting in the home, the full use of optical aids including magnifying glasses, large print, and special glasses; and the elder is referred to a low vision clinic if possible. Family physicians should remember that the key to preserving vision is early recognition of ophthalmologic problems.

Hearing

Hearing loss is the most common sensory impairment in the elderly. The prevalence of hearing impairment increases with advancing age and approaches 60% during the ninth decade. Hearing impairment results in social isolation, reduced mobility, decreased self-assessment of well-being, and increased risk of depression and psychosis.[12] It is also suspected that hearing impairment may accelerate the cognitive losses seen with dementing disorders.[13]

Most hearing loss in the elderly is of the sensorineural type, including presbycusis. Conductive hearing losses are less common. An important treatable cause of hearing loss is cerumen impaction, which is found in up to 30% of elderly people.

Because of the many adverse consequences of progressive hearing loss, family physicians should be alert to patients with varying degrees of hearing impairment and refer them for audiometric evaluation and hearing aids when appropriate. Although screening all elderly patients with pure tone audiometry would be costly, relying on a self-report of hearing impairment is insensitive. Simple office screens for hearing loss include the whisper test or finger friction rub, either of which can be reliably used for screening purposes.[14] With the whisper test, the examiner keeps his or her face out of direct view and tests each ear by whispering a short easily answered question, such as "What is your name?" With the finger rub test, the examiner gently rubs his or her fingers to determine whether the patient can detect the noise at a distance of 8 cm.

Laboratory and Other Testing

Laboratory and other testing should be used, although sparingly, for patients who are likely to benefit from early detection (e.g., the well, functionally able elder). Because many women have been inadequately screened for cervical and breast cancer, the use of the Papanicolaou smear and mammography should be strongly considered. The role of lipid screening is particularly controversial, but lipid levels remain predictors of coronary events; unfortunately, the effect of lipid lowering on all-cause mortality in the elderly remains unclear.[5-7] Tuberculosis screening should be undertaken for patients at high risk, such as nursing home residents.[5-7]

Tertiary Prevention

Case-finding, early detection, functional assessment, and rehabilitation are important tertiary preventive services for older adults. "Screening" for depression, incontinence, falls, and abuse are important activities that may improve a patient's life far more than any medication or disease therapy. Likewise, support for the caregiver, screening for burden, modification of disease effects, and rehabilitation can be rewarding.

Assessment

One of the most important aspects of geriatric care is preservation of functional ability. As part of a well-rounded preventive approach to the elder, functional screening should be entertained. Two levels of function are often alluded to: activities of daily living (ADL), such as bathing, self-care, and continence, and instrumental activities of daily living (IADL), such as balancing one's checkbook, shopping, cleaning, and cooking. Limitations in function increase with age: Almost 50% of elders 85 or older report an ADL deficit.[15] Particular attention to function should be paid to the old-old, those with multiple medical problems, and patients recently discharged from acute care. When choosing a tool for functional assessment, the physician should consider the goals of the evaluation and the characteristics of the population to be assessed. For a frail nursing home patient who may have multiple functional deficits of the ADLs, an instrument such as the Katz Index of Independence in Activities of Daily Living is sensitive to these deficits.[16] For the more functionally intact, home-dwelling elder, the Lawton or Fillenbaum instrument, which measures IADLs, would be more appropriate.[17] By having an accurate baseline functional picture, changes may be ascertained accurately—often the first signs of significant illness or disease. Moreover, specific treatment and rehabilitation goals may be set in functional terms.

Measure of mental status such as Pfeiffer's Short Portable Mental Status Questionnaire[18] or Folstein's Mini-Mental State Examination[19] are easily completed in the office setting and possess reasonable screening properties. It must be remembered, however, that these tests are not diagnostic, and common problems such as depression and delirium may significantly affect the results. Nonetheless, functional and mental status assessment instruments can point to correctable problems, which can significantly improve quality of life.

Common Clinical Problems

Atypical Presentations

Many precepts of medicine are unreliable in older patients, who often present with multiple multifactorial problems with complicated interrelations or atypical presentations of more common diseases or illnesses. The average older individual has multiple diseases, with complex interactions. Often the "obvious diagnosis" (e.g., a ventricular dysrhythmia causing a "spell") may be totally unrelated or only partially account for the presenting complaint. Nonspecific presentations are also common. Falls, loss of function, fatigue, and incontinence may be the only clue to a significant underlying problem. Furthermore, symptoms may point to a system unrelated to the true causative pathology. For example, dyspnea in conjunction with atrial fibrillation may be related to thyroid dysfunction. Other presentations may be "silent," such as the myocardial infarction that presents without chest pain or the bacteremia that presents without fever. Moreover, elders often underreport symptoms, especially when related to stigmatized problems such as incontinence, depression, or dementia. Finally, the typical busy physician's office impedes the optimal history and physical examination of the elder. Remaining alert to significant medical problems presenting in nonspecific fashion or as apparently innocuous symptoms is important when evaluating the elder.[20,21]

Drug Use in Elders

Older adults are disproportionate consumers of drugs and thus are at significant risk for medication-related problems. At any given time, the average elder uses 4.5 prescriptions and 3.5 over-the-counter medications. Sixty percent of visits to the doctor result in a prescription. The elderly account for 30% of the drug expense and 25% of prescription use, or $10 billion annually.[22]

Although the effect of increasing age on the likelihood of an adverse drug reaction is controversial, it is clear that the chance of a drug–drug interaction or iatrogenic problem is increased with the number of drugs used.[23] If an elder uses only one or two medications, the chance of a problem is approximately 2%; with 10 medications, the chance of problems increases to 10%. As many as 17% of hospital admissions are attributable to inappropriate medication use, and 1 in 1000 hospitalized geriatric patients dies because of a medication problem.[24] Thus, older adults use disproportionately more drugs and are at significant risk for drug-related problems.

What can be done to decrease drug-related problems in the older person? First, it is helpful to understand physiologic changes with aging that may influence drug-related problems. As with all physiologic processes, there tends to be significant interindividual variability as a patient ages. Nonetheless, several general principles are worth remembering. Changes in absorption of medications are usually clinically inconsequential, whereas alterations in their distribution, metabolism, and clearance are often important. Because there is usually increased body fat and decreased body water in the older adult, the volume of distribution for lipophilic agents increases and that for water-soluble drugs decreases. Therefore, lipophilic drugs such as diazepam (Valium) or chlordiazepoxide (Librium) may have significantly increased elimination half-lives. Drugs such as digoxin (Lanoxin) and ethyl alcohol are significantly increased in the serum, increasing the potential for toxicity. Protein binding may also be altered because of a decrease in albumin, leading to increased serum concentrations of highly protein-bound drugs such as phenytoin (Dilantin) and digoxin. In terms of metabolism, phase I oxidative reduction in the liver by the cytochrome P-450 system is decreased; therefore, serum levels of such drugs as diazepam and chlordiazepoxide are increased. In contrast, phase 2 conjugation reactions are usually unaffected by age. Thus, agents such as alprazolam (Xanax) and temazepam (Restoril) have less altered metabolism. There is also decreased first-pass effect, hepatic blood flow, and hepatic mass. Thus, agents that are predominantly metabolized by the liver, such as propranolol and lidocaine, tend to reach increased serum concentrations. Renal clearance of medications also tends to decrease with decreasing renal plasma flow and glomerular filtration rate. The creatinine clearance may be predicted by the serum creatinine and the patient's gender, age, and weight.[25]

There are also pharmacodynamic changes that occur with aging. With these effects, certain drugs (e.g., β-blockers) have altered biochemical or physiologic actions. Other physiologic changes with aging can have unsuspected interactions with medication use. For example, drugs with anticholinergic effects may be more likely to cause blurring of vision because of the eye's decreased ability to accommodate. Postural hypotension may be a significant problem for older adults. A diuretic therefore may increase the risk for falls or serious injury. Moreover, concomitant diseases may radically

TABLE 5.1. Tips for improving drug use in the elderly

1. Use medications only when necessary; many problems in the older adult (e.g., cognitive impairment) are more safely treated nonpharmacologically. When in doubt, cut the drug out!
2. Record and update regularly all medications (including over-the-counter, topical, and nonprescription drugs). A brown bag test ("Bring *all* your medications to me at your next visit in a brown paper bag") is often the most significant intervention a physician can take (see tip 1).
3. When beginning medications, start at a low initial dose and titrate carefully.
4. Look explicitly for drug–disease interactions.
5. Ask specific questions concerning side effects; do not treat drug side effects with another drug—stop the offending agent.
6. Explicitly set outcome goals including expectations regarding function and well-being.
7. Help elders with adherence: Give careful written instructions that are comprehensible to the patient; enlist family support; and ask about drug usage at every visit.

affect appropriate therapy, for example, the need to avoid β-blockers in patients with significant chronic obstructive pulmonary disease. Drug–drug interactions should be anticipated; and the use of manual or computerized interaction guides should be routine. Special care must be taken in the frail elder and those with cognitive impairment. Even minimal doses of medications usually thought to be free of central nervous system (CNS) effects can cause delirium. Tips for improving drug use in the elderly are outlined in Table 5.1. Drug use in the older adult can never be without risk; however, the family physician is in an ideal position to make informed management decisions using science, the patient, and the patient's family as allies.

Sexuality

Sexual functioning of older patients is an area in which the family physician is often asked for advice or assistance. As the average life-span increases, male and female patients are concerned about aspects of their sexuality that may not have affected them at a younger age. The family physician should be familiar with the normal changes of aging that affect sexuality, including a slower, weaker erection, increased anejaculatory orgasm, and increased refractory period in men, and reduced secretions, reduced vulval and vaginal size, and possible atrophic changes in women.[26] The most common cause of decreased frequency of sexual intercourse is impotence for men and lack of a suitable partner for women.

Male impotence is a frequent source of concern for both men and their partners but needs to be carefully distinguished from normal aging changes. A thorough interview exploring the patient's urologic history, medication and substance use (particularly alcohol), and mental state frequently points out the best direction for pursuing additional diagnostic and therapeutic modalities, if indicated. Nocturnal penile tumescence can be determined with simple snap gauges that the patient applies at bedtime. Sophisticated Doppler devices can measure penile blood flow when vascular insufficiency is suspected.

Trauma, degenerative neurologic disorders, or prostate surgery may prompt the decision to pursue erection devices. External vacuum assist devices provide an adequate erection for many who can manage the technique and have limited risks. The cost is moderate at approximately $500. Implantable devices offer a range of options and costs but should be implanted by a surgeon skilled in both preoperative counseling and operative techniques. The cost of an implant is between $5000 and $10,000.

Pharmacotherapy for sexual dysfunction has limited application. Depression frequently causes decreased libido, and many antidepressants cause sexual dysfunction. Trazodone (Desyrel) has been associated with priapism. Testosterone is indicated only for those few patients who may be hypoandrogenic. Bromocriptine (Parlodel) has also been used with some success in the presence of hyperprolactinemia.

The older female patient may also have concerns about sexual functioning that stem from medical conditions. For the postmenopausal woman, the salutary benefits of estrogen cannot be overemphasized. Estrogen provides excellent protection against vaginal atrophy and dryness. It can enhance a woman's sense of well-being while protecting her from osteoporosis and atherosclerotic vascular disease, as well as potentially reducing her risk of ovarian and breast cancer. For a patient in whom vaginal stenosis has developed, vaginal dilation may be appropriate.

As with all sexually active patients, some attention should be directed at protection from sexually transmitted diseases. If monogamy is not acceptable, condoms should be recommended. Sexuality may remain an important aspect of the older patients' lives, and many opportunities are available to positively affect this area of aging.

Pain Management

Pain is one of the more common symptoms facing the clinician who cares for elders. It is useful to decide at the onset whether the pain is acute and self-limited or chronic. Acute pain is generally thought of as lasting less than 6 weeks (e.g., surgical pain), whereas chronic pain lasts longer. Pain from malignancy is a special type of chronic pain that prompts a specific approach to treatment.

Rest or immobilization is a mainstay for treating acute painful syndromes. Use of ice, compression, and elevation, if appropriate, also has salutary effects for acute pain. Brief periods (<72 hours) of rest may also be useful for acute flairs of chronic pain; but generally early mobilization and activity reduce the morbid complications of prolonged disease. Exercise has been demonstrated to raise levels of endorphins, which may account for the observed benefits of exercise in patients with chronic painful syndromes such as arthritis.

Analgesics are frequently prescribed for painful syndromes, but their use requires particular care because of their associated effects on the CNS, kidneys, and liver. Nonsteroidal antiinflammatory drugs (NSAIDs) have demonstrated efficacy in reducing pain comparable with mild narcotics, but most must be given orally. Exceptions include ketorolac (Toradol), which is available for oral and intramuscular use, and aspirin, acetaminophen, and indomethacin (Indocin), which may be given as rectal suppositories. Fentanyl also is available as a transdermal patch, but its 24-hour onset of action makes it unsuitable for most acute pain syndromes. NSAIDs interfere with the generation of prostaglandins and should be carefully monitored in patients with compromised renal function or a history of upper gastrointestinal bleeding. Chronic acetaminophen use has been implicated in hepatotoxicity.

Acute painful syndromes in the hospital setting (especially after surgery) are often best managed by patient-controlled analgesia (PCA) if the patient is cognitively intact.[27] Administering frequent doses of potent analgesics usually results in lower total doses of narcotics and less chance of dependence. Morphine sulfate has a relatively short duration of action and can be reversed quickly. Operative pain usually peaks at 24 hours and steadily subsides over the ensuing days assuming no new insult is added to the clinical picture. If PCA is unavailable, administering morphine sulfate or equivalent on a schedule sufficient to maintain the patient at a level to avoid over- or underdosing is ideal. Equipotent doses of parenteral narcotic analgesics include oxymorphone (Numorphan) 1 mg, hydromorphone (Dilaudid) 1.5 mg, morphine 10 mg, and meperidine (Demerol) 100 mg.[27]

Nonnarcotic analgesics, psychotropic agents, and adjunctive therapies are helpful for chronic pain syndromes. It is important that the physician validate the patient's symptom of pain and remain optimistic in the face of sometimes challenging patients. Antidepressants in doses of 25 to 50 mg at bedtime often correct disordered sleep architecture and improve patients' tolerance of pain. Antidepressants with low postural, cardiac, and anticholinergic effects, such as trazodone (Desyrel), nortriptyline (Pamelor), or desipramine (Norpramin), are preferred.

Regular exercise, either alone or in organized groups, also often improves patients' pain tolerance. Acupuncture, prayer, transcutaneous nerve stimulation, and chiropractic manipulation may be helpful as well.

Chronic pain due to malignancy deserves special mention. These patients are particularly vulnerable and need the full measure of our abilities as family physicians. Encouraging independence while not isolating or distancing ourselves from the dying patient is crucial. Patients may be reassured to know that although there may be no hope for recovery, the physician stands ready to allay pain with a variety of modalities. PCA and continuous epidural morphine may be useful for some patients, especially where service is provided by a home health agency. Alcohol blocks combined with local injections of steroids can also help carefully chosen patients. Finally, radiation therapy may provide substantial relief for patients with metastatic bone pain. In summary, acute and chronic pain syndromes are distinct and require distinct management approaches.[28]

Incontinence

Urinary incontinence affects 15% to 30% of community-dwelling elders and more than 50% of those who are institutionalized.[29] Incontinence has significant medical, psychosocial, and economic consequences. From a medical standpoint, incontinent individuals are predisposed to perineal rashes and ulcers, urinary tract infections, falls, and fractures. Psychologically, they suffer from embarrassment, social isolation, and depression. Incontinence is often the "last straw," leading to placement in a nursing home. In 1987 Americans spent nearly $10 billion on urinary incontinence.[29]

Because of the stigmatization of incontinence, afflicted individuals seldom seek medical attention; and if they do, the problem is often inadequately evaluated. Incontinence has been referred to as a "conspiracy of silence." It is unfortunate because urinary incontinence is curable in many cases, especially in those who have adequate mobility and mental functioning. Relying on patients to self-report incontinence leaves most cases undetected. It is up to the family physician to ask patients, "Do you ever lose urine and get wet?"

The first step in the evaluation of urinary incontinence is to properly identify the cause. Incontinence can be caused by pathologic, anatomic, or physiologic factors that directly and indirectly affect the urinary tract. A focused patient history usually indicates whether the incontinence is transient or an established condition. The causes of transient incontinence can be remembered with the use of the mnemonic DIAPERS (delirium, infection, atrophic vaginitis/urethritis, pharmaceuticals, excessive urinary output, restricted mobility, stool impaction). The source of most of these causes of transient incontinence lies outside the urinary tract, and with appropriate management the incontinence usually resolves.

Once it is determined that potential transient conditions associated with urinary incontinence are not responsible, attention should be focused on identifying its cause. Causes of established urinary incontinence can be divided into difficulties with bladder activity (detrusor hyperactivity or hypoactivity) or with bladder outlet functions (outlet incompetence or obstruction) (Table 5.2). A focused interview is the most important part of an incontinence evaluation. Augmenting the clinical history are two indispensable tools that can help the clinician determine the type of incontinence: the voiding record and the postvoid residual (PVR) urine volume determination. The patient's voiding record provides information about the magnitude of the problem and an estimate of functional bladder capacity (the amount of urine voided each time). The PVR determination helps the clinician determine if the patient is emptying his or her bladder adequately. On completion of voiding, a patient should have less than 100 ml of urine in the bladder. PVR volumes of less than 50 to 100 ml are suggestive of urge or stress incontinence, and PVR volumes greater than 100 ml are consistent with overflow or reflex incontinence.

Urge Incontinence

Urge incontinence is the most common type of incontinence affecting older adults. Also known as detrusor hyperactivity, urge incontinence is the involuntary loss of urine associated with the key symptom of an abrupt strong desire to void (urgency). Urge incontinence is frequently associated with neurologic disorders such as cerebrovascular disease or Alzheimer's disease, where there is disruption of the tonic inhibitory control that is normally exerted via cortical connections to the pontine micturition center in the brainstem. On occasion, however, there are local factors such as tumor or genitourinary tract stones within the bladder that cause it to be unstable. When it is determined that these local factors are not responsible for the bladder instability, the clinician should proceed with treatment modalities that attempt to improve bladder storage. The first step is behavior modification using routine 2-hour toileting and urge control techniques. Because the duration of a typical bladder contraction is less than 60 seconds, patients can often learn to sit still to "wait out" a contraction until after the sensation of urgency passes. Then, under less hurried conditions, the patient can proceed to the toilet. In addition to the above behavioral strategies, patients often gain substantial relief with anticholinergic medications such as oxybutynin (Ditropan) or imipramine (Tofranil), each of which decreases the intensity of bladder contractions.

Stress Incontinence

Stress incontinence is also a common form of incontinence, particularly in elderly women, and can be thought of as bladder outlet incompetence. It is defined as the involuntary loss of urine during coughing, sneezing, laugh-

TABLE 5.2. Diagnosis and treatment of incontinence

Type	Predominant symptoms	Postvoid residual	Volume of urine lost	Nocturnal bed wetting	Management
Hyperactive bladder (urge, detrusor instability)	Urge or warning	Low	Large	± (depends on severity and mobility)	Routine toileting Urge control Oxybutynin or propantheline
Hypoactive bladder (neurogenic bladder)	Inability to void voluntarily; often wet without warning	High	Small volumes but nearly continuous	+	Intermittent straight catheterization
Outlet incompetence (stress incontinence)	Urine loss with coughing, sneezing, changing positions	Low	Small	−	Estrogen α-Adrenergic agonists Pessary Kegel exercises Surgical correction
Outlet obstruction (overflow incontinence)	Hesitancy, often wet without warning; "dribbling"	High	Small volumes but nearly continuous	+	Avoid α-agonists and anticholinergic drugs α-Blockers Surgical correction

ing, or any other maneuver that increases intraabdominal pressure. Unlike urge incontinence, stress incontinence is not accompanied by a sensation of urgency. When the patient with a full bladder is in a standing position and is asked to bear down, the result is likely an immediate loss of urine, which is essentially pathognomonic of stress incontinence. Treatment should be directed toward improving outlet strength. Kegel exercises, estrogen preparations, and α-adrenergic medications such as phenylpropanolamine can be useful measures to improve outlet function. Because the internal urethral sphincter muscle is largely responsible for maintaining outlet competence and is under α-adrenergic influence, medications such as phenylpropanolamine are often effective. Surgical correction is also appropriate in selected cases.

Overflow Incontinence

Overflow incontinence is the involuntary loss of urine associated with overdistension of the bladder; it is seen predominantly in older men. This type of incontinence is usually the result of bladder outlet obstruction secondary to prostatic enlargement. There may be a variety of presenting symptoms, but usually there is a history of continuous dribbling and a sensation of incomplete voiding and hestitancy. The physical examination may or may not be helpful because prostate size does not necessarily correlate with the presence of obstruction. It may be possible to palpate a distended urinary bladder on abdominal examination. A postvoid residual urine volume of more than 100 ml provides corroborating evidence of overflow incontinence. It may be appropriate to determine a prostate-specific antigen level to help identify patients likely to have prostatic carcinoma. Treatment of overflow incontinence is targeted at relieving the obstruction. α-Adrenergic blocking agents such as terazosin (Hytrin) and doxazosin (Cardura) have been used successfully to decrease the resistance of the internal urethral sphincter and may even reduce the amount of prostate tissue. New 5α-reductase inhibitors (e.g., Proscar) may prove effective in reducing prostate size and relieving obstructive symptoms. Transurethral resection of the prostate and related surgical techniques remain viable treatment options in many individuals.

Bladder Hypoactivity

Bladder hypoactivity accounts for another form of overflow incontinence and represents the fourth major type of incontinence. With this type of incontinence, the family physician should search for potentially reversible causes of hypoactive bladder, such as strongly anticholinergic medicines and stool impaction. When treating potentially reversible causes of hypoactive bladder, it may be necessary to decompress the bladder with the use of an indwelling catheter for 7 to 14 days. Once decompressed, the bladder may again resume its contractile function. Bladder hypoactivity may also be associated with CNS lesions, especially of spinal cord, and occasionally is seen in patients with neuropathy, as in diabetes or vitamin B_{12} deficiency. This form of incontinence is difficult to manage with pharmacologic measures but can be managed successfully with intermittent self-catheterization or, less preferably, chronic indwelling catheterization.

In summary, even if an established lower urinary tract abnormality is present, urinary incontinence can be improved or cured by improving the patient's functional status, treating co-morbid medical conditions, discontinuing potentially offending medications, adjusting the hydration status, reducing environmental barriers that prevent timely toileting, and using targeted behavioral and pharmacologic treatments.

Falls and Gait Disorders

Falls represent a prototypic problem in geriatrics: They are common, often the result of multiple causes, and frequently a challenge to prevent or evaluate. One-third of the community dwelling elderly fall each year; and each nursing home patient falls, on average, almost twice each year. Falls may result in serious injury including fractures, soft tissue trauma, subdural hematoma, burns, aspiration, and hypothermia. Perhaps equally important, falls are markers for underlying problems. Falls are more likely in patients with cognitive impairment, multiple medical problems, or multiple medications, and in those who are frail and functionally impaired. Physiologic changes predispose the elderly to falls, including muscle weakness, stiffness in the joints, decreased coordination, increased reaction time, and decreased ability to autoregulate cerebral blood flow. Couple these changes of aging with predisposing medications, diseases, and environmental factors, and it becomes apparent why falls comprise most accidents suffered by the elderly; they are the sixth leading cause of mortality.[30,31]

When confronted with the older patient who has fallen, obtaining a complete history is imperative, including a history from any observers of the episode. Many people say, "I must have tripped," but it is important to ascertain if an environmental factor precipitated the incident and what other contributing causes might be present (Table 5.3). The physical examination should include orthostatic vital signs, vision and hearing screening, neck range of motion and movements, a thorough cardiovascular examination, and a careful neurologic examination including an assessment of muscle strength, gait, and the Nylen-Barany or Hallpike maneuver.[32] The orthopedic examination should include a careful inspection of the feet and an assessment of gait. The "get up and go test" is quick and simple: The patient gets up from a chair, walks, turns around, walks, and sits down.[33] The sternal tap, performed by gently but firmly tapping

TABLE 5.3. Important factors and common problems associated with falls by older adults

Factor	Associated problem
Position during fall or change in posture	Orthostatic hypotension, carotid sinus hypersensitivity, cervical disc spondylosis
Other symptoms during fall	Look for signs/symptoms of cardiac disease, association with cough, micturition, exercise
Neurologic symptoms/disease	Parkinsonism, stroke, or other disease affecting gait, neuropathy, tinnitus, vertigo
Environmental factors	Loose carpets, wires, obstacles, pets, poor lighting, unsafe bathrooms, stairs, having to carry objects such as groceries
Medications	Predisposition to delirium, postural hypotension, gait instability, disruption of vision/hearing
Musculoskeletal problems	Gait problem, osteoarthritis or other rheumatologic disorder, foot deformity, decreased strength
Cognitive impairment	Dementia, delirium, depression

the patient on the sternum while standing also helps assess stability. After a complete history and physical examination have been performed, judicious laboratory and ancillary testing should be undertaken. Although a "cookbook" approach is to be spurned, consideration of a hemoglobin assay to rule out anemia, a blood glucose assay in diabetics if hypoglycemia is suspected, and roentgenography on the basis of the physical examination may be justified. Underlying medical problems should be addressed and elimination of potentially predisposing medications attempted. Preventive counseling is in order. A home visit and discussion with caregivers can often uncover environmental factors associated with falls that are readily correctable. Falls are common and associated with significant morbidity. The occurrence of a fall should prompt a thorough evaluation of the patient and the environment, as well as correction of reversible problems.

Long-Term Care and End-of-Life Decision Making

Although approximately 5% of Americans older than 65 live in nursing homes, fewer than one-half of all practicing physicians ever visit nursing homes. As part of the Omnibus Budget Reconciliation Act of 1987 (OBRA), Congress mandated that all nursing homes focus on residents' rights and their physical, mental, and psychosocial well-being. OBRA has also targeted polypharmacy as an area of emphasis and has established guidelines for the appropriate use of psychotropic medications. Additional guidelines have been directed toward the management of behavior problems with the intent to curtail the excessive use of physical restraints. It is of note that antipsychotic drugs cannot be used for wandering, restlessness, unsociability, or uncooperative behavior.[34] More recent regulations also require physicians to visit their nursing home patients at a minimum of every 60 days.

Family physicians who provide care to nursing home patients are faced with many ethical issues.[35] These issues often center around end-of-life medical decision making. Although not limited to nursing home patients, the issue of advance directives is an especially critical one for this population. The Patient Self Determination Act was enacted to ensure that patients entering hospitals and nursing homes are informed of their right to self-determination. Patients are also being educated about advance directives, such as living wills and durable powers of attorney for health care. Living wills are documents for patients to direct their medical care in the event of terminal, sudden, or catastrophic illness, when it would be impossible for them to participate in medical decision making. Durable powers of attorney for health care can augment the living will, as a person is designated to make medical decisions on the patient's behalf (proxy) when the patient loses decision making capacity.

It has been long established that patients have the right to accept or reject any proposed medical treatment. It is only recently, though, that this right has been made widely known to patients. As a result, medical decision making by patients will likely increase. It in no way diminishes the responsibility of physicians to advocate for their patients. Increasing technologic advancements in medicine are in many ways a double-edge sword replete with potential benefits and burdens. Are patients prepared to make "high tech" decisions to direct their care? Will their directives cover all possible contingencies? The answer to these questions in most cases is no, which emphasizes the important role physicians will continue to play. Physicians need to be actively involved in advance directive decision making to improve the likelihood that patients will make choices consistent with their personal values. The days of unilateral decision making by the physician are appropriately over. What remains is an advocacy role for the family physician who cares for the elderly person in the nursing home. The nursing home physician must have an awareness of patient and family wishes, an awareness of benefits and burdens of treatment, and the wisdom to appropriately integrate the two to serve as a patient advocate.

References

1. US Bureau of the Census, US Department of Commerce. Projections of the population of the United States by age, sex, and race: 1988–2080. Current Population Reports, Population Estimates and Projections, series p-25, no. 1018, 1989.

2. Fowles DG. A profile of older Americans: 1990. Washington, DC: American Association of Retired Persons, Administration on Aging; 1990:4. DHHS publication PF 3029 (1290) D996.
3. Atchley R. Social forces and aging. 6th ed. Belmont, CA: Wadsworth, 1991.
4. Gornick M, Greenberg JN, Eggers PW, et al. Twenty years of Medicare and Medicaid: covered populations, use of benefits, and program expenditures. HCF Review 1985 Annual Supplement, December 1985.
5. US Preventive Services Task Force. Guide to clinical preventive services. Baltimore: Williams & Wilkins, 1989.
6. Zazove P, Mehr DR, Ruffin MT, et al. A criterion-based review of preventive health care in the elderly. Part 2. A geriatric health maintenance program. J Fam Pract 1992;34:320–47.
7. Lavizzo-mourey R, Day SC, Diserens D, Grisso JA. Practicing prevention for the elderly. Philadelphia: Hanley & Belfus, 1989.
8. Larson EB, Bruce RA. Health benefits of exercise in an aging society. Arch Intern Med 1987;147:353–6.
9. Posner JD. Optimal aging: the role of exercise. Patient Care 1992;26:35–52.
10. Paffenbarger RS, Hyde RT, Wing AL, Hsien CC. Physical activity, all-cause mortality and longevity of college alumni. N Engl J Med 1986;314:605–13.
11. Thomson JR, Gibson JM, Jagger C. The association between visual impairment and mortality in elderly people. Age Ageing 1989;18:83–88.
12. Herbst KG. Psycho-social consequences of disorders of hearing in the elderly. In: Hinchcliffe R, editor. Hearing and balance in the elderly. London: Churchill Livingstone, 1983:182–3.
13. Malloy TR, Potter JF. Relationship of hearing impairment to dementia. Geriatr Med Today 1991;10:16–20.
14. Uhlman RF, Rees TS, Psaty BM, Duckert LG. Validity and reliability of auditory screening tests in demented and non-demented older adults. J Gen Intern Med 1989;4:90–96.
15. Dawson R, Hendershott G, Fulton J. Aging in the eighties: functional limitations of individuals age 65 and over. Advance Data No. 133. Washington, DC: National Center for Health Statistics, June 10, 1987.
16. Katz S, Downs TD, Cash HR, Grotz RC. Progress in development of the index of ADLs. Gerontologist 1970;10:20–30.
17. Fillenbaum GG. Screening the elderly: a brief instrumental activities of daily living measure. J Am Geriatr Soc 1985;33:698–706.
18. Pfeiffer E. A short portable mental status questionnaire for assessment of organic brain deficit in elderly patients. J Am Geriatr Soc 1975;23:433–41.
19. Folstein MF, Folstein SE, McHugh PR. Mini-mental state: a practical method for grading the cognitive state of patients for the clinician. J Psychiatr Res 1975;12:186–98.
20. Fried LP, Storer DJ, King DE, Lodder F. Diagnosis of illness presentation in the elderly. J Am Geriatr Soc 1991;39:117–23.
21. Levkoff SE, Cleary PD, Wetle T, Besdine RW. Illness behavior for clinicians: implications for clinicians. J Am Geriatr Soc 1988;36:622–9.
22. Vestal RE. Drug use in the elderly: a review of problems and special considerations. Drugs 1978;16:358–82.

23. Carboni P, Pahor PM, Bernabei R, Sgadari A. Is age an independent risk factor of adverse drug reactions in hospitalized medical patients? J Am Geriatr Soc 1991;39:1093–9.
24. Roberts J, Tumer N. Pharmacodynamic basis for altered drug action in the elderly. Clin Geriatr Med 1988;4:127–49.
25. Cockcroft DW, Gault MH. Predication of creatinine clearance from serum creatinine. Nephron 1976;16:31–41.
26. Ham RJ. Sexuality. In: Ham RJ, Sloan PD, editors. Primary care geriatrics: a case-based approach. St. Louis: Mosby Year Book, 1992:444–55.
27. Acute Pain Management Guideline Panel. Acute pain management in adults: operative procedures: quick reference guide for clinicians. AHCPR Publ. No. 92-0019. Rockville, MD: AHCPR, PHS, US DHHS, 1992.
28. Foley KM, Sundaresan N. Management of cancer pain. In: Devita A, Hellman S, Rosenberg SA, editors. Principles and practice of oncology. Philadelphia: Lippincott, 1985:1940–1.
29. Urinary Incontinence in Adults Guideline Panel. Urinary incontinence in adults: quick reference guide for clinicians. AHCPR Publ. No. 92-0038. Rockville, MD: AHCPR, PHS, US DHSS, 1992.
30. Tinetti ME, Speechley M, Ginter SF. Risk factors for falls among elderly persons living in the community. N Engl J Med 1988;319: 1701–7.
31. Tamarin FM. Falls in the elderly: risks and prevention. Geriatr Med Today 1988;7:83–86.
32. Sloan PD. Dizziness. In: Ham RJ, Sloan PD, editors. Primary care geriatrics: a case-based approach. St. Louis: Mosby Year Book, 1992:336–61.
33. Mathias S, Nayak UL, Isaacs B. Balance in elderly patients: the "get up and go test." Arch Phys Med Rehabil 1986;67:387–9.
34. Beck JC, editor. Geriatric review syllabus, 1991–1992. New York: American Geriatric Society, 1991:494–6.
35. Goldstein MK. Ethics. In: Ham JH, Sloan PS, editors. Primary care geriatrics: a case-based approach. St. Louis: Mosby Year Book, 1992:209–37.

CASE PRESENTATION

Subjective

PATIENT PROFILE

Harold Nelson is a 76-year-old married white male retired welder.

PRESENTING PROBLEM

"I can't control my urine."

PRESENT ILLNESS

There is a 2-day history of urinary incontinence, and on three occasions, the patient has lost control of his urine, wetting his clothing. This follows a several-month history of urinary hesitancy and difficulty initiating the stream. There has been no dysuria, but the patient has been out of bed several times to pass urine during each of the past few nights.

PAST MEDICAL HISTORY

Mr. Nelson has had type 2 diabetes mellitus for 24 years and is now taking glyburide. He has had osteoarthritis of multiple joints for 20 years and underwent a lumbar laminectomy at age 60.

SOCIAL HISTORY

Mr. Nelson lives with his wife, aged 71.

HABITS

He does not smoke. He takes "a few drinks" each evening and drinks 2 cups of coffee daily.

FAMILY HISTORY

Both parents died in their mid-80s of "old age."

REVIEW OF SYSTEMS

He has had a recent cold with nasal congestion and cough.

- What additional medical history might be useful, and why?
- What more might you ask about his alcohol intake? How would you address this issue?
- What might be pertinent about his "cold?"
- What might be pertinent about the family's reaction to his recent incontinence, and how would you inquire about this issue?

Objective

VITAL SIGNS

Height, 5 ft 7 in; weight, 156 lb; blood pressure, 150/84; pulse, 90; temperature, 37.4°C.

EXAMINATION

The abdomen has no mass or organ enlargement. There is mild suprapubic tenderness. No costovertebral angle tenderness is present. His genitalia are normal for age, and there is no hernia. The prostate is 3 plus enlarged, smooth, and symmetric.

LABORATORY

A urinalysis shows 4 to 6 white blood cells per high-powered field; no glucose is present.

- What more—if anything—would you include in the physical examination, and why?
- Are there any diagnostic maneuvers that may be helpful today?
- What—if any—additional laboratory tests might be helpful in evaluating today's problem?
- What—if any—diagnostic imaging studies should be obtained today?

Assessment

- What seems to be Mr. Nelson's problem, and how would you describe this to the patient and the family?

- What are likely causes of the problem?
- What might be the meaning of this illness to the patient and the family?
- What might be unspoken concerns of the patient regarding today's problem? How might these concerns relate to his age?

Plan

- What therapeutic recommendations would you make today?
- How would you advise the patient and his family regarding the possibility of future urinary problems?
- What is the appropriate locus of care for this patient's problem? Is a consultation with a urologist likely to be needed now or in the future?
- What follow-up would you recommend to Mr. Nelson?

6

Domestic Violence

VALERIE J. GILCHRIST AND MELINDA STROUSE GRAHAM

"Domestic violence is an extensive, pervading, and entrenched problem in the United States. It is an outrage to women and the entire American family."[1] Although "domestic violence" sometimes refers to all aspects of family violence—child abuse, spouse abuse, and elder abuse—this chapter focuses on violence within an intimate relationship either past or present. Ninety-five percent of such abuse involves a man abusing his female partner. Although several studies have shown an almost equal number of episodes of violence perpetrated by men and women, the context, intent, and outcome of these episodes result in injury and fear in the female partner.[2–4] There is little published information concerning the remaining 5% of incidents, the majority of which occur between homosexual partners (male or female) and which are even more likely than heterosexual abuse to be unreported by victims and unrecognized by clinicians.[2]

The goal of the abuse is power and control by the perpetrator. Dominance may manifest in several spheres, as indicated in Figure 6.1, but is always reinforced by sexual and physical violence. Ultimately, ongoing ego-battering erodes the victim's self-image. She comes to believe that she is somehow to blame for the violence she suffers and that she is worthless, helpless, and incapable of survival without her abuser.[2,4–7]

Violence within families, and especially toward women, has long been sanctioned. Blackstone's 1768 codification of English common law asserted that a husband had the legal right to "physically chastise" his wife, provided that the stick he used was no thicker than his thumb. Thus was born the familiar phrase *rule of thumb*.[2] Before the mid-1970s, spouse abuse was a misdemeanor, whereas the same assault committed against a stranger was a felony.[8] Until the 1980s, marital rape was not considered a crime.[2]

Prevalence

A conservative estimate is that in the United States 2 million to 4 million women per year are assaulted by their partners and that nearly one-fourth of the women in the United States are abused by a current or former

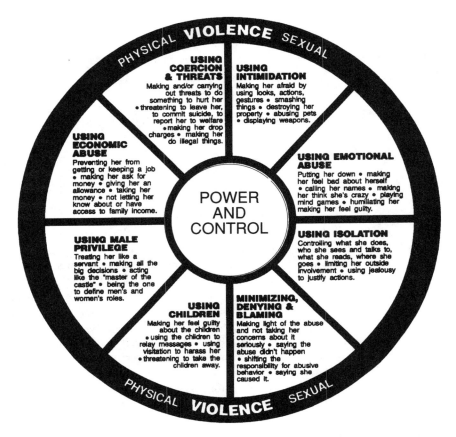

FIGURE 6.1. Spectrum of domestic violence. (Developed by the Duluth Domestic Abuse Intervention Project. Reprinted with permission.)

partner at some time in their lives.[1,8] Walker estimated that fully one-half of all women in an intimate relationship are battered during their lifetimes.[5] Battery is the single greatest cause of injury to women.[2] According to FBI statistics, 52% of female murder victims in 1990 were killed by a current or former partner.[8]

Cycle of Violence

The cycle of violence characterizes abusive relationships. Over time, this cycle increases in frequency and severity. After an abusive episode comes the *honeymoon phase.* The abuser is apologetic, promising that he will never hurt the victim again. He often "courts" her with gifts and romantic behavior. The woman wants to believe him. She becomes convinced that it is her responsibility to maintain peace and harmony because her partner tells her so repeatedly. This phase invariably shifts into the *tension-building phase.* During this period, the most destructive battering occurs—the erosion of the woman's self-esteem. She lives in an atmosphere of extreme tension and fear as her partner threatens and isolates her. She is systematically stripped of the resources that would allow her to leave: her self-respect, pride, career, money, friends, and family. The tension-building phase ultimately culminates in the *violent phase* of battery and abuse. The cycle then starts again. With repetition, the tension-building phase grows shorter and the violent phase more brutal and disfiguring. There may be no honeymoon phase.[5,6,9]

Clinical Presentation

Battered women present with repeated, increasingly severe physical injuries, self-abuse, and psychosocial problems that include depression, drug or alcohol abuse, and suicide attempts. It is estimated that one-half the victims of assaults by intimates are seriously injured.[8] Twenty-five percent of battered women report receiving medical care, and 10% require hospital treatment.[8]

Domestic violence is underrecognized. As many as 35% of women who visit emergency departments are battered, but fewer than 5% of these women are recognized as such.[1,8] Teenagers, elderly women, and never-married women are also at risk for battery.[10,11] Battered women are far more likely to present for routine medical care than for emergency care.[2,7,8] Two surveys in family practice settings revealed current abuse in 25% to 48% of women, with a lifetime prevalence of 38.8%.[12,13] Only 6 of 394 women surveyed in one study had been asked about abuse by their physician, and only 3 of the 139 patients giving a history of abuse had this recorded as a problem.[11,13] The lack of recognition of domestic violence within all areas of medicine resulted in the Joint Commission for the Accreditation of Health Care Organizations mandating policies in emergency departments and ambulatory centers for the identification, assessment, documentation, and referral of victims of violence.[8]

Battering injuries are often bilateral, may be found only in areas covered by clothing, or may be confined to the face, head, or neck. There may be contusions, lacerations, abrasions, pain without obvious tissue injury, evidence of injuries of different ages, and evidence of rape. Most of the injuries do not require hospitalization.[2,14]

Women who experience serious assault averaged almost double the number of days in bed due to illness compared with other women.[15]

Abused women often present with multiple somatic symptoms and show an increase in surgical procedures, pelvic pain, functional gastrointestinal problems, chronic headaches, and chronic pain problems in general.[2,8,14]

Pregnancy may incite the initial episodes of abuse or cause ongoing abuse to increase.[16] One in six women are abused during pregnancy. Abused women are twice as likely to delay seeking prenatal care, twice as likely to miscarry, and four times as likely to have a low-birth-weight infant; these infants are 40% more likely to die during the first year of life.[17–19]

One-third to one-half of women presenting to mental health centers have been battered.[20] They suffer higher levels of depression, anxiety disorders, substance abuse, and somatic complaints.[15,20,21] The diagnosis of borderline personality disorder and substance abuse are particularly common, although in a family practice center study, depression was the strongest indicator of domestic violence.[9,11,20] Domestic violence is a cause of posttraumatic stress disorder.[2,17]

Studies of battered women reported concurrent use of alcohol and drugs during 25% to 80% of the battering episodes.[2,12,21] After battery, victims have demonstrated a ninefold increased risk for drug abuse, and the use of alcohol increased 16-fold.[21] Substance abuse may be used to excuse or rationalize violent behavior. To be effective, prevention and education must address both substance abuse and interpersonal violence.[2,7,22] The presence of one problem should initiate questions about the other.

One in 10 victims of abuse attempts suicide, and of those individuals, 50% try more than once.[21] Battery is the major factor in 50% of suicide attempts by black women and in 25% of attempts by all women.[2,8,21]

In 45% to 60% of child abuse cases, there is concurrent domestic violence.[23] Research on the children of battered women is complicated by the fact that there are often concurrent issues such as poverty, drug use, and frequent moves.[24] Child abuse should stimulate the clinician to investigate domestic violence.

Diagnosis

Although there may be cues to domestic violence (Table 6.1), the single most important step medical professionals can take is to ask every woman if she is being or has been abused. Domestic violence cuts across all ages and socioeconomic, racial, ethnic, religious, and professional groups; however, social and ethnic backgrounds may influence both the victim's and perpetrator's perception of domestic violence. Domestic violence occurs at a frequency comparable with that of breast cancer and is more common than other conditions for which screening is routine, such as colon cancer, thyroid problems, and hypertension.[2] Questioning communicates to the

TABLE 6.1. Clues to identification of the battered woman

Multiple injuries
Evidence of old injuries
Injuries that are minimized or an explanation that fails to account for the type or pattern
    of injuries
Sexual assault
Injuries during pregnancy
Child abuse
Elder abuse
Low self-esteem, self-blame, guilt
Stress-related symptoms
Anxiety
Depression
Drug and alcohol abuse
Suicide attempt(s)
Multiple visits to the emergency department or office
Noncompliance
Chronic pain—abdominal, pelvic, musculoskeletal, headache
Multiple or vague complaints without physiologic abnormalities and with negative
    workups

patient that the problem is not trivial, shameful, or irrelevant. It conveys to all women the physician's belief that it is important to talk about the problem of abuse.[7]

Physicians should *begin with general questions and then become more specific.* Ask about the relationship ("How are things going at home?"), then ask about conflict resolution ("How do you and your spouse resolve differences?"). Next ask about nonviolent but psychologically abusive acts ("Are you insulted, threatened?" "Are you afraid of him?"). Ask next about the use of force such as grabbing or restraining, pushing, throwing objects (be specific about the type of objects thrown). Finally, ask about more serious violence—forced sex, clubbing, beating, choking, and the use of weapons. Negative responses to lower levels of violence do not preclude positive responses to more severe violence. Physicians must not only diagnose domestic violence but establish its severity and the risk to the patient.[2,8,14,21]

There is no characteristic premorbid personality profile of the abused woman. The abuse itself creates fear, confusion, and a sense of powerlessness. Victims have been compared with prisoners of war. In both situations, there is isolation, humiliation, degradation, and physical abuse, followed by kindness with the threat of return to the degraded state.[6,9,21] This pattern leads the victim to bond to the abuser and explains part of why battered women struggle to separate themselves emotionally from their abusers, why they may return if they leave, and why they may develop borderline personality characteristics. Bonding to one's tormentor may be a universal response to inescapable violence.[6,7,9]

Ninety percent of men who batter have no criminal record. Commonalities in the lives of men who batter include a strong belief in the traditional role of women, the belief that women are inferior to men and should be submissive to them, the desire for control, the belief that violence is acceptable, and refusal to accept responsibility for battering.[2,4,25] Men who have witnessed domestic violence in their family of origin display a 1000% greater rate of wife abuse.[4] Physicians should question men as well as women about conflict resolution. Men who assault their spouses are four times more likely to have assaulted someone outside of the family.[15]

Battered women may lack money for or transportation to medical facilities, or they may be prevented by their abuser from seeking medical care. Once with a clinician, victims may fear retribution for any disclosure. The woman may feel ashamed, humiliated, or that her injuries are not serious. She may not admit to the abuse in an effort to protect her partner or her children. She may not recognize the behavior as abuse or may believe she deserved it.[2,14,21] Nonetheless, if asked directly in a nonjudgmental manner, most women give a full history.

Physicians have not been taught to recognize domestic violence, nor have they learned the skills necessary to help battered women. Physicians may avoid asking about domestic violence because they believe they are "opening a can of worms." They cite lack of time and believe themselves powerless to effect change. Clinicians themselves may have witnessed or been victims of abuse. They may fear for their personal safety. They may blame the victim.[8,26,27] Family physicians who appreciate a systems perspective may believe they should maintain a neutral stance. Candib has criticized this reluctance as reinforcing the status quo and allowing perpetuation of the abuse.[28] Physicians may also be reluctant to interfere in the private domain of the family. The American Medical Association (AMA) has clearly outlined a physician's responsibility to intervene and to prevent the associated morbidity and mortality.[29] Female physicians and physicians who have treated victims diagnose domestic violence more readily.[27,30]

Management

The quality of medical care a battered woman receives often determines if she will follow through with referrals to legal, social service, and health care agencies.[7] Women are more likely to turn to their primary physicians for help than to psychiatrists, police officers, or lawyers.[4,5,7]

Once domestic violence has been recognized, the *immediate danger* must be assessed. The best way to ascertain the woman's risk is to ask: "Are you safe tonight? Can you go home now? Are your children safe? Where is your batterer now?" If she says she is in immediate danger, believe her and begin to explore safer options.[2,8,12,14,21]

The physicians must review with the battered woman the *features associated with increasing risk*. They include (1) an increasing frequency of violence; (2) severe injuries; (3) the presence of weapons; (4) substance abuse; (5) threats and overt forced sexual acts; (6) threats of suicide or homicide; (7) surveillance; (8) abuse of children, pets, other family members, or the destruction of treasured objects; (9) increased isolation; (10) extreme jealousy and accusations of infidelity; (11) failure of multiple support systems; (12) a decrease or elimination of remorse expressed by the batterer.[2,14,21]

The battered woman needs to develop a *safe plan* so she can escape quickly. It may save her life. A safe plan consists not only of consideration of where to flee but includes such things as a set of clothes packed for her and her children; an extra set of keys to home and car; evidence of abuse, such as names and addresses of witnesses, pictures of injuries, and medical reports; cash, checkbook, and other valuables; legal documents such as birth certificates, social security cards, driver's license, insurance policies, protection orders, prescriptions; something meaningful for each child (blanket, toy, book); a list of important telephone numbers and places to stay.[2,8,14,21]

Principles of Management

It is critical for the physician to breach the battered woman's isolation and to validate her view of reality.[7,9,28] The battered woman needs a place to tell her story in privacy and safety. She needs to know that her records are confidential unless she decides to use them. It is important to remain nonjudgmental and relaxed because abused women are extremely sensitive to nonverbal cues.[2,8,14,21]

There are several "Do's and Don'ts" for treating abused women (Table 6.2). Scheduled follow-up visits provide opportunities to acknowledge the validity of her experiences, the difficulties in her situation, and the chance to reassess her options. Has the violence changed? The battered woman must be reminded that she can take civil actions, which include filing a protective order, injunction, or restraining order, which direct the batterer to stop his abuse. She may also choose to file criminal charges including prosecution for assault and battery, aggravated assault or battery, harassment, intimidation, or attempted murder. The physician must be cautious about prescribing psychoactive drugs because of the battered woman's risk for suicide. Finally, the health care professional should be cognizant of the pitfalls of rescuing.[2,8,14,21]

Continued support, validation, risk assessment, and documentation comprise the physician's "treatment" of domestic violence. Separation from an abusive partner is an ongoing process. Abused women report that it was often "easier" to return to the abusive relationship than to confront poverty, isolation, and continued threats from their spouse.[31]

TABLE 6.2. Do's and don'ts of treating domestic violence

Do

Ask all women patients about violence in the home.

Tell her domestic violence is a crime. There is nothing she did to deserve the abuse. It is not her fault.

Tell the patient things can improve and that her feelings of defeat are a result of the abuse.

At each visit, assess safety, establish and review a "safe plan," review high-risk factors, and remind her of the cycle of violence.

Give practical advice such as the local women's shelter or crisis number. Caution her that she may encounter prejudices. Direct patients to support groups.

Use neutral but precise and descriptive language in the medical record.

Don't

Assume domestic violence is not occurring in your neighborhood or among your patients.

Question the patient's sense of danger.

Rationalize, minimize, or excuse the abuser's violence.

Recommend family therapy. Separation from and treatment for the abuser must be accomplished first.

Insist that the patient terminate the relationship—she alone can make that decision.

Use judging statements and questions.

Underestimate her risk. Women are at even more risk when attempting to leave; most of the murders happen then.

Ask why she does not leave. (Ask, instead, why does he batter.)

Documentation

The physician's documentation provides the history and evidence of abuse. Notes should be nonjudgmental, precise, and document the chronology. The chief complaint and a description of the abusive event should use the patient's own words. Include a complete description of the injuries—including type, number, size, location, age, and the explanation offered (with body diagrams). Photographs should be taken before medical treatment if possible and the consent forms included. Document the results of diagnostic procedures, referrals, recommended follow-up, and record any contact with the abuser. The number of the investigating officer, if the police are notified, is important.[2,8,14,21]

Prevention

Primary prevention of domestic violence will be achieved only by challenging the roles of violence and patriarchy in society.[4] Secondary prevention can be achieved by the interruption and elimination of intergenerational abuse of all kinds. Tertiary prevention can be achieved by identifying victims and their abusers and helping each one. Arrest can be a deterrent to further abuse; however, in only one state (Kentucky) is there mandatory reporting of suspected domestic violence.[19] Only 7% of domestic assaults are reported to police.[15] Court-ordered programs for male batterers have had some success in the reduction of battery.[25] When available, battered women's shelters are effective, although fewer than one-fourth of the women in need can access them.[2] Many communities and states operate toll-free 24-hour domestic violence hotlines. Other resources include the National Council on Child Abuse and Family Violence (800-222-2000), the National Coalition against Domestic Violence (303-839-1852), and the National Coalition of Physicans against Violence (312-464-5000).

Family and Community Issues

"Our desire to idealize family life is partly responsible for a tendency either not to see family violence or to condone it as being a necessary and important part of raising children, relating to spouses, and conducting other family transactions."[4] This statement is substantiated by the number of physicians who condone corporal punishment[32] and the number of people who think it is appropriate for a husband to hit his wife under certain conditions.[4] Families who engage in one form of family violence are likely to engage in others.[4] Family physicians are in a unique position to interrupt the cycle of violence and to effect positive change in the lives of victims, abusers, and children involved in domestic violence.

References

1. Novello AC, Shosky J. From the Surgeon General, US Public Health Service: a medical response to domestic violence. JAMA 1992;267:3132.
2. Sassetti MR. Battered women. In: Violence education: toward a solution. Kansas City, MO: Society of Teachers of Family Medicine, 1992;31–53.
3. Council on Scientific Affairs, American Medical Association. Violence against women: relevance for medical practitioners. JAMA 1992;267: 3184–9.
4. Gelles RJ, Cornell CP. Intimate violence in families. 2nd ed. Newbury, CA: Sage Publications, 1990.
5. Walker LE. The battered woman syndrome. New York: Springer, 1984.
6. Graham DLR, Rawlings E, Rimini N. Survivors of terror: battered women, hostages and the Stockholm syndrome. In: Yllo K, Bograd M, editors. Feminist perspectives on wife abuse. Newbury Park, CA: Sage Publications, 1988:217–33.
7. Burge SK. Violence against women as a health care issue. Fam Med 1989;21: 368–73.
8. American Medical Association. Diagnostic and treatment guidelines on domestic violence. Chicago: American Medical Association, 1992.
9. Herman JL. Trauma and recovery. New York: Basic Books, 1992.
10. McLeer SV, Anwar R. A study of battered women presenting in an emergency department. Am J Public Health 1989;79:65–66.

11. Saunders DG, Hamberger K, Hovey M. Indicators of woman abuse based on a chart review at a family practice center. Arch Fam Med 1993;2:537–43.
12. Rath GD, Jarratt LG, Leonardson G. Rates of domestic violence against adult women by men partners. J Am Board Fam Pract 1989;2:227–33.
13. Hamberger LK, Saunders DG, Hovey M. Prevalence of domestic violence in community practice and rate of physician inquiry. Fam Med 1992;24:283–7.
14. Flitcraft A. Battered women in your practice? Patient Care 1990;Oct 15:107–18.
15. Straus MA, Smith C. Family patterns and primary prevention of family violence. Trends Health Care Law Ethics 1993;8:17–25.
16. Newberger EH, Barkan SE, Lieberman ES, et al. Abuse of pregnant women and adverse birth outcome: current knowledge and implications for practice [commentary]. JAMA 1992;267:2370–2.
17. McFarlane J. Abuse during pregnancy: the horror and the hope. Clin Issues Perinatal Women's Health Nursing 1993;4:350–61.
18. McFarlane J, Parker B, Soeken K, Bullock L. Assessing for abuse during pregnancy: severity and frequency of injuries and associated entry into prenatal care. JAMA 1992;267:3176–8.
19. Domestic violence: a policy statement of the American Public Health Association. Am J Public Health 1993;83:458–63.
20. Carmen EH, Rieker PP, Miles T. Victims of violence and psychiatric illness. Am J Psychiatry 1984;141:378–83.
21. McLeer SV, Anwar RAH. The role of the emergency physician in the prevention of domestic violence. Ann Emerg Med 1987;16:1155–61.
22. Schwartz I. Alcohol and family violence [letter]. JAMA 1989;262:351–2.
23. McKibben L, De Vos E, Newberger EH. Victimization of mothers of abused children: a controlled study. Pediatrics 1989;84:531–5.
24. Jaffe PG, Hurley DJ, Wolfe D. Children's observations of violence. I. Critical issues in child development and intervention planning. Can J Psychiatry 1990;35:466–70.
25. Hamberger LK. Identifying and intervening with men who batter. In: Violence education: toward a solution. Kansas City, MO: Society of Teachers of Family Medicine, 1992:55–66.
26. Sugg NK, Inui T. Primary care physicians' response to domestic violence: opening Pandora's box. JAMA 267:3157–60.
27. Brown JC, Lent B, Sas G. Identifying and treating wife abuse. J Fam Pract 1993;36:185–91.
28. Candib LM. Violence against women: no more excuses [editorial]. Fam Med 1989;21:339–42.
29. Council on Ethical and Judicial Affairs, American Medical Association. Physicians and domestic violence. JAMA 1992;267:3190–3.
30. Saunders DG, Phillips K. Predictors of physician's response to woman abuse: the role of gender, background, and brief training. J Gen Int Med 1993;8:606–9.
31. Newman KD. Giving up: shelter experiences of battered women. Public Health Nursing 1993;10:108–13.
32. McCormick K. Attitudes of primary care physicians toward corporal punishment. JAMA 1992;267:3161–5.

CASE PRESENTATION

Subjective

PATIENT PROFILE

Ann Martino-Priestley is a 22-year-old married white female nursery school teacher found to be pregnant on her last visit 6 weeks ago.

PRESENTING PROBLEM

"Routine prenatal visit."

PRESENT ILLNESS

The patient is now 13 weeks pregnant and no longer has nausea and urinary frequency. There is no vaginal spotting. She feels well and is "excited about this first pregnancy." Her appetite is good, and she is taking prenatal vitamins.

PAST MEDICAL HISTORY, SOCIAL HISTORY, HABITS, AND FAMILY HISTORY

These are unchanged since her first prenatal visit (see Chapter 3).

REVIEW OF SYSTEMS

While taking the history, you noticed a bruise below her left eye, although this was not mentioned by the patient. When questioned, the patient reports that she walked into a partially opened bathroom door while going to the toilet at night.

- The husband insists on being present throughout the examination and the following consultation. How do you respond to this request?
- What additional information about the progress of the pregnancy would be important today?
- What might be the patient's goals for today's visit?
- What more would you like to know about the bruise below the left eye? How would you frame the question(s)?

Objective

VITAL SIGNS

Weight, 131 lb; blood pressure, 120/72; pulse, 74; temperature, 37.2°C.

EXAMINATION

There is no abdominal tenderness. The uterus is palpable at a 3 months' size. In addition to the fading ecchymosis below the left eye, there is a recent-appearing ecchymosis 2 to 4 cm in size of the left lower abdomen and another bruise 2 by 3 cm of the lateral right breast. The patient was apparently unaware of these bruises and reports that she does not know the cause.

LABORATORY

On laboratory examination, the urine is negative for protein and glucose.

- What additional information derived from the physical examination would be useful in regard to the pregnancy?
- What additional physical examination data might help clarify the cause of the bruising?
- What laboratory specimens—if any—should you obtain today?
- What diagnostic imaging—if any—would you obtain today?

Assessment

- What are the diagnostic possibilities, and how will you share these with the patient?
- What might be the significance of the pregnancy to the patient and her husband?
- What may be the patient's concerns, and how would you elicit these?
- What physical diseases could explain the bruising? What drugs might contribute to the bruising? How readily will you accept these possible explanations?

Plan

- What is your recommendation to the patient and her husband?
- What community agencies might become involved, and how should they be contacted?
- The patient expresses concern about the cost of prenatal care, hospital confinement, and delivery. How would you respond?
- As you are concluding the visit, the patient begins to cry and says, "I'm afraid." What would you do next?

7
Headache

ANNE D. WALLING

Headache is an almost universal experience. Few individuals claim never to have suffered from headache; conversely, more than 40% of North American adults have experienced severe headache[1] and up to 10% of this population report headache as a severe, recurrent, and periodically disabling symptom.[2] Headaches are most prevalent among young adults. Nearly 60% of men and 76% of women aged 12 to 29 years report headache within any 4-week period.[3] Although most headaches are not brought to medical attention, the condition still leads more than 40 million Americans to consult physicians annually[4] and is the seventh leading presenting complaint in ambulatory care settings.[3] Family practice studies consistently find headache to be one of the most frequently presented problems.[5] The costs of headache, including expenditure on treatments and investigations and the disruption of personal and family life style, are enormous. Many of these costs are hidden. Headache is the single largest cause of lost work days in the United States—some 155 million work days annually.[6]

Headache can result from many causes. The classic view that cephalic pain could result only from the brain linings and blood vessels has been challenged, and it now seems likely that certain types of headache are generated within the brain itself.[1] Headache is, however, rarely an objectively definable symptom. The pain sensation is interpreted by each patient in terms of experience and culture; thus, a relatively minor headache may lead one patient to seek emergency care and thorough neurologic assessment, whereas a patient with a personal and family history of migraine may manage several days of severe symptoms without seeking medical intervention.

Physicians are also influenced by many factors in their approach to headache patients.[5] Headache is one of the conditions most frequently identified by physicians as "heartsink," i.e., the patient evokes "an overwhelming mixture of exasperation, defeat, and sometimes plain dislike."[7] Accurate diagnosis and effective management of headaches requires the development of a "therapeutic alliance" between physician and patient based on objectivity and mutual respect.[8]

Clinical Approach to the Headache Patient

With so many potential causes and complicating circumstances, a systematic approach to the headache patient is essential for objective, effective, efficient management. It can be achieved in four stages.

1. Clarification of the reasons for the consultation
2. Diagnosis (classification) of the headache
3. Negotiation of management
4. Follow-up

In addition to those patients who give headache as the presenting or principal complaint, it is common in practice to discover a significant headache history on systematic inquiry of a patient presenting for other reasons. The clinical approach in these patients reverses the first question to identify why the patient avoided seeking medical help for headache symptoms.

Clarification of the Reasons for Consultation

As only a small proportion of all headaches lead to medical consultation, those that do have particular significance. It is important to have the patient articulate his or her beliefs about the symptoms and expectations of treatment.[8] Reasons for consultation range from fear of cancer to seeking validation that current use of over-the-counter medications is appropriate. Headache is frequently used as a "ticket of admission" symptom by the patient who wishes to discuss other medical or social problems. In practice, a change in the coping ability of the patient, family, or coworkers is as frequent a cause of consultation as any change in the severity or type of headache. Patients may also consult when they learn new information, particularly concerning situations in which a severe illness in a friend or relative presented as headache.

All headache patients should be directly asked what type of headache they think they have and what causes it. These issues must be addressed during the management even if they are inaccurate. Patients should also be asked about expectations of management. With rare exceptions, headaches can be expected to recur, and clinical goals are of management rather than cure. Successful management avoids dependency by emphasizing the patient's role in reducing the frequency and severity of headaches and increasing his or her ability to cope with a recurrent condition.

Background information from relatives and friends may give useful insights concerning the impact of headaches on the patient's daily life. Disruptive headaches lead to highly charged situations, and the physician must remain objective and avoid becoming triangulated between the patient and others. With good listening and a few directed questions, the background to the consultation can be clarified and the groundwork laid for accurate diagnosis and successful management. This short time is well invested. In headache patients presenting to family practitioners, "listening" time makes significantly greater contributions to diagnosis and management than time spent in physical examination or other investigations,[9] although all are appropriate.

Diagnosis

The International Classification of Headaches, developed in 1988,[10] established diagnostic criteria for 13 major types of headache with approximately 70 subtypes. Table 7.1 lists major headache types, according to whether they are primary, secondary to other causes, or unclassifiable. A useful grouping in family practice uses five categories.

1. Migraine (all types)
2. Cluster headaches
3. Tension/stress (or muscle contraction) headaches
4. Headaches secondary to other pathology
5. Specific headache syndromes (e.g., cough headache)

Table 7.1. Headache types

Primary headaches	Secondary headaches
Migraine	*Associated with*
Without aura	Head trauma
With aura	Vascular disorders
Ophthalmoplegic	Intracranial disorders
Retinal	Substance use or withdrawal
Childhood syndromes	Systemic infections
Migraine complications	Metabolic disorders
Other	Structural disorder of head or neck
Tension type	Neuralgia syndromes
Episodic	
Chronic	**Unclassifiable headaches**
Other	
Cluster	
Episodic	
Chronic	
Chronic paroxysmal hemicrania	
Other	
Miscellaneous	
"Ice-pick"	
External compression	
Cold stimulus (including ice cream)	
Cough	
Exertional	
Coital	

These categories are broad with considerable overlap. "Mixed headaches," where the clinical picture contains elements of more than one headache category, are common. Individual patients may also describe more than one type of headache (e.g., migraineurs experience tension headaches on occasion). The individual categories are discussed below.

The diagnosis of headache syndromes (Table 7.2) is an excellent example of the clinical reasoning process in which a systematic approach and judicious use of investigations determines the probable diagnosis. A particular feature of headache is the potential to use the diagnostic process to build patient understanding of the condition and prepare the patient to play the major role in long-term management.

History

The essential element in headache diagnosis is the history. An open-ended approach such as, "Tell me about your headaches," supported by specific questioning to elucidate essential features usually indicates which of the diagnostic categories is most probable. The history should clarify the following.

Duration: age at onset, any change in nature or pattern over time

Pattern: frequency of attacks, precipitating or associated factors

Type: prodromes, location in the head, radiation, nature of the pain, associated symptoms, relieving behaviors or response to medication, duration of pain, postheadache symptoms

History: personal history or vulnerability to medical, occupational, or other "secondary" causes of headache, especially head trauma; family history, especially of migraine; history of previous investigations for headache

The specific headache profile that emerges from the history provides a high probability of correctly classifying the headache[8,9,11] based on these data alone. In addition to eliciting information on the headache, it is important to establish a general impression of the patient, particularly his or her affect and behavior. Although subjective, the general impression of the patient should correlate with the headache story such that a highly probable diagnosis is made for each patient. Certain types of headache are more common in certain types of patient; for example, cluster headache is most frequently seen in middle-aged men, whereas migraine is more prevalent in young women. By the end of the history-taking process, the physician should have the answer to two questions: "Which of the five headache groups best fits the story?" "Is it a likely diagnosis for this particular patient?"

TABLE 7.2. Diagnostic criteria for common primary headaches[a]

Headache	Duration	Characteristics	Associated symptoms	Other
Migraine	4–72 hours	*At least two:* Unilateral Pulsating Moderate–severe Aggravated by activity	*At least one:* Nausea/vomiting Photophobia *and* phonophobia	No neurologic source for symptoms Multiple types (Table 7.1) At least 5 attacks for diagnosis
Cluster	15–180 minutes (individual attacks) 1–8 attacks/day for 7 days to 1 year or longer (cluster episodes)	Unilateral orbital/temporal stabbing Severe–very severe	*At least one:* Conjunctival injection Lacrimation Nasal congestion Rhinorrhea Sweating Miosis Ptosis Eyelid edema	No neurologic source for symptoms At least 5 attacks for diagnosis
Tension/stress	30 minutes–7 days (individual headaches) Headaches <15 days/month or <180/year	*At least two:* Pressure/tightness Bilateral Mild–moderate Not aggravated by activity	No nausea Photophonia and photophobia: absent or only one present, not both	No neurologic source for symptoms At least 10 episodes for diagnosis

[a]Developed using data in ref. 10.

Physical Examination

The physical examination continues the dual processes of confirming a specific diagnosis and laying the groundwork for successful management. Unless the consultation coincides with an attack, many migraine, cluster, and other headache patients can be expected to have no abnormal findings on physical examination. This situation has led some authors to recommend that only a targeted examination be performed, focusing on causes of secondary headache elicited from the history,[9] whereas others emphasize the importance of complete physical and neurologic examination of every headache patient.[11,12] In practice, headache is seldom a situation covered by pure logic. The time devoted to a complete examination may be a wise investment, as it documents both positive and negative physical findings, contributes to the "therapeutic alliance," and is in many instances therapeutic. This therapeutic effect is seen most dramatically when the patient has a particular concern (e.g., fear of a brain tumor).

The diagnostic power of physical examination is most apparent for headaches secondary to other pathology. As literally thousands of physical and psychological conditions can include headache as a symptom, the evaluation cannot be a "blind search" but is complementary to a careful history and clinical acumen. The physical examination targets the most probable diagnoses based on the symptoms presented by the patient and the physician's knowledge of conditions relevant to the individual. For example, severe occipital pain and neck stiffness in a child suggests meningitis, whereas similar symptoms in his or her mother might indicate subarachnoid hemorrhage, and in the grandmother, they could originate from osteoarthritis of the cervical spine.

Other Investigations

Targeted laboratory and radiologic investigations are best used to confirm the etiology of secondary headaches. The most striking example of a helpful diagnostic laboratory test is the erythrocyte sedimentation rate in elderly patients with temporal arteritis. One or more tests ranging in complexity from white blood cell counts to biochemical markers for pheochromocytoma may be indicated in individual patients. Tests, however, are often performed to relieve either physician or patient distress and uncertainty. If the patient or family insists on tests the physician does not believe appropriate, the contributions and limitations of the test in question should be reviewed with the patient and family. Similarly, the physician experiencing the WHIMS (*what have I missed syndrome*) must review the data and attempt to make a rational decision as to the potential contribution of additional testing.

Most debate over the appropriate role of testing currently involves radiologic investigation, specifically computed tomography (CT) and magnetic resonance imaging (MRI). Both modalities have high sensitivity (e.g., CT has a more than 90% capability to detect an enhancing brain tumor[13]), but the role of CT and MRI for diagnosing headaches that present to family physicians is limited by the rarity of such conditions in practice. Intracranial lesions accounted for only 0.4% of headache patients in two large studies[9,14] of headache in family practice populations. When deciding to refer a patient for advanced radiologic testing, the family physician must seriously consider the probability of such a rare diagnosis and balance the potential benefits of the test against cost and radiation exposure. CT has a high probability of detecting intracranial lesions, provided they are enhancing lesions of sufficient size and are situated clear of tissues such as bone, which can interfere with visualization. MRI also has high sensitivity and is in many respects complementary to CT examination, as MRI can visualize infiltrating tumors, is less influenced by bone artifacts, and is particularly good at detecting vascular structures. MRI does not carry any risk of radiation exposure but is significantly more expensive than CT.

Family physicians should refer a patient for CT and MRI only when the history and physical examination indicate that an intracranial lesion is the probable diagnosis. This protocol is in general agreement with the National Institutes of Health (NIH) Consensus Development Panel, which recommended CT investigation of patients whose headaches were "severe, constant, unusual, or associated with neurological symptoms."[15] This recommendation cannot be strictly followed in practice, however, as more than half the patients describe their headaches as severe.[9] The other elements of the NIH recommendations, particularly the presence of neurologic signs, are more useful; but the final decision to refer for CT or MRI remains a clinical judgment based on the characteristics of the patient and his or her symptom complex and risk factors for intracranial pathology.

Negotiation of Management

Migraine, cluster, tension/stress, and many secondary headaches are recurrent; hence, the emphasis is on enabling the patient to successfully manage a life style that includes headaches. The physician who sets a goal of abolishing headaches is being unrealistic in almost all cases.[8,9] More appropriate goals are effective treatment of individual headache episodes and minimizing the number and severity of these episodes. Most headache patients are open to the concept that they carry a vulnerability to headaches and are willing to learn how to manage this tendency. Patients who strongly resist this management approach are often highly dependent personalities who may have drug-seeking behavior or may change to another chronic-pain symptom complex when offered aggressive treatment of headaches. The complete management plan includes patient education, treatment plans for both prophylaxis and acute management, and follow-up.

Patient education is essential for the patient and family to manage headaches. They must understand the type of headache and its treatment and natural history. In addition to providing information, the physician must address hidden concerns. Many myths and beliefs are associated with headaches, and patients are greatly empowered to deal with their headaches once these beliefs are addressed. Patients may be embarrassed by their fears: For example, almost all migraine patients have feared cerebral hemorrhage during a severe attack.

With headaches, patient education and treatment overlap as the patient and family become responsible for identifying and managing situations that precipitate or exacerbate headache. These situations range from avoiding foods that trigger migraine attacks to practicing conflict resolution. Stress is implicated in almost all headaches; even the pain of secondary headaches is less easy to manage in stressful situations.

There are few "absolutes" in the pharmacologic treatment of headaches, and the large number of choices can be bewildering to both physicians and patients. In general, first-line analgesics and symptomatic treatment are effective, and narcotic use should be avoided. A common mistake is to appear tentative about therapy. The exasperated physician who uses phrases such as, "We'll try this," may convey the message that the medication is not expected to work. Conversely, implying to patients that one has selected a medication specific to their situation and based on an understanding of the headache literature recruits the placebo effect and is much more likely to succeed. Patients gather information about headaches and their treatment from a wide variety of sources, including news media and the experience of friends. Patient knowledge and opinions of specific treatments should be established before issuing a prescription.

Nonpharmacologic advice is a powerful factor in building the placebo effect and therapeutic alliance. Physicians gather experiences from many patients and can pass on "tips" for headache management. There are many examples.

1. Lamaze-type breathing exercises for tension headaches
2. Getting into a cold environment during cluster attacks
3. Cold washcloth over the eyes during migraine
4. Occipital pressure and heat during migraine
5. Vigorous exercise at the start of migraine, cluster, or tension headaches

Including such information in the overall treatment plan enhances the physician's credibility and reinforces the message that the patient and family are the primary managers of the headache problem.

Follow-up

With the exception of headaches secondary to acute self-limiting conditions, headaches tend to be recurrent problems. Unless follow-up is well managed, the patient returns only at times of severe symptoms or exasperation at the failure of treatment. This pattern implies the risk of emergency visits at difficult times and consultations complicated by hostility or disappointment. In practice, patients manage well given scheduled appointments, particularly if it is combined with the expectation that the patient will come to the consultation well prepared (i.e., with information on the number, pattern, response to treatment, and any other relevant information about headaches since the last visit). Some authors recommend a formal headache diary.[9] This model, similar to that used for diabetic patients, is a clinical metaphor that can be used to discourage the dependent patient. The patient is encouraged to believe he or she has a condition despite which a successful life can be expected; and, furthermore, the patient is primarily responsible for management of his or her medical problem.

Clinical Types of Headache

Migraine

Migraine is a common disorder with an overall estimated prevalence in the population of 10%.[16] It is more common in women at all ages, and the peak prevalence is during young adulthood. Up to 30% of women aged 21 to 34 report at least one migraine headache per year, but this figure declines to 10% by age 75.[1,13] Up to 90% of migraine patients have a first-degree relative, usually a parent, also affected by migraine[1]; and perhaps because of familiarity with the condition, significant numbers of migraine sufferers (up to 50%) do not seek medical assistance.[13,17] Several classifications of migraine have been suggested. As shown in Table 7.1, the current international classification is based on clinical features, particularly the presence of aura. In practice, it is seldom useful to subclassify migraine, except for childhood migraine syndromes and to distinguish some forms from more sinister causes of transient neurologic signs.

Patients in the "classic" subgroup (approximately 20% of all migraineurs) experience a characteristic aura before the onset of migraine head pain. This aura may take many forms, but visual effects such as scotomas, zigzag lines, photopsia, or visual distortions are the most common. A much larger proportion of patients describe prodromal symptoms, which may be visceral, such as diarrhea or nausea, but are more commonly alterations in mood or behavior. Food cravings, mild euphoria (or, conversely, yawning), and heightened sensory perception, particularly of smell, are surprisingly common.

The headache of migraine is severe, usually unilateral, described as "throbbing" or "pulsating," and aggravated by movement. The pain usually takes 30 minutes to 3 hours to reach maximum intensity, and it may last several hours. The eye and temple are the most frequent centers of pain, but occipital involvement is common. Each patient describes a characteristic group of associated symptoms among which nausea predominates. Either nausea or photophobia and phonophobia are required for diagnosis along with the characteristic headache. During attacks, migraine patients avoid movement and sensory stimuli, especially light. They may use pressure and either heat or cold over the areas of maximal pain. The attack usually terminates with sleep. Vomiting appears to shorten attacks, and some patients admit to self-induced vomiting. Many patients report "hangover" on waking after a migraine, but others report complete freedom from symptoms and a sense of euphoria. The cause of migraine remains unknown; research indicates that the migraine process begins in neurons as a biochemical process and that vascular phenomena are secondary effects.[16]

The treatment of migraine typifies the approach of enabling patients to manage their own condition. A bewildering variety of therapies are available, and management should be individualized. The treatment plan has three aspects: avoidance of precipitants, aggressive treatment of attacks, and prophylactic therapy if indicated. Patients and their families can usually identify triggers of migraine attacks. The role of specific foods has probably been exaggerated,[17] although red wine and cheese continue to have a significant reputation as migraine triggers. Disturbances in routine, particularly missed meals, excessive sleeping, and relaxation after periods of stress, are notorious precipitants of migraine attacks. Women often correlate migraines with the onset of menstruation each month, but the effect of oral contraception is unpredictable. Migraines commonly disappear during pregnancy.

In addition to planning to minimize exposure to precipitants, patients should be encouraged to recognize their own aura or prodrome, as early treatment may abort the attack. The classic treatment is ergotamine, which may be given by any route. The fastest practical route for self-administration is by inhaler, but in clinical situations, intravenous or intramuscular forms may be used. Metoclopramide is often also given early in the attack as an antiemetic and to promote gastric emptying. The use of ergotamine is limited by its side effect, nausea. In certain patients, vasoconstriction is also a contraindication. Many patients are better treated with adequate dosages of analgesics to which antiemetics can be added. Nonsteroidal antiinflammatory drugs (NSAIDs), especially the naproxen group, appear particularly effective; and the injectable NSAID ketorolac (Toradol) is useful. Patients appear to derive considerable benefit from an individual analgesic for several months but then need to change. Many combination medications are available that generally contain an analgesic, antiemetic, and sedative. These agents should be used with prudence, as patients may try to drive or work despite the migraine. Also, use of a butabarbital-containing medication may worsen the migraine hangover.

A completely new class of medications is available directed at the possible underlying abnormality of serotonin metabolism. The first of this class, sumatriptan (Imitrex), is available as self-administered subcutaneous injections.[18] The first experience should be under observation to assess effectiveness and monitor adverse effects, especially elevation of blood pressure. Migraine symptoms may reoccur several hours after injection.

When negotiating management with patients, more than one medication may be used (i.e., ergotamine or analgesic for situations when they need to "keep going" and a combination including a sedative for situations when they can "crash").

Narcotics have almost no place in migraine therapy. Even in the emergency department situation, controlled studies have shown that adequate analgesia, use of injections of antiemetics, or injectable ergotamines are superior to narcotics.[1] The migraine patient who demands narcotics or claims allergies to alternative treatments may be a drug abuser. Rarely, patients develop dehydration and "status migrainous" when the attack lasts several days. These patients may require hospitalization and steroids in addition to fluids, intravenous ergotamines, and antiemetics.[19]

If patients find normal life impossible because of the frequency and severity of migraine attacks, prophylactic treatment should be considered.[20] β-Blockers are the most widely studied agents. Those without intrinsic sympathomimetic activity (e.g., propranolol, nadolol, timolol, atenolol, metoprolol) are effective, but the dosage at which individual patients benefit must be established by clinical trial.[1,20] Amitriptyline is also effective and appears to prevent migraine at lower dosages than used for treatment of depression. Effective dosages to prevent migraine range from 25 to 150 mg/day. β-Blockers and amitriptyline are synergistic if used together. Many other drugs have been recommended, but studies are often small and difficult to interpret because of placebo effect and patient selection.[20] A serotonin agonist, pizotifen, and a calcium channel blocker, flunarizine, are widely used in other countries[17] but are not yet approved for use in the United States. Conversely, methysergide, which has largely fallen out of use in the United States because of fears of retroperitoneal fibrosis, is returning to use in other countries at low dosages and with monitoring for side effects.[17,20] Migraine patients can usually be assisted to find regimens that enable them to minimize attacks and deal effectively with those that do occur. They can be consoled that the condition wanes with age, has been associated with lower rates of cerebrovascular and ischemic heart disease than expected,[16] and has afflicted a galaxy of famous people.

Cluster Headache

The cluster headache, a rare but dramatic form, occurs predominantly in middle-aged men. The estimated prevalence is 69 per 100,000 adults[1] with a 6:1 male preponderance.[21,22]

The headache is severe, unilateral, centered around the eye or temple, and accompanied by lacrimation, rhinorrhea, red eye, and other autonomic signs on the same side as the headache. Symptoms develop rapidly, reaching a peak intensity within 10 to 15 minutes, and last up to 2 hours. During the attack, the patient is frantic with pain and may be suspected of intoxication, drug-induced behavior, or hysteria.[8] This behavior, including talk of suicide because of the severity of the pain, is characteristic, but patients may be too embarrassed to volunteer this information. The diagnosis is based on the description of attacks, especially their severity, and is confirmed by the unique time pattern described by the patient. During a "cluster" period, which typically lasts 4 to 8 weeks, the patient experiences attacks at the same time or times of day with bizarre regularity. Approximately half these attacks wake the patient and are particularly frequent around 1 a.m. Most patients experience one or two cluster periods per year and are completely free from symptoms at other times; however, up to 10% of patients develop chronic symptoms, with daily attacks over several years. During a cluster period, drinking alcohol almost inevitably precipitates an attack. It is speculated that the cluster headache is due to a disorder of serotonin metabolism or circadian rhythm (or both), but the cause remains unknown.[1]

Management strategies aim to provide relief from attacks and prophylactically to shorten cluster episodes (Table 7.3). Acute treatment must be of rapid onset and capable of administration by the patient or family. Conventional analgesics do not act quickly enough to provide relief, and all the current treatments of acute cluster headaches are difficult to administer in a patient who is restless and distracted with pain. Inhalation of oxygen is the traditional treatment, but inhalation or instillation of local anesthetics into the nostril on the affected side may also be effective. The only ergotamines likely to be effective during the acute attack are those delivered by inhaler or injection. European studies indicate that self-administered injections of sumatriptan are effective.[22]

The mainstay of cluster headache management is to suppress headaches during a cluster period. As shown in Table 7.3, several drugs are effective. Treatment should be initiated as soon as a cluster period begins and continued for a few days beyond the expected duration of the cluster. Only the previous experience of each patient can be used to judge duration of therapy. Each patient has a set length for his or her cluster period as well as a tendency to repeat the same time and symptom pattern of individual headaches. It is particularly important in the age group usually affected by cluster headache to monitor prophylactic drugs such as lithium, pred-

TABLE 7.3. Pharmacologic treatment of primary headaches

Headache type	Acute attack[a]		Prophylactic therapy	
	Dose	Comment	Dose	Comment
Migraine	Ergotamines Inhalation (0.36 mg/dose) Oral, sublingual, rectal (1–2 mg) IM or IV (0.2–0.5 mg)	Many formulations and combination drugs available Side effects: nausea, vasoconstriction	β-Blockers Propranolol (40–320 mg) Nadolol (40–240 mg) Timolol (10–60 mg) Atenolol (50–200 mg) Metoprolol (50–250 mg)	Dosage individualized; side effects are fatigue, GI upset; contraindicated with asthma, heart failure
	Analgesics Aspirin (650–1000 mg) Acetaminophen (<1000 mg) Ibuprofen (<600 mg) Naproxen (<550 mg)	Many analgesics and NSAIDs effective Dosage individualized Combinations available with sedatives and antiemetics Side effects: mainly gastric upset	Amitriptyline (10–175 mg hs)	Sedation, weight gain, dry mouth; synergistic with β-blockers
	5HT agonist Sumatriptan (6 mg SC) Oral and other forms (100 mg)	FDA approval for SC only	Phenelzine (MAOI) (30–75 mg)	Insomnia, hypotension; interacts with tyramine in food

	Treatment	Comments
	Calcium channel blockers Flunarizine (10 mg hs) Verapamil	Pending FDA approval; dosage individualized
	Serotonin-receptor antagonists Pizotifen (0–5 mg hs) Methysergide (0.5–2.0 mg)	Pending FDA approval; sedation, weight gain, cramping; vasoconstriction, fibrosis
	Prednisone (10–80 mg daily) Lithium (300–900 mg daily) Ergotamine (1–2 mg for attacks) Indomethacin (120 mg daily) Nifedipine (40–120 mg daily)	
Cluster	Oxygen 100% 8–10 l/min for 10 min Ergotamine 0–36 mg/puff × 1–3 Lidocaine 4% 1 ml into nostril Methoxyflurane inhale 10 drops	
Tension-stress	Analgesics and NSAIDs (as for migraine but at lower dosages) Amitriptyline (50–100 mg hs) Imipramine (25–75 mg)	

[a]Treatment must be of rapid onset. (1) All therapy should be started at first sign of attack. (2) Other symptomatic relief may be added, especially antiemetics and sedatives. (3) Encourage patients to find abortive therapy (e.g., caffeine, exercise, cold ± pressure over the site of pain) to use in addition to above. (4) Narcotics are rarely necessary for migraine.

nisone, ergotamine, indomethacin, calcium channel blockers, and methysergide for side effects.

Tension-Stress (Muscle Contraction) Headaches

Tension-stress headaches are the most frequent of all headaches.[1,13,23] In one study of family practice consultations, they accounted for 70% of all new headache patients.[9] These patients represent a select sample of all tension headache patients, as most sufferers are believed to manage their symptoms using simple analgesics or other strategies.[24] Although physicians are familiar with the condition, it is difficult to define it because it presents in myriad forms. The formal definition (Table 7.2) contains both positive and negative criteria, but a common problem is to diagnose "tension headaches" only after searching for more "interesting" etiologies for the symptoms.

The etiology and pathophysiology of tension headaches are poorly understood. Stress, psychological abnormalities, muscle contraction, and abnormalities of neurotransmitters have all been implicated. The clinical syndrome may represent more than one entity, and in many cases, there is considerable overlap with migraine.[1]

As with migraine, more than 70% of tension headaches occur in women,[1] and a substantial proportion of patients (40%) give a family history of similar symptoms. Tension headaches, however, tend to have their onset at an older age (70% after 20 years) and to produce symptoms daily or on several days per week, rather than occur as episodic attacks.

The clinical story is characterized by several years of almost daily headaches that vary in intensity throughout the day. Most patients "keep going" with daily activities, but going to bed early is characteristic. The pain may be described in many ways, of which "pressure," "tight band," and "aching" predominate. Patients usually express exhaustion, and the patient's affect and body language convey weariness and frustration. Sleep disturbances are common.

Physical examination may be negative with tension headaches but is important for confirming the diagnosis (particularly to rule out causes of secondary headache) and for establishing the therapeutic relationship. Attempts to treat the headaches with analgesics before establishing patient confidence in the diagnosis risk failure despite escalating use of analgesics including narcotics.

The treatment of tension headaches is frequently unsatisfactory.[23,24] Success depends on treatment of any underlying condition (particularly depression), patient education about the nature of the condition, and the control of symptoms without creating either dependency or other adverse effects. Tension headache patients frequently take large quantities of analgesics, leading to gastrointestinal and other complications, or they use combination medicines containing sedatives. A wise investment during the history is to clarify all medication use, including over-the-counter medications, and to explore previous encounters with physicians. Patients may have been extensively investigated previously, and prior medical experiences color expectations and evaluation of management approaches.

Acute episodes of headache are best managed by first-line analgesics, such as acetaminophen, aspirin, or ibuprofen.[24,25] Narcotics and combination drugs, especially those that contain barbiturates or caffeine, should be avoided. NSAIDs may be more effective than other analgesics,[23-25] especially if prescribed on a regular schedule for several days rather than on an as-needed basis. It is useful to teach the patient and family simple massage and relaxation techniques and to explore methods to resolve conflicts and enhance self-esteem. Not all patients require extensive counseling or biofeedback. The most significant predictor of symptom resolution after 1 year has been shown to be patient confidence that the problem had been fully discussed with a physician.[9] In addition to treating underlying depression, amitriptyline and other tricyclic drugs raise pain thresholds and play a significant role in enabling patients to manage symptoms. The effective dosage may be lower than that required for depressive illnesses.

Secondary Headaches

Headache is part of the clinical picture of many conditions. Particularly in children, frontal headache is a common accompaniment of fever. In all age groups, almost any condition of the head and neck and several systemic conditions can present as headache. A careful history, combined with physical examination and other investigations when appropriate, can almost always differentiate secondary from primary headache.[5]

There is particular concern in family practice not to miss the rare but serious intracranial condition, especially brain tumor. The symptoms of an intracranial lesion depend on its size, location, and displacement effect on other tissues. No single characteristic headache story can therefore be given. Suspicion should be raised about headaches of recent onset that appear to become steadily more severe, do not fit any of the primary classifications, and do not respond to first-line treatment. Close follow-up and repeated physical examinations may detect the earliest neurologic abnormalities; but if there is a high degree of suspicion, early radiologic investigation or specialist consultation should be obtained. With intracranial vascular lesions, the first symptom may be a catastrophic hemorrhage.

Specific Headache Syndromes

The literature describes several specific primary headache syndromes that are uncommon but may be encountered in practice. These syndromes seem to be more common in men and are characterized by the severity of the pain and the potential for confusion with serious intracranial conditions. Despite the dramatic history, these conditions are generally benign and respond well to indomethacin. CT scans may be necessary to confirm the diagnosis. Explanation, reassurance, and symptom control are usually effective.

References

1. Raskin NH. Headache. 2nd ed. New York: Churchill Livingstone, 1988.
2. Hansotia P. Evaluation and treatment of headache. Postgrad Med 1986;79: 75–84.
3. Diamond S, Feinberg DT. The classification, diagnosis and treatment of headaches. Med Times 1990;118:15–27.
4. Greer T, Katon W, Christman N, et al. Headache and chronic pain in primary care. J Fam Pract 1988;27:477–82.
5. Baker RM. Headache. In Sloane PD, Slatt LM, Baker RM, editors. Essentials of family medicine. Baltimore: Williams & Wilkins, 1988:112–17.
6. Diamond S. Treatment of chronic headache. Postgrad Med 1987;81:91–96.
7. O'Dowd TC. Five years of heartsink patients in general practice. BMJ 1988; 297:528–30.
8. Graham JR. Headaches. In: Noble J, editor. Textbook of general medicine and primary care. Boston: Little, Brown, 1987:1521–60.
9. McWhinney IR. A textbook of family medicine. New York: Oxford University Press, 1989.
10. International Headache Society. Classification and diagnostic criteria for headache disorders, cranial neuralgias and facial pain. Cephalgia 1988;8 (Suppl7):1–96.
11. Diamond S, Dalessio DJ, editors. The practicing physician's approach to headache. 4th ed. Baltimore: Williams & Wilkins, 1986.
12. Gunderson CH, editor. Essentials of clinical neurology. New York: Raven Press, 1990.
13. Dalessio DJ, editor. Wolff's headache and other head pain. 5th ed. New York: Oxford University Press, 1987.
14. Becker L, Iverson DC, Reed FM, et al. Patients with new headache in primary care: a report from ASPN. J Fam Pract 1988;27:41–47.
15. NIH Consensus Development Panel. Computer tomographic scanning of the brain. In: Proceedings from NIH Consensus Development Conference, NIH, Bethesda. Washington, DC: Government Printing Office 1982;4:2.
16. Blau JN. Migraine: theories of pathogenesis. Lancet 1992;339:1202–7.
17. Lance JW. Treatment of migraine. Lancet 1992;393:1207–9.
18. Bateman X. Sumatriptan. Lancet 1993;341:221–4.
19. Kunkel RS. Abortive treatment of migraine. In: Diamond S, editor. Migraine headache prevention and management. New York: Marcel Dekker, 1990:45–55.
20. Walling A. Drug prophylaxis for migraine headaches. Am Fam Physician 1990;42:425–32.

21. McKenna JP. Cluster headaches. Am Fam Physician 1988;37:173–8.
22. Walling AD. Cluster headaches. Am Fam Physician 1993;47:1457–63.
23. Clough C. Non-migrainous headaches [editorial]. BMJ 1989;299:70–72.
24. Kunkel RS. Tension-type (muscle-contraction) headaches: evaluation and treatment. Mod Med 1989;57:60–68.
25. Elkind AH. Muscle contraction headache. Postgrad Med 1987;81: 203–17.

CASE PRESENTATION

Subjective

PATIENT PROFILE

Lois Nelson Martino is a 44-year-old divorced white woman who works as a paralegal.

PRESENTING PROBLEM

Headaches.

PRESENT ILLNESS

For 6 months, Lois has had headaches that occur two or three times a month. The headaches are sometimes preceded by a sense of feeling a little "mentally fuzzy," and there may be slightly blurred vision. The headache pain, which begins about 20 to 30 minutes after the onset of the initial symptoms, is severe, throbbing, and generally right-sided, although it sometimes is on the left or spreads to involve the whole head. Lois reports that nausea often accompanies the pain but that she has never vomited during a headache. When the headache is present, she is especially sensitive to noise or bright lights, and she generally retreats to a dark room for the duration of the pain, which is usually some 3 to 6 hours. The patient has used aspirin and ibuprofen (Advil) for pain, but these afford little relief. She is concerned because the headaches sometimes occur during the day and are interfering with her work.

PAST MEDICAL HISTORY

She had an appendectomy at age 16 and is the mother of one child, aged 22.

SOCIAL HISTORY

Mrs. Martino has been employed with the same law firm for 8 years. She left her previous job at the time of her divorce 10 years ago; her ex-husband, Ralph Martino, is an attorney. She lives alone in an apartment not far from the home of her daughter Ann and son-in-law Luke Priestley.

HABITS

She has never smoked and uses alcohol only rarely. She takes no daily medications. Her meals are often at irregular times, and she drinks approximately six cans of diet cola each day.

FAMILY HISTORY

Her father, aged 76, has osteoarthritis and type 2 diabetes mellitus. Her mother, aged 71, has hypertension and sometimes takes medication for depression. She has three siblings.

REVIEW OF SYSTEMS

The patient believes that she sometimes feels excessively tired at the end of the day and sometimes awakes in the middle of the night and has trouble getting back to sleep.

- What more do you wish to know about the patient's headaches?
- How would you inquire to learn more about events in her personal life and at work?
- What else would you ask about the family history? Why?
- What would you ask about her diet and health habits, and how might these be related to her headaches?

Objective

GENERAL

Mrs. Martino seems slightly anxious. She uses notes and a calendar while describing her symptoms.

VITAL SIGNS

Height, 5 ft 6 in; weight, 133 lb; blood pressure, 126/82; pulse, 74; temperature, 37.1°C.

EXAMINATION

The eyes, ears, nose, and throat are normal, including an unremarkable funduscopic examination. There are no abnormalities of the neck and thyroid. Cranial nerves II to XII are normal. The finger-to-nose test, deep tendon reflexes, and Romberg test are all normal.

LABORATORY

No office laboratory tests are performed at this visit.

- What more—if anything—would you include in the physical examination, and why?
- What additional neurologic tests might be useful?
- What laboratory tests—if any—might be helpful?
- What diagnostic imaging—if any—might be important and cost-effective?

Assessment

- What appears to be Mrs. Martino's problem, and how would you explain it to her?
- What do you think is the patient's chief concern about her headaches? Explain.
- How are her headaches likely to be affecting her life at home and at work?
- What is the possible significance of her tiredness and sleep disturbance?

Plan

- What medical therapy would you recommend today? Why did you choose this regimen?
- What diet and life-style changes would you advise?
- How might you involve the family and employer in management of the problem?
- If the headaches become more severe or more frequent over the next few months, what would you do then?

8
Hypertension

STEPHEN A. BRUNTON AND RITA K. EDWARDS

Despite widespread efforts to improve education and enhance public awareness, up to 33% of persons with hypertension remain undiagnosed, and only about 50% of those known to have hypertension are adequately controlled. However, the percentages of patients who are aware that they have hypertension, who are treated, and who are controlled have increased over the past 20 years (Table 8.1). Most have stage 1 hypertension, and controversy still exists concerning the appropriate approach to these patients. Nonpharmacologic therapy is often the first choice, and this approach continues to evolve.[1] Of the 20 million to 30 million hypertensives who receive pharmacologic therapy, fewer than 50% adhere to their therapeutic regimen for more than 1 year, and 60% of these patients reduce the dosage of their drug owing to adverse effects. A negative impact on the patient's quality of life may occur as a result of just making the diagnosis. Effects such as increased absenteeism, sickness behavior, hypochondria, and decreased self-esteem have been noted in cohorts of previously well individuals who have been told they were hypertensive.[2] A 1987 survey of physicians revealed that they regarded quality of life changes to be the primary impediment to effective pharmacologic treatment of hypertension.

The challenge to the clinician is to provide patient education and develop a hypertensive regimen that effectively lowers blood pressure or reduces cardiac risk factors, minimizes changes in concomitant disease states, and maintains or improves quality of life. Putting the patient first necessitates integrating the individual patient's life style and current disease states with a thorough understanding of the effect of drug and nondrug therapy on quality of life. This chapter reviews nonpharmacologic and pharmacologic therapy, with special emphasis on individualizing patient regimens to improve adherence.

Detection

The diagnosis of hypertension should not be based on any single measurement but should be established on the basis of at least three readings with an average systolic blood pressure of 140 mm Hg and a diastolic pressure

TABLE 8.1. Hypertension[a] awareness, treatment, and control rates

Factor	1971–72[b]	1974–75[b]	1976–80[c]	1988–91[d]
Aware: percentage of hypertensives told by physician	51	64	(54) 73	(65) 84
Treated: percentage of hypertensives taking medication	36	34	(33) 56	(49) 73
Controlled: percentage of hypertensives with blood pressure <160/95 mm Hg on one occasion and reported currently taking antihypertensive medication	16	20	(11) 34	(21) 55

Source: National Institutes of Health.[1]

[a]Defined as 160/95 mm Hg or more on one occasion or reported currently taking antihypertensive medication. Numbers in parentheses are percentages at 140/90 mm Hg or more.

[b]Source: National Health and Nutrition Examination Survey I.

[c]Source: National Health and Nutrition Examination Survey II.

[d]Source: National Health and Nutrition Examination Survey III (unpublished data provided by the Centers for Disease Control and Prevention, National Center for Health Statistics).

TABLE 8.2. Classification of blood pressure for adults aged 18 years and older[a]

Category	Systolic (mm Hg)	Diastolic (mm Hg)
Normal[b]	<130	<85
High normal	130–139	85–89
Hypertension[c]		
Stage 1 (mild)	140–159	90–99
Stage 2 (moderate)	160–179	100–109
Stage 3 (severe)	180–209	110–119
Stage 4 (very severe)	≥210	≥120

Source: National Institutes of Health.[1]

Note: In addition to classifying stages of hypertension based on average blood pressure levels, the clinician should specify the presence or absence of target organ disease and additional risk factors. For example, a patient with diabetes and a blood pressure of 142/94 mm Hg plus left ventricular hypertrophy should be classified as "stage 1 hypertension with target organ disease (left ventricular hypertrophy) and with another major risk factor (diabetes)." This specificity is important for risk classification and management.

[a]Not taking antihypertensive drugs and not acutely ill. When systolic and diastolic pressures fall into different categories, the higher category should be selected to classify the individual's blood pressure status. For instance, 60/92 mm Hg should be classified as stage 2, and 180/120 mm Hg should be classified as stage 4. Isolated systolic hypertension is defined as systolic pressure of 140 mm Hg or more and diastolic pressure of less than 90 mm Hg and staged appropriately (e.g., 170/85 mm Hg is defined as stage 2 isolated systolic hypertension).

[b]Optimal blood pressure with respect to cardiovascular risk is systolic pressure <120 mm Hg and diastolic pressure <80 mm Hg. However, unusually low readings should be evaluated for clinical significance.

[c]Based on the average of two or more readings taken at each of two or more visits after an initial screening.

of 90 mm Hg. Mechanisms should be established to standardize the measurement process: (1) The patient should be seated comfortably with the arm positioned at heart level. (2) Caffeine or nicotine should not have been ingested within 30 minutes before measurement. (3) The patient should be seated in a quiet environment for at least 5 minutes. (4) An appropriate sphygmomanometer cuff should be used (i.e., the rubber bladder should encircle at least two-thirds of the arm). (5) Measurement of the diastolic blood pressure should be based on the disappearance of sound (phase V Korotkoff sound).

Table 8.2 describes the classification of blood pressure for adults.

Evaluation

Evaluation is directed toward establishing the etiology of hypertension, identifying other cardiovascular risk factors, and evaluating the possibility of target organ damage. Although most hypertension is considered "essential," primary, or idiopathic, it is necessary to eliminate secondary causes of hypertension, including renovascular disease, polycystic renal disease, aortic coarctation, Cushing syndrome, and pheochromocytoma. It is important to ensure that the patient is not on medications that may result in increased blood pressure, such as oral contraceptives, nasal decongestants, appetite suppressants, nonsteroidal antiinflammatory drugs, steroids, and tricyclic antidepressants.

Medical History

The medical history should include a review of the family history for hypertension and cardiovascular disease, previous measurements of blood pressure, symptoms suggestive of secondary causes of hypertension, and other cardiovascular risk factors including smoking, hyperlipidemia, obesity, and diabetes. Also, environmental and psychosocial factors that may influence blood pressure control or the ability of the individual to comply with therapy should be considered.

Physical Examination and Laboratory Tests

The examination should include more than one blood pressure measurement in both standing and seated positions with verification in the contralateral arm. (If a discrepancy exists, the higher value should be used.) The rest of the physical examination includes (1) an evaluation of the optic fundi with gradation of hypertensive changes; (2) examination of the neck for bruits and thyromegaly; (3) a heart examination to evaluate for hypertrophy, arrhythmias, or additional sounds; (4) abdominal examination to search for evidence of aneurysms or kidney abnormalities; (5) examination of the extremities to check the pulses; and (6) a careful neurologic evaluation.

Some baseline laboratory tests may be helpful for the initial evaluation. They might include urinalysis and serum potassium, blood urea nitrogen, and creatinine levels. A lipid panel may help evaluate cardiovascular risk.

Treatment

The goal of therapy is not just to bring the blood pressure lower than 140 mm Hg systolic and 90 mm Hg diastolic but, rather, to prevent the morbidity and mortality associated with hypertension. As such, the decision to treat hypertension is based on documentation that blood pressure has remained elevated and the assessment of the individual risk for that particular patient.

In general, individuals with diastolic blood pressure ranges considered borderline high (i.e., 85–89 mm Hg) should have their blood pressures rechecked within 1 year. Blood pressures in the mild range should be confirmed within 2 months by repeated measurements; however, certain life-style approaches are appropriate even at this level. Blood pressures that are markedly elevated (e.g., 115 mm Hg) or those associated with evidence of existing end-organ damage may require immediate pharmacologic intervention. In general, whether pharmacologic intervention is initiated, a nonpharmacologic approach should be the foundation of any management strategy.[1]

Nonpharmacologic Therapeutic Approaches

Information concerning dietary modifications, exercise and weight reduction, the role of cations, and the possible role of relaxation and stress management techniques for reducing blood pressure have opened the door for greater acceptance of multiple nonpharmacologic approaches to the treatment of hypertension. The 1988 report of the Joint National Committee (JNC) on the Detection, Evaluation, and Treatment of High Blood Pressure recommended that "Nonpharmacological approaches be used both as definitive intervention and as an adjunct for pharmacological therapy and should be considered for all antihypertensive therapy."

Several studies have shown positive correlation of increased blood pressure with alcohol consumption of more than 2 ounces/day.[3] Although smoking has not been shown to cause sustained hypertension, it is associated with increased cardiovascular, pulmonary, and hypertension risks and therefore should be eliminated.[4]

Weight reduction has a strong correlation with decreased blood pressure in obese individuals. Stamler et al. reported that a 10-pound weight loss maintained over a 4-year period allowed 50% of participants previously on pharmacologic management to remain normotensive and free of medication.[5]

Sodium restriction has been a mainstay of hypertension control, as a 100-mEq drop in daily intake can result in a 2- to 9-mm Hg decline in systolic blood pressure in salt-sensitive individuals. This is one of the easiest goals for a patient to accomplish, as moderate restriction can be accomplished by eliminating table salt for cooking, avoiding salty foods, and using a salt substitute.[6]

Regular aerobic exercise not only assists with weight reduction but also appears to lower diastolic blood pressure. Cade and associates reported a decline from 117 mm Hg to 97 mm Hg diastolic blood pressure after 3 months of daily walking or running for 2 miles. This effect appeared to be independent of weight loss, and some benefit persisted even if the patient became sedentary.[7]

Vegetarian diets high in polyunsaturated fats, potassium, and fiber result in lower blood pressures than diets high in saturated fats. Dietary fat control also contributes to the reduction of cholesterol and coronary artery disease risk.[8] The role of cations such as potassium, magnesium, and calcium in lowering blood pressure has now been investigated. High potassium intake (>80 mEq/day) may result in a modest decline in blood pressure while offering a natriuretic and cardioprotective effect. These effects are more pronounced in hypokalemic individuals.[9] Magnesium and calcium supplementation of more than 300 mg/day and 800 mg/day, respectively, have been shown to lower the relative risk of developing hypertension in a large cohort of women. However, the impact of individual supplementation is less clear, and the role of these substances is still controversial.[10]

Stress management and relaxation techniques over a 4-year period have been shown to reduce systolic blood pressure 10 to 15 mm Hg and diastolic blood pressure 5 to 10 mm Hg. However, these results are variable and are largely dependent on the instructor–patient relationship.[11]

The effects of nonpharmacologic approaches can be additive and certainly are beneficial even if the patient requires drug therapy. Stamler and associates documented that reducing weight and lowering salt and alcohol intake allowed 39% of patients previously on therapy to remain normotensive without medication over a 4-year period. In the mildly hypertensive individual, these life-style modifications should be tried for at least 6 months before initiating pharmacologic therapy.[12]

Pharmacologic Therapy

Pharmacologic therapy is considered when the diastolic blood pressure remains greater than 90 to 94 mm Hg despite life-style modifications. The decision to initiate drug therapy requires consideration of individual pa-

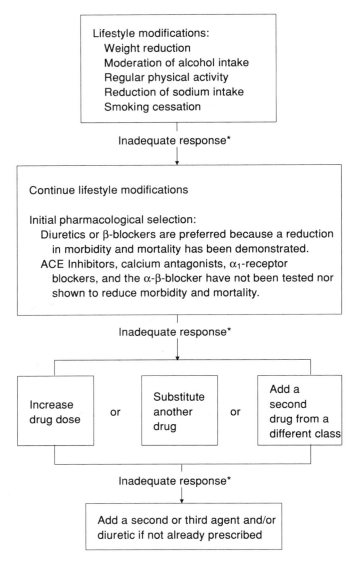

FIGURE 8.1. Treatment algorithm. *Response means achieved goal blood pressure, or patient is making considerable progress toward this goal. (From National Institutes of Health.[1])

tient characteristics, such as age, race, sex, family history, cardiovascular risk factors, concomitant disease states, compliance, and ability to purchase the prescribed therapeutic agent. Treatment of moderate to severe hypertension (diastolic pressure >104 mm Hg) has reduced cardiovascular morbidity and mortality dramatically over the past 30 years. Controversy still exists regarding treatment of milder hypertension (diastolic pressure 90–94 mm Hg) due to adverse drug reactions compromising quality of life, cost of therapy, and little change in coronary heart disease morbidity and mortality. Decreased incidence of stroke, congestive heart failure, and left ventricular hypertrophy has occurred in treated mild hypertensives, and therapy is recommended if the patient has one or more cardiovascular risk factors.

The ideal antihypertensive agent would improve quality of life, reduce coronary heart disease risk factors, maintain normal hemodynamic profiles, reduce left ventricular hypertrophy, have a positive impact on concomitant disease states, and reduce end-organ damage while effectively lowering blood pressure on a convenient dosing regimen at minimal cost to the patients. This "magic bullet" has yet to be synthesized, but several of the newer antihypertensive classes offer many of these positive outcomes. The selection of an appropriate antihypertensive agent may be based on the recommendations of the JNC on the Detection, Evaluation, and Treatment of High Blood Pressure individualized to the specific medical, social, psychological, and economic situation of each patient.[1] The previous stepped care approach has been modified by the JNC into an algorithm that permits an individualized approach to the patient (Fig. 8.1).

Major Antihypertensive Classes

ACE Inhibitors

Angiotensin-converting enzyme (ACE) inhibitors (Table 8.3) block the conversion of angiotensin I to angiotensin II, resulting in decreased aldosterone production with subsequent increased sodium and water excretion. Renin and potassium levels are usually increased as a result of this medication. The hemodynamic response includes decreased peripheral resistance, increased renal blood flow, and minimal changes in cardiac output and glomerular filtration rate. There is little change in insulin and glucose levels or in the lipid fractions. The adverse effects of ACE inhibitors include cough (1–30%), headache, dizziness, first-dose syncope in salt- or volume-depleted patients, acute renal failure in patients with renal artery stenosis, angioedema (0.1–0.2%), and teratogenic effects in the human fetus. Captopril (Capoten) has a higher incidence of rash, dysgeusia, neutropenia, and proteinuria than others, owing to a sulfhydryl group in the ring structure.[13]

The ACE inhibitors are good first-line agents for patients with diabetes, congestive heart failure, peripheral vascular disease, elevated lipids, and renal insufficiency. This class is effective in all races and ages, although black patients respond better with the addition of a diuretic.[14,15]

Table 8.3. Major antihypertensive drugs

Drug class	Available doses (mg)	Usual dosing schedule (mg/day)	Half-life (hr)	Peak (hr)	Pregnancy class
ACE inhibitors					
Benazepril (Lotensin)	5, 10, 20, 40	10–40 qd	10	2–4	X
Captopril (Capoten)	12.5, 25, 50, 100	25–100 bid–tid	2	1–2	X
Enalapril (Vasotec)	2.5, 5, 10, 20	5–40 qd	11	4	X
Fosinopril (Monopril)	10, 20	10–40 qd	12	2–6	X
Lisinopril (Prinivil, Zestril)	5, 10, 20, 40	10–80 qd	12	6	X
Quinapril (Accupril)	5, 10, 20, 40	10–80 qd	2	2–4	X
Ramipril (Altace)	1.25, 2.5, 5, 10	2.5–20.0 qd	2	3–6	X
β-Blockers				*Selectivity*	
Atenolol (Tenormin)	25, 50, 100	50–100 qd	9	β_1	C
Acebutolol (Sectral)	200, 400	200–600 bid	4	β_1, ISA	B
Betaxolol (Kerlone)	10, 20	10–40 qd	22	β_1	C
Carteolol (Cartrol)	2.5, 5	2.5–20.0 qd	6	β_1, β_2, ISA	C
Nadolol (Corgard)	20, 40, 80, 120, 160	40–240 qd	24	β_1, β_2	C
Metoprolol (Lopressor)	50, 100	100–450 qd	3	β_1	C
Penbutolol (Levatol)	20	20–80 qd	5	β_1, β_2, ISA	C
Pindolol (Visken)	5, 10	5–30 bid	4	β_1, β_2, ISA	B
Propranolol (Inderal)	60, 80, 120, 160 SR	80–160 SR qd	10	β_1, β_2	C
	10, 20, 40, 60, 80, 90	20–120 bid	4	β_1, β_2	C
Timolol (Blocadren)	5, 10, 20	10–30 bid	4	β_1, β_2	C
Calcium entry antagonists				*Peak (hr)*	
Amlodipine (Norvasc)	2.5, 5, 10	2.5–10 qd, 30–50	6–12		C
Diltiazem (Cardizem)	SR 90, 120	SR 60–120 bid		6–11	
	CD 240, 310	CD 240–300 qd	6	12	C
	30, 60, 90, 120	30–90 qid		2–3	
Felodipine (Plendil)	SR 5,10	5–20 qd	16	2–5	C
Isradipine (Dynacirc)	2.5, 5.0	2.5–5.0 bid	8	1.5	C
Nicardipine (Cardene)	SR 30, 45, 60	SR 30–60 bid			
	20, 30	10 tid	4	0.5–2	C
Nifedipine (Procardia)	SR 30, 60, 90	30–120 qd	5	0.5–6	C
Verapimil (Calan, Isoptin)	SR 120, 180, 240	SR 120–240 bid	7	1–2	C
α_1-Blockers					
Doxazosin (Cardura)	1, 2, 4, 8	1–16 mg qd	22	2–3	B
Prazosin (Minipress)	1, 2, 5	1–5 bid–tid	3	3	C
Terazosin (Hytrin)	1, 2, 5, 10	1–10 qd	12	1–2	C

Table 8.3. *(continued)*

Drug class	Available doses (mg)	Usual dosing schedule (mg/day)	Half-life (hr)	Peak (hr)	Pregnancy class
αβ-Blocker					
Labetolol (Normodyne)	100, 200, 300	100 mg–1.2 g bid	6	β_1, β_2, α	C
Central α_2-agonists					
Clonidine (Catapres)	0.1, 0.2, 0.3	0.1–1.2 bid	16	3–5	C
	TTS 1, 2, 3	1 patch weekly	19	2–3 days	
Guanabenz (Wytensin)	4, 8	4–8 bid	6	2–4 days	C
Guanafacine (Tenex)	1	1–3 qd	17	3	B
Methyldopa (Aldomet)	125, 250, 500	250–500 tid–qid	2	2–4	B
Vasodilators					
Hydralazine (Apresoline)	10, 25, 50, 100	10–50 qid	7	0.5–2	C
Minoxidil (Loniten)	2.5, 10.0	10–40 qd	4	2–3	C
Selected thiazide diuretics					
Chlorothiazide (Diuril)	250–500	500–2000 qd	6–12	4	
Hydrochlorothiazide (Hydrodiuril)	25, 50, 100	25–50 qd	6–12	4–6	
Chlorthalidone (Hygroton)	25, 50, 100	25–100 qd	24–72	2–6	
Indapamide (Lozol)	2.5	2.5–5.0 qd	36	2	B
Metolazone (Zaroxolyn)	0.5, 2.5, 5, 10	2.5–10 qd	12–24	2.6	B
Loop diuretics					
Bumetamide (Bumex)	0.5, 1, 2	0.5–2.0 qd	4–6	1–2	C
Furosemide (Lasix)	20, 40, 80	20–40 qd–bid	6–8	1–2	C
Torsemide (Demadex)	5, 10, 20, 100	2.5–10 qd	3.5	1	B
Potassium-sparing diuretics					
Amiloride (Midamor)	5	5–20 qd	24	6–10	B
Spironolactone (Aldactone)	25, 50, 100	50–100 qd	48–72	48–72	X
Triamterene (Dyrenium)	50, 100	100 bid	12–16	6–8	B

ISA = intrinsic sympathomimetic activity. X = Fetal abnormalities may occur. Use is contraindicated in pregnancy. C = Fetal risk documented in animals. B = Fetal risk is low.

Calcium Entry Antagonists

Calcium entry antagonists inhibit the movement of calcium across cell membranes in myocardial and smooth muscles. This action not only dilates coronary arteries, but additional peripheral arteriole dilation reduces total peripheral resistance resulting in decreased blood pressure. Although the mechanism of action for lowering blood pressure is similar for these agents, structural differences result in varying effects on cardiac conduction and adverse effect profiles. Verapamil (Calan, Isoptin) and diltiazem (Cardizem) slow atrioventricular (AV) node conduction and prolong the effective refractory period in the AV node. Cardiac output is increased by nifedipine (Procardia), nicardipine (Cardene), isradipine (Dynacirc), and felodipine (Plendil).

The calcium entry antagonists are contraindicated for heart block, cardiogenic shock, or acute myocardial infarction (diltiazem). Common adverse effects include peripheral edema, dizziness, headache, asthenia, nausea, constipation, flushing, and tachycardia. Calcium entry antagonists have no significant impact on lipid profiles or glucose metabolism.[13] These agents are effective in all ages and races and are good choices for patients with diabetes, angina, migraine, chronic obstructive pulmonary disease (COPD) or asthma, peripheral vascular disease, renal insufficiency, and supraventricular arrhythmias.[14,15]

Diuretics

Thiazide and loop and potassium-sparing diuretics have been the mainstay of antihypertensive therapy for 30 years. They remain as first-line agents in the stepped care approach, although the ACE inhibitors and calcium entry antagonists are rapidly replacing diuretics as monotherapy for hypertension. Thiazide diuretics increase renal excretion of sodium and chloride at the distal segment of the renal tubule, resulting in decreased plasma volume, cardiac output, and renal blood flow, and increased renin activity. Potassium excretion is increased, whereas calcium and uric acid elimination is decreased.[13] Thiazides adversely affect lipid metabolism by increasing total cholesterol 6% to 10% and low-density lipoprotein cholesterol 6% to 20% and by causing a possible 15% to 20% rise in triglycerides.[15] Plasma glucose levels increase secondary to a decrease in insulin sensitivity. Clinical adverse effects include nausea, vomiting, diarrhea, dizziness, headache, fatigue, muscle cramps, gout attacks, and impotence. Thiazides are inexpensive choices for initial therapy, but caution must be exercised in patients with preexisting cardiac dysfunction, lipid abnormalities, diabetes mellitus, and gout. The lowest effective dose is recommended to minimize these potential adverse effects. Suggested daily doses are hydrochlorothiazide (Hydrodiuril) 25 mg, chlorthalidone (Hygroton) 500 mg, and indapamide (Lozol) 2.5 mg. Indapamide is unique among thiazides in that it has a minimal effect on glucose, lipids, and uric acid. Thiazides are good choices for volume-dependent, low-renin hypertensive individuals. Thiazides improve blood pressure control when added to ACE inhibitors, β-blockers, vasodilators, and α-blockers.

The loop diuretics furosemide (Lasix), torsemide (Demadex), and bumetanide (Bumex) inhibit sodium and chloride reabsorption in the proximal and distal tubules and the loop of Henle. These diuretics are effective in patients with decreased renal function. The primary adverse effects include ototoxicity with high doses in patients with severe renal disease and, in combination with an aminoglycoside, photosensitivity, excess potassium loss, increased serum uric acid, decreased calcium levels, and impaired glucose metabolism. Patients may experience nausea, vomiting, diarrhea, headache, blurred vision, tinnitus, muscle cramps, fatigue, or weakness. Furosemide and bumetanide are used in patients with compromised renal function or congestive heart failure (CHF); they are used as adjuncts to volume-retaining agents such as hydralazine (Apresoline) and minoxidil (Loniten).

The potassium-sparing diuretics spironolactone (Aldactone), triamterene (Dyrenium), and amiloride (Midamor) are useful for preventing potassium wastage from thiazide and loop diuretics. Spironolactone competitively inhibits the uptake of aldosterone at the receptor site in the distal tubule, thereby reducing aldosterone effects. It is used for treatment of primary aldosteronism, CHF, cirrhosis with ascites, hypertension, and hirsutism. Triamterene is used in combination with hydrochlorothiazide (Dyazide, Maxzide) and effectively prevents potassium loss. Amiloride inhibits potassium excretion at the collecting duct. Adverse reactions of spironolactone include gynecomastia, nausea, vomiting, diarrhea, muscle cramps, lethargy, and hyperkalemia. Triamterene and amiloride have adverse effects similar to those of the thiazide diuretics.[13–15]

Antiadrenergic Agents

β-Blockers

β-Adrenergic blocking agents compete with β-agonists for β_1-receptors in cardiac muscles and β_2-receptors in bronchial and vascular musculature, inhibiting vasodilator, inotropic, and chronotropic effects of β-adrenergic stimulation.

Clinical response to β-adrenergic blockade include decreased heart rate, cardiac output, blood pressure, renin production, and bronchiolar constriction; there is also an initial increase in total peripheral resistance that returns to normal with chronic use.

β-Blockers are contraindicated for sinus bradycardia, second- or third-degree heart block, cardiogenic shock, cardiac failure, and severe COPD or asthma. The adverse effect profile of β-blocking agents is partially dependent on their receptor selectivity (Table 8.3). Acebutolol (Sectral), pen-butolol (Levatol), carteolol (Cartrol), and pindolol (Visken) have intrinsic sympathomimetic activity (ISA) resulting in less effect on cardiac output and the lipid profile. β-Blockers without ISA slow the heart rate, decrease cardiac output, increase peripheral vascular resistance, and cause broncho-spasm. Common adverse effects include fatigue, impotence, depression, shortness of breath, cold extremities, cough, drowsiness, and dizziness. The more lipid-soluble agents, such as propranolol and metoprolol, have a higher incidence of central nervous system effects. In diabetic patients, β-blockers may mask the usual symptoms of hypoglycemia, such as tremor, tachycardia, and hunger.[13] Increased triglycerides (30%) and decreased high-density lipo-protein cholesterol (1–20%) occur with non-ISA agents.[15] β-Blockers are effective agents in the young and white populations. Elderly and black patients may not respond as well to monotherapy as a result of lower beta responsiveness. β-Blockers are good choices for patients with supra-ventricular tachycardia, high cardiac output, angina, migraine, and glau-coma. Caution should be exercised in the presence of diabetes, CHF, peripheral vascular disease, COPD, asthma, and elevated lipid profiles.[14]

Central Acting Agents

Methyldopa (Aldomet), clonidine (Catapres), guanfacine (Tenex), and guana-benz (Wytensin) are central α_2-agonists. These agents decrease dopamine and norepinephrine production in the brain, resulting in a decrease in sympathetic nervous activity throughout the body. Blood pressure declines with the decrease in peripheral resistance. Methyldopa exhibits a unique adverse effect profile as it induces autoimmune disorders such as positive Coombs' and antinuclear antibody tests, hemolytic anemia, and hepatic necrosis. The other agents produce sedation, dry mouth, and dizziness. Abrupt clonidine withdrawal may result in rebound hypertension. These drugs are good choices for patients with asthma, diabetes, a high choles-terol level, peripheral vascular disease, and old age.

Peripheral Acting Agents

Guanadrel (Hylorel), reserpine (Serpasil), and guanethidine (Ismelin) are peripheral antiadrenergic agents. Their mechanism of action is at the storage granule level of norepinephrine release. They are infrequently chosen because of their significant side effects, which include profound hypotension, sedation, depression, and impotence.

α_1-Blockers

α_1-Receptor blockers have an affinity for the α_1-receptor on vascular smooth muscles, thereby blocking the uptake of catecholamines by smooth muscle cells. This action results in peripheral vasodilation. The currently available agents are prazosin (Minipress), terazosin (Hytrin), and doxazosin (Cardura). There is a marked reduction in blood pressure with the first dose of these drugs. It is recommended that they be started with 1 mg at bedtime and then titrated slowly upward over 2 to 4 weeks. When adding a second antihypertensive the α-blocker dose should be decreased and titrated upward again. Often a diuretic is added to α_1-blocker therapy to reduce sodium and water retention. The primary adverse effects of these three drugs are dizziness, sedation, nasal congestion, headache, and postural effects. They do not significantly affect lipids, glucose, electrolytes, or exercise tolerance. α_1-Blockers are good choices for young, active adults and for patients with diabetes, renal insufficiency, CHF, peripheral vascular disease, COPD or asthma, or elevated lipids.

Vasodilators

The two direct vasodilators, hydralazine (Apresoline) and minoxidil (Loniten), dilate peripheral arterioles, resulting in a significant fall in blood pressure. A sympathetic reflex increase in heart rate, renin and catecholamine release, and venous constriction occurs. Renal response includes sodium and water retention. The patient may also experience tachycardia, flushing, and headache. Addition of a diuretic and a β-blocker to therapy relieves the major adverse effects of the vasodilators. Hydralazine may cause a lupus-like reaction with fever, rash, and joint pain. Chronic use of minoxidil often results in hirsutism, with increased facial and arm hair. These drugs are third- or fourth-line agents due to their adverse effect profile.[13–15]

Quality of Life Issues

The necessity of life-style changes and probable drug therapy increases the possibility that the patient's quality of life will be altered. The adverse physical, mental, and metabolic effects of antihypertensive therapy results in significant nonadherence to prescribed regimens. In 1982, Jachuck and associates investigated the effect of medications on their patients by asking the patients, their closest relatives, and their physicians a series of questions concerning quality of life since initiating blood pressure medications. The physicians and the patients thought there was either no change or an improvement, whereas 99% of the relatives thought the patients were worse. They cited side effects such as memory loss, irritability, decreased libido, hypochondria, and decreased energy as major effects.[16] Other studies during the 1980s confirmed that nonselective β-blockers, diuretics, and methyldopa compromised quality of life to a far greater extent than ACE inhibitors or calcium entry antagonists.[17,18] Further research in this area is necessary to assist the physician to determine the optimum strategy for blood pressure control to improve adherence and quality of life.

Antihypertensive Selection

It is important to consider the patient's life style, economic status, belief systems, and concerns with treatment when selecting an antihypertensive agent. Therapy should be initiated with one drug in small doses to minimize adverse effects. The patient should understand the long-term benefits of therapy, including decreased incidence of stroke and renal and cardiac disease. Adequate follow-up visits should be scheduled to assess adherence and adverse effects. During these visits, the patient should be encouraged to describe the mental, physical, and emotional changes that have occurred as a result of therapy. If adverse effects are bothersome, consider an alternative selection from a different drug class and attempt to maintain monotherapy. If a second drug is needed, agents can be combined to improve efficacy without significantly increasing the adverse effects (e.g., a diuretic to an ACE inhibitor).

There are some *special considerations* when prescribing medications. Concomitant disease states should be considered and drugs selected that either improve or at least maintain the current clinical solution. Hypertension is a major risk factor for thrombotic and hemorrhagic strokes; and smoking, CHF, diabetes, and coronary artery disease increase the risk. Patients with coronary artery disease may benefit from a calcium entry antagonist or β-blocker with ISA to decrease anginal pain while causing minimal changes in lipid profiles. Congestive heart failure and hypertension respond well to ACE inhibitors and diuretic therapy. Diabetes may be adversely affected by thiazide diuretics and β-blockers. ACE inhibitors, calcium entry antagonists, and central α_2-agonists are appropriate choices.

Patients with severe renal disease are most effectively treated with loop diuretics, whereas ACE inhibitors and calcium entry antagonists may decrease proteinuria and slow the progress of renal failure. As renal function declines, ACE inhibitors must be used with some caution as increased potassium and decreased renal perfusion may occur. With a few agents, such as methyldopa, clonidine, atenolol, nadolol, and captopril, the dosage must be reduced in patients who develop renal failure.

Asthma and COPD patients may be effectively treated with calcium entry antagonists, central α_2-agonists, and α_1-blockers. β-Blockers and possibly diuretics should be avoided owing to possible exacerbation of bronchospasm.

The elderly are of special concern when selecting an antihypertensive agent because of their decreased receptor sensitivity, changing baroreceptor response, atherosclerosis, decreased myocardial function, declining total body water, decreased renal function, and memory loss. Blood pressure should be lowered cautiously, using smaller than normal doses that are slowly titrated upward. Calcium entry antagonists, ACE inhibitors, and diuretics are possible choices for the elderly.

β-Blockers are not usually effective in normal doses owing to decreased β-receptor sensitivity in the elderly. Larger doses result in declining mental function, depression, fatigue, and impotence. α_1-Blockers and central α_2-agonists may be used but with caution. First-dose syncope and sedation are the major concerns.

Black patients may not respond as well to ACE inhibitors or β-blockers as other races. Their poorer response may be due in part to low renin or volume-dependent hypertension. Thiazide diuretics may adversely affect diabetes, gout, and lipids and may not be the best choice for a black patient. Calcium entry antagonists, α_1-blockers, central α_2-agonists, and ACE inhibitors are possible choices.

Young women with hyperdynamic hypertension may respond best to a β-blocker for slowing the heart rate and relieving symptoms of stress. A physically active young man would be better served with an ACE inhibitor, calcium entry antagonist, or α-blocker; β-blockers and diuretics may cause impotence and exercise intolerance.[14]

Severe Hypertension and Emergencies

Patients with a diastolic pressure of more than 115 mm Hg must be treated on diagnosis. Blood pressure should be lowered in increments of 5 to 10 mm Hg, with a goal of less than 100 mm Hg after several weeks of therapy. Often more than one drug must be used initially to control the blood pressure. A hypertensive emergency exists if the diastolic pressure is greater than 130 mm Hg and evidence of end-organ damage exists, such as retinal hemorrhage, encephalopathy, pulmonary edema, myocardial infarction, or unstable angina. Drugs available for treatment in this situation include sodium nitroprusside, nitroglycerin, hydralazine, phentolamine, labetolol, and methyldopa. Patients must be hospitalized for appropriate monitoring. A hypertensive urgency exists when the diastolic pressure is more than 115 mm Hg without evidence of end-organ damage. Oral agents such as nifedipine, clonidine, captopril, and minoxidil may be used to lower the pressure 10 to 15 mm Hg over several hours.[1]

Conclusion

Pharmacologic management of hypertension challenges the physician to understand the patient's social, psychological, and economic status in order to select an antihypertensive regimen that can effectively lower blood pressure, improve concomitant disease states, and allow easy adherence. Continual assessment of therapy is necessary to determine the effectiveness of the regimen, adverse side effects, and the patient's quality of life issues.

References

1. The Fifth Report of the Joint National Committee on Detection, Evaluation, and Treatment of High Blood Pressure. National High Blood Pressure Education. National Institutes of Health. National Heart, Lung and Blood Institute. NIH Publication No. 93-1088. January 1993.
2. Haynes RB, Sackett DL, Taylor DW, et al. Increased absenteeism from work after detection and labeling of hypertensive patients. N Engl J Med 1978; 297:741–4.
3. Gordon T, Doyle JT. Alcohol consumption and its relationship to smoking, weight, blood pressure, and blood lipids. Arch Intern Med 1986;146: 262–5.
4. Pooling Project Research Group. Relationship of blood pressure, serum cholesterol, smoking habit, relative weight and ECG abnormalities to incidence of major coronary events. J Chronic Dis 1978;31:201–6.
5. Stamler J, Farinaro E, Majonnier LM, et al. Prevention and control of hypertension by nutritional-hygienic means. JAMA 1980;243:1819–23.
6. Rose G, Stamler J. The Intersalt Study: background, methods and main results; Intersalt Cooperative Research Group. J Hum Hypertens 1989;3: 283–8.
7. Cade R, Mars D, Wagemaker H, et al. Effect of aerobic exercise training on patients with systemic arterial hypertension. Am J Med 1984;77:785– 90.
8. Margetts BM, Beilin LJ, Armstrong BK. A randomized control trial of a vegetarian diet in the treatment of mild hypertension. Clin Exp Pharmacol Physiol 1985;12:263–6.
9. Kaplan NM. Non-drug treatment of hypertension. Ann Intern Med 1985; 102:359–73.
10. Witteman JC, Willett WC, Stampfer MJ, et al. A prospective study of nutritional factors and hypertension among US women. Circulation 1989;80: 1320–7.
11. Patel C, Marmot MG. Stress management, blood pressure and quality of life. J Hypertens 1987;5(Suppl1):521–8.
12. Stamler R, Stamler J, Grimm R, et al. Nutritional therapy for high blood pressure. JAMA 1987;257:1484–91.
13. American Hospital Formulary Service Drug Information. Bethesda: American Society of Hospital Pharmacists, 1990.
14. Kaplan NM. Clinical hypertension. 5th ed. Baltimore: Williams & Wilkins, 1993.
15. Houston MC. New insights and new approaches for the treatment of essential hypertension: selection of therapy based on coronary heart disease, risk factor analysis, hemodynamic profiles, quality of life and subsets of hypertension. Am Heart J 1989;117:911–51.

16. Jachuck SJ, Brierly H, Jachuck S, et al. The effect of hypotensive drugs on quality of life. J R Coll Gen Pract 1982;32:103–5.
17. Croog SH, Levine S, Testa MA, et al. The effects of antihypertensive therapy on the quality of life. N Engl J Med 1986;314:1657–64.
18. Steiner SS, Friedhoff AJ, Wilson BL, et al. Antihypertensive therapy and quality of life: a comparison of atenolol, captopril, enalapril and propranolol. J Hum Hypertens 1990;4:217–25.

CASE PRESENTATION

Subjective

PATIENT PROFILE

Mary Nelson is a 71-year-old married white female retired teacher.

PRESENTING PROBLEM

High blood pressure.

PRESENT ILLNESS

Mrs. Nelson is here for continuing care of hypertension, which has been present since age 61. She currently takes 50 mg hydrochlorothiazide daily and feels well. Her last periodic health examination with laboratory tests and x-ray was 2 years ago.

PAST MEDICAL HISTORY

She had an abdominal hysterectomy for fibroids at age 50 and is currently taking no estrogen replacement. She has been treated for depression at times but is taking no medication now.

SOCIAL HISTORY

She retired as a middle school history teacher at age 62. She lives with her husband, Harold, aged 76, and son Samuel, aged 48.

HABITS

She does not use alcohol or tobacco. She drinks one cup of coffee daily.

FAMILY HISTORY

She is an orphan, adopted in infancy, and her biological parents are unknown. She and her husband, Harold, had four children. Three are living and have no serious illnesses; their son Samuel, aged 48, has COPD.

She sleeps poorly and wakes early in the morning, unable to fall asleep again. She feels tired throughout the day and occasionally is inappropriately sad.

- What additional medical history might be helpful, and why?
- What questions might help elucidate target organ damage related to hypertension or problems with medication?
- What more would you like to know about her tiredness and sleep disturbance?
- What are possible reasons why the patient is not taking antidepressant medication, and how would you address this issue?

Objective

VITAL SIGNS

Height, 5 ft 3 in; weight, 122 lb; blood pressure, 162/84; pulse, 72.

EXAMINATION

The patient's affect seems somewhat dull and flat compared with previous visits. The head, eyes, ears, nose, and throat are normal. The neck and thyroid gland are normal. Her chest is clear to percussion and auscultation. The heart has a regular sinus rhythm with no murmurs.

- Is there any additional information regarding the physical examination that might be helpful, and why?
- What other areas of the body—if any—should be examined today?
- What—if any—laboratory tests should be obtained today?
- What—if any—diagnostic imaging should be obtained today?

Assessment

- What is the current status of Mrs. Nelson's hypertension? How would you explain this to the patient?
- Describe the pathophysiology of hypertension in the elderly patient. How might this influence your choice of therapy?
- What is the apparent status of her recurrent depression, and how would you explain this to the patient?

- What are some possible adaptations of this patient to her illnesses, and how might these be important in care?

Plan

- What would be your therapeutic recommendations today regarding diet and medication?
- What are possible interrelationships of Mrs. Nelson's problems and the medications that might be used to treat them?
- If Mrs. Nelson is your patient in a capitated plan for which you are a case manager, how might this influence your thinking and actions?
- What continuing care would you recommend for this patient?

9
Sinusitis and Pharyngitis

BARBARA D. REED

Sinusitis and pharyngitis are infectious syndromes commonly seen in the outpatient setting in which short- and long-term morbidity may be decreased by appropriate recognition and treatment. However, the clinical diagnosis of both entities relies on a high index of suspicion, an understanding of the limitations and benefits of the clinical examination and available tests, and an awareness of the treatment options available.

Sinusitis

Although sinusitis accounts for almost 16 million outpatient office visits per year in the United States, the diagnosis and treatment of this infection continues to present many dilemmas to the practicing physician. Sinusitis in children has now been found to be commonly underdiagnosed and may complicate 5% to 10% of the upper respiratory infections of childhood.[1] Therefore, suspicion of the diagnosis and knowledge of up-to-date diagnostic and treatment methods are needed if morbidity is to be decreased.

The paranasal sinuses are air cells lined with pseudostratified ciliated columnar epithelium that develop in the frontal, maxillary, ethmoid, and sphenoid bones of the face. The frontal, anterior ethmoidal, and maxillary sinuses drain into the middle meatus via an area known as the osteomeatal complex, whereas the posterior ethmoidal and sphenoidal sinuses drain into the superior meatus. The osteomeatal area is thought to be critical in the development of most cases of sinusitis, and hence management that affects this area has been most successful. Inadequate drainage of the sinus cavities and increased risk of sinusitis is associated with obstruction of the sinus ostia, impaired function of the cilia, and abnormal quality of sinus secretions. Each of these abnormalities may be produced or exacerbated by swelling or inflammation of the upper respiratory tract due to infection or allergy, resulting in sinus obstruction and infection.

Clinical Presentation

Symptoms

Sinus infections can be divided into two groups based on their clinical presentation and microbiology: acute sinusitis (that which has been present for <30 days) and chronic sinusitis (that of longer duration). The classic presentation of acute sinusitis in adults consists of facial pain, headache (often around or behind the eyes), mucopurulent nasal drainage and fever, and pain radiating to the affected sinus (Table 9.1). However, many patients with infected sinuses, particularly those with chronic disease, do not have marked symptoms. Symptoms and signs of sinusitis in infants and children are often lacking, and infected children may not appear ill (Table 9.1). Therefore, diagnosis in these cases depends on a high index of suspicion followed by diagnostic testing when appropriate.

Children with sinusitis also have a higher prevalence of other respiratory ailments, such as otitis media, allergic rhinitis, and asthma. Children with allergic rhinitis and asthma have abnormal sinus radiographs in at least

TABLE 9.1. Clinical features of sinusitis

Infants
  Irritability
  Chronic rhinorrhea/congestion
  Fever of unknown origin

Children
  Persistent rhinorrhea or postnasal drip (>10 days) of any character
  Severe symptoms of an upper respiratory infection
  Cough, often worse at night
  Allergic rhinitis, asthma, or otitis media
  Fever
  Headache
  Lack of smell, presence of metallic taste
  Bad breath
  Discomfort below or behind the eyes or on eye movement
  Toothache or temporal pain
  Pain in the glabellar and medial canthal regions
  Pain in the occipital, temporal, postauricular, or frontal areas
  Painless morning eye swelling

Adults
  Headache and/or facial pain: site dependent on sinus affected
    Periorbital, temporal, maxillary, teeth, deep-seated
    Pain may worsen with position (supine or upright)
  Nasal congestion or obstruction
  Fever

half the cases.[2] At least half the children with sinusitis have positive allergy tests, and half have otitis media.[3] Aggressive therapy of sinusitis may result in a decreased requirement for bronchodilators and steroids, improved pulmonary function testing in adults and children, and subjective improvement in adults.[4]

Physical Findings

Clinical findings in acute sinusitis vary from none at all to marked tenderness or erythema over the affected sinus, drainage visible under the middle turbinate, fever, or any combination thereof (Table 9.1). Periorbital edema is occasionally seen. Patients with chronic disease may have less distinctive findings. However, because patients with few signs may have sinus infection, auxiliary testing may be needed to make the correct diagnosis.

Diagnosis

The diagnosis of acute and chronic sinusitis depends on interpretation of historical and physical findings, with appropriate addition of adjunctive tests, radiographs, or cultures in specific situations, as described below.

Transillumination

Although lack of transillumination is associated with a fluid- or tissue-filled cavity, the accuracy of this procedure is controversial. Some authors have found it to have no diagnostic value,[3] whereas others find that grossly abnormal or totally normal transillumination is predictive of sinus disease as determined by antral puncture.[5,6] Findings that are less extreme are much less accurate, and the use in children younger than 10 years of age is not reliable.

Plain Radiographs, Computed Tomography, Ultrasonography

Standard x-ray films, including the anteroposterior, lateral, and occipitomental (Waters) views, are used as an adjunct to the office examination of patients with persistent or recurrent disease and of those with suspected sinusitis accompanied by a nonclassic presentation. Abnormal findings of diffuse opacification, mucosal thickening of at least 4 mm, or an air–fluid level may be seen in association with persistent or severe respiratory symptoms; and when both are present, a high density of bacteria is found in the maxillary-sinus aspirate 75% of the time.[7]

The accuracy of plain radiographs of the sinuses in children is controversial.[6,8,9] Results of plain radiographs that are grossly abnormal (opaque or air–fluid levels) or totally normal are associated with results of sinus aspirates and computed tomography (CT) scan findings, but less extreme roentgenographic findings are not.[6,9] One study indicated that plain films of the sinuses did not correlate with CT findings in 74% of children with symptoms compatible with chronic sinusitis; 45% of those with normal plain films had abnormal CT findings, and 34% of those with abnormal plain films had normal CT scans.[9] Therefore, plain films of the sinuses are predictive of disease status only when grossly abnormal; but when less abnormal, they may lead to both over- and underdiagnosis. Furthermore, infection is commonly present in multiple sinuses and is more common in the anterior ethmoidal sinuses—an area that is better visualized with CT scans than by physical examination and plain radiographs. Associations are good between CT scan results and intraoperative findings of the sinuses using endoscopic visualization, with false-negative and false-positive rates of 7% and 20%, respectively.[3]

Ultrasonography is also being evaluated as a diagnostic tool in cases of suspected sinusitis, but results are conflicting. Further study is needed to document the reliability of ultrasonography for diagnosis.[7]

Nasopharyngeal Cultures and Antral Puncture

Cultures taken from the nose or nasopharyngeal mucus do not correlate well with those taken from the sinus by aspiration or antrostomy,[5–7,10] and the bacteriologic yield using biopsy samples of sinus mucosa was double that obtained from sinus secretions alone.[11] Furthermore, culture results of aspiration of one sinus may not be indicative of organisms in other sinuses.

Therefore, because of the invasiveness of the procedures and the limitations of the results, microbiologic information is usually not obtained in uncomplicated cases of sinusitis. Hence, antimicrobial choice is based on the known prevalences of infecting organisms and outcomes of treatment trials.

Microbiology

Bacterial Findings

Acute Sinusitis

The classic definition of bacterial infection of a sinus is the presence of more than 10^4 organisms per milliliter or the observation of any organism on Gram stain in the aspirate fluid.[7] Most adults and children with acute sinusitis are infected with *Streptococcus pneumoniae*, *Haemophilus influenzae*, or *Moraxella catarrhalis* (formerly known as *Neisseria* or *Brahamella catarrhalis*).[6,7] However, many other organisms have been isolated, including group A or C β-hemolytic *Streptococcus*, *Streptococcus viridans*, peptostreptococci, and *Eikenella corrodens*.

Chronic Sinusitis and Anaerobes

Patients with chronic sinusitis are more likely to have *Staphylococcus aureus* and anaerobes present in the sinus fluid than are those with acute sinusitis.[10,12] In both adults and children, anaerobic bacteria have been found in approximately 0% to 12% of cases of acute sinusitis[6,7,13] and in 28% to 100% of patients with chronically inflamed sinuses,[10,12] although other investigators have found anaerobes to be less common in children.[5] Furthermore, almost half the anaerobes produced β-lactamase, suggesting that antimicrobial resistance may be a more common factor in these persistent cases.[10,12]

β-Lactamase-Producing Organisms and Susceptibility Testing

Organisms producing β-lactamase are reported with increasing frequency, with 18% to 41% of *H. influenzae*, most *M. catarrhalis*, and half of anaerobes producing this enzyme.[10,12] Furthermore, the prevalence of β-lactamase-producing organisms may increase after treatment with other antibiotics.[14] Theoretically, the production of β-lactamase by these organisms at the site of infection could have an inhibitory effect on susceptible antibiotics, such as the penicillins and some cephalosporins.[15,16] Although several investigators have found an association between clinical efficacy and the in vitro susceptibility of pathogens isolated,[5,13] the findings of others illustrate that clinical improvement is often not directly related to the in vitro susceptibility found.[17]

Nonbacterial Causes of Sinusitis

Viral isolates, such as adenovirus, parainfluenza virus, rhinovirus, and influenza virus, may also be present in approximately 10% of patients with acute sinusitis.[6] A higher percentage is found if diagnostic aspiration is done earlier in the course of respiratory symptoms, although research in this area is limited.[7] Fungal infections of the paranasal sinuses, such as *Aspergillus fumigatus* infection or mucormycosis, may also occur, usually in patients with chronic infection, in diabetic patients, and in other immunocompromised individuals. Diagnosis is obtained via antrostomy and tissue biopsy.

Sinusitis Associated with Nasotracheal Intubation

Patients with nasotracheal tubes are at increased risk of sinusitis, and this diagnosis should be considered in intubated patients with unexplained signs of infection. Cultures indicate that these infections are often polymicrobial, with *Staphylococcus aureus* most common (16%), followed by *Enterobacter* species (13%), *Pseudomonas aeruginosa* (13%), *Bacteroides fragilis*, and *Bacteroides melaninogenicus* (13%).[18]

Treatment

The goal of treatment for sinusitis is to reverse infection and inflammation and reestablish ventilation and drainage of the sinus cavities. Medical treatment is initially attempted unless severe intraorbital or intracranial complications exist, with surgical treatment reserved for resistant and severe cases. Potential medical therapies include antibiotics, decongestants, topical steroids, systemic liquefying agents, humidification, and occasionally antihistamines.[3] More than 80% of children and adults with acute sinusitis respond to medical treatment.[8]

Antibiotics

The backbone of medical treatment for sinusitis is antibiotics that have antimicrobial activity against the prevalent organisms. The common antibiotics recommended are shown in Table 9.2.

Amoxicillin is the first-line antimicrobial used for acute uncomplicated sinusitis because of its efficacy, low cost, and safety profile, with cure rates for children ranging from 67% to 100%. Although approximately 35% of *H. influenzae* and 75% of *M. catarrhalis* strains produce β-lactamase, clini-

TABLE 9.2. Antimicrobial therapy for acute and chronic sinusitis in children and adults

Drug	Dose	
	Children	Adults
Ampicillin	100 mg/kg/day in 4 divided doses	2 g in 4 divided doses
Amoxicillin	40 mg/kg body weight/day in 3 divided doses	1.5 g in 3 divided doses
Erythromycin-sulfisoxazole	50–150 mg/kg/day in 4 divided doses	Not applicable
Trimethoprim-sulfamethoxazole	8–40 mg/kg/day in 2 divided doses	320–1600 mg in 2 divided doses
Cefaclor	40 mg/kg/day in 3 divided doses	2 g in 4 divided doses
Loracarbef	Not applicable	800 mg in 2 divided doses
Resistant, persistent, and recurrent cases		
Amoxicillin-clavulanate potassium	40–100 mg/kg/day in 3 divided doses	1.5 g in 3 divided doses
Cefuroxime axetil	250 or 500 mg/day in 2 divided doses	0.5 g in 2 divided doses

cal cure rates when using amoxicillin have not been substantially different from those seen with drugs resistant to this enzyme.[19]

Many other antimicrobials may be used for acute sinusitis with similar clinical response. Studies in adults with acute sinusitis indicated a microbiologic cure in 84% to 100% of cases in which ampicillin, amoxicillin, trimethoprim-sulfamethoxazole, cefaclor, cefuroxime axetil, cyclacillin, loracarbef, and amoxicillin-clavulanate potassium were used.[19] Results with cefaclor have been variable, often related to the dosing schedule, with some studies finding lower efficacy if used at 500 mg bid or tid,[20] and others finding comparable bacteriologic cure rates when used at high doses and frequent intervals (2 g in four divided doses).[6]

For patients who fail to improve and for those with more complicated infections (high fever or periorbital swelling), the broader-spectrum regimens that cover β-lactamase-producing bacteria, such as amoxicillin-clavulanate potassium, erythromycin-sulfisoxazole, and cefuroxime axetil, are appropriate.[8,19] Using antimicrobials with activity against anaerobes has not been well studied but needs evaluation owing to the high prevalence of anaerobes in chronic sinusitis.

The duration of treatment may be an important determinant of clinical response, but few comparative data are available. If the clinical response to treatment is rapid (3–4 days), a 10-day course of antimicrobials may be sufficient, although the trend is to treat the patient a minimum of 14 days. If resolution is slower antibiotics should be continued until 7 days after symptoms resolve[19] or for 21 or more days.[3,8]

Decongestants, Antihistamines, and Nasal Steroids

Drugs that may decrease the engorgement of the nasal and sinus mucosa would be expected to decrease the obstruction to sinus drainage and aid in the resolution of acute sinusitis. Decongestants increase the patency of the maxillary sinus ostium and decrease nasal airway resistance in patients with chronic sinusitis and in normal controls,[21] but their effect on the clinical course of acute sinusitis has not been well studied.[19] Decongestant nasal sprays may be helpful for promoting drainage and aeration of sinuses but should be used for only 3 to 5 days to avoid potential rebound. Steroid nasal sprays may also reduce mucosal edema and reestablish ostial patency; they may be used in patients who do not respond to initial therapy or in those with concomitant allergy.[3] There is no evidence that histamines are increased in patients with sinusitis, and no studies have reported improved response when antihistamines are used. Therefore, these agents should be reserved for patients with recognized allergies.[19]

Surgical and Endoscopic Management

Surgical management is recommended for resistant or chronic sinusitis to relieve obstruction of the natural ostia, resect inflammatory or infected tissue, and provide an airway with drainage for all the nasal and sinus compartments. Many procedures have been used based on the location and severity of the disease. Tonsillectomy and adenoidectomy have been used as a method to remove tissue blocking the sinus ostia and may be beneficial if such obstruction is documented by endoscopy, although controlled studies on the efficacy are lacking. Procedures that address drainage of the sinuses more directly include antral lavage, intranasal antrostomy, the Caldwell-Luc sublabial procedure, intranasal sphenoethmoidectomy, transantral ethmoidectomy, and endoscopic surgery. Selected procedures are discussed below.

Antral Lavage

Antral lavage of the sinus has been a standard treatment for chronic sinusitis, but efficacy studies are conflicting, with the preponderance of evidence suggesting no clear advantage over the use of antibiotics alone.

Nasoantral Window

The nasoantral window or fistula in the maxillary sinus has been used to attempt to facilitate gravitational drainage of the sinuses because of its safety, relative simplicity, and need for only local anesthesia. However, few data exist regarding the efficacy of this procedure. Furthermore, the cilia still transport secretions toward the natural meatus.[19] After this procedure, only 27% of patients had improved at the 6-month follow-up.[22] This fact, along with increased recognition that the obstruction in the area of the osteomeatal complex plays a major role in the pathogenesis of chronic sinusitis, has led to the development of other surgical techniques.

Functional Endonasal Sinus Surgery

Functional endonasal sinus surgery is an endoscopic procedure that is performed under direct visualization to enlarge the *natural* meatus of the maxillary outflow tract by excising the uncinate process and the ethmoidal bullae and performing an anterior ethmoidectomy. In one pediatric study, 71% of patients were considered normal by their parents 1 year after this operation,[23] and effectiveness of 85% to 96% has been documented by others.[24,25] Reported complications have been minimal.

Recurrent Sinusitis

Children may be predisposed to recurrent sinus infections due to allergic inflammation, cystic fibrosis, immunodeficiency disorders, ciliary dyskinesia, or anatomic problems.[19] In children with recurrent disease, additional evaluation includes allergy evaluations, a sweat chloride test, immunoglobulin measurement, or a mucosal biopsy to assess ciliary function and structure, with therapy directed at the abnormalities found.

The use of antimicrobial prophylaxis[19] for children with recurrent disease may be considered. Although this modality has proved useful for reducing recurrent symptomatic episodes of acute otitis media,[26] it has not yet been well studied in recurrent sinusitis. Hence response to such prophylaxis should be carefully documented and periodic cessation of therapy attempted.

Chronic disease in adults, despite antimicrobial and surgical therapy, is more common in those with sinusitis related to dental disease, nasal allergy, and nasal polyps. Hence the presence of these contributing factors should also be assessed and addressed.[27]

Complications of Sinusitis

Approximately 80% of children with sinusitis respond to treatment without complications. However, because of the lack of diagnosis of the acute infection in a larger proportion of affected children, complications may be the presenting symptoms.

Risks of orbital and intracranial complications are increased in patients with acute frontal or sphenoidal sinusitis, and hence infections with prominent findings of increased pain in the supine position, frontal headache and tenderness, or deep-seated headache with multiple foci should be treated as a medical emergency with aggressive treatment and close follow-up. Orbital complications of sinusitis include inflammatory edema of the orbit, orbital cellulitis, subperiosteal abscess of the orbit, orbital abscesses, and cavernous sinus thrombosis. Intracranial complications also occur, including meningitis, epidural abscess, subdural empyema, venous sinus thrombosis, and cerebral abscess. Orbital complications should be suspected if eye swelling, exophthalmos, or impaired extraocular eye movements occur. Intracranial complications may present with increased intracranial pressure, meningeal irritation, or focal neurologic deficits. Evaluation by the CT scan is essential for diagnosis in these cases, and emergent antibiotic therapy and surgical drainage are usually required for successful treatment.[19]

Pharyngitis

More than 30 million patients with pharyngitis present yearly to outpatient settings in the United States.[28] Some present because of marked symptoms and the desire for treatment, others because of their concern about "strep throats" and the associated potential complications.

Pharyngitis caused by group A β-hemolytic streptococci (GABHS) is associated with several complications that have decreased dramatically since the 1960s, including suppurative sequelae (retropharyngeal and peritonsillar abscesses and otitis) and immunologically mediated sequelae (rheumatic fever and poststreptococcal glomerulonephritis). Although the prevalence of rheumatic fever has declined from 20 in 100,000 to 1 in 100,000 since the early 1900s, clusters of cases have now been reported in the United States, indicating that the risk remains.[29] Rheumatic fever occurs in 0.3% to 3.0% of those with untreated streptococcal infection[30] and is associated with specific subtypes of GABHS that exhibit increased virulence and rheumatogenicity.[29] Treatment of GABHS pharyngitis within 10 days of onset prevents this complication[31]; however, approximately one-third of cases follow asymptomatic infection. Furthermore, although the incidence of acute rheumatic fever has declined, that of streptococcal pharyngitis has not. Hence recognition of pharyngeal infections and appropriate treatment of those caused by GABHS is indicated if complications are to be minimized.

Clinical Presentation

Group A β-Hemolytic Streptococcal Pharyngitis

GABHS is the most common bacterial cause of pharyngeal infections, occurring in one-third to one-half of cases of pharyngitis in children aged 2 to 14 years; more than one-third of children with infection are within the 6- to 8-year age group.[32] In contrast, only 1 in 10 adults with pharyngitis are culture-positive for GABHS. Patients with signs and symptoms of pharyngitis are more likely than are those who are asymptomatic to have a predominant growth of an individual bacterial microorganism,[32] to be infectious, and to develop subsequent rheumatic fever.[31]

Pharyngitis caused by GABHS classically presents with an acute onset of sore throat with fever and anterior neck tenderness, and occasionally with headache and abdominal pain. Typically, prominent cough, rhinorrhea, or hoarseness is not present. Children younger than the age of 3 years are less likely to have overt GABHS pharyngitis and may present with decreased appetite, irritability, fever, and a history of contact with schoolage children.[32] Signs of pharyngitis include erythema or swelling of the posterior pharynx or tonsillar pillars, pharyngeal exudate, enlarged tender anterior cervical adenopathy, palatal petechiae, and fever. A characteristic rash of scarlet fever with a red blanching appearance and sandpaper texture may be present.

Several of these symptoms and signs are associated with GABHS pharyngitis, but none is highly predictive of culture results.[33] Risk factor scoring systems have been developed to predict the probability of GABHS infection in patients with pharyngitis, and some have been fairly successful. However, even with the more accurate systems, one-fifth of the culture-positive patients were missed among the patients scoring in the low-risk group, whereas 22% of patients in the high-risk group were culture-negative.[34] Hence the clinical diagnosis of GABHS pharyngitis is inexact and requires confirmatory testing for accurate diagnosis.

Other Bacterial Pathogens

Pharyngeal infections may also be associated with other microorganisms. Non-GABHS appears not to be a common cause of pharyngitis,[32] although epidemics of groups C and G have been reported. Group C β-hemolytic streptococci may cause a mild form of pharyngitis, but it is not known if treatment of patients who are symptomatic with non-GABHS is beneficial.[35]

Corynebacterium diphtheria is an uncommon cause of pharyngitis in the United States due to the DPT immunization program of children but continues to be a cause of serious pharyngeal infections in the world. The diagnosis is suggested by the presence of a gray-green membrane adhering to the tonsils and pharyngeal mucosa, occasional hoarseness and stridor, tender anterior cervical lymphadenopathy, or inflammatory edema creating a "bull-neck" appearance.

Evidence suggests that *Corynebacterium hemolyticum* is associated with pharyngitis and a scarlatiniform rash, primarily in older children and adults.[31] It may respond clinically and microbiologically to treatment with a 10-day course of erythromycin. The role of other bacteria, such as *Streptococcus pneumoniae, Staphylococcus aureus, Moraxella catarrhalis,* and *Neisseria meningitidis,* in pharyngitis is not clear, with comparable rates of colonization/infection found in symptomatic and asymptomatic patients.[31] Whether *Haemophilus influenzae* causes pharyngeal symptoms is also unclear. Although studies suggested it may be an opportunistic organism in an inflamed pharynx, it is usually not considered a pharyngeal pathogen, and treatment is not currently recommended. However, epiglottitis caused by *H. influenzae* may present as a sore throat and is a life-threatening emergency. Associated symptoms may include high fever, dysphagia, and characteristic drooling in a patient sitting forward in the chair or hesitating to lie down. Immediate evaluation with a lateral neck radiograph is required to further assess this complex of symptoms.

Viral Pharyngitis

Viral infections are a common cause of pharyngitis in children and young adults, occurring in approximately half of infants younger than 2 years, 10% of children aged 2 to 11, and one-third of university students with signs of pharyngitis, compared with the uncommon presence of viruses in asymptomatic controls.[32] Viral pathogens include adenovirus, parainfluenza virus, rhinovirus,[32] herpes simplex virus, and coxsackie A virus. Pharyngitis caused by adenovirus is often associated with a pharyngeal exudate and may clinically mimic GABHS infection. Mononucleosis, caused by the

Epstein-Barr virus, typically presents with a cheesy, creamy-white exudate or membrane confined to the tonsils, generalized lymphadenopathy, abnormal liver function tests, and a peripheral blood lymphocytosis with atypical mononuclear cells; there is occasional periorbital edema and a rash. However, if symptoms of throat discomfort persist over a period of 2 to 3 days, GABHS infection should be ruled out.

Chlamydia trachomatis and Mycoplasma pneumoniae Pharyngitis

Although *Chlamydia trachomatis* and *Mycoplasma pneumoniae* have been reported to be common causes of pharyngitis in adults as determined by serologic evidence,[36] other studies in adults[37,38] and children[32,39] have indicated that these organisms are uncommon pharyngeal pathogens. *M. pneumoniae* is present in 3% to 15% of children with pharyngitis, being more common in young teens and adults and rare in children younger than the age of 6 years. Although seen more commonly in those with symptoms of pharyngitis than in controls,[32] it too has not been associated with specific pharyngeal symptoms, signs, or subsequent complications. Hence testing for and treatment of this organism is not recommended unless lower respiratory symptoms coexist.

Other Organisms Isolated from the Pharynx

Patients may have pharyngeal infections with organisms that are usually sexually transmitted, including *Neisseria gonorrhoeae, Trichomonas vaginalis, Mycoplasma hominis,* and *Ureaplasma urealyticum.*[40,41] Symptomatic infection from these organisms is, however, uncommon. *Candida albicans* is more common in patients with exudative pharyngitis who were not infected with a bacterial or viral pathogen than in normal controls.[42] Immuno-compromised individuals are also more likely to have *Candida* pharyngitis; thus patients with recurrent pharyngeal candidiasis should be evaluated for acquired immunodeficiency syndrome and other immunosuppressed states.

For more than half of adults and a smaller percentage of children, there is no discernible cause for the pharyngitis.[32] Although not distinguished accurately by symptoms and signs, patients with hoarseness and those without physical findings are more likely to fit into this group.

Diagnostic Testing

Because the symptoms and signs of pharyngitis are not good predictors of the presence of GABHS infection, further diagnostic testing is often needed to improve diagnostic accuracy. Common methods used to identify of the GABHS organism are culture and rapid in-office diagnostic tests.

Bacterial Cultures

Identification of GABHS by culture methods can be performed at minimal cost (<$10) in the outpatient setting or in a central laboratory. Although false-negative results occur, culture on sheep blood agar media or selective media incubated in an anaerobic environment for 24 to 48 hours results in sensitivities higher than 90%.[33] Treatment of the patient, or discontinuation of medication if empirically started, can then be initiated as indicated by the results.

Rapid In-Office Tests

Rapid diagnosis of GABHS infection at the time of the initial visit is desired by patients and physicians to initiate therapy, minimize symptoms, limit contagiousness, and avoid uncertainty about the treatment plan. Many in-office tests for detecting GABHS antigens have been developed, most of which have specificities of 85% to 100% but sensitivities of only 31% to 95%.[43,44] Thus, a positive test is fairly predictive of GABHS infection, and culture documentation may be omitted; but a negative test should be followed by a culture to identify those who are falsely negative on the direct test.[29,33]

Treatment

GABHS Infection

Antimicrobial treatment of patients with symptomatic GABHS infection has been found to decrease the risk of subsequent rheumatic fever and may prevent suppurative complications.[31] Evidence suggests that treatment results in more rapid clinical improvement and may reduce the risk of recurrence and the duration of infectivity.[31] Whether early treatment results in a blunted immunologic response to the organism, with an increase in recurrence rates, is unclear.[45-47] At this time, treatment of symptomatic GABHS infection is recommended, with minimal risk of delaying treatment pending culture results when the probability of infection is low, and potential shortening of the symptomatic and infectious period via early treatment when the probability of infection is high.

The GABHS organism is sensitive to penicillin, and it has remained the antibiotic of choice for GABHS pharyngitis. Parenteral long-acting penicillin also effectively eradicates the organism, is inexpensive, and removes the need for patient adherence to the drug regimen. However, treatment with penicillin results in adverse reactions in 1% to 2% of patients, and 1 in 100,000 patients may die from a reaction to the drug.[48] Parenteral treatment should be considered for patients who are very ill, vomiting, or unable to take oral medication. Also, patients in whom compliance is anticipated to be especially problematic, those with frequent recurrences despite adequate therapy, and children with rheumatic heart disease in whom persistent GABHS infection should be avoided are candidates for parenteral therapy.[31]

Studies suggest that penicillin may not be as effective against GABHS infections as in the past.[29] One explanation could be the protection of the GABHS organism from antibiotics that are inactivated by the presence in the pharynx of β-lactamases produced by other organisms,[15] such as *Staphylococcus aureus, Haemophilus influenzae, Moraxella catarrhalis,* and anaerobes.[49] Treatment of patients with persistent or recurrent disease may benefit from treatment with antibiotics resistant to β-lactamase activity, but further research is needed.

Patients who are allergic to penicillins may be treated with other antimicrobials, as shown in Table 9.3. Erythromycin has traditionally been used as an alternative treatment and is effective in most cases. However, data from Finland suggest new resistance to this antibiotic of 20% of isolates of GABHS in the pharynx, with a corresponding decrease in clinical response to treatment in these patients.[50]

Treatment for 10 days with oral penicillin is associated with lower treatment failure and recurrence rates than are seen with 5- and 7-day courses.[31] However, compliance with four daily doses of medication is difficult, and fewer than 60% of patients complete the prescribed course.[51] Other treatment regimens have therefore been evaluated (Table 9.3). A meta-analysis found that cephalosporins (e.g., cephalexin, cefadroxil, and cefuroxime) produce bacteriologic and clinical cure rates superior to those seen with penicillin.[52] The development of antimicrobials that can be prescribed on a once- or twice-daily schedule has further expanded the options available for treatment. A 5-day course of azithromycin once daily eradicates the GABHS organism in 91% of patients,[53] and 10 days of clarithromycin given twice a day cured 99% of patients.[54] Although it is assumed that eradication of the GABHS organism by any antimicrobial can prevent suppurative and nonsuppurative sequelae, studies on this point are lacking.

Treatment of Other Causes of Pharyngitis

There are few other causes of pharyngitis for which treatment is recommended. *Corynebacterium diphtheriae* infection is treated with antitoxin and clindamycin or erythromycin, and *Corynebacterium haemolyticum* infection may respond clinically and microbiologically to a 10-day course of erythromycin. Viral infections are treated symptomatically with oral or pharyngeal analgesics (e.g., sprays or lozenges) to minimize symptoms. Patients with mononucleosis should be cautioned to avoid trauma due to possible splenic enlargement and risk of rupture. Patients with culture-proved gonococcal or chlamydial pharyngitis should be treated according to Cen-

Table 9.3. Treatment for group A β-hemolytic streptococcal pharyngitis

Antibiotic	Dose[a] Children	Adults
Benzathine penicillin	<60 pounds 600,000 units IM ≥60 pounds 1.2 million units IM	Same
Penicillin V	40 mg/kg/day in 4 divided doses or 250 mg 4 times a day 500 mg twice a day	Same
Erythromycin estolate	20–40 mg/kg/day in 2–4 divided doses (max., 1 g/day)	250 mg 4 times daily
Erythromycin ethylsuccinate	40 mg/kg/day in 2–4 divided doses (max., 1 g/day)	400 mg 4 times daily
Clarithromycin	Not yet approved	250 mg twice a day
Azithromycin	Not yet approved	500 mg on day 1; then 250 mg daily on days 2–5
Cephalosporins		
Cephalexin	25–50 mg/kg/day in 2 or 4 divided doses	1 g/day in 2–4 divided doses
Cefadroxil	25–30 mg/kg in 2 or 3 divided doses	1 g/day in 1 or 2 doses
Cefuroxime	250 mg bid (older than age 13)	250 mg twice a day
Cefprozil (Cefzil)	Not yet approved	500 mg daily
Cefaclor	20 mg/kg/day divided tid	250 mg 3 times a day
Persistent carrier state		
Clindamycin	20 mg/kg/day in 3 or 4 divided doses	150 mg 4 times a day
Amoxicillin/clavulanate potassium	20 mg/kg/day in 3 divided doses	250 mg 3 times a day

[a]Duration of treatment is 10 days unless otherwise stated.

ters for Disease Control guidelines.[55] No current recommendations suggest treatment of culture-proved *Mycoplasma pneumoniae, Ureaplasma urealyticum, Haemophilus influenzae,* non-GABHS, or *Staphylococcus aureus* infections. Patients with symptoms and signs of pharyngitis who fail to improve after 48 hours of therapy require further evaluation, including a repeat clinical assessment, to look for less common types of pharyngitis and for symptoms of concomitant infections (e.g., sinusitis, otitis media, pneumonia).

Cost-Benefit of Treatment Strategy

Studies have evaluated the costs of various combinations of testing and treating patients with possible GABHS infection. Unfortunately, no single decision strategy minimizes untreated cases, unnecessary treatment, costs, and potential side effects; and hence the priorities of the physician and patient must be understood. Several concepts have emerged. As the pretest probability of disease increases owing to a high prevalence of disease in the community (>20%, for example), treating all patients with symptoms or signs of disease without culture confirmation may be rational.[56] When the risk of disease is low based on the community prevalence of GABHS and clinical risk factors (<5%, for example), the costs of evaluation, risk of reaction to an unnecessary medication, and high proportion of positive cultures arising from carriers are greater than those associated with missed infection, resulting in a recommendation that no testing or treatment be pursued. For situations with risk of disease somewhere between these two extremes, reliance on the clinical findings alone leads to high rates of untreated infection and unnecessary medication. Therefore, testing with culture or an in-office test with culture confirmation when the in-office test is negative is recommended.[33,56] Whether to treat presumptively with antibiotics pending culture confirmation is controversial. Factors to consider in this decision include the severity of illness, the physician's perception of risk of disease, risk of transmission to large numbers of individuals, and the patient's willingness to accept risks of disease sequelae versus risks of unnecessary antimicrobial therapy.

Treatment of the Carrier State

Treatment recommendations for asymptomatic patients who have a positive culture for GABHS are controversial. Prevalence rates of carriage vary, with reports of 45% to 60% of third- and fourth-graders being culture-positive[57] to 11% of children 14 years of age or younger, and 0.6% of adults at least 45 years old.[58] The rationale for treating these patients is to reduce the recurrence rates, the transmission of organisms to other individuals, and the risk of subsequent rheumatic fever. Data suggest that the degree of infectivity of carriers of GABHS is low compared with that of symptomatic patients, as is their risk of developing rheumatic fever.[31] Therefore, treatment is primarily recommended in patients with recurrent disease and in those with a personal or family history of rheumatic fever.[31]

Using clindamycin or amoxicillin/clavulanate potassium has improved short-term eradication of the GABHS from the pharynx in patients who failed traditional therapy with penicillin or erythromycin (Table 9.3).[31] Follow-up at 18 to 24 months after treatment with clindamycin indicated that recurrence of GABHS infection is rare.[59] These antibiotics, each of which is resistant to β-lactamase in the pharynx, suggest a potential role of β-lactamase producers in antimicrobial failure rates.

Follow-up Cultures

Because treatment of GABHS carriers is recommended only in the limited instances described above, routine cultures of patients who respond clinically to antimicrobial therapy are not warranted.

Tonsillectomy

Tonsillectomy has been recommended for patients with recurrent severe episodes of pharyngitis, although little information is available regarding the efficacy of this treatment compared with medical management. One randomized clinical trial in which children had at least seven episodes of a throat infection within 1 year, five episodes during each of 2 years, or three during each of 3 years suggested that patients undergoing tonsillectomy were less likely to have moderate or severe pharyngitis during the year after surgery (8%) compared with controls (66%), although one-third of those in the medical management group eventually had a tonsillectomy.[31] Nevertheless, most of the other medically treated children had only mild courses of illness. Fourteen percent of those undergoing tonsillectomy had complications, but all were readily managed or self-limited. Hence tonsillectomy after unsuccessful medical management may be considered in children with this severity of recurrent infections.

Prevention

Currently, secondary prevention of complications of GABHS infections is attempted by the diagnosis and treatment of infections. However, primary prevention of infection during times of high infection rates has been found to decrease infection rates.[60] Prophylaxis with 1.2 million units of penicillin G benzathine (or erythromycin for those who are penicillin-allergic) may be considered during epidemics for groups of people having close contact, such as those in day care centers, camps, schools, and prisons.[61]

Prophylaxis with penicillin for children with recurrent infections has not been well studied, although it has been shown to be effective in preventing recurrent GABHS infection and recurrent rheumatic episodes in patients with rheumatic fever.[31] A trial of antimicrobial prophylaxis may be reasonable before consideration of tonsillectomy in patients who respond to medical therapy but relapse when antimicrobials are discontinued.

References

1. Wald ER, Guerra N, Byers C. Upper respiratory tract infections in young children: duration of and frequency of complications. Pediatrics 1991;87: 129–33.
2. Rachelefsky GS. Sinusitis in children—diagnosis and management. Clin Rev Allergy 1984;2:397–408.
3. Younis RT, Lazar RH. The approach to acute and chronic sinusitis in children. Ear Nose Throat J 1991;70:35–39.
4. Slavin RG. Sinusitis in adults. J Allergy Clin Immunol 1988;81:1028–32.
5. Evans FO Jr, Sydnor JB, Moore WE, et al. Sinusitis of the maxillary antrum. N Engl J Med 1975;293:735–9.
6. Gwaltney JM Jr, Sydnor A Jr, Sande MA. Etiology and antimicrobial treatment of acute sinusitis. Ann Otol Rhinol Laryngol Suppl 1981;90:68–71.
7. Lusk RP, Lazar RH, Muntz RH. The diagnosis and treatment of recurrent and chronic sinusitis in children. Pediatr Clin North Am 1989;36:1411–21.
8. Wald ER, Milmoe GJ, Bowen A, et al. Acute maxillary sinusitis in children. N Engl J Med 1981;304:749–54.
9. McAlister WH, Lusk R, Muntz HR. Comparison of plain radiographs and coronal CT scans in infants and children with recurrent sinusitis. AJR 1989;153:1259–64.
10. Brook I. Bacteriologic features of chronic sinusitis in children. JAMA 1981; 246:967–9.
11. Karma P, Jokippi L, Sipila P, et al. Bacteria in chronic maxillary sinusitis. Arch Otolaryngol 1979;105:386–90.
12. Brook I. Bacteriology of chronic maxillary sinusitis in adults. Ann Otol Rhinol Laryngol 1989;98:426–8.
13. Hamory BH, Sande MA, Sydnor A Jr, et al. Etiology and antimicrobial therapy of acute maxillary sinusitis. J Infect Dis 1979;139:197–202.
14. Reed BD, Huck W, Zazove P. Treatment of beta-hemolytic streptococcal pharyngitis with cefaclor or penicillin: efficacy and interaction with beta-lactamase producing organisms in the pharynx. J Fam Pract 1991;32:138–44.
15. Simon HJ, Sakai W. Staphylococcal antagonism to penicillin-G therapy of hemolytic streptococcal pharyngeal infection: effect of oxacillin. Pediatrics 1963;31:463–9.
16. Brook I, Yokum P. In vitro protection of group A beta-hemolytic streptococci from penicillin and cephalothin by Bacteroides fragilis. Chemotherapy 1983; 29:18–23.
17. Wald ER, Chiponis D, Ledesma-Medina J. Comparative effectiveness of amoxicillin and amoxicillin-clavulanate potassium in acute paranasal sinus infections in children: a double-blind, placebo-controlled trial. Pediatrics 1986;77:795–800.

18. Linden BE, Aguilar EA, Allen SJ. Sinusitis in the nasotracheally intubated patient. Arch Otolaryngol Head Neck Surg 1988;114:860–1.
19. Wald ER. Sinusitis in children. N Engl J Med 1992;326:319–23.
20. Sydnor A Jr, Gwaltney JM Jr, Cocchetto DM, Scheld M. Comparative evaluation of cefuroxime axetil and cefaclor for treatment of acute bacterial maxillary sinusitis. Arch Otolaryngol Head Neck Surg 1989;115:1430–3.
21. Melen I, Friberg B, Andreasson L, et al. Effects of phenylpropanolamine on ostial and nasal patency in patients treated for chronic maxillary sinusitis. Acta Otolaryngol (Stockh) 1986;101:494–500.
22. Muntz HR, Lusk RP. Nasal antral windows in children: a retrospective study. Laryngoscope 1990;100:643–6.
23. Lusk RP, Muntz HR. Endoscopic sinus surgery in children with chronic sinusitis: a pilot study. Laryngoscope 1990;100:654–8.
24. Gross CW, Lazar RH, Gurucharri MJ, et al. Pediatric functional endonasal sinus surgery. Otolaryngol Clin North Am 1989;22:733–8.
25. Davis WE, Templer JW, Lamear WR, et al. Middle meatus anstrostomy: patency rates and risk factors. Otolaryngol Head Neck Surg 1991;104:467–72.
26. Perrin JM, Charney E, MacWhinney JB Jr, et al. Sulfisoxazole as chemoprophylaxis for recurrent otitis media: a double-blind crossover study in pediatric practice. N Engl J Med 1974;291:664–7.
27. Melen I, Lindahl L, Andreasson L. Short- and long-term treatment results in chronic maxillary sinusitis. Acta Otolaryngol (Stockh) 1986;102:282–90.
28. Schappert SM. National ambulatory medical care survey: 1989 summary, United States. Vital Health Stat [13] 1992;110:49.
29. Bisno AL. Group A streptococcal infections and acute rheumatic fever. N Engl J Med 1991;325:783–93.
30. Kaplan EL, Top FH Jr, Dudding BA, Wannamaker LW. Diagnosis of streptococcal pharyngitis: differentiation of active infection from the carrier state in the symptomatic child. J Infect Dis 1971;123:490–501.
31. Paradise JL. Etiology and management of pharyngitis and pharyngotonsillitis in children: a current review. Ann Otol Rhinol Laryngol Suppl 1992;155:51–57.
32. Glezen WP, Clyde WA Jr, Senior RJ, et al. Group A streptococci mycoplasmas, and viruses associated with acute pharyngitis. JAMA 1967;202:455–60.
33. Reed BD, Huck W, French T. Diagnosis of group A beta-hemolytic streptococcus using clinical scoring criteria, directigen 1-2-3 group A streptococcal test, and culture. Arch Intern Med 1990;150:1727–32.
34. Breese BB. A simple scorecard for the tentative diagnosis of streptococcal pharyngitis. Am J Dis Child 1977;131:514–17.
35. Meier FA, Centor RM, Graham L Jr, Dalton HP. Clinical and microbiological evidence for endemic pharyngitis among adults due to group C streptococci. Arch Intern Med 1990;150:825–9.
36. Komaroff AL, Aronson MD, Pass TM, et al. Serologic evidence of Chlamydia and mycoplasmal pharyngitis in adults. Science 1983;222:927–9.
37. Jones RB, Rabinovitch RA, Katz BP, et al. Chlamydia trachomatis in the pharynx and rectum of heterosexual patients at risk for genital infection. Ann Intern Med 1985;102:757–62.

38. Huss H, Jungkind D, Amadio P, Rubenfeld I. Frequency of Chlamydia trachomatis as the cause of pharyngitis. J Clin Microbiol 1985;22:858–60.
39. Reed BD, Huck W, Lutz LJ, Zazove P. Prevalence of Chlamydia trachomatis and *Mycoplasma pneumoniae* in children with and without pharyngitis. J Fam Pract 1988;26:387–92.
40. Terezhalmy GT. Oral manifestations of sexually related diseases. Ear Nose Throat J 1983;62:287–96.
41. Sackel SG, Alpert S, Fiumara NJ, et al. Orogenital contact and the isolation of Neisseria gonorrhoeae, Mycoplasma hominis, and Ureaplasma urealyticum from the pharynx. Sex Transm Dis 1979;6:64–68.
42. Moffet HL, Siegel AC, Doyle HK. Nonstreptococcal pharyngitis. J Pediatr 1968;73:50–60.
43. Huck W, Reed BD, French T, Mitchell RS. Comparison of the directigen 1-2-3 group A strep test with culture for detection of group A beta-hemolytic streptococci. J Clin Microbiol 1989;27:1715–18.
44. Wegner DL, Witte DL, Schrantz RD. Insensitivity of rapid antigen detection methods and single blood agar plate culture for diagnosing streptococcal pharyngitis. JAMA 1992;267:695–7.
45. Pichichero ME, Disney FA, Talpey WB, et al. Adverse and beneficial effects of immediate treatment of group A beta-hemolytic streptococcal pharyngitis with penicillin. Pediatr Infect Dis J 1987;6:635–43.
46. El-Daher NT, Hijazi SS, Rawashdeh NM, et al. Immediate vs. delayed treatment of group A beta-hemolytic streptococcal pharyngitis with penicillin V. Pediatr Infect Dis J 1991;10:126–30.
47. Gerber MA, Randolph MF, DeMeo KK, Kaplan EL. Lack of impact of early antibiotic therapy for streptococcal pharyngitis on recurrence rates. J Pediatr 1990;117:853–8.
48. Idsoe O, Guthe T, Willcox RR, de Weck AL. Nature and extent of penicillin side-reactions with particular reference to fatalities from anaphylactic shock. Bull WHO 1968;38:159–88.
49. Brook I. The role of beta-lactamase-producing bacteria in the persistence of streptococcal tonsillar infection. Rev Infect Dis 1984;6:601–7.
50. Seppala H, Nissinen A, Jarvinen H, et al. Resistance to erythromycin in group A streptococci. N Engl J Med 1992;326:292–7.
51. Charney E, Bynum R, Eldrege D, et al. How well do patients take oral penicillin? A collaborative study in private practice. Pediatrics 1967;40:188–95.
52. Pichichero ME, Margolis PA. A comparison of cephalosporins and penicillins in the treatment of group A beta-hemolytic streptococcal pharyngitis: a meta-analysis supporting the concept of microbial copathogenicity. Pediatr Infect Dis J 1991;10:275–81.
53. Hooton TM. A comparison of azithromycin and penicillin V for the treatment of streptococcal pharyngitis. Am J Med 1991;91:23S–26S.
54. Stein GE, Christensen S, Mummaw N. Comparative study of clarithromycin and penicillin V in the treatment of streptococcal pharyngitis. Eur J Clin Microbiol Infect Dis 1991;10:949–53.
55. Sexually transmitted diseases treatment guidelines. MMWR 1989;38:1–43.

56. Tompkins RK, Burnes DC, Cable WE. An analysis of the cost-effectiveness of pharyngitis management and acute rheumatic fever prevention. Ann Intern Med 1977;86:481–92.
57. Quinn RW, Denny FW, Riley HD. Natural occurrence of hemolytic streptococci in normal school children. Am J Public Health 1956;47:995–1007.
58. Hoffmann S. The throat carrier rate of group A and other beta-hemolytic streptococcal among patients in general practice. Acta Pathol Microbiol Immunol Scand 1985;93:347–51.
59. Brook I, Leyva F. The treatment of the carrier state of group A beta-hemolytic streptococci with clindamycin. Chemotherapy 1988;27:360–7.
60. Gray GC, Escamilla J, Hyams KC, et al. Hyperendemic Streptococcus pyogenes infection despite prophylaxis with penicillin G benzathine. N Engl J Med 1991;325:92–7.
61. Denny FW. The streptococcus saga continues [editorial comment]. N Engl J Med 1991;325:127–8.

CASE PRESENTATION

Subjective

PATIENT PROFILE

Luke Priestley is a 22-year-old married white male graduate student.

PRESENTING PROBLEM

Sore throat.

PRESENT ILLNESS

For 2 days, Mr. Priestley has had a sore throat and fever. There has been slight pain in both ears and a mild cough. He is taking aspirin for the symptoms and has continued to attend classes.

PAST MEDICAL HISTORY

He had a positive tuberculin skin test on entering college 5 years ago. This finding followed a year as an exchange student in Korea.

SOCIAL HISTORY

Mr. Priestley is in his first year as a graduate student in a MBA program. He and his wife, Ann, are expecting their first child in 5 months.

HABITS

He uses no tobacco, alcohol, or recreational drugs.

FAMILY HISTORY

His father died of heart failure at age 55. His mother is living and well at age 57. His sister, aged 26, has mitral valve prolapse.

- What more would you like to know about the history of the present illness, and why?
- What further information would you like to know about Mr. Priestley's school work? Why?

• What family history might be pertinent, and why?
• What additional information might be pertinent about his positive tuberculin skin test?

Objective

Vital Signs

Blood pressure, 120/78; pulse, 88; respirations, 26; temperature, 38.8°C.

Examination

The patient's face appears flushed, and the pitch of his voice seems altered by throat swelling. The tympanic membranes are both mildly injected but not retracted. The throat and tonsils are swollen bilaterally and erythematous. There is bilateral, tender cervical adenopathy. The thyroid is not enlarged. The chest examination reveals a few rhonchi at the bases bilaterally, but no wheezes are heard. The heart has a regular sinus rhythm without murmurs.

Laboratory

A rapid screening test for β-hemolytic streptococcus is positive.

• What more—if anything—would you include in the physical examination, and why?
• Are there other areas of the body that should be examined, and why?
• What might cause you to be concerned about airway obstruction, and how would you address this concern?
• What—if any—laboratory or diagnostic imaging studies would you obtain today? Why?

Assessment

• What is your diagnostic impression, and how would you explain this to Mr. Priestley?
• What might be the meaning of this illness to the patient? To his wife?
• Mr. Priestley asks if he might develop complications of this illness. How would you respond?

- What are the risks that Mr. Priestley's wife or classmates might develop streptococcal pharyngitis, and what—if anything—should be done regarding this risk?

Plan

- Describe your therapeutic recommendations for the patient.
- If the patient were worse in 48 hours, what would you suspect? What would you do?
- Mrs. Priestley asks if there is any risk to the pregnancy. How would you respond?
- What follow-up would you advise?

10
Viral Infections of the Respiratory Tract

GEORGE L. KIRKPATRICK

Viral infections of the respiratory tract are responsible for large amounts of time lost from the workplace and significant morbidity and mortality in the very young and the very old. The worldwide pandemic of influenza in 1918 was alone responsible for nearly 30 million deaths in excess of those expected for influenza. Studies have demonstrated the importance of a variety of viruses, including respiratory syncytial virus (RSV) and parainfluenza virus, which can both cause significant disease in high risk populations. Garibaldi and Brodine[1] reported prevalence rates from 3.0% to 4.6% for all viral respiratory infections in long-term care facilities.

Viruses Involved with Upper Respiratory Tract Infections

Three studies, compared in Table 10.1, reflect similar prevalence rates for the most common upper respiratory tract viruses. A 12-month epidemiologic study of viral respiratory infections in Croatia from September 1, 1986, until August 31, 1987, studied 527 patients.[2] An Indian hospital-based study conducted from 1986 to 1989 on 736 children younger than the age of 5 years proved viral respiratory infections in 22% of the cases by using nasopharyngeal cultures.[3] Finally, in a geriatric setting of institutionalized elderly, Falsey and Treanor found 149 nursing home residents with upper respiratory tract illnesses during a 3-month period.[4]

Respiratory Syncytial Virus

RSV, a single-stranded RNA paramyxovirus, is the leading cause of pneumonia and bronchiolitis in infants and children. Two antigenically distinct groups of RSV (A and B) are recognized. Community outbreaks of RSV usually appear during the winter and spring in temperate climates. The diagnosis of RSV in the acute setting is usually obtained by viral culture of

TABLE 10.1. Prevalence of common upper respiratory tract viruses

Virus	Croatia study		Indian hospital study		Nursing home study	
	Patients	Prevalence (%)	Patients	Prevalence (%)	Patients	Prevalence (%)
Respiratory syncytial virus	177	33.6	37	5	18	12
Rhinoviruses					14	9.4
Herpes simplex	8	1.3			6	4
Parainfluenza (types 1, 2, 3)	12	2.3	38	5	3	2
Influenza (types A and B)	3	0.6	45	6	0	0
Adenoviruses	40	7.6	22	3		
Coronaviruses						
Enteroviruses	18	4.0				
Measles virus			23	3		
Mixed infections	9	1.5			2	1.3

nasopharyngeal secretions. A rapid diagnostic test (Abbott test pack RSV; Directigen RSV by Becton Dickinson) using antigen detection in nasal secretions is relatively sensitive and specific in both children and elderly.

The spectrum of illness associated with RSV is broad, ranging from mild nasal congestion to high fever and respiratory distress. RSV tends to peak during early January most years. Evidence suggests that in infants group A viruses are associated with more severe infections than group B viruses.[5] Modes of spread are primarily via large droplet inoculation (requiring close contact) and self-inoculation via contaminated fomites or skin. RSV is recoverable from countertops for up to 6 hours from the time of contamination; from rubber gloves for up to 90 minutes; and from skin for up to 20 minutes. Viral shedding of RSV in infants is a prolonged process averaging 7 days. Strategies for controlling spread of RSV should be aimed at interrupting hand carriage of the virus and self-inoculation of the eyes and nose. Masks commonly used for respiratory viruses have not been shown to be an effective measure in curtailing RSV outbreaks on pediatric wards. Hand washing is probably the single most important infection control measure for RSV.

Influenza Viruses

Influenza, often considered a benign disease today, has ravaged human populations recently enough that there are still those living who can recall the 1918 worldwide pandemic called the "Spanish flu." This particular influenza was described as beginning with what appeared to be an ordinary attack of influenza and rapidly developing into severe pneumonia. Two hours after admission, the patients would have mahogany-colored spots over the cheek bones; within a few hours, cyanosis would begin spreading over the face. Shortly, death would overcome patients as they struggled for air and suffocated. The second documented pandemic of influenza occurred in 1957, when an outbreak of type A (antigenic determinant H2N2) from South Central China encircled the globe. Eleven years later, another epidemic emerged from eastern Asia caused by an H3N2 influenza type A. Both epidemics were associated with extensive morbidity and a marked increase in mortality, but neither was as vicious as the epidemic of 1918.

During 1977 to 1978, the National Health Survey estimated that 101 million acute respiratory illnesses caused by all types of respiratory viruses were medically attended in the United States. As many as 20 million cases could have been prevented by effective influenza prophylaxis. In addition to the predominant influenza virus that invades an area each season, many types, subtypes, or variants are identified during each epidemic period. These antigenically distinct viruses produce "herald waves." For several successive years, a relatively small wave of infections with an antigenically distinct virus can occur during the second half of an epidemic and herald the epidemic virus for the following year. For example, during the influenza A/Victoria epidemic of 1976, a few infections with influenza type B/Hong Kong were detected. This virus became epidemic the following year. A small wave of influenza type A (H3N2) infections during the second half of the influenza type B/Hong Kong epidemic in 1977 became epidemic during the following season. These herald waves are useful to epidemiologists for predicting what viral antigens should be included in each new season's vaccine. During the early stage of an epidemic, a disproportionate number of cases involve school-age children, 10 to 19 years old. Later in the epidemic, more cases are diagnosed in younger children and adults. This age shift suggests that the early spread of influenza viruses in a community is concentrated among school-age children.

Another characteristic of influenza virus is the decreased rate of infection in children living in urban areas compared with those living in rural areas. In 1974, the rate of influenza B was four times greater for children living in rural areas of Michigan than in the urban areas. Children of low income families in urban areas tend to become infected earlier in life and have milder illnesses. When these children experience intensive exposure to influenza type B during their school years, they may have immunity that is relatively more protective than that of children in the rural areas, who had less prior exposure.[6]

Parainfluenza Viruses

Parainfluenza is a single-strand RNA virus of which four serotypes and two subtypes are recognized (parainfluenza types 1, 2, 3, 4A, and 4B). Peak activity of parainfluenza illness tends to occur in the fall and spring. These viruses can cause acute bronchitis and pneumonia in young children. Most persons have been infected with parainfluenza virus by age 5 years. Immunity to parainfluenza is incomplete; and as with RSV, reinfection occurs throughout life. Parainfluenza types 1 and 2 tend to peak during the autumn of the year, whereas parainfluenza type 3 shows an increased prevalence during late spring. Adult infection results in mild upper respiratory tract symptoms, although pneumonia occasionally occurs. Outbreaks of parainfluenza types 1 and 3 have been reported from long-term care facilities.[7] Illness was characterized by fever, sore throat, rhinorrhea, and cough. The rate of pneumonia was relatively high. With parainfluenza type 1, the rate was 17%, and with parainfluenza type 3, the rate was 29% including several deaths.

Most studies suggest direct person-to-person transmission. Parainfluenza is stable in small-particle aerosols at the low humidity found in hospitals. However, outbreaks tend to proceed more slowly than influenza or other aerosol-spread infections.[8] Infection control policies should emphasize hand washing and isolation of patients.

Rhinoviruses

Rhinovirus is the most frequent cause of upper respiratory tract infections in adults. More than 100 antigenic types have been identified, and reinfection occurs throughout life. In temperate climates, rhinovirus infection shows spring and fall peaks of activity.[9] Diagnosis of a rhinovirus infection is made by viral culture of nasopharyngeal secretions. In the healthy adult, rhinovirus infection is self-limited and characterized by sneezing, rhinorrhea, and a mild sore throat. Although cough is common, direct viral invasion of the respiratory tract is rare. Unlike other respiratory viruses, such as influenza or adenoviruses, rhinovirus infections produce relatively minor damage to the nasal epithelium and probably no damage to the tracheal mucosa. Because rhinovirus replication is reduced at elevated body temperatures, direct invasion of the lower respiratory tract is unusual at all ages.

In one study, rhinovirus infections produced the first seasonal peak of respiratory infections in a long-term care facility.[10] Seasonal peaks occur most frequently between September and November. Rhinoviruses are easily transmitted by contact with infected secretions. The most efficient modes of spread are hand-to-hand contact or direct contact with a contaminated surface followed by inoculation of the nose or conjunctiva. Rhinoviruses remain infectious for as long as 3 hours on nonporous surfaces. Transmission can be decreased by hand washing and disinfection of environmental surfaces.

Coronaviruses

Coronaviruses are single-stranded RNA viruses that have been identified as a major cause of colds in the general population. Epidemics occur during the winter and early spring.[11] Infections in volunteers produced an illness similar to rhinovirus infection. Those infections produced malaise, headaches, and sore throat. Low-grade fever was present in approximately 20% of the patients. Upper respiratory tract infection is the most common result of coronavirus invasion. Coronaviruses have also been associated with exacerbations of chronic pulmonary diseases.

Diagnosis is difficult because the organism is not easy to isolate, and serology is generally not available. In a study of 11 long-term care facilities by Nicholson and Baker,[12] patients with respiratory illnesses were analyzed for evidence of coronavirus infections. Antibodies to the two most well-studied antigenic strains of coronavirus (229 E and OC43) were detected by enzyme-linked immunosorbent assay (ELISA). It was noted that illnesses were indistinguishable from RSV and influenza infections. Lower respiratory complications, such as pneumonia, occurred on one-fourth of the infected residents.

Adenoviruses

Adenoviruses are double-stranded DNA viruses, with 41 recognized serotypes that most commonly cause infections in children. Coryza, pharyngitis, pneumonia, pharyngoconjunctival fever, and epidemic keratoconjunctivitis are all attributable to adenoviruses. Transmission can occur by aerosolized droplets, fomites, and hand carriage as well as the fecal–oral route. The virus can be isolated for prolonged periods from respiratory secretions, conjunctival secretions, and stools of infected patients. The identification of adenoviruses can be confirmed by viral cultures, but the genetic heterogeneity of adenoviruses makes the information of little value. Studies have failed to show a significant incidence of infection in long-term care facilities for children or elderly patients. However, should an outbreak of adenovirus occur, strategies for control should take into account the various modes of transmission.

Herpes Simplex and Measles Viruses

Herpes simplex and measles viruses are rarely cultured from nasopharyngeal secretions. In one study,[3] measles virus was found in 3% of nasopharyngeal cultures. The study also showed a case-fatality rate of 43% among patients from whom the measles virus was cultured. Similarly, herpes simplex virus showed a prevalence of 1.3% in nasopharyngeal cultures. There was no speculation about its involvement as a causative agent in the upper respiratory symptomatology.

Disease Presentations

Common Cold

The common cold, a disease of antiquity, is characterized by objective signs and subjective symptoms that are usually self-limited. Symptoms that occur with common colds include sneezing, watering of the eyes, nasal stuffiness, nasal obstruction, postnasal discharge, sore throat, hoarseness, cough, and sputum production. The common cold is a clinical diagnosis and lacks specificity because other ailments such as allergies and early effects of more serious illnesses mimic common cold symptoms.

Diagnosis

Rhinoviruses, coronaviruses, and RSV are most likely to produce the clinical findings of the common cold. These viruses are identifiable on culture. Neutralization tests with specific rabbit serum identify the rhinoviruses and the coronaviruses. RSV may be identified by immunofluorescence staining of cultured cells or ELISA studies. It is also possible to use specific immunoglobulin G assays to identify rhinoviruses and coronaviruses. These tests take time, require nasopharyngeal washings or blood samples, and are an expensive way to make a definitive diagnosis.

In one study,[13] 420 subjects were exposed to one of a variety of respiratory viruses, including rhinoviruses types 2, 9, and 14, RSV, and coronavirus, or in a control sample simply containing saline drops. Results showed that 82% of the subjects who received intranasal drops containing virus became infected and showed signs and symptoms typical of the common cold.

Management

There are as many ways to manage the common cold as there are physicians. The use of antibiotics for the treatment of a common cold is of no proved value, as antibiotics have no effect on the viruses involved. Berkowitz and Tinkelman[14] studied the effects of a nonsedating antihistamine for treating rhinitis symptoms associated with the common cold and concluded that neither the symptoms nor the signs of the common cold were alleviated to any degree. Rest, adequate hydration, and time to recover should be stressed during management of the common cold.

Complications and Sequelae

When the diagnosis of the common cold is accurate, complications and sequelae are minimal. Those cases of the common cold caused by RSV are associated with significantly more fever and respiratory distress. More children than adults die as a result of RSV infections, although some deaths are reported in most studies. There are few if any deaths from rhinoviral or coronaviral common colds.

Control and Prevention

Hand washing is the most important way to prevent transmission of these viruses. With rhinoviruses and RSV, direct contact with a contaminated surface followed by inoculation of the nose or conjunctiva can result in infection. Use of masks and gloves and isolation of infected persons are the most effective ways to limit the spread of cold viruses. With minimal symptoms and multiple sources of infection in the community, however, these measures are not practical.

Influenza

Influenza has one of the more characteristic sets of clinical findings. Onset is usually sudden, with shivering, sweating, headache, aching in the orbits, and general malaise and misery. Cough is often found early in the course, aggravating headaches and causing generalized aching. Onset is generally explosive with fever in adults ranging up to 102°F. In children, the fever may be higher than 102°F, and sore throat may be an early sign. The most consistent signs are the presence of polymyalgias, weakness, and malaise.

Diagnosis

Not surprisingly, the diagnosis of influenza is more accurate during epidemics and less accurate during nonepidemic periods. Influenza in the United States usually occurs during December, January, and February. Some years, epidemics have begun earlier or continued beyond February. Successful presumptive diagnosis requires appropriate clinical symptomatology at the right time of the year and a knowledge of the pattern of influenzal illness around the world. Virologic studies, including cultures from throat swabs and nasopharyngeal washings, cells from nasopharyngeal washings stained with monoclonal antibody fluorescence stains, and complement fixation studies on paired serum samples can confirm the diagnosis. The hospital virology laboratory can suggest the most appropriate test for each case.

Management

Management of influenza is generally symptomatic. If the family physician is fairly sure that the virus in question is type A influenza, the patient may benefit greatly from the use of amantadine. Amantadine (Symmetrel) in a dose of 200 mg/day has long been known to be excellent prophylaxis against type A influenza.[15] It is most effective if started early in the course of the disease, although it does reduce symptoms and shortens the course of illness even if started 3 to 5 days into the disease process. The dose of amantadine is 100 mg two times a day except for patients who have compromised renal function, for whom dosage adjustment is necessary. Because of the severity of the myalgias and headache associated with influenza, physicians should prescribe appropriate analgesics adequate to relieve discomfort. Aspirin and nonsteroidal antiinflammatory drugs may not suffice and a narcotic-containing product is frequently indicated. With good instructions, the patient can get double benefit from codeine or hydrocodone by reducing not only the myalgias but the cough.

Amantadine is not effective for treating influenza type B. Preparing cultures or determining complement fixation titers does not provide information early enough on which to base the decision to use amantadine. Epidemiologic information is more useful.

Complications and Sequelae

Most statistical methods for assessing excess morbidity and mortality are based on an index of influenza complicated by pneumonia, which may produce an underestimation of the serious morbidity and mortality. Twice as many deaths during an influenza epidemic are attributable to ischemic heart disease than to pneumonia.[16] Glezen[16] studied hospital admissions with the diagnosis of acute respiratory disease during the period 1975 to 1976. From July 1, 1975, through June 30, 1976, 3301 hospitalized patients were assessed with the admission diagnosis of acute respiratory disease. Pneumonia was the most frequent reason for admission (52.5%). Acute bronchitis and bronchiolitis caused admission 18.9% of the time. Influenza and other respiratory disease were the cause 21.4% of the time.

Glezen also noted that the rate of hospitalization with acute respiratory disease during the influenza A/Victoria epidemic varied by age group. Infants younger than age 1 year had a hospitalization rate of 160 per 10,000 patients. Patients between age 1 and 65 years had low hospitalization rates, whereas those older than 65 had a rate of 167 per 10,000. Other studies have shown that the rate of infection is highest in the school-age population. In Glezen's study, the rates of hospitalization were low in the school-age group that normally would have had the highest rates of infection.

Family Issues

Because of the considerably higher rates of infection in school-age children, families with such children are much more likely to form clusters of influenza cases. The spread of infection goes from the child attending school to young children in the home and elderly family members.

Control and Prevention

Important epidemiologically are the facts that (1) influenza vaccine is produced each year, and (2) amantadine can be used prophylactically. The problem practitioners have using amantadine is knowing when to start and stop prophylaxis. Influenza vaccine is produced on the recommendation of the Food and Drug Administration Vaccines and Related Biologicals Advisory Committee. Antigenic choices are based on (1) the viruses that have been seen during the previous year, (2) the viruses that are being seen in other parts of the world during the current year, and (3) the estimated antibody response in persons previously infected or vaccinated to these viruses. For example, the vaccine for the 1992 to 1993 influenza season[17] contained A/Texas, which is an H1N1 virus. It also contained A/Beijing, which is an H3N2 influenza virus, and the third viral component was a B/Panama-like influenza virus.

There are two basic strategies for the use of vaccines and chemotherapy. A current strategy is to immunize high-risk groups (the elderly and children with underlying conditions including heart, pulmonary, malignant, and some metabolic diseases).[18] Unfortunately, the level of acceptance by patients and the overall delivery of vaccines to high-risk children has been consistently poor. This approach leaves most of the population unvaccinated, which produces a large "at risk" population who can be infected. Healthy persons who become infected spread their infection to non-immunized high-risk children. Another approach to the control of influenza is to immunize all schoolchildren, children in day care, college students, military personnel, and employees of large companies. These groups have the highest susceptibility and, because of the nature of their activities, are the principal vectors of influenza virus in the community. They are also an accessible population with a structured environment that permits effective distribution of influenza vaccine. Efforts should also be directed toward immunizing as many high-risk patients as possible or to start them on amantadine at the first evidence of an epidemic.

Bronchitis

Diagnosis

Bronchitis is an inflammation of the major and minor bronchial branches. It is characterized by a cough that is frequently productive of sputum, depending on the inflammatory cause. Bacterial causes of bronchitis generally produce purulent-looking sputum. Viral causes of bronchitis can cause purulent-appearing sputum but more commonly produce either clear sputum or there is a nonproductive cough. On physical examination, a patient with bronchitis has a noticeable cough but is usually normal to auscultation except for a few scattered rhonchi. Rales, dullness to percussion, egophony, and other lower respiratory findings are usually absent. Cigarette smoking, other air pollutants, and chemical exposures that cause bronchial irritation may prolong an episode of bronchitis. Systemic lupus erythematosus can be a cause of persistent bronchitis in a few affected patients.[19]

Spectrum of Infection

Studies indicate that viral causes of acute bronchitis tend to be more common with influenza (types A and B), parainfluenza of all four serotypes, and RSV. Coronavirus and adenoviruses cause bronchitis less commonly. RSV and parainfluenza viruses are found more commonly in the younger population, and coronaviruses and adenoviruses occur in older patients. Influenza causes bronchitis in all ages. Rhinovirus is the most frequent cause of upper respiratory tract infection in adults and can be a cause of coughing.

Complications and Sequelae

Liou and colleagues[18] studied an influenza type B outbreak in Philadelphia from December 1985 through April 1986 and found that all patients who had positive cultures for influenza type B were younger than the age of 3 years. Fifty percent of these patients had cough and fever associated with their symptoms. Glezen,[16] in a study of hospitalized patients with acute respiratory diagnoses, found acute bronchitis in 18.9%. Glezen also found that adult admissions for bronchitis showed an appreciable increase only during the influenza A/Victoria epidemic, and pediatric admissions for bronchitis increased during the autumn parainfluenza types 1 and 2 epidemic and the RSV outbreak in December. Falsey and Treanor[4] reported that in institutionalized elderly patients RSV was likely to cause bronchitis, whereas rhinovirus was more likely to cause rhinorrhea with cough as a secondary symptom. Sputum production was considerably less frequent with the rhinovirus infection than with RSV infection. Bronchitis due to parainfluenza virus is common in young children. Reinfection by parainfluenza in young healthy adults typically presents as an upper respiratory infection including bronchitis. In the elderly, parainfluenza virus is not as common a cause of bronchitis and is much more likely to cause rhinorrhea, pharyngitis, and lower respiratory tract infections.

Viral Croup

Although croup is a frightening family experience, especially for new parents of very young children, it is a self-limited illness. Patients usually respond to breathing cool air (or in some cases, warm mist in a steamed bathroom) and require little additional therapy. Those cases of croup that are not resolved by the time the family comes to the office or emergency department usually respond to racemic epinephrine administered as an aerosol. Physicians should look for the coexistence of underlying illnesses and reassure the family that croup is a manageable illness. Croup is a viral illness caused by several upper respiratory viral agents. In fact, during the outbreak of influenza type B in Philadelphia in 1985 and 1986, Liou et al.[18] found that 4% of the children in their study younger than 3 years of age had croup. Croup is common in young children and is due to parainfluenza during the fall and spring. Croup is not commonly associated with rhinovirus infections but is associated with coronavirus infections. Adenovirus is a common cause of croup in children and occurs sporadically throughout the year, being most common during the winter and spring.

Bronchiolitis

Clinical Picture

Bronchiolitis is an acute viral respiratory disease generally found in children younger than 2 years old. The typical clinical presentation is an upper respiratory infection with cough that progresses to a more severe cough and tachypnea. Respirations become rapid and shallow with a prolonged expiratory phase. Because the infants are not able to breathe well, they are also unable to suck or drink and so can become dehydrated.

Diagnosis

Physical findings include intercostal retractions and nasal flaring, which may suggest pneumonia. A chest roentgenogram shows only hyperinflation with no infiltrates. Tight respiratory sounds (not entirely typical of wheezes found with asthma) are usually present, as are some rhonchi. Rales and dullness to percussion suggest the coexistence of pneumonia.

Bronchiolitis is most commonly caused by RSV, occurring predominantly during the winter and spring. Parainfluenza viruses, particularly types 1 and 2, can cause bronchiolitis during early winter. The most severe cases of bronchiolitis are usually caused by influenza viruses, especially type A. The virus involved can be identified by culture of nasopharyngeal secretions. Serologic techniques such as the ELISA and complement fixation studies are available for retrospective diagnosis, if needed.

Management

Management of bronchiolitis depends on the progression of signs and symptoms. Hospitalization may be necessary to correct hypoxemia or dehydration. If fever is significant, pneumonia must be ruled out. Cases that appear to be recurrent bronchiolitis may be asthma, even if the child is younger than 1 year old.

Outpatient treatment is generally supportive, with careful attention to hydration. If hospitalization becomes necessary to correct hypoxemia or dehydration, treatment is focused on oxygenation, mist, and mechanically clearing the upper airway.

Complications and Sequelae

The most serious complication of bronchiolitis is respiratory failure requiring ventilatory assistance. It is best managed with continuous positive airway pressure and oxygen. Steroids and antibiotics are of questionable benefit for treating even the most severe cases of bronchiolitis. Ribavirin (Virazole) is useful as a continuous aerosol when RSV causes bronchiolitis. Ribavirin (6 g in 300 ml of water) is aerosolized in a small croup tent 16 to 20 hours a day for a minimum of 3 days up to 6 days.

Family Issues

Family support is particularly important when infants require hospitalization. Many children subsequently wheeze with other viral respiratory illnesses, which alarms the family. The family needs to know that the long-term prognosis is excellent. Some research suggests that pulmonary function remains impaired in these children, especially those who have serious underlying respiratory or cardiovascular diseases.

Pharyngoconjunctival Fever

Pharyngoconjunctival fever is an upper respiratory illness that affects teenagers and adults. It manifests as pharyngitis, cough, fever, headache, myalgias, malaise, and particularly conjunctivitis. This is a syndrome caused by adenoviruses, particularly serotypes 3 and 7. These viruses are frequently found in natural bodies of water and reservoirs.

Symptoms may be similar to those of influenza. Conjunctivitis is generally not present with influenza but is always found with pharyngoconjunctival fever and usually at an early stage. There is a spring and summer seasonal prevalence. It can be diagnosed by viral cultures of nasopharyngeal and throat swabs or paired complement fixation antibody studies for adenovirus.

Management of pharyngoconjunctival fever is symptomatic. There is no indication for systemic antibiotic treatment or ophthalmic antibiotics. There are no long-term complications or sequelae. Recovery is generally complete within 1 week.

Laryngitis

There are six distinct causes of laryngitis, the most common being viral infections of the upper respiratory tract. Vocal cord tumors can cause laryngitis; allergies are a frequent cause; and strain of the vocal cords caused by long periods of loud talking produces laryngitis. A fairly frequent cause of laryngitis is hard coughing associated with either an upper or lower respiratory tract infection. The least frequent cause is a bacterial infection of the throat.

Most of the causes of laryngitis are obvious. Viral laryngitis is difficult to distinguish from the less frequent bacterial laryngitis that might require antibiotic treatment.

Children older than age 2 years and adults rarely have significant swelling of the throat that would put them at risk of airway obstruction. Children younger than age 2 years are more likely to develop airway obstruction. Viral causes of laryngitis include the parainfluenza viruses, rhinoviruses, adenoviruses, and the influenza viruses.

Voice rest makes the greatest impact on recovery. Patients who are able to gargle with warm, very weak saline solution sometimes find it soothing. Being a fairly common complaint in the family physician's office, patients should be told that it is not a serious disease and that adequate time to recover is the only therapy in most cases.

Viral Respiratory Tract Infections in Very Young and Old Patients

Patients younger than age 2 years present some special problems. Perhaps as many as two-thirds of pediatric emergency department visits for respiratory infections are inappropriate.

Mayefsky and El-Shinaway[20] studied the pediatric emergency department at Cook County Hospital in Chicago, where 60,000 children between the ages of birth and 16 years of age were seen annually. Mayefsky and El-Shinaway concluded that parents using the emergency department for evaluation of their children's colds have reasonable concerns for the health of their children. More than 50% of the parents needed only reassurance that their child was not seriously ill.

Mullooly and Barker[21] studied the impact of type A influenza on children at the Kaiser-Permanente Medical Care Program in Oregon from 1968 to 1973. They compared excess morbidity with excess rates of hospitalization for influenza-related conditions. Excess hospitalization rates for the younger-than-age-4 group during influenza epidemics were three to five times higher than the rates for children older than age 4 years.

TABLE 10.2. Patterns of viral illness in children and elderly patients

Virus	Signs and symptoms		
	Young children	Adults	Elderly
Respiratory syncytial virus	Wheezing, bronchiolitis pneumonia, bronchitis	Nasal congestion and cough	Nasal congestion, cough, fever, pneumonia, wheezing, bronchitis
Influenza	Sore throat, high fever, myalgias, bronchitis, croup, bronchiolitis, rhinorrhea, otitis media	Fever, headache, myalgias, malaise, cough, weakness, bronchitis, laryngitis	Bronchitis, low-grade fever, sore throat, pneumonia
Parainfluenza	Croup, bronchitis, pneumonia, sore throat, bronchiolitis	Common cold, laryngitis	Rhinorrhea, sore throat, cough, pneumonia, fever
Rhinoviruses	Sore throat, rhinorrhea	Rhinorrhea, sneezing, cough, sore throat, laryngitis	Rhinorrhea, cough, sneezing
Coronaviruses	Croup, sore throat	Common cold, malaise, headache, sore throat, low-grade fever	Exacerbation of chronic pulmonary disease, pneumonia, bronchitis
Adenoviruses	Croup, sore throat	Coryza, sore throat, pneumonia, pharyngoconjunctival fever, keratoconjunctivitis, laryngitis	Bronchitis rarely

The study by Sugaya and Nerome[22] in Japan during the winter of 1989 and spring of 1990, where the epidemics of influenza type A H3N2 and influenza type B viruses were severe, showed a remarkable increase in the number of pediatric admissions.

Although most respiratory virus infections in children appear to be self-limited and without complications or sequelae, mortality statistics in 1976 showed that infections of the respiratory tract rank third among the leading causes of death in infants 28 days to 1 year of age and second in children between 1 and 4 years of age. Table 10.2 details the patterns of viral illness found in young children, adults, and elderly patients.[23, 24]

The institutionalized elderly represent a subgroup of older people who are prone to excess morbidity and mortality from respiratory tract infections. Each year many elderly persons living in long-term care facilities become ill with respiratory illnesses that are mistakenly attributed to bacterial pneumonia or influenza. The respiratory tract viruses seen in

Table 10.2 (particularly RSV, parainfluenza virus, and influenza virus) are a significant cause of disease in this high-risk population. Large epidemiologic studies have found a predominance of noninfluenza agents responsible for respiratory tract disease. RSV ranks second to influenza as the most common cause of serious viral respiratory infections in long-term care facility patients. A significant number of reported deaths are of cardiovascular origin, related to the viral infection rather to pneumonia.[16] The pattern of reported outbreaks of RSV in a long-term care facility is usually a steady trickle of cases over several months—distinctly different from outbreaks of influenza, which tend to be explosive. Parainfluenza virus is a common cause of croup and bronchitis in young children; however, because full immunity does not develop, reinfection is common in the older population. In the institutionalized elderly, parainfluenza presents as rhinorrhea, pharyngitis, cough, and pneumonia.

References

1. Garibaldi RA, Brodine S. Infections among patients in nursing homes: policies, prevalence, and problems. N Engl J Med 1982;305:731–5.
2. Mlinaric G. Epidemiological picture of respiratory viral infections in Croatia. Acta Med Iugosl 1991;45:203–11.
3. Jain A. An Indian hospital study of viral causes of acute respiratory infection in children. J Med Microbiol 1991;35:219–23.
4. Falsey AR, Treanor JJ. Viral respiratory infections in the institutionalized elderly; clinical and epidemiology findings. J Am Geriatr Soc 1992;40:115–9.
5. McConnochie KM, Hall CB. Variation in severity of respiratory syncytial viruses with subtype. J Pediatr 1990;117:52–58.
6. Glezen WP. Consideration of the risk of influenza in children and indications for prophylaxis. Rev Infect Dis 1980;2:408–20.
7. Public Health Laboratory Service Communicable Disease Surveillance Center. Parainfluenza infections in the elderly 1976–1982. BMJ 1983;287:1619.
8. Graman PS, Hall CB. Epidemiology and control of nosocomial viral infections. Infect Dis Clin North Am 1989;3:815–41.
9. Gwaltney JM, Mandell GL, Douglas RG Jr. Principles and practices of infectious diseases, 3rd ed. New York: Churchill Livingstone, 1989:1399–1404.
10. Grose PA, Rodstein M. Epidemiology of acute respiratory illness during an influenza outbreak in a nursing home: a prospective study. Arch Intern Med 1988;148:559–61.
11. Larsen HE, Reed JE. Isolation of rhinoviruses and coronaviruses from 38 colds in adults. J Med Virol 1980;5:221–9.
12. Nicholson KG, Baker DJ. Acute upper respiratory tract illness and influenza immunizations in homes for the elderly. Epidemiol Infect 1990;105:609–18.
13. Cohen S, Tyrrell DAJ. Psychological stress and susceptibility to the common cold. N Engl J Med 1991;29:606–11.

14. Berkowitz RB, Tinkelman DG. Evaluation of oral terfenadine for treatment of the common cold. Ann Allergy 1991;67:593–7.
15. Kobayashi JM. Control of influenza A outbreaks in nursing homes: amantadine as an adjunct to vaccine—Washington, 1989–90. MMWR 1991;40: 841–4.
16. Glezen WP. Serious morbidity and mortality associated with influenza epidemics. Epidemiol Rev 1982;4:25–43.
17. Nerome K, Chakraverty M. Update: influenza activity—United States and worldwide, and composition of the 1992–1993 influenza vaccine. MMWR 1992;41:316–7.
18. Liou YS, Barbour SD, Bell LM. Children hospitalized with influenza B infection. Pediatr Infect Dis J 1987;6:541–3.
19. Raz E, Bursztyn M. Severe recurrent lupus laryngitis. Am J Med 1992;92: 109–10.
20. Mayefsky JH, El-Shinaway Y. Families who seek care for the common cold in a pediatric emergency department. J Pediatr 1991; 119:933–4.
21. Mullooly JP, Barker WH. Impact of type A influenza on children: a retrospective study. Am J Public Health 1982;72:1008–16.
22. Sugaya N, Nerome K. Impact of influenza virus infection as a cause of pediatric hospitalization. J Infect Dis 1992;165:373–5.
23. Bardin PG, Johnston SL, Pattemore PK. Viruses as precipitants of asthma symptoms. Clin Exp Allergy 1992;22(9):809–22.
24. Busse WW, Lemanske RF, Dick EC. The relationship of viral respiratory infections and asthma. Chest 1992;101:3855–85.

Case Presentation

Subjective

Patient Profile

Kendra Nelson is a 16-year-old single white female high school sophomore.

Presenting Problem

Fever and weakness.

Present Illness

For the past day-and-a-half, Kendra has felt weak and achy. She has had a temperature of 103°F at home. There is a generalized headache, a mild cough, and a decreased appetite. A few of her schoolmates have had similar symptoms.

Past Medical History

No prior hospitalization or serious injury.

Social History

Kendra lives with her parents. She is a "good student" and has had a steady boyfriend for the past year.

Habits

She uses no tobacco, alcohol, or coffee.

Family History

Her parents are living and well. She has one sibling, aged 19, who is away from home in the Army.

- What additional historical information might be useful, and why?
- What might be the meaning of this illness to the patient?
- Would further information regarding her classmates or boyfriend be helpful? Why?

- What are likely adaptations of this teenager to her illness? Why might this be pertinent?

Objective

VITAL SIGNS

Blood pressure, 104/60; pulse, 86; respirations, 22; temperature, 38.6°C.

EXAMINATION

The patient is alert and ambulatory but looks "ill." The tympanic membranes are normal. The pharynx is mildly injected. The neck is supple without adenopathy, and the thyroid gland is normal. Her chest is clear. The heart has a normal sinus rhythm with no murmurs present.

- What further information about the physical examination might be useful, and why?
- What other areas of the body—if any—should be examined? Why?
- What—if any—laboratory tests should be obtained today? Why?
- What—if any—diagnostic imaging studies should be obtained today?

Assessment

- What is the likely diagnosis, and how would you explain this to the patient and her parents?
- Kendra's mother asks if Kendra is likely to be even worse during the next few days and what to do if this occurs. How would you reply?
- If the patient also had a rash, what diagnoses would you consider?
- What are the family/community implications of this illness?

Plan

- What would be your therapeutic recommendation to Kendra regarding medication, diet, pain relief, and return to school?
- Kendra asks about the possibility of others catching her illness. How would you reply?
- Kendra's mother asks about preventing such an illness in the future. How would you respond?
- What continuing care would you recommend?

11

Otitis Media and Externa

Jo Ann Rosenfeld

Otitis Media

Otitis media is one of the most frequent illnesses that affects children. Although family physicians see patients with this diagnosis repeatedly and it has been studied extensively, there are still basic controversies concerning its treatment. Infection and inflammation in the middle ear has been called by many names. Acute otitis media (AOM) is short-lived, purulent, and infectious in origin. Infection can recur or persist. Serous otitis media is usually inflammatory and chronic, although it may be infectious. The latter has also been called otitis media with effusion, chronic otitis media, or chronic mucoid otitis media ("glue ear").

Incidence

Otitis media is the most frequent reason parents bring their children into physicians' offices and the most common diagnosis made by physicians who care for children.[1–3] It is virtually a universal experience; by the age of 3 years approximately two of three children have experienced at least one episode of AOM, and one-third have had three or more episodes.[2–4] In the United States, AOM accounts for one-third of all visits to a physician during the first year of life for illness—approximately 30 million office visits per year.[1,3–6] More than one-fourth of the prescriptions written per year for antibiotics are for the treatment of AOM.[1,3] Two billion dollars is spent annually on medical and surgical treatment of otitis media in United States.[2]

Acute Otitis Media in Children

Epidemiology

Certain groups of children are more likely to acquire AOM and its complications. AOM is seasonal, more common during the winter than the summer.[2,7,8] Bottle-fed children, especially those put to bed with bottles,

223

are more likely to develop AOM.[9,10] Boys have AOM more often than girls.[2,7,11] Premature infants and children younger than age 2 years are more likely to have ear infections. The incidence of AOM decreases with advancing age, becoming much less common after age 7 years.[2,4,6,7,12–14] American Indians and Eskimos are much more likely to experience severe, prolonged, and repetitive otitis. Children who attend day care centers, those living with siblings with otitis media, those in a home with many children or in a home with smokers, and those of lower socioeconomic levels are more likely to have more episodes of AOM.[2,6,7] Because of developmental and anatomic abnormalities of the upper respiratory tract and ear, children who have cleft lip or palate (or both) or Down syndrome are much more likely to develop early repeated AOM.[2,15]

Etiology

The most important factor that contributes to AOM is abnormal functioning of the eustachian tube. A dysfunctional eustachian tube may allow reflux aspiration of fluid and bacteria from the nasopharynx into the middle ear.[2,16] Other possible etiologies are extension of infection from nearby sites, hematogenous spread of bacteria, and primary mucosal disease of the middle ear as a result of allergy.[2]

Approximately 3.5 cm in length in adults, the eustachian tube has an hourglass shape and is lined with respiratory mucosa. The middle section is bony, and the nasopharyngeal section is cartilaginous. In children, significant lymphoid tissue is present underneath the lining of the eustachian tube and in the middle ear. The eustachian tube has three functions: (1) regulation of pressure in the middle ear; (2) protection of the middle ear from nasopharyngeal secretions; and (3) clearance of secretions from the middle ear into the nasopharynx.[2,17] These functions are accomplished by intermittent active opening of the tube by contraction of the veli palatini muscles.[3,17–19]

The eustachian tube can malfunction two ways. The more common way is a functional abnormality, occurring in small children and infants. The eustachian tube is more flexible in younger children than it is in older children, causing moderate negative pressures, which may allow fluid to accumulate. Children also have shorter eustachian tubes; it is proposed that the same volume of secretions that may be stopped by the longer adult tubes may reach the middle ear in children. Fluid is more likely to accumulate in the middle ear in the supine position, a position that is more likely to occur, and for longer periods, in infants and young children.[17] Even in apparently otologically normal children, the eustachian tube does not work as efficiently as it does in adults. Children are less able to equilibrate negative intratympanic pressure by swallowing. Studies have shown that the veli palatine muscles are relatively small in children and may not function efficiently to clear the eustachian tube until after age

6 years. Function improves with age; children ages 7 to 12 years had more efficiently functioning eustachian tubes than those aged 3 to 6 years.[17]

Mechanical dysfunction of the eustachian tube may also be caused by congenital or acquired physical abnormalities, as in children with cleft lip or palate, Down syndrome, or acquired extrinsic masses such as inflammation of the nasal mucosa due to infection, allergy, or tumors. In children with cleft palate, the palatal muscles are underdeveloped and often inserted incorrectly, predisposing the child to otitis.[17,20] Thousands of adenoidectomies were performed to correct hypertrophy of the adenoid tissues, which was thought to cause extrinsic pressure on the eustachian tube, and to prevent recurrent AOM and chronic serous otitis media (CSOM).[21–26] In 1979, approximately 634,000 adenoidectomies were performed, making adenoidectomy at that time the most common pediatric surgical procedure requiring anesthesia.[4]

Many factors complicate already poor eustachian tube function, predisposing the child to AOM. Upper respiratory tract infections (URIs) and AOM occur more frequently during fall, winter, and spring and less often in summer.[17,27] Viruses that cause URIs, such as respiratory syncytial virus (RSV), type 2 parainfluenza viruses, rhinoviruses, and adenoviruses, have been recovered from middle ear fluid. In one study, both bacteria and viruses were cultured from the middle ear fluid in 18% of children with AOM. One-half to three-fourths of children who develop a URI develop abnormal eustachian tube dysfunction.[27–30]

Allergies also play a role. Some children have a genetically determined inability to produce adequate antibacterial antibodies against bacteria at levels that are sufficient to either protect the child against bacterial infection in the middle ear or to eradicate the bacteria once they have arrived there.[31,32] There is a decrease in specific humoral antibody (i.e., immunoglobulin G_2 [IgG_2] directed against some bacteria, especially those against *Streptococcus pneumoniae* in otitis-prone children).[32] Many otitis-prone children have allergic rhinitis, elevated IgE levels, and other symptoms of allergic disease.[31,32] Intranasal challenges with histamine or prostaglandin D_2 can cause eustachian tube dysfunction.[33]

Clinical Presentation and Diagnosis

AOM presents with fever, otalgia, or purulent discharge from the ear. In young children, any of the following may be the only signs of AOM: irritability, sleep disturbances, lethargy, fussiness, anorexia, nausea, vomiting, or diarrhea. A history of the child's pulling on his or her ears may be a clue to the diagnosis of AOM.

The diagnosis is clinical and made by otoscopy. The canal may be dry or wet (with exudate), pink or red, and swollen. Observation of the tympanic membrane is conclusive. Unlike its usual pearl-gray color and translucent appearance, a tympanic membrane with AOM appears red or dark and bulging or retracted with pus, fluid, or air bubbles behind it. The presence of an abnormal tympanic membrane confirms the diagnosis of otitis media.[3]

Pneumatic otoscopy (inspection of the tympanic membrane while varying air pressure) is necessary for diagnosis. A good seal must be present, and air is introduced by blowing from the mouth or by bulb. The membrane moves rapidly away from the examiner when positive pressure is applied gently in the normal ear. The examiner should determine if the tympanic membrane's motion is bidirectional and brisk (normal), in an outward direction only (negative middle ear pressure), or sluggish or absent (as when fluid is present). When fluid is present, mobility is inhibited.[34,35] Assessing tympanic membrane mobility may be difficult in a restless child. If there is a perforation, pneumatic otoscopy may be painful.[36]

Otoscopy can be difficult in infants: The child may be crying, causing coincidental erythema of the tympanic membrane. The infant's external auditory canal is narrow, and the canal wall itself can move with pneumatic insufflation. The physician may need to pull back the pinna gently to open the external auditory canal, allowing observation of the tympanic membrane. There have been many suggestions as to the best way to examine the infant; sitting the child on the mother's lap, with or without the mother restraining him or her against her body with her two hands, one on the head, one over his or her arms, or laying the infant down on the table while the child is given a bottle have been recommended. The mobility of tympanic membrane in the infant is decreased. Pneumatic otoscopy and tympanometry may not be reliable in infants younger than 7 months.[37]

Causative Organisms

The bacterial organisms that infect the middle ear in children are similar to those found in the nasopharynx: *Streptococcus pneumoniae, Haemophilus influenzae, Moraxella catarrhalis,* and β-hemolytic streptococci. The incidence of types of bacterial infection are age-related. From 6 weeks of age until 4 years, *S. pneumoniae* and *H. influenzae* are the most common organisms. Above the age of 4 years, *H. influenzae* is less likely to cause AOM.[38] In infants younger than 6 weeks of age, approximately 15% of cases of AOM are caused by gram-negative enterobacteria, specifically *Escherichia coli* and *Klebsiella.* These infections are usually caused by hematogenous spread; hence sepsis and meningitis, although rare, are more likely sequelae than in older children.[5]

The sensitivities of the bacterial organisms causing AOM have changed, as have the relative incidences of infection by organism. Up to 30% of *H. influenzae* strains and up to 90% of the *M. catarrhalis* strains are β-lactamase producers (BLPs). These are insensitive to amoxicillin and other penicillins. *M. catarrhalis* has become a more frequent cause of otitis media, causing up to 22% of AOM. AOM caused by *M. catarrhalis* is less likely to be associated with fever and earache.[1-3,39]

Viruses may also cause AOM. RSV accounted for 10 of 13 viruses identified.[29] RSV, type 2 parainfluenza viruses, rhinoviruses, and adenoviruses have been recovered from middle ear fluid.[28]

Treatment

Whereas diagnosis is relatively straightforward, there are differing opinions as to the best treatment of those with otitis media and its complications. The goals of treatment are to correct the eustachian tube dysfunction, provide symptomatic relief, eliminate infectious organisms, drain fluid from the middle ear, and prevent complications and future problems. Some of the therapies used in the past are not always effective, especially with changing patterns of bacterial sensitivity. Otitis may resolve without any pharmacologic intervention. Thus, each therapy must be examined as to efficacy and side effects.

Antibiotics

Antibiotic therapy has been the foundation of treatment of AOM. Yet, there are questions as to whether antibiotics are necessary, how long they need to be used, and which ones are most efficacious and have the fewest side effects.

AOM resolves spontaneously, sometimes without the use of antibiotics.[5,40] In up to one-third of cases of AOM, culturing the middle ear fluid produces no organisms.[40] Eichenwald reported that spontaneous resolution of AOM may occur in up to 60% of cases within 10 days of illness.[5] In 1958, Fry found that 85% of children cleared their AOM without antibiotics and without an increase in the number of recurrences or in the number of children whose hearing worsened.[41] In 1981, van Buchem, studying 171 children, found that reduction of pain, temperature, duration of discharge, and otoscopic appearances were unrelated to any of four therapeutic methods: no treatment, myringotomy, antibiotics, or myringotomy and antibiotics.[18,41] The definition of AOM, cure, and selection of patients in these studies has been questioned. Few other studies have had a "no treatment" group, so prevalent is the conviction that antibiotics are necessary and even that it would be malpractice not to use antibiotics. A recent meta-analysis of primary AOM in 5400 children in 33 randomized controlled studies showed an 81% cure without any antibiotics and a 13.7% additional cure with antibiotics.[42]

Howie and Ploussard, studying 280 children with AOM in 1972, found that 3 to 5 days of antibiotics was superior to placebo for bacterial sterilization of the middle ear and resolution of the illness.[43] Although some studies suggest that symptomatic treatment alone may be sufficient for some children with AOM, most investigators believe that the clinical response is improved with antibiotic therapy until further evidence proves the inefficacy of antibiotics.

Choice of Antibiotics

The antibiotic of choice for AOM (Table 11.1) is amoxicillin. Ampicillin can be used, but it has fallen into disfavor because it produces more drug reactions and side effects than amoxicillin.[1] Amoxicillin is active against many strains of *H. influenzae* and *S. pneumoniae,* is not affected by food intake, and is relatively inexpensive. It can be given in three daily doses.[1,14] Amoxicillin had the highest levels of penetration into middle ear fluid, making it the preferred treatment for AOM.[44]

There are several other choices for primary or secondary treatment of AOM. If the patient is allergic to penicillin, fixed combinations of trimethoprim/sulfa (TMX/sulfa: Bactrim, Septra) or erythromycin/sulfa (Pediazole) can be used. TMX/sulfa combinations are fairly inexpensive, are given only twice a day, and are effective against many organisms. They are not effective against *Streptococcus pyogenes* and should not be used if there is coexistent streptococcal pharyngitis.[1,35] The liquid preparations of TMX/sulfa are available in well-tolerated grape, fruit-licorice, or strawberry flavors. TMX/sulfa had the highest concentrations in middle ear effusions of the drugs used for BLP organisms.[44] It should not be used in children with glucose-6-phosphate dehydrogenase (G6PD) deficiency or who are folate-deficient. The erythromycin/sulfa combination has a wide spectrum of activity, but combinations should be used cautiously in children with asthma because erythromycin use can interfere with theophylline levels. It is moderately expensive and has a strawberry-banana taste. It can cause nausea, epigastric distress, and hemolysis in persons with G6PD deficiency. It should be given with food four times a day.[1,35] This combination may have less penetration into middle ear effusions than some of the other drugs.[44]

β-Lactamase production by strains of *H. influenzae* and *M. catarrhalis* has become an increasing problem (Table 11.2). If amoxicillin has been used and is ineffective or a BLP organism is suspected, another antibiotic should be chosen. Erythromycin/sulfa, TMX/sulfa, and cephalosporins are effective against BLPs. Cephalexin (Keflex; a first-generation cephalosporin), cefaclor (Ceclor) or cefuroxime (Ceftin) (second-generation cephalosporins), or cefixime (Suprax; an oral third-generation cephalosporin)—all significantly more expensive than amoxicillin—can be used as alternatives.

Cephalexin, less expensive than the other cephalosporins, is prescribed four times a day. It has a bubble-gum flavor.[14] Cefaclor is well absorbed, moderately expensive, reaches good levels in the middle ear, and has two well-tolerated flavors (grape and cherry); moreover, food does not decrease its absorption.[14,35] Cefaclor was as effective in eliminating symptoms and producing sterility of the middle ear as amoxicillin.[45]

TABLE 11.1. Some common antibiotics used for acute otitis media

Agent	Dosing and flavors	Spectrum of activity	Comments
Penicillins			
Amoxicillin	20–40 mg/kg/day tid	Covers *H. influenzae*, *S. pneumoniae*, some staphylococci	Drug of choice; chewable tablets
Amoxicillin/clavulanate (Augmentin)	20–40 mg/kg/day tid; banana, orange	Similar to amoxicillin with activity against β-lactamase producers (BLP)	Chewable tablets; may cause diarrhea
Cephalosporins			Use with caution in penicillin-allergic patients
Cefaclor (Ceclor)	40 mg/kg/day tid/bid; grape, cherry	Effective against staphylococci, group A streptococci, *H. influenzae* including some BLPs	Second-line therapy; may be drug of choice in infants <6 weeks old
Cefuroxime axetil (Ceftin)	bid	Efficacy like that of cefaclor	Only available as a tablet, which may be crushed but has a bitter taste
Cephalexin (Keflex)	qid; bubble-gum	Spectrum like that for cefuroxime	Can be generic
Cefixime (Suprax)	qd or bid; strawberry	Effective only against group A β-hemolytic streptococci, *S. pneumoniae*, and *H. influenzae*, including some strains of BLPs	Once-daily dosing may help compliance
Others			
Erythromycin ethylsuccinate/ sulfisoxazole (Pediazole)	50 mg/kg/day Eryth. qid; strawberry, banana	Effective against staphylococci, group A β-hemolytic streptococci, and *H. influenzae*	Contraindicated in infants <2 months; often used in patients allergic to penicillin
Trimethoprim/sulfa (Bactrim; Septra)	8 mg/kg/day/40 mg/kg/day bid; strawberry, grape, fruit-licorice	Effective against *S. pneumoniae* and *H. influenzae* including some BLPs	Contraindicated in infants <2 months; often used as second line; may be generic
Sulfisoxazole (Gantrisin)	qid; strawberry	Effective against many gram-positive and gram-negative organisms; not totally effective against staphylococci or *H. influenzae* alone	Used for prophylaxis; may be generic
Sulfamethoxazole (Gantanol)	bid; cherry	As with sulfisoxazole	Used for prophylaxis; may be generic

Source: Rosenfeld.[35] With permission.

TABLE 11.2. Efficacy of selected antimicrobial agents on
common pathogens for acute otitis media

Antibiotic	*Streptococcus*	*H. influenzae*	*B. catarrhalis*	*S. pyogenes*	*S. aureus*
Ampicillin/amoxicillin	+	+/−	+/−	+	+/−
Erythromycin/sulfa	+	+	+	+	+
Trimethoprim/sulfa	+	+	+	−	−
Cefaclor	+	+	+	+	+
Cefixime	+	+	+	+/−	−

Cefuroxime, although effective, is not presently available in liquid form, limiting its use in children. Although the tablet can be crushed, it has a bitter taste.[1,3,14] Cefixime is the only oral third-generation cephalosporin and the only oral drug with once-daily dosing, which may help compliance. It is effective against BLPs and many gram-negative bacilli, but not *Staphylococcus aureus*. It is moderately expensive and has a greater associated incidence of diarrhea than cefaclor or amoxicillin, but not as much as amoxicillin/clavulanate.[1,3,14]

A fixed combination of amoxicillin with clavulanic acid (Augmentin), which inactivates β-lactamase production, can be used. Its side effects include diarrhea and abdominal pain. It is fairly expensive but is not affected by food intake; it is given three times a day.[1,14,35]

Which antibiotic should be used as the second choice is up to the physician's personal preference, cost, the patient's allergies or sensitivities to penicillins, and the dosing interval desired. A drug effective against BLPs is probably a good second choice.[3] Cefaclor, TMX/sulfa, erythromycin/sulfa, amoxicillin/clavulanate, or cefixime are all reasonable choices. Studies have shown few significant differences in compliance, symptom resolution, cure, sterilization of middle ear fluid, outcome, or number or type of complications between cefaclor and TMX/sulfa.[45-50] Erythromycin/sulfa was as efficacious as amoxicillin, and children who used it had fewer recurrences.[51,52]

With appropriate therapy, most children with AOM improve within 48 to 72 hours. If signs and symptoms progress despite use of antibiotics, the patient should be reevaluated. Persistent or recurrent pain or fever suggests continued infection; if it occurs, a different antibiotic should be chosen that is effective against BLP bacteria.[1,3]

Usually, treatment is prescribed for 10 days.[3] A randomized double-blind controlled trial compared 3- and 10-day courses of amoxicillin in 84 children. There was little difference in speed of resolution of symptoms and signs, the number of primary treatment failures, or the frequency of recurrent ear infections between the 3- and 10-day courses. There were no complications in either group. Future studies are needed to determine if shorter courses of antibiotics are advisable.[53] Compliance may be a problem. In one study, nearly 40% of patients did not complete the entire course of antibiotics.[14] Compliance can be improved by using an antibiotic with fewer daily doses, by giving the parent verbal and written instructions, and by dispensing medications with calibrated measuring devices.[54,55] Many early treatment failures are caused by lack of compliance of medication. Compliance was better in low-income groups if the patient was seen by his or her own doctor and not by partners or emergency department doctors. Compliance is also improved, especially in children, by using those liquid preparations that have more acceptable flavors. However, liquids can spill and may be difficult to measure accurately.[54]

In infants 6 weeks or younger, primary therapy may be cefaclor or amoxicillin/clavulanate, rather than amoxicillin, as 10% to 15% of organisms causing AOM in this age group are gram-negative enteric bacilli and *S. aureus,* which may be resistant to amoxicillin.[1,14] These infants may need hospitalization and parenteral antibiotics, as AOM may be a sign of systemic infection. Continuing fever despite antibiotic therapy, dehydration, vomiting, toxic appearance, lethargy, anorexia, or severe diarrhea are indicators of the need for hospitalization.

There are times when immediate referral or admission to the hospital is recommended. Hospitalization may be indicated for children with AOM who are toxic or seriously ill, who have cystic fibrosis or Down syndrome, who have a continued severe febrile course despite antibiotics, in whom suppurative complications occur, who are younger than 6 months old, or who are immunocompromised. When a child treated for AOM presents with persistent headache, lethargy, malaise, irritability, continued severe otalgia, facial pain, stiff neck, focal seizures, ataxia, blurred vision, papilledema, diplopia, hemiplegia, aphasia, dysdiadochokinesia, intention tremor, dysmetria, hemianopsia, or persistent unremitting fever, suppurative intracranial complication should be suspected. Although rare, these cases can be dangerous if not treated early and adequately.[15]

There is no place for surgical treatment of AOM. Although myringotomy (incision of the tympanic membrane) may provide symptomatic relief, it provides no improvement over antibiotics in terms of resolution, response, or audiometric tests and may, in fact, be ineffective for curing AOM.[38,56,57]

Adjuvant Measures to Provide Comfort

It has been common practice to prescribe antihistamines and decongestants for AOM to relieve pain and alleviate discomfort. They do not alter the course or improve the cure rate of AOM. There was no difference between children with AOM treated with antihistamines and decongestants and untreated children in regard to clinical course, tympanometry, audiometry, degree of parental concerns, or incidence of recurrences of AOM.[14,36,58–61] For otalgia, analgesic otic drops may be of benefit.[14]

Acute Otitis Media in Adults

AOM presents differently in adults than in children. The initial symptoms are usually pain, hearing loss, and otorrhea but not fever.[62] The hearing loss is primarily conductive and usually mild to moderate. The physical examination may reveal a red ear drum or a nonhealing perforation of the drum. There is often intermittent or recurrent discharge that is usually mucopurulent but can also be green and fetid.[63] URIs usually accompany AOM.

The bacteriology of adult AOM is also unlike than that of children. *S. pneumoniae* is slightly less likely. *H. influenzae* has been found in increased frequency in older children and adults: in 10% to 33% of AOM episodes.[43,64–66] Treatment should provide coverage for *S. pneumoniae, H. influenzae,* and other gram-positive organisms.[64]

Amoxicillin is still the drug of choice. Tetracycline, doxycycline, cephalexin, or cefaclor can be used; erythromycin or penicillin alone are inadequate. If there is a high incidence of BLPs in the community or if patients are at high risk, diabetic, or immunocompromised, cefuroxime axetil, amoxicillin/clavulanic acid, cefixime, or TMX/sulfa may be a better first choice.[64]

Chronic Otitis Media

Chronic otitis media encompasses a variety of disease processes, with many differences in recommendations for treatment. AOM can persist or recur, becoming chronic. Moreover, fluid can form and remain in the middle ear, producing what can be called serous otitis media, otitis media with effusion, or chronic effusion. CSOM may have a profound impact by producing hearing loss, language delay, and school difficulties. Whether the treatment of CSOM is medical or surgical and when to treat it surgically are controversial.

Persistent Infectious Otitis Media

After a course of antibiotics, the child should be reexamined within 10 to 30 days. If the tympanic membrane still is affected, an alternate antibiotic active against BLPs should be prescribed for another 10-day course.

It may be that the original organism was not sensitive to the antibiotic given or that the drug was not taken as prescribed. In many cases, compliance is a problem, and an antibiotic that has fewer daily dosings should be prescribed with detailed directions given to the patient's parents, perhaps in writing.

Studies using biotyping suggest that early recurrent AOM may be a result of relapse with initial infecting *H. influenzae* strain or noncompliance.[67] Only a few organisms obtained by tympanocentesis have been found to be resistant to the antibiotic initially chosen.[36,38] Another antibiotic should be tried for another course. The child should be reexamined to document cure after another 10 to 30 days. If no improvement or worsening occurs, referral to an otolarnyngologist for surgical drainage for therapy and culture might be indicated.

Recurrent Otitis Media

There are a group of children who clear one episode of AOM, with a documented cure, only to have the AOM recur soon after. The flora of children with recurrent AOM, when episodes are separated by 1 month or more, is similar to that found during the first episode.[21] Thus, second episodes of AOM should be treated in the same manner as the first episode. In these children, chronic antibiotic prophylaxis may prevent recurrences of AOM.[36,68,69] Young children and those in day care profit more by prophylaxis.[70]

Daily prophylactic antibiotics should be considered if there are three or four episodes within 6 to 18 months.[3,36] Sulfisoxazole has proved effective in preventing recurrent symptomatic AOM and is safe for long-term use.[69-71] Doses suggested for children younger than age 2 years are 250 mg bid and for those aged 2 to 5 years 500 mg bid or 75 mg/kg/day bid.[69,71,72] It can be given once or twice a day. In a cross-over double-blind study of 35 children aged 6 months to 5 years with recurrent infectious otitis media, sulfisoxazole reduced the rate of AOM recurrences by 40%.[73] Treatment should continue for up to 6 months.[14] Erythromycin in doses of 20 mg/kg/day bid or amoxicillin 20 mg/kg/day bid can be used for prophylaxis.[3,36,72] TMX/sulfa, in doses of TMX 12 mg/kg/day, has also been studied and has been found safe for long-term use and prophylaxis.[49,70,74] There are certain children in whom TMX/sulfa should be used with caution or avoided: those with folate deficiency, prematurity, G6PD deficiency, or known sensitivity to trimethoprim or sulfas.[71]

If episodes of otitis media are frequent, prevention of further attacks should be attempted. A search is made for respiratory allergies or a physical abnormality of the pharynx. In older children, sinusitis is ruled out by roentgenography and treated if present. In some children, immunologic studies may be warranted, especially if other infections are present. Children with recurrent AOM should be examined for evidence of chronic middle ear effusions.[4]

There have been a few studies on the effectiveness of vaccination to prevent AOM. The first studies in Finland, using pneumococcal vaccine, showed a positive effect of vaccination on decreasing the incidence of AOM recurrences.[75] One study in the United States showed that in black infants the incidence of subsequent AOM after vaccination was lowered.[76] However, other studies failed to show a statistical difference in the incidence of AOM after vaccination with pneumococcal vaccine.[75] Viral vaccination has been proposed as a method of decreasing the incidence of recurrent otitis media and CSOM as up to 50% of AOM episodes are preceded by URIs. The seasonal incidence of colds and otitis media parallel each other. Viruses have been recovered from patients with AOM and CSOM. Yet, vaccines are available for only about 10% of viruses.[27]

Chronic Serous Otitis Media

Diagnosis and Etiology

CSOM is the persistent presence of fluid in the middle ear. It can be painful, cause decreased hearing, or be asymptomatic, detected only on a follow-up visit for AOM or by chance. The diagnosis is suggested by pneumatic otoscopy. Air bubbles, an air–fluid level, or decreased motion of the tympanic membrane with insufflation are diagnostic.

Tympanometry is 85% accurate for diagnosing CSOM.[55] Tympanometry is the measurement of acoustic impedance across the tympanic membrane. The middle ear functions as a transformer, and its function can be measured by its impedance. Any disease process, including fluid in the middle ear, either increases or decreases the impedance across the tympanic membrane, interfering with sound transmission. Acoustic impedance is measured by a tympanometer. A plug is placed in the external auditory canal and seals the ear. There is a pressure gauge and a source of pure tone. Intensity of pure tone reflected from the tympanic membrane is plotted against a range of pressures. This graph is called a tympanogram. Normal tympanograms have a peaked appearance. Children with decreased middle ear pressure but no fluid have peaked tympanograms that are shifted. Flat tympanograms, showing decreased impedance across the tympanic membrane, suggest fluid behind the membrane and serous otitis media.[19]

Diagnosis of CSOM is also suggested by an acquired conductive hearing loss. Pure tone hearing tests are difficult and may be unreliable in children younger than the age of 4 years. Younger children can be tested by "baby-grams," where the infant is placed on a movable surface that is connected to a graphing mechanism. When a sound is heard, the infant moves, causing a change in the graph. This test is used only for screening. A much more sophisticated hearing test is for auditory evoked potentials. The infant's electro-encephalogram is recorded while different sounds are produced in one head-phone. Computer averaging is necessary. This method can determine hearing loss in very young infants or mentally retarded children who cannot cooperate.

The etiology of CSOM is complex and not completely understood. Eustachian tube dysfunction, AOM and bacterial infection, allergies, passive smoke inhalation, and URIs can contribute to CSOM. Younger children are more likely to develop effusions. In as many as 40% of patients, serous effusions may be found 4 to 6 weeks after AOM.[5] There is a higher incidence of CSOM in children with allergy.[77] Cigarette smoking in the home has been found to be related to the incidence of URIs and CSOM.[78–81] CSOM is likely to be associated with frequent URIs[82,83]; in one study up to 76% of children with CSOM had had prior URIs.[84]

Effect of CSOM

Fear that CSOM produces hearing loss and learning disabilities has driven physicians to great lengths to eradicate the fluid from the middle ear. Many believe that rapid and adequate treatment, with normalization of hearing, is essential for normal growth and development. More surgery is performed on children to correct CSOM than for any other reason. However, the natural course of the effusions in many cases may be spontaneous resolution.[4,15,21,36,77,78,82] There are only two reasons for treating effusions: to alleviate symptoms and to reduce occurrence of complications and sequelae.[83]

Long-term persistent fluid in the middle ear definitely can produce a hearing loss, which is usually conductive.[4,83,85] This loss is the most common complication of middle ear disease. Sensorineuronal involvement can also occur.[4] The degree of loss is variable; approximately 10% show a hearing loss of less than 10 decibels (dB), approximately 90% have losses of 10 to 49 dB, and fewer than 1% have losses greater than 50 dB.[4,86–88]

Bilateral hearing loss that continues throughout infancy and early childhood may affect many aspects of development.[4,83,85,89,90] The determination of when and how long effusions in the middle ear can cause severe enough hearing loss to affect growth and development is disputed. There have been several studies that have shown developmental abnormalities in children with CSOM, but many were retrospective.[56,85,91,92] Moreover, many subjects in these studies were not representative; they were either deprived or referral populations. There were several studies in which the associations between CSOM and later developmental impairment were not found.[93–96]

Some researchers have suggested that there is a critical period during infancy when CSOM is more disabling, especially if it is bilateral.[7,37,83] One critical time may be within the first 6 months of life.[4,37] A small decrease in hearing in a younger child may be more disabling than in older children.[7,97] Others believe that the evidence suggests acquisition of language is not limited to specific and fixed periods of brain development, and most children catch up with their peers once the effusion resolves and hearing is restored.[5]

More than 6 months of CSOM, if bilateral, may cause the development of hearing deficits and subsequent chronic language delays.[83] Children who have recurrent otitis media with resulting periods of effusion may have developmental abnormalities of speech.[4,7,85,89,90,98,99] Children with a history of recurrent CSOM may have normal-sounding spontaneous speech with a history of delay rather than deviance in acquisition, but they have problems reading and have limited vocabularies and syntax compared with children without CSOM.[4] One well-controlled but retrospective study of a few children found that their subjects with a history of CSOM had deficits in auditory and language skills including reception, processing, and production of verbal responses, but the visual learning abilities were unaffected.[90] A study that followed 205 children from birth to school age and recorded the number of episodes of AOM and number of months of CSOM also found that children who spent prolonged periods with middle ear effusions scored lower in language and speech tests. The effect was more pronounced if the children had ear disease at 6 to 12 months. The correlation was strongest in children from high socioeconomic levels. A prolonged period was defined specifically as more than 130 days over 3 years.[100] Other studies seemed to agree that children with persistent CSOM (>12 weeks), even when normal hearing was regained, scored less well on standardized verbal and language tests.[56,89]

Thus, long-term effusions in the middle ear, especially in young children, should be aggressively treated. The definition of "long term" is controversial, although many researchers suggest 6 months as an acceptable period after which more aggressive treatment is necessary. Those children younger than 2 years of age may deserve more aggressive treatment sooner. Short periods (3–4 months) of middle ear effusions are probably harmless developmentally. How invasive treatment should be is the most common question.[56,95] Certainly, for children older than 2 years of age and with CSOM present less than 6 months, either no treatment or medical treatment alone should be sufficient.[3,4,7,91,92] In children with severe disease or disease that persists more than 6 months despite medical treatment, surgical treatment should be considered.

Treatment of CSOM in Children

No treatment is an option for CSOM that has been present less than 6 months. Many effusions resolve spontaneously within 2 to 6 months with no treatment, especially if they were discovered after AOM.[4,5,22,36,77,78] In one study that looked at private pediatric practices, 70% of children had middle ear effusions at the conclusion of antimicrobial therapy at 2 weeks. However, only 40% continued to have effusions at 1 month, 20% had effusions at 2 months, and 10% had effusions at 3 months.[4]

Antibiotics are commonly suggested as treatment for CSOM. Early studies showed the fluid to be sterile, but some later studies showed that in one-half to two-thirds of patients with CSOM bacteria have grown from the fluid. The pathogens growing were similar to those in AOM. Although antibiotics sterilize the middle ear space during treatment for AOM, middle ear effusions may persist for weeks to months after an acute episode of otitis media.[4] In several studies, antibiotics were judged to be generally superior to no therapy in terms of alleviation of symptoms and healing of tympanic membranes. However, findings were not consistent, the differences were modest, and the response to therapy was difficult to quantify.[101,102] In one study, all children scheduled for myringotomy with tympanostomy and tube placement (MTTP) were randomized into two groups. One group received erythromycin 20 to 30 mg/kg/day for 10 days. Of the children so treated, the CSOM resolved in 45%, and their surgery was cancelled.[51] One study has disputed the efficacy of antibiotics for treatment of CSOM.[103]

The addition of antihistamines to antibiotics is suggested to eradicate middle ear effusions.[3] Some randomized studies treated children with antibiotics and antihistamines or antibiotics and placebo. The addition of antihistamines to antibiotics hastened the recovery symptomatically and reduced the presence of persisting effusions 2 weeks after the start of treatment.[83,104] Antihistamines alone have been proved to be no better than placebo in reducing the symptoms or occurrences or in improving the hearing or school performance of children with CSOM, treated for 3 months and followed for 1 year.[59,60,83,105,106]

A search for causes of respiratory allergy and then treatment or avoidance may also decrease middle ear effusions. Middle ear fluid from patients with chronic or recurrent middle ear effusions has high histamine levels.[32,78] There is a definite decrease in specific humoral antibodies against certain bacteria in the otitis-prone child. In one study, children who were otitis-prone were more likely to have lower antibody levels to *S. aureus, Pseudomonas aeruginosa, E. coli, S. pneumoniae, S. epidermidis,* and *H. influenzae.*[32] Deficiency of IgG2, which is important to the development of specific antibodies against the capsular antigen of pneumococcus, has been found in some children with CSOM.[107]

Steroids have been suggested for treatment of CSOM without proof of efficacy.[36] Oral dexamethasone and beclomethasone nasal spray have been equally disappointing for clearing CSOM.[83,108]

Treatment for CSOM thus should include, first, a 10-day course of antibiotics, with perhaps a second course of another antibiotic after failure of the first. If effusions persist, an antihistamine can be added to the antibiotic. If these measures fail, a search for respiratory allergy may be the next step. Finally, despite treatment and follow-up of CSOM, there remains a small percentage of children who continue to have fluid in the middle ear. These children may be treated surgically. Surgery should be considered if effusions persist more than 3 months after treatment of a child younger than 6 months of age or if they persist more than 6 months in an older child despite aggressive medical treatment without satisfactory resolution of effusion.[2,3,86]

Children with cleft palate or an abnormal pharynx may require surgical treatment sooner. One study[95] matched 24 children with cleft palates who underwent myringotomy and tube placement with 24 children who did not. At 5 to 11 years old, the two groups were similar otoscopically, tympanometrically, and audiometrically. However, early pressure-equalizing (PE) tube placement resulted (at all ages) in slightly better hearing and substantially better articulation than in the non-early-placement groups. There was no detectable differences between the two groups in terms of cognitive, linguistic, or social and emotional development.

Surgical procedures for the treatment of CSOM have been the most common operations in children for generations. MTTP is currently the most common surgical procedure that requires general anesthesia in children. Each year, 1 million children get tympanostomy tubes, and 600,000 children have tonsillectomies.[3,4]

Surgical treatment of otitis was first performed in 1760 for relief of deafness. In 1870, Meyer noted that enlarged adenoids may be associated with serous fluid in ears. In 1902, Politzer commented on this fact and suggested adenoidectomy with or without tonsillectomy for treatment of CSOM.[23] Subsequently, tonsillectomy with adenoidectomy became one of the most common operations in children. In disagreement, Marshak and Neriah[24] and Roydhouse[25] condemned adenoidectomy as primary or secondary treatment for CSOM. Few studies have reported that adenoidectomy with or without tonsillectomy improves CSOM.[83]

Ventilating tubes were used near the end of the nineteenth century, but they were abandoned because they were eventually expelled from the ears. In 1954, Armstrong reintroduced tympanostomy with plastic ventilator tubes (or pressure equalizing tubes) as a treatment for CSOM and suggested that they had good short-term effects.[1,109–111] Studying 500 children retrospectively, success was defined as the need for only one surgical intubation to restore hearing function to thresholds of 20 dB; 75% of children required only one intubation.[22,110] It was suggested that MTTP allowed the middle ear mucous membrane to return to normal and prevented short-term accumulation of effusion and short-term improvement of hearing. Bluestone suggested that there exist a group of children with diminished eustachian tube compliance who might benefit from adenoidectomy.[111] Proposed in 1976 by Cantekin and Bluestone, the efficacy of MTTP was studied in a pilot project in 20 patients and was found effective for curing CSOM.[111,112]

Although MTTP cures CSOM immediately, because the tubes extrude within 4 to 8 months there is continuing controversy as to whether there is any long-term improvement in hearing or a decrease in the recurrence or persistence of CSOM. Recurrence of middle ear effusions after extrusion of PE tubes is likely in as many as 20% to 40%.[83] Few studies are available to determine if tympanotomy benefits or harms the patient in the long run. Tympanograms in children 3 to 5 years after placement of PE tubes were no different from those in children who were not treated with surgery.[113] Twenty years ago, middle ear effusions were rarely diagnosed. Yet, prolonged deafness occurred infrequently, and permanent language defects were no more common than they are now.[5] Tube placement results in normalization of hearing, but this effect is transient. Little difference in hearing has been found with children treated surgically or not with 3 to 6 months follow-up.[36] PE tubes seem to gain 3 to 6 months of improved hearing before the child's hearing improves on its own.[22,36,110,111]

In addition to the continuing and ever-present risks of anesthesia, there are complications of MTTP. The death rate is 1 per 3,000 to 1 per 27,000.

Otorrhea is the desired outcome, but the discharge may become profuse and cause eczematoid external otitis. Moreover, persistent perforation, atrophic scars or tympanosclerosis, and scarring of the tympanic membrane are possible complications.[4,83] Although rare, other complications include hearing loss, perforation or retraction pocket of the tympanic membrane, adhesive otitis media, ossicular discontinuity and fixation, chronic suppurative otitis media, cholesteatoma, mastoiditis, labyrinthitis, facial paralysis, and cholesterol granulomas. Cholesteatomas, accumulation of desquamating keratinizing stratified squamous epithelium within the middle ear or temporal bone, are also rare, occurring in 6 per 100,000.[4] Only 1.9% children in one study had long-term ear problems from MTTP. In one study of 6429 children referred for MTTP, only 42% were referred for appropriate indications; many MTTPs may be performed for inappropriate indications.[115]

Thus, surgical treatment of CSOM, which in the past included adenoidectomy with or without tonsillectomy, is now MTTP. Although MTTP has a constant complication rate caused by anesthesia, the complications related to the procedure itself are rare, and there is less than a 2% incidence of chronic discharge. The short-term efficacy of MTTP is definite: It cures CSOM immediately and restores hearing. The effect, however, is temporary, allowing improved hearing until the eustachian tube function matures and improves. This period may be a critical time for language acquisition and may be sufficient time that further CSOM does not occur in the older child. There is little proof of any long-term efficacy of MTTP, but the short-term gain may be sufficient.

There is no consensus about treatment of CSOM in adults. Treatment should be medical, as in children, with antibiotics and antihistamines. Unless there is demonstrable conductive hearing loss, surgery is probably not indicated. MTTP has been used in adults with some short-term improvement of hearing.[114]

Otitis Externa

Otitis externa (OE) is inflammation or infection of the external ear canal. The external auditory canal (EAC) is a cartilaginous canal lined with squamous epithelium. It communicates through the meatus to the outside, and there are small fissures of Santorini that allow some communication anteriorly with the parotid gland. The facial nerve is close to the parotid gland and the EAC.[116]

OE can be acute or chronic and can involve many disease processes. Acute OE is usually irritative, with or without superimposed infection. In children, foreign body irritation must always be suspected in acute OE. Acute OE is often caused by prolonged swimming and is then called swimmer's ear. Chronic OE can be caused by chronic bacterial or fungal infections or any chronic inflammation that affects other skin areas. Eczema, psoriasis, or seborrhea can affect the EAC.

Acute Otitis Externa

In children, a common cause of acute OE is foreign bodies. All must be removed on detection. All varieties of objects have been found in the ears of children: toys, paper, jewelry, dirt, and so on. Some potentially serious objects include watch batteries, which must be removed immediately. These objects can be removed by simple grasping instruments, irrigation, or suction.[117]

Children and adults with abnormal or congenitally defected ears are more likely to develop OE.[116] Congenital cysts and sinuses are not uncommon. These cysts may be anterior and inferior to the ear.[117]

Traumatic injury can cause otitis. A laceration or hematoma can result from a fall, person-to-person violence, or ear piercing and can become infected. Human bites to the pinna are usually infected and often serious; often the infection extends into the canal. Treatment includes simple closure of wounds if they are clean. More complex injuries must be meticulously débrided with conservation of tissue. Any hematomas should be drained by needle or incision, repeatedly if fluid reaccumulation occurs. Some kind of pressure bandage should also be used: fluffed gauze, Ace wrap, or a tie-through suture.[117]

Prolonged exposure to swimming has been correlated with the development of *swimmer's ear,* or *acute inflammatory OE.* The inflammation is often accompanied by infection, making treatment somewhat more complicated than just avoidance of swimming. Swimmers who developed OE were more likely to have been swimming longer, more frequently, and with more frequent submersion of their head than swimmers without OE, independent of the type of water. OE was more likely associated with swimming in fresh water than with ocean and pool water, and it increased with 1 month of exposure, but only in those who swam frequently.[118] Swimmer's ear is more likely in hot, humid climates and 10 to 20 times more likely during the summer.[119]

Those features of the EAC that protect the ear against invasion from infection and foreign bodies—tortuosity of the canal, spatial orientation, and external hairs—also prevent water from escaping. Clinically, the patient complains of pain and itch for 1 to 2 days after prolonged swimming. There can be a history of local trauma, scratching or rubbing the canal, or prolonged occlusion of the canal.[119]

Clinical symptoms include otorrhea, which can be white, green, or foul-smelling, otalgia, pinna pain, and even hearing loss. Examination reveals a swollen canal that is often red with discharge. Pulling the pinna upward and backward often elicits discomfort.

Repeated exposure to water removes the protective waxy coating of the EAC, allowing it to become macerated and predisposed to infection by gram-negative bacteria. *Pseudomonas aeruginosa,* the universal inhabitant of moist environments, is the most likely bacterial cause of OE, in one study growing in two of every three infected ears.[118,120] Other pathogens include *E. coli, Aerobacter, S. aureus,* streptococci, and some *Proteus* species.[117]

Once the EAC is infected and swollen, treatment includes gentle cleaning of the canal if possible. Topical medication is the treatment of choice. The topical medications can include acid/alcohol drops, which reduce inflammation and are antifungal (Otic Domeboro—aqueous, or VoSol Otic with propylene glycol).[119] A 1:1 mixture of vinegar and rubbing alcohol is less expensive and probably just as effective, although it can be painful and thus difficult to administer to children.[117] An antibiotic/steroid liquid preparation can be used to reduce inflammation and infection.[121] The antibiotic preparations used can be a combination of polymyxin B and neomycin or colistin sulfate to provide gram-negative and gram-positive coverage; or gentamicin alone may be used. Both preparations—gentamicin and colistin/neomycin/hydrocortisone otic—produce few side effects. However, gentamicin is more likely to eradicate the organism, whereas the others relieve inflammation over a shorter period. Gentamicin drops can produce systemic allergies. Hydrocortisone is added to decrease inflammation[121] (Table 11.3).

Topical medication should be given three or four times a day. If the canal is too swollen to allow easy access of the drops, a wick of 0.25-inch gauze or cotton may be inserted into the swollen external canal for 24 to

TABLE 11.3. Commonly used otic drops

Preparation name	Principal agents	Dosage
Colymycin S otic	Colistin Neomycin Hydrocortisone	3–4 drops 3–4 times a day
Cortisporin otic solution and suspension	Polymyxin B Neomycin Hydrocortisone	3–4 drops 3–4 times a day
Otic Domeboro	Acetic acid in aluminum acetate	4–6 drops q2–3h
VoSol Otic solution	Acetic acid in propylene glycol	5 drops 3–4 times a day
VoSol HC Otic solution	Acetic acid Hydrocortisone in propylene glycol	5 drops 3–4 times a day

36 hours. Medication can then be dropped onto the wick. Alternately, although used infrequently, powdered antibiotics or boric acid powder can be instilled into the external canals through a nebulizer. Treatment should be continued 7 to 10 days and the ear canal protected from water for 2 weeks.[117] Systemic antibiotics are seldom needed.

Most episodes of swimmer's ears can be prevented. Children or adults who develop OE frequently can avoid prolonged exposure to moisture and use preventive antiseptics or water-repellent skin coatings. Eardrops such as VoSol or Otic Domeboro can be used after swimming. Treating predisposing skin conditions such as eczema can minimize the incidence of swimmer's ear.[119]

Chronic Otitis Externa

Chronic OE is either inflammatory, caused by conditions that affect other skin surfaces, or infectious. Psoriasis, eczema, and seborrhea can cause chronic OE. Some people have chronically itching ears with dry, scaly skin. Chronic OE is usually associated with dry skin elsewhere on the body and with aging. If it occurs only in the patient's ears, it may be a self-inflicted problem of habitual cleaning or picking at the ears. Treatment is education and a change of habits. The patient must be told to keep everything out of the EAC. Two or three drops of baby oil in the external ear canal on a daily or weekly basis provides excellent relief.[122]

Some adults have excessive accumulation of cerumen, which may lead to conductive hearing loss, impaction with or without secondary infection, and pain and frustration when it has to be removed. Such excessive cerumen is worsened by patients who use cotton-tipped applicators, which irritate the canal and push the cerumen farther back. Treatment includes prior installation of a wax softener, such as olive oil or mineral oil, or use of carbamide peroxide (which should be used cautiously because it can cause dermatitis itself). Irrigation is then used if the tympanic membrane is intact. After removal of wax, hearing function should be evaluated. Often a steroid-containing otic solution is given for 7 to 10 days to reduce subsequent swelling. Acetic acid drops may prevent further accumulation.

Psoriasis can cause persistent OE. It presents with dry, itchy, flaky skin and is treated with steroid cream or lotion.[123] Seborrhea can cause a scaly inflammation in the EAC and behind external ears. Usually it is accompanied by seborrhea in the eyelids, forehead, and face. It can be controlled by antiseborrheic shampoos daily and topical steroids.[117] Allergic reactions can occur in the EAC as well as anywhere. A common cause of allergy is a nickel-plated earring. Eczema and atopic disease can affect the external ear as well. Symptoms include chronically itching ears.[117,124]

Treatment of most forms of chronic inflammatory OE includes removal of debris and reduction of swelling. Steroid otic solutions may help reduce swelling.[122] A few drops of oil can be used to reduce pruritus. A wick can be placed daily with Domeboro Otic. The patient should be counseled to avoid using anything to scratch the EAC.[117,124] Systemic antibiotics are almost never used unless there is evidence of OM. If the patient has diabetes mellitus or arteriosclerosis, close observation is necessary for other infectious complications.

Chronic infection may be caused by recurrent infection of congenital cysts or sinus tracts. Treatment may include antibiotic therapy and local treatment such as hot packs. Incision of cysts may be necessary.[116] Fungal infections of the external ear can be persistent and difficult to cure.[124] They are more likely in adults, diabetic patients, and immunocompromised hosts. The discharge can be green or white or have white and black amorphous debris caused by *Aspergillus niger.* Fungi are an unusual cause of chronic OE in temperate climates, although common in the tropics. The fungi recovered are saprophytes; *Aspergillus, Penicillium, Rhizopus,* and *Alternaria* are the most common species. *Candida* and *Tinea dermatophytes* can cause a low-grade infection and inflammation.[119] Treatment must be thorough. The canal must be cleaned well, possibly with an operating microscope, removing all loose surface skin. Sulfanilamide powder may be used.

Malignant Otitis Externa

Malignant OE was first reported in 1968 as an infection caused by *Pseudomonas aeruginosa.* Rare but potentially lethal, it is a rapidly progressive necrotizing serious infection that begins in the EAC.[116] Of 150 reported cases, nearly all were in elderly patients (average age, 68); 90% were in diabetic patients. Eight cases were reported in children with Stevens-Johnson syndrome, leukopenia, malnutrition, chemotherapy, or diabetes mellitus.[119] Malignant OE spreads to soft tissue underneath the temporal bone and may lead to facial nerve palsy, mastoiditis, multiple cranial nerve palsies, meningitis, and occasionally death.[117] Recognized early and treated appropriately, sometimes with surgical débridement, the consequences of malignant OE have decreased in severity since the 1980s.[124] Before combined carbenicillin/gentamicin therapy was common, the overall mortality was 50% to 63%; and it was higher if the patient developed nerve palsies.[124,125] In children, malignant OE has not carried as severe a prognosis.[119]

The symptoms include an intensely inflamed ear filled with granulation tissue pus. On examination, there is erythema, swelling, and tenderness of auricular and preauricular tissue, sometimes with a unilateral facial palsy, which is almost always permanent.[119] Examination of the ear canal with SPECT bone scintigraphy may allow early distinction of malignant OE from severe OE in diabetic patients.[126] The standard therapy is aggressive parenteral aminoglycoside and carbenicillin plus surgical débridement.

Long-term therapy with outpatient tobramycin and either an anti-pseudomonal cephalosporin or carbenicillin decreases its severity.[116,124,126]

References

1. Bluestone CD. Management of otitis media in infants and children: current role of old and new antimicrobial agents. Pediatr Infect Dis 1988;7:S129–36.
2. Bluestone CD. Otitis media in children: to treat or not to treat. N Engl J Med 1982;306:1399–1404.
3. Bluestone CD. Modern management of otitis media. Pediatr Clin North Am 1989;36:1371–87.
4. Bluestone CD, Klein JO, Paradise JL, et al. Workshop on effects of otitis media on the child. Pediatrics 1983;71:639–52.
5. Eichenwald HE. Developments in diagnosing and treating otitis media. Am Fam Physician 1985;31:155–64.
6. Howie VM, Schwartz RH. Acute otitis media. Am J Dis Child 1983;137:155–8.
7. Kirkwood DR, Kirkwood ME. Otitis media and learning disabilities. J Fam Pract 1983;17:219–27.
8. Lim DJ, Demaria TF. Bacteriology and immunology: pathogenesis of otitis media. Laryngoscope 1982;92:278–84.
9. Shaefer O. Otitis media and bottle feeding. Can J Public Health 1971;62:478–83.
10. Biles RW, Buffer PA, O'Donnell AA. Epidemiology of otitis media: a community study. Am J Public Health 1980;70:593–8.
11. Baine DJ. Acute otitis media in children: diagnostic and therapeutic dilemmas. J Fam Pract 1978;6:259–63.
12. Warren WS, Stool SE. Otitis media in low birth weight infants. J Pediatr 1971;79:740–5.
13. Berman SA, Balkany TJ, Simmons MA. Otitis media in the neonatal intensive care unit. Pediatrics 1978;63:198–203.
14. Zenk KE, Ma H. Pharmacological treatment of otitis media and sinusitis in pediatrics. J Pediatr Health Care 1990;4:297–303.
15. Bluestone CD. Otitis media and sinusitis: management and when to refer to the otolaryngologist. Pediatr Infect Dis J 1987;6:100–6.
16. Holmquist J, Renvall U. Middle ear ventilation in secretory otitis media. Ann Otol Rhinol Laryngol 1976;85:178–82.
17. Bluestone CD, Doyle WJ. Anatomy and physiology of eustachian tube and middle ear related to otitis media. J Allergy Clin Immunol 1988:81:997–1003.
18. Van Buchem FL, Dunk JH, Van't Hof MA. Therapy of acute otitis media: myringotomy, antibiotics or neither? Lancet 1981;2:883–7.
19. Ruben RJ. The ear. In: Rudolph AM, editor. Pediatrics. 16th ed. Norwalk, CT: Appleton-Century-Crofts, 1977:952–65.
20. Drake-Lee AB, Casey WF, Ogg TW. Anaesthesia for myringotomy. Anaesthesia 1983;38:314–8.

21. Jahn AF, Abramson M. Medical management of chronic otitis media. Otolaryngol Clin North Am 1984;17:673–7.
22. Smyth GD. Management of otitis media with effusion: a review. Am J Otol 1984;5:344–9.
23. Ballin MJ, Heller CL, editors. A textbook of the disease of the ear. 4th ed. London: Ballière, Tindall & Cox, 1902.
24. Marshak G, Neriah ZB. Adenoidectomy versus tympanostomy in chronic secretory otitis media. Ann Otol Rhinol Laryngol 1980; 89:316–8.
25. Roydhouse N. Adenoidectomy for otitis media with mucoid effusion. Ann Otol Rhinol Laryngol 1980;89:312–5.
26. Gates GA, Avery DA, Prihoda TJ, Cooper JR. Effectiveness of adenoidectomy and tympanostomy tubes in the treatment of chronic otitis media with effusion. N Engl J Med 1987;317:1444–51.
27. Gwaltney JM. Viral vaccines in the control of otitis media. Pediatr Infect Dis J 1989;8:S78–S79.
28. Chonmaitree T, Howie VM, Truant AL. Presence of respiratory viruses in middle ear fluids and nasal wash specimens from children with acute otitis media. Pediatrics 1986;77:698–702.
29. Klein BS, Dollete FR, Yolken RH. The role of respiratory syncytial virus and other viral pathogens in acute otitis media. J Pediatr 1982;101:16–20.
30. Henderson FW, Collier AM, Clyde WA, Denny FW. Respiratory syncytial virus infections, reinfections and immunity: a prospective, longitudinal study in young children. N Engl J Med 1979;300:530–5.
31. Rubin W, Jacob RD. Allergy and the immunologic aspects of otitis media with effusion. Am J Otol 1986;7:373–8.
32. Bernstein JM. Recent advances in immunologic reactivity in otitis media with effusion. J Allergy Clin Immunol 1988;81:1004–9.
33. Fireman P. The role of antihistamines in otitis. J Allergy Clin Immunol 1990;86:638–41.
34. Gates GA, Northern JL, Ferrer HP, et al. Diagnosis and screening. Ann Otol Rhinol Laryngol 1989;98:39–41.
35. Rosenfeld JA. Managing middle ear inflammation: a review. Fam Pract Recert 1990;12:49–68.
36. Legler JD. An approach to difficult management problems in otitis media in children. JABFP 1991;4:331–9.
37. Marchant CD, Shurin PA, Turczyk VA, et al. Course and outcome of otitis media in early infancy: a prospective study. J Pediatr 1984;104:826–31.
38. Roddey OF, Earle R, Haggerty R. Myringotomy in acute otitis media. JAMA 1966;197:849–53.
39. Marchant CD. Spectrum of disease due to Branhamella catarrhalis in children with particular reference to acute otitis media. Am J Med 1990;88:15S–19S.
40. Frenkel M. Acute otitis media: does therapy alter its course? Postgrad Med 1987;82:84–86.
41. Fry J. Antibiotics in acute tonsillitis and acute otitis media. BMJ 1958;2:883–6.
42. Rosenfeld RM, Vertrees JR. Clincal efficacy of antimicrobial drugs for acute otitis media: a meta-analysis of 5400 children from thirty-three randomized trials. J Pediatr 1994;124(3):355–67.

43. Howie VN, Ploussard JH. Efficacy of fixed combination antibiotics versus separate components in otitis media. Clin Pediatr (Phila) 1972;11:205–14.
44. Krause PJ, Owen NJ, Nightingale CH, et al. Penetration of amoxicillin, cefaclor, erythromycin-sulfisoxazole, and trimethoprim-sulfamethazole into the middle ear fluid of patients with chronic serious otitis media. J Infect Dis 1982;145:815–21.
45. Giebink GS, Batalden PB, Russ JN, Le CT. Cefaclor v. amoxicillin in treatment of acute otitis media. Am J Dis Child 1984;138:287–92.
46. Marchant CD, Shurin PA, Turcyzk FA, et al. A randomized controlled trial of cefaclor compared with trimethoprim-sulfamethoxazole for treatment of acute otitis media. J Pediatr 1984;105:633–8.
47. Feldman W, Richardson H, Rennie B, Dawson P. A trial comparing cefaclor with cotrimazole in the treatment of acute otitis media. Arch Dis Child 1982;57:594–6.
48. Tarpay M, Marks MI, Hopkins C, et al. Cefaclor therapy twice daily for acute otitis media. Am J Dis Child 1982;136:33–35.
49. Cunningham MJ. Chemoprophylaxis with oral trimethoprim-sulfamethoxazole. Clin Pediatr (Phila) 1990;29:273–7.
50. Marchant CD, Shurin PA, Johnson CE, et al. A randomized controlled trial of amoxicillin plus clavulanate compared with cefaclor for treatment of acute otitis media. J Pediatr 1986;109:891–5.
51. Ernstson S, Sundberg L. Erythromycin in the treatment of otitis media with effusion. J Laryngol Otol 1984;98:767–9.
52. Rodriguez WJ, Schwartz RH, Sait T, et al. Erythromcyin-sulfisoxazole v. amoxicillin in the treatment of acute otitis media in children. Am J Dis Child 1985;139:766–70.
53. Chaput de Saintonge DM, Levine DF, Savage IT, et al. Trial of three day and ten day courses of amoxycillin in otitis media. BMJ 1982;284:1078–81.
54. Reed BD, Lutz LJ, Zazove P, Ratcliffe SD. Compliance with acute otitis media treatment. J Fam Pract 1984;19:627–32.
55. Mattar MD, Markello J, Yaffee SJ. Pharmaceutic factors affecting pediatric compliance. Pediatrics 1975;55:101–8.
56. Paradise JL. Secretory otitis media: what effects on children's development? Adv Otol Rhino Laryngol 1988;40:89–98.
57. Lorentzen P, Haugsten P. Treatment of acute suppurative otitis media. J Laryngol Otol 1977;91:331–40.
58. Browning GG, Gatehouse S, Calder IT. Medical management of active chronic otitis media: a controlled study. J Laryngol Otol 1988;102:491–5.
59. O'Shea JS, Langenbrunner DJ, McCloskey DE, et al. Childhood serous otitis media. Clin Pediatr (Phila) 1982;21:150–3.
60. Cantekin EI, Mandel EM, Bluestone CD, et al. Lack of efficacy of a decongestant-antihistamine combination for otitis media with effusion in children: results of a double blind randomized trial. N Engl J Med 1983;308:297–301.
61. Bhambhani K, Foulds DM, Swamy KN, et al. Acute otitis media in children: are decongestants or antihistamines necessary? Ann Emerg Med 1983;12:37–41.
62. Froom J, Mold J, Culpepper L, Boisseau V. The spectrum of otitis media in family practice. J Fam Pract 1980;10:599–605.

63. Jahn AF. Chronic otitis media: diagnosis and treatment. Med Clin North Am 1991;75:1277–91.
64. Celin SE, Bluestone CK, Stephenson X, et al. Bacteriology of acute otitis media in adults. JAMA 1991;266:2249–53.
65. Schwartz RH, Rodriguez WJ. Acute otitis media in children eight years old and older: a reappraisal of the role of Haemophilus influenzae. Am J Otolaryngol 1981;2:19–21.
66. Sugita R, Fujimaki Y, Deguchi K. Bacteriologic features and chemotherapy of adult acute purulent otitis media. J Laryngol Otol 1985;99:629–35.
67. Barenkamp SJ, Shurin PA, Marchant CD, et al. Do children with recurrent Haemophilus influenzae otitis media become infected with a new organism or reacquire the original strain? J Pediatr 1984;105:533–7.
68. Teele DW, Pelton SI, Klein JO. Bacteriology of acute otitis media unresponsive to initial antimicrobial therapy. J Pediatr 1981;98:537–9.
69. Varsano I, Volovitz, Mimouni F. Sulfisoxazole prophylaxis of middle ear effusion and recurrent acute otitis media. Am J Dis Child 1985;139:632–5.
70. Prinicipi N, Marchisio P, Massironi E, et al. Prophylaxis of recurrent otitis media and middle ear infections. Am J Dis Child 1989;143:1414–18.
71. Liston TE, Foshee WS, Pierson WD. Sulfasoxazole chemoprophylaxis for frequent otitis media. Pediatrics 1983;71:524–30.
72. Lampe RM, Weir MR. Erythromycin prophylaxis for recurrent otitis media. Clin Pediatr (Phila) 1986;25:510–15.
73. Schwartz RH, Puglise J, Rodriguez WJ. Sulphamethoxazole prophylaxis in the otitis-prone child. Arch Dis Child 1982;57:590–3.
74. Gaskins JD, Holt RJ, Kyong CU, et al. Chemoprophylaxis of recurrent otitis media using trimethoprim sulfamethoxazole. Drug Intell Clin Pharm 1982;16:387–90.
75. Makela PH, Karma P. Vaccination trials in otitis media: experiences in Finland since 1977. Pediatr Infect Dis J 1989;8:S79–S82.
76. Howie VM, Ploussard J, Sloyer JL, Hill JC. Use of pneumococcal polysaccharide vaccine in preventing otitis media in infants: different results between racial groups. Pediatrics 1984;73:79–82.
77. Fireman P. Otitis media and nasal disease: a role for allergy. J Clin Immunol 1988;82:917–26.
78. Fireman P. Otitis media and its relationship to allergy. Pediatr Clin North Am 1988;35:1075–90.
79. Kraemer MJ, Richardson MA, Weiss NS, et al. Risk factors for persistent middle-ear effusions. JAMA 1983;249:1022–5.
80. Schenker MB, Samet JM, Speizer FE. Risk factors for childhood respiratory disease: the effect of host factors and home environmental exposures. Am Rev Respir Dis 1983;128:1038–43.
81. Ferris BG, Ware JH, Berkey CS, et al. Effects of passive smoking on health of children. Environ Health Perspect 1985;62:289–95.
82. Tos M, Holm-Jensen S, Sorensen CH, Mogenson C. Spontaneous course and frequency of secretory otitis in 4 year old children. Arch Otolaryngol 1982;108:4–10.
83. Paradise JL. Management of secretory otitis media. Adv Otol Rhinol Laryngol 1988;40:99–109.

84. Pukander J. Clinical features of acute otitis media among children. Acta Otolaryngol (Stockh) 1983;95:117–22.
85. Callahan CW, Lazoritz S. Otitis media and language development. Am Fam Physician 1988;37:186–90.
86. Cohen D, Sade J. Hearing in secretory otitis media. Can J Otolaryngol 1972;1:27–29.
87. Bluestone CD, Beery QC, Paradise JL. Audiometry and typanometry in relations to middle ears in children. Laryngoscope 1973;83:594–604.
88. Bluestone CD. Morbidity, complications and sequelae of otitis media. In: Harford ER, Bess FH, Bluestone CD, et al, editors. Impedance screening in middle ear disease in children. Orlando, FL: Grune & Stratton, 1978:17–22.
89. Klein JO. Otitis media and the development of speech and language. Pediatr Infect Dis 1984;3:389–91.
90. Holm VA, Kunze LH. Effect of chronic otitis media on language and speech development. Pediatrics 1969;43:833–9.
91. Rapin I. Conductive hearing loss effects on children's language and scholastic skills: a review of the literature. Ann Otol Rhinol Laryngol Suppl 1979;88:3–12.
92. Paradise JL. Otitis media during early life; how hazardous to development? A critical review of the evidence. Pediatrics 1981;68:869–73.
93. Bennett FC, Ruuska SH, Sherman R. Middle ear function in learning disabled children. Pediatrics 1980;66:254–60.
94. Hoffman-Lawless K, Keith RW, Cotton RT. Auditory processing abilities in children with previous middle ear effusions. Ann Otol Rhinol Laryngol 1981;90:543–5.
95. Hubbard TW, Paradise JL, McWilliams BJ, et al. Consequences of unremitting middle ear disease in early life: otologic, audiologic, and developmental findings in children with cleft palate. N Engl J Med 1985;312:1529–34.
96. Roberts JE, Sanyal MA, Burchinal MR, et al. Otitis media in early childhood and its relationship to later verbal and academic performance. Pediatrics 1986;78:423–30.
97. Merluzzi E, Henchcliffe R. Threshold of subjective auditory handicap. Audiology 1973;12:65–68.
98. Fry J, Dillane JB, McNab-Jones RF, Kalton G. The outcome of acute otitis media. Br J Prev Soc Med 1969;23:205–9.
99. Bax M. The intimate relationship of health, development, and behavior in the young child. In: Brown CC, editor. Infants at risk: pediatric roundtable 5. New Brunswick, NJ: Johnson & Johnson, 1981:106–13.
100. Teele DW, Klein JO, Rosner BA, et al. Otitis media with effusion during the first three years of life and development of speech and language. Pediatrics 1984;74:282–7.
101. Halstead C, Lepow ML, Balassanian AI, et al. Otitis media: clinical observations, microbiology and evaluation of therapy. Am J Dis Child 1968;115:542–51.
102. Laxdal OE, Merida J, Jones RHT. Treatment of acute otitis media: a controlled study of 142 children. Can Med Assoc J 1970;102:263–8.
103. Cantekin EI, McGuire TW, Griffith TL. Antimicrobial therapy for otitis media with effusion (secretory otitis media). JAMA 1991;266:3309–17.

104. Moran DM, Mutchie KD, Higbee MD, Paul LD. The use of an antihista-mine-decongestant in conjunction with an anti-infective drug in the treat-ment of acute otitis media. J Pediatr 1982;101:132–6.
105. Mandel EM, Rockette HE, Bluestone CD, et al. Efficacy of amoxicillin with and without decongestant-antihistamine combination for otitis media with effusion in children: results of a double blind randomized trial. N Engl J Med 1987;316:432–7.
106. Thomsen J, Sederbert-Olsen J, Balle V, et al. Antibiotic treatment of children with secretory otitis media: a randomized, double blind, placebo controlled study. Arch Otolaryngol Head Neck Surg 1989;115:447–51.
107. Dagoo B, Freijd A. Immune deficiency and otitis media. In: Bernstein JM, Ogra PL, editors. Immunology of the ear. New York: Raven Press, 1987:363–80.
108. Lindholdt T, Kortholm B. Beclamethasone nasal spray in the treatment of middle ear effusion. Int J Otorhinolaryngol 1982;4:133–7.
109. Smyth G, Patterson C, Hall S. Tympanostomy tubes: do they significantly benefit the patient? Otolaryngol Head Neck Surg 1982;90:783–6.
110. Bonding P, Tos M. Grommets versus paracentesis in secretory otitis media: a prospective controlled study. Am J Otol 1985;6:455–60.
111. Cantekin EI, Bluestone CD. Membrane ventilating tube for the middle ear. Ann Otol Rhinol Laryngol 1976;85:270–6.
112. Donaldson JA. Surgical management of otitis media (recurrent and non-suppurative). J Allergy Clin Immunol 1988;81:1020–4.
113. Gates G, Wachtendorf C, Hearne E, Holt G. Treatment of chronic otitis media with effusion: results of tympanostomy tubes. Am J Otolaryngol 1985;6:249–53.
114. Brenman AK, Meltzer CR, Milner RM. Myringotomy and tube ventilation in adults. Am Fam Physician 1982;26:181–4.
115. Kleinman LC, Kosecoff J, Dubois RW, Brook RH. The medical appropri-ateness of tympanostomy tubes proposed for children younger than 16 years in the United States. JAMA 1994;271(16):1250–5.
116. Johnson JT, Rood SR, Newman RK. Abnormalities in and around the ear. Postgrad Med 1982;72:123–30.
117. Amundson LH. Disorders of the external ear. Prim Care 1990;17:213–31.
118. Springer GL, Shapiro ED. Fresh water swimming as a risk factor for otitis externa: a case controlled study. Arch Environ Health 1985;40:202–6.
119. Marcy SM. Infections of external ear. Pediatr Infect Dis 1985;4:192–201.
120. Mitchell RB. Rapid microbiological methodology in military medicine. Milit Med 1955;116:85–89.
121. Reich JJ. Ear infections. Emerg Med Clin North Am 1987;5:227–42.
122. Keim RJ. How aging affects the ear. Geriatrics 1977;12:97–99.
123. Kopstein E. Otitis externa: unorthodox but effective treatments. Laryngo-scope 1984;94:1248.
124. Strauss M, Aber RC, Conner GH, Baum S. Malignant external otitis: long-term (months) antimicrobial therapy. Laryngoscope 1982;92:397–406.
125. Meyerhoof WL, Gates GA, Montalbo PJ. Pseudomonas mastoiditis. Laryngoscope 1977;87:483–92.
126. Hardoff R, Gips S, Uri N, et al. Semiquantitative skull planar and SPECT bond scintigraphy in diabetic patients; differentiation of mectotizing ma-lignant external otitis from severe external otitis. J Nucl Med 1994;35(3):411–5.

CASE PRESENTATION

Subjective

PATIENT PROFILE

Jason Harris is a 4-year-old white male child.

PRESENTING PROBLEM

Earache.

PRESENT ILLNESS

For 2 days, Jason has complained of a left earache. There has been a low-grade fever, sore throat, and nasal congestion. Jason has had three prior episodes of earache over the past 6 months.

PAST MEDICAL HISTORY

No serious illness or hospitalization since birth.

SOCIAL HISTORY

Jason attends day care 5 mornings per week.

FAMILY HISTORY

His parents are both living and well. There is a 1-year-old sibling.

- What other historical information might be pertinent, and why?
- What might be the significance of having had three prior episodes of ear infection?
- What—if anything—might be pertinent about the child's day care experience?
- What more might you like to know about the family history, and why?

Objective

VITAL SIGNS

Pulse, 78; respirations, 22; temperature, 38.0°C.

EXAMINATION

Patient is alert but in pain with a left earache. The left tympanic membrane is injected but not retracted or bulging. There is mild injection of the pharynx without tonsillar swelling or exudate. There are few enlarged left cervical lymph nodes. The chest is clear, and the heart is normal.

- What more—if anything—would you include in the physical examination, and why?
- How might you evaluate the child's hearing?
- What—if any—laboratory tests might you order today?
- If there were thick purulent drainage from the ear, what would be its significance?

Assessment

- What is the probable diagnosis? Describe the likely etiologic agent(s).
- How would you explain this diagnosis to the family?
- The parents ask if Jason needs a referral to an ear, nose, and throat specialist. How would you respond?
- What are the family implications of this illness?

Plan

- What therapeutic recommendations would you make regarding medication for relief of pain?
- When can Jason return to day care? What might influence your decision?
- If Jason's mother calls tonight to report that there is purulent drainage from the left ear, what would you advise?
- What follow-up would you advise for this illness?

12

Ischemic Heart Disease

Jim Nuovo

Cardiovascular disease remains the most significant cause of morbidity and mortality in the United States. In 1990, 1.5 million Americans experienced a myocardial infarction; approximately 500,000 of them died.[1] It is estimated that 6.1 million Americans are alive today with a history of myocardial infarction, angina, or both. The financial impact of this disease is enormous. The cost estimate for cardiovascular disease in 1992 was $108.9 billion. It is important for all primary care providers to implement screening and preventive care programs to reduce the burden of cardiovascular disease for the population in general and for the individual patient. Because of the high morbidity and mortality, it is also important to recognize the early manifestations of this disease.

Unfortunately, in up to 20% of patients, the first manifestation of ischemic heart disease (IHD) is sudden cardiac arrest.[2] Most deaths from IHD occur outside the hospital and within 2 hours of onset of symptoms.[3,4] For the past 30 years, a great deal of effort has been directed toward the practice of cardiopulmonary resuscitation and emergency cardiac care. These efforts have been directed toward minimizing the number of cardiac deaths.[5] Furthermore, there has been an enormous undertaking to identify and treat those individuals with significant cardiovascular risk factors with the goal of lowering morbidity and mortality. This effort has been successful as noted by the decline in death rates from myocardial ischemia and its complications. The purpose of this chapter is to discuss three issues relevant to the family physician regarding IHD: the evaluation of patients with chest pain, the diagnosis and management of angina pectoris, and the diagnosis and management of myocardial infarction.

Chest Pain

Chest pain is one of the common reasons for patients visiting primary care physicians.[6] The major diagnostic considerations for chest pain are listed in Table 12.1. Of the diagnostic considerations, which are the ones most

TABLE 12.1. Some common causes of
chronic and recurrent chest pain

Cardiac causes
  Hypertrophic cardiomyopathy
  Ischemic heart disease
  Mitral valve prolapse
  Pericarditis

Chest wall problems
  Costochondritis
  Myofascial syndrome

Gastrointestinal causes
  Esophageal motility disorders
  Gastroesophageal reflux

Neurologic causes
  Radiculopathy
  Zoster (postherpetic neuralgia)

Psychiatric causes
  Anxiety
  Depression
  Hyperventilation
  Panic disorder

---

commonly seen by primary care physicians? A Family Practice Research Network recently investigated this issue. Over 1 year, the Michigan Research Network prospectively collected information on 399 patients with episodes of chest pain.[6] The most common diagnostic findings included (1) musculoskeletal pain (20.4%), (2) reflux esophagitis (13.4%), (3) costochondritis (13.1%), and (4) angina pectoris (10.3%). The highest priority is generally given to distinguishing cardiac from noncardiac chest pain. Of the many diseases listed, the most common differential diagnostic considerations are of esophageal and psychiatric etiologies.

Noncardiac Chest Pain

Studies have demonstrated that 10% to 30% of patients with chest pain who undergo coronary arteriography have no arterial abnormalities.[7–9] Follow-up studies of these patients have shown that the risk of subsequent myocardial infarction is low.[10–17] Fifty to seventy-five percent of these patients have persistent complaints of chest pain and disability.[12,14] The most common noncardiac problems in the differential are esophageal disorders, hyperventilation, panic attacks, and anxiety disorders.

Esophageal Chest Pain

Of the patients who have undergone coronary arteriography and have been found to have normal coronary arteries, as many as 50% have demonstrable esophageal abnormalities.[17-19] Richter et al.[20] critically reviewed 117 articles on recurring chest pain of esophageal origin to clarify issues related to this disease. They paid specific attention to the following controversial issues: the potential mechanisms of esophageal pain, differentiation of cardiac and esophageal causes, evaluation of esophageal motility disorders, use of esophageal tests for evaluating noncardiac chest pain, usefulness of techniques for prolonged monitoring of intraesophageal pressure and pH, and the relation of psychological abnormalities to esophageal motility disorders. They concluded that (1) specific mechanisms to produce chest pain are not well understood; (2) esophageal chest pain has usually been attributed to the stimulation of chemoreceptors (acid and bile) or mechanoreceptors (spasm and distension); (3) studies performed to confirm direct associations between these factors and pain have not been consistent in their findings; and (4) it appears that the triggers for esophageal chest pain are multifactorial and often idiosyncratic to a particular patient.

Differentiating cardiac from esophageal disease can often be frustrating. As many as 50% of patients with coronary artery disease have esophageal disease.[21] There are many case reports of esophageal disorders producing pain that mimics myocardial ischemia.[22] Areskog et al.[23] have shown that esophageal abnormalities are common in patients who are admitted to a coronary care unit and are later found to have no evidence of cardiac disease. The clinical history frequently does not differentiate between cardiac and esophageal chest pain, although some features may be helpful in this process. Features suggesting an esophageal origin include pain that continues for hours, pain that interrupts sleep or is meal-related, pain relieved by antacids, or the presence of other esophageal symptoms (heartburn, dysphagia, regurgitation).[24] Conversely, it is well documented that gastroesophageal reflux may be triggered by heavy exercise and may produce exertional chest pain mimicking angina even during treadmill testing.[22]

Tests that can be performed to determine the presence of esophageal disease include esophageal motility testing and provocative testing (e.g., acid perfusion and balloon distension). Although findings from these tests have produced a better understanding of the pathologic conditions leading to the development of chest pain with esophageal disorders, there is no consensus as to the usefulness of these tests for the specific patient with chest pain. As noted by Pope,[25] "What is needed is a simple and safe provocative esophageal maneuver to turn on chest pain that possesses a high degree of sensitivity."

There is clearly an interaction between psychological abnormalities and esophageal disorders. Patients with esophageal disorders have been shown to have significantly higher levels of anxiety disorders, somatization, and depression.[26,27] It is not clear if there is a cause-and-effect relation. Given the aforementioned difficulties in the diagnosis of esophageal chest pain, the differentiation of this pain from cardiac disease, and the close relation between cardiac, esophageal, and psychiatric disease, it is wise to maintain a consistent approach to the evaluation of these patients. Richter et al.[20] developed a stepwise approach for patients with recurring chest pain. They recommended the exclusion of cardiac disease, with the subsequent evaluation to rule out structural abnormalities of the upper gastrointestinal tract (barium swallow, upper gastrointestinal series, and endoscopy). Also recommended is a trial of antireflux therapy for 1 to 2 months. In those patients who fail to respond, specialized testing may then be appropriate (esophageal motility, 24-hour pH monitor, provocative testing, and psychological evaluation).

Psychiatric Illness

There has long been a connection with psychiatric disorders that can produce chest pain. Katon et al.[28] reported the results of an evaluation of 74 patients with chest pain and no history of organic heart disease. Each patient underwent a structured psychiatric interview immediately after coronary arteriography. Patients with chest pain and negative coronary arteriograms were significantly younger, more likely to be female, more apt to have a higher number of autonomic symptoms (tachycardia, dyspnea, dizziness, paresthesias) associated with chest pain, and more likely to describe atypical chest pain. These patients also had significantly higher scores on indices of anxiety and depression that met DSM-III criteria for panic disorder, major depression, and phobias. Waxler et al.[29] concluded that 40% of women with chest pain who had normal coronary arteries had hypochondriacal or neurotic behavior. Specific medical therapy directed at the anxiety and depression may help these patients. Cannon et al. recently published a study on a group of patients with chest pain despite normal coronary angiograms. Imipramine was shown to improve their symptoms. Patients who were given 50 mg nightly had a statistically significant mean reduction of 52% in episodes of chest pain.[30] Iatrogenic uncertainty may also contribute to persistent pain.

Cardiac Chest Pain: Angina Pectoris

Angina is not simply one type of pain; it is a constellation of symptoms related to cardiac ischemia. The description of angina may fit several patterns.

1. *Classic angina.* It presents as a ill-defined pressure, heaviness (feeling like a weight), or squeezing sensation brought on by exertion and relieved by rest. The pain is most often substernal and left-sided. It may

radiate to the jaw, interscapular area, or down the arm. Angina usually begins gradually and lasts only a few minutes.

2. *Atypical angina.* Similar symptoms are experienced but with the absence of one or more of the criteria for classic angina. For example, the pain may not be consistently related to exertion or relieved by rest. Conversely, the pain may have an atypical character (sharp, stabbing), but the precipitating factors are clearly anginal.

3. *Anginal equivalent.* The sensation of dyspnea is the sole or major manifestation.

4. *Variant (Prinzmetal's) angina.* This angina occurs at rest and may manifest in stereotyped patterns, such as nocturnal symptoms or symptoms that appear only after exercise. It is thought to be caused by coronary artery spasm. Its symptoms often occur periodically, with characteristic pain-free intervals, and are associated with typical electrocardiographic (ECG) changes, most commonly ST segment elevation.[31,32]

5. *Syndrome X (microvascular angina).* Some patients with the clinical diagnosis of coronary artery disease have no evidence for obstructive atherosclerosis. Several reports investigating this population have found a subset with metabolic evidence for ischemia (myocardial lactate during induced myocardial stress as evidence for ischemia). Kemp reported this group to have "syndrome X."[33] It has been suggested that some of these patients have microvascular angina.[34]

Confounding Problems in the Differential Diagnosis

It is important for clinicians to recognize the factors that may confound the clinical diagnosis of angina pectoris. Some of these factors are as follows: (1) The severity of pain is not necessarily proportional to the seriousness of the underlying illness. (2) The physical examination is not generally helpful for differentiating cardiac from noncardiac disease. A normal examination cannot be counted on to rule out significant cardiac disease. (3) The ECG is normal in more than 50% of patients with ischemic cardiac disease. A normal ECG cannot be used to rule out significant cardiac disease. (4) Denial is a significant component in the presentation of chest pain caused by myocardial infarction. (5) Some of the diseases common in the differential diagnosis of chest pain may present concurrently. Major depressive disorder and panic disorder are known to be prevalent in patients with esophageal disorders.[27] Colgan et al.[35] reported that of 63 patients with chest pain and normal angiograms, 32 (51%) had evidence of an esophageal disorder, and 19 of the 32 (59%) had a current psychiatric disorder (anxiety or depression). Patients with concurrent disorders will be particularly challenging to a clinician in sorting out the cause of their chest pain.

Can the presence of one of these concurrent disorders precipitate myocardial ischemia? A recent study by Lam et al. looked specifically at the question of esophageal dysfunction as a cause of angina. The phenomenon of reflux and/or esophageal motility disorder causing myocardial ischemia has been called "linked angina." In a study of 30 patients, there was no evidence of this phenomenon.[36]

Clinical Tools Used to Distinguish Cardiac from Noncardiac Chest Pain

Despite the difficulties noted above, there are important clinical tools that can be used to distinguish cardiac from noncardiac chest pain.

History

Despite the mentioned difficulties, the history is key to distinguishing cardiac from noncardiac etiologies of chest pain. Noncardiac chest pain is often fleeting, brief, sharp, or stabbing. The pain may be reproduced by palpating the chest wall. The duration of pain is also important. Symptoms that last many hours or days are not likely to be anginal. A great deal of work has been done to assess the probability of IHD in a given patient based on clinical presentation. In 1979, Diamond and Forrester[37] presented such an approach. Using data from the clinical presentation correlated with autopsy and angiographic information, they presented a pretest likelihood of coronary artery disease in symptomatic patients according to age, sex, and type of chest pain (nonanginal, atypical angina, or typical angina); several observations can be made from this chart (Table 12.2): Men have a substantially greater risk than women for any given type of chest pain and for any given age. A middle-aged man with atypical chest pain has a high chance of having significant coronary artery disease. Young women (aged 30–40) with classic angina have a relatively low chance of having significant coronary artery disease.

TABLE 12.2. Pretest likelihood of significant ischemic heart disease based on symptoms

Age (years)	Nonanginal chest pain	Atypical angina	Typical angina
30–39	5% M/0.8% F	22% M/4% F	69% M/26% F
40–49	14% M/3% F	46% M/13% F	87% M/55% F
50–59	21% M/8% F	59% M/32% F	92% M/79% F
60–69	28% M/18% F	67% M/54% F	94% M/90% F

Source: Diamond and Forrester.[37] Reprinted by permission of the New England Journal of Medicine.

Diagnostic Testing

After establishing a pretest probability of IHD, there are a variety of tests available to help establish an accurate diagnosis. Although many tests are now firmly established in clinical practice, none is particularly suited to wide-scale, cost-effective application because each has limitations concerning sensitivity and specificity.

Exercise Tolerance Testing

In 1986, the American College of Cardiology and the American Heart Association Task Force on Assessment of Cardiovascular Procedures set guidelines for exercise treadmill testing (ETT).[38] For patients with symptoms suggestive of coronary artery disease, there are five basic indications for undertaking exercise stress testing: (1) as a diagnostic test in patients with suspected IHD; (2) to assist in identifying those patients with documented IHD who are potentially at high risk due to advanced coronary disease or left ventricular dysfunction; (3) to evaluate patients after coronary artery bypass surgery; (4) to quantify a patient's functional capacity or response to therapies; and (5) to follow the natural course of the disease at appropriate intervals. The purpose of the ETT for the patient with chest pain is to help establish whether the pain is indeed IHD.

Although there are many exercise protocols available, the protocols proposed by Bruce in 1956 remain appropriate.[39] A review of the ETT for family physicians has been published.[40,41] With one standard ETT (*Bruce protocol*), the patient is asked to exercise for 3-minute intervals on a motorized treadmill device while being monitored for the following: heart rate and blood pressure response to exercise, symptoms during the test, ECG response (specifically ST segment displacement), dysrhythmias, and exercise capacity. Contraindications to ETT include unstable angina, myocardial infarction (MI), rapid atrial or ventricular dysrhythmias, poorly controlled congestive heart failure, severe aortic stenosis, myocarditis, recent significant illness, and an uncooperative patient. A significant (positive) test includes an ST segment depression of 1.0 mm below the baseline. Many factors influence the results of an ETT and can lead to false-positive or false-negative results. Factors leading to false-positive results include the following: (1) the use of medications such as digoxin, estrogens, and diuretics; and (2) conditions such as mitral valve prolapse, cardiomyopathy, and hyperventilation. Factors leading to false-negative results include the following: (1) the use of medications such as nitrates, β-blockers, calcium channel blockers; and (2) conditions such as a prior MI or a submaximal test.[38,39] The sensitivity of the ETT has been estimated to range from 56% to 81% and the specificity to range from 72% to 96%.[42] The key point is that given the vagaries of the ETT for diagnosing IHD (generally low sensitivity and specificity), a patient with a high pretest likelihood of IHD (e.g., a 50-year-old man with typical angina) still has a high probability of significant disease even in the face of a normal (negative) test. Furthermore, a patient with a low probability of IHD (e.g., a 40-year-old woman with atypical chest pain) still has a low chance of significant disease even if the test is positive.[37] The optimal use of diagnostic testing is for those patients with moderate pretest probabilities (e.g., a 40- to 50-year-old man with atypical pain).

In addition to the diagnostic implications of an ETT, there are prognostic implications. The following are considered to be parameters associated with poor prognosis or increased disease severity: failure to complete stage II of a Bruce protocol, failure to achieve a heart rate greater than 120 beats/min (off β-blockers), onset of ST segment depression at a heart rate of less than 120 beats/min, ST segment depression greater than 2.0 mm, ST segment depression lasting more than 6 minutes into recovery, ST segment depression in multiple leads, poor systolic blood pressure response to exercise, ST segment elevation, angina with exercise, and exercise-induced ventricular tachycardia.[38]

Radionuclide ETT

There are patients in whom the standard ETT is not a useful diagnostic tool and in whom a radionuclide procedure would be more appropriate. Patients with baseline ECG abnormalities due to digitalis or left ventricular hypertrophy with strain or those with bundle branch block (especially left bundle branch block) cannot have proper evaluation of the ST segment for characteristic ischemic changes. In these patients, a thallium 201 stress test is appropriate. The thallium ETT has the advantage of increased sensitivity (80–87%) and specificity (85–90%).[43] Unfortunately, the cost of this procedure is almost four times as great as a standard ETT ($175–$250 versus $1000–$1400).[40]

Response to Nitroglycerin

Another approach uses clinical information to determine the probability of coronary artery disease based on response to treatment. One such study involved the use of sublingual nitroglycerin to determine likelihood of disease. Horwitz et al.[44] evaluated the usefulness of nitroglycerin as a diagnostic aid for IHD. They found a sensitivity of 76% and a specificity of 80% in 70 patients with chest pain of anginal type. It was concluded that 90% of patients with recurrent, angina-like chest pain who exhibit a prompt response to nitroglycerin (within 3 minutes) have IHD; however, a delayed or absent response paradoxically indicates either an absence of IHD or unusually severe disease. Therefore, failure to respond to nitroglycerin should not be used to exclude the diagnosis of IHD.

Angina Pectoris

Once the diagnosis of angina is established, there are several important management considerations for this disease. The first is related to disease prognosis, the second to drug therapy, and the third to further investigative tests and invasive therapeutic interventions.

Prognosis

Three major factors determine the prognosis of patients with angina pectoris: the amount of viable but jeopardized left ventricular myocardium, the percentage of irreversibly scarred myocardium, and the severity of underlying coronary atherosclerosis. There have been several studies published before invasive therapies were available that assess the prognosis of patients with stable antina. Most of them were published between 1952 and 1973 and reported an annual mortality of 4%.[45,46] Since cardiac catheterization has come into general use, the prognosis has been modified and based on the number of diseased vessels. During the 1980s, annual mortality for patients with one-vessel disease, two-vessel disease, three-vessel disease, and left main coronary artery disease (CAD) was 1.5%, 3.5%, 6.0%, and 8.0% to 10.0%, respectively.[47]

ETT has been used to establish prognosis in patients with symptomatic IHD. The exercise test parameters associated with a poor outcome have been described above.[38] There are no randomized studies available to assess the impact of medical therapy on the prognosis of patients with stable angina. Of interest is the impact of percutaneous transluminal coronary angioplasty (PTCA). It is unclear from this point that PTCA significantly improves the prognosis in patients with stable angina. A study of the Coronary Artery Surgery Study registry patients who were potentially suitable for PTCA revealed a 4-year survival of 96%.[48] A similar study of medically treated patients suitable for PTCA revealed a 5-year survival of 97%.[49] When does angina signal severe coronary disease? Pryor et al.[50] developed a nomogram based on a point scoring system to help answer this question. They based the nomogram on the following factors: type of chest pain (typical, atypical, or nonanginal), sex, selective cardiovascular risk factors (hypertension, smoking, hyperlipidemia, and diabetes mellitus), anginal duration (months), and the presence of carotid bruits. By applying the nomogram for the individual patient, one can determine the probability of severe disease (i.e., 75% narrowing of the left main coronary artery or three-vessel disease).

Drug Therapy

In patients with stable exertional angina who do not have severe disease, the prognosis is excellent, and there is no difference between medical and surgical treatment as far as long-term mortality is concerned.[51] The goal of therapy is to abolish or reduce anginal attacks and myocardial ischemia and to promote a normal life style. For the relief of angina, the treatment strategy is to lower myocardial oxygen demand and increase coronary blood flow to the ischemic regions. Patients should be screened for the presence of significant cardiovascular risk factors and should be advised to modify any that are present. Three classes of antianginal drugs are commonly used: nitrates, β-blockers, and calcium channel blockers. Each reduces myocardial oxygen demand and may improve blood flow to the ischemic regions. The mechanisms by which these agents reduce myocardial oxygen demand or increase coronary blood flow to ischemic areas differ from one class of drug to another. No greater efficacy in relieving chest pain or decreasing exercise-induced ischemia has been shown for one or another group of drugs.

Nitrates

Nitrates are potent venous and arterial dilators. At low doses venous dilation predominates, and at higher doses arterial dilation occurs as well. Nitrates decrease myocardial oxygen demand in the following ways: decreased venous return reduces left ventricular end-diastolic volume and ventricular wall stress. Increased arterial compliance and cardiac output lowers systolic blood pressure and decreases peripheral resistance (afterload). It also enhances myocardial oxygen supply by preventing closure of stenotic coronary arteries during exercise, dilating epicardial coronary arteries, and decreasing left ventricular end-diastolic pressure, thereby enhancing subendocardial blood flow and inhibiting coronary artery spasm. Nitrates are inexpensive and have a well-documented safety record. Both short- and long-acting nitrates are available. Short-acting preparations are used for the relief of an established attack, whereas long-acting nitrates are used for prevention.[52] The most significant concern about the long-acting nitrates is tolerance. Most studies have shown that tolerance develops rapidly when long-acting nitrates are given for anginal prophylaxis.[53] With nitroglycerin patches, tolerance can develop within 24 hours, and further therapy can lead to complete loss of the antianginal effect.[54] Various dosing strategies with oral and transdermal formulations have been used to overcome the development of nitroglycerin tolerance. Patch-free intervals of 10 to 12 hours are commonly used to retain the antianginal effectiveness.[55] For oral nitroglycerin, isosorbide dinitrate three times daily at 7 a.m., noon, and 5 p.m. appears to prevent the development of tolerance.[53] Because of the concern for intervals during which patients remain unprotected, it is common to add another antianginal agent to the nitroglycerin regimen. Other problems with nitroglycerin include the fact that 10% of patients do not respond and 10% have associated intolerable headaches that may necessitate discontinuation.[56]

β-Blockers

The antianginal effect of β-blockers is well established.[57,58] These agents improve exercise tolerance and reduce myocardial ischemia. The effect produces a reduction in myocardial oxygen demand through a reduction in heart rate and contractility. Many β-blockers are available; they may be divided into those that are nonselective (β_1 and β_2) (i.e., propranolol, timolol, nadolol), those that are β_1-selective (i.e., atenolol, metoprolor, acebutolol), and those that are nonselective and produce vasodilatory effects through the ability to block α_1-receptors and dilate blood vessels directly (i.e., labetolol, pindolol). All β-blockers, irrespective of their selective properties, are equally effective in patients with angina.[58] Some 20% of patients do not respond to β-blockers. Those who do not respond are more likely to have severe IHD. Furthermore, some patients do not tolerate the adverse side effects, such as fatigue, depression, dyspnea, and cold extremities. Other concerns include a small but significant aggravation of hyperlipidemia and precipitation of congestive heart failure and bronchospasm in susceptible individuals. Generally, β-blockers are dose-adjusted to achieve a heart rate of 50 to 60 beats/min. Patients should be cautioned to not stop β-blockers abruptly, thereby avoiding a rebound phenomenon.

Calcium Channel Blockers

Calcium channel blockers are a diverse group of compounds, all of which impede calcium ion influx into the myocardium and smooth muscle cells.[59] These agents relieve myocardial ischemia by reducing myocardial oxygen demand secondary to decreased afterload and myocardial contractility. Also, these agents dilate coronary arteries. There are three classes of calcium channel blockers: papaverine derivatives (verapamil), dihydropyridines (nifedipine, nicardipine), and benzothiazepines (diltiazem). Each of the drugs in the three classes has different effects on the atrioventricular node, heart rate, coronary vasodilation, diastolic relaxation, cardiac contractility, systemic blood pressure, and afterload. All three classes are effective for the management of patients with stable angina.[60] Most studies have shown them to have effects equal to those of β-blockers. Calcium channel blockers may be preferred in patients with obstructive airway disease, hypertension, peripheral vascular disease, or supraventricular tachycardia. In general, they are well tolerated. The most troublesome side effects include constipation, edema, headache, and aggravation of congestive heart failure.

Combination Therapy

It is important to maximize therapy with any one class of antianginal drug before considering it a failed trial. If monotherapy fails, it is appropriate to add another agent. Generally, β-blockers and nitrates or calcium channel blockers and nitrates complement each other. Because nitrates and nifedipine may increase the heart rate, it is advisable to use a combination of nitrates plus verapamil or diltiazem.[56] Calcium channel blockers and β-blockers can be used together. Combination therapy may be more effective than either agent alone.[61] It is important to be cautious, as some combinations produce deleterious effects. For example, verapamil and β-blockers may produce extreme bradycardia or heart block.

Aspirin

Aspirin is effective for primary and secondary prevention of myocardial infarction, presumably by inhibiting thrombosis.[62–64] There is no evidence to support the idea that aspirin is effective for primary prevention of angina.[65] Although there is controversy as to the ideal therapeutic dose, "low-dose" therapy (80–300 mg) is generally recommended.[64]

Invasive Testing

Cardiac catheterization is not routinely recommended for initial management of patients with stable angina. Patients who warrant such an evaluation are those who exhibit evidence for severe myocardial ischemia on noninvasive testing or who have symptoms that are refractory to antianginal medications. In patients who undergo catheterization, the most important determinant of survival is left ventricular function followed by the number of diseased vessels. Patients with left main artery disease or three-vessel disease with diminished left ventricular function are candidates for a coronary artery bypass graft procedure. Others (those with one- or two-vessel disease) are managed medically or considered for PTCA.

Unstable Angina Pectoris

Unstable angina manifests clinically either as an abrupt onset of ischemic symptoms at rest or as an intensification or change in the pattern of ischemic symptoms in a patient with a history of IHD. This intensification may be manifested by an increase in the frequency, severity, and duration of symptoms as well as an increasing ease of provocation (symptoms at rest or with minimal effort). Recurrence of ischemic symptoms soon after an MI (usually within 4 weeks) is also considered a sign of unstable angina. The diagnosis of unstable angina is generally made on clinical grounds alone. Because of the episodic nature of ischemia in unstable angina, however, transient ECG abnormalities (ST segment depression or elevation or T-wave abnormalities, i.e., inversion, flattening, or peaking) may not be documented in 50% to 70% of patients with the clinical diagnosis of unstable angina. In studies in which prolonged Holter monitoring was used during the in-hospital phase of unstable angina, transient ischemic ST segment deviations have been described in 60% to 70% of cases, more than 70% of them being clinically unsuspected or silent.[66,67]

Prognosis

The prognosis of patients with unstable angina is clearly not as good as those with chronic stable angina. During the precatheterization era, the mortality rate was estimated to be 12% to 15% for 3 months.[47] The rate of nonfatal MI is about 8% to 10% during the first 2 weeks. Mortality is increased in those who fail to respond to initial therapy, who have severe left ventricular dysfunction, and who have multivessel CAD (particularly left main artery disease).

Management Strategy

The most important recent development in the management of unstable angina has been the 1994 report of the Agency for Health Care Policy and Research.[68] This report includes clinical practice guidelines that are based on a consensus panel of experts. The guidelines allow physicians to consider outpatient management for a select subgroup of patients with this problem, specifically those who are thought to be at low risk for myocardial infarction. According to the report, in the initial management, physicians should use the information in Table 12.3 to determine whether a particular patient has a high, intermediate, or low likelihood of having significant CAD. For example, the patient with a low likelihood will be nondiabetic, have atypical chest pain, be younger (<60 for men, 70 for women), and have a normal ECG. The next step is to determine the level of risk of MI. The information in Table 12.4 allows for a similar stratification of risk. For example, a low-risk patient is one with a history of angina that is now provoked at a lower threshold yet not at rest, and the ECG is normal or unchanged. Low-risk patients may be treated with aspirin, nitroglycerin, and/or β-blockers. Follow-up should be no later than 72 hours. High- or moderate-risk patients should be admitted for intensive medical management. Intensive medical management includes consideration of aspirin, heparin, nitrates, β-blockers, calcium channel blockers (if the patient is already on adequate doses of nitrates and β-blockers or unable to tolerate these), and morphine sulfate.

Once the patient is stable, he or she should be considered for noninvasive exercise testing to further define the prognosis and direct the treatment plan. Low-risk patients can be medically managed. Those of intermediate risk should be considered for additional testing (either a cardiac catheterization or a radionuclide stress test or echocardiographic stress test). Those of high risk should be referred for cardiac catheterization.[68]

TABLE 12.3. Likelihood of significant CAD in patients with
symptoms suggesting unstable angina

High likelihood	Intermediate likelihood	Low likelihood
Any of the following features:	*Absence of high likelihood features and any of the following:*	*Absence of high or intermediate likelihood features but may have:*
Known history of CAD	Definite angina: males <60 or females <70 years	Chest pain, probably not angina
Definite angina: males ≥60 or females ≥70 years	Probable angina: males >60 or females >70 years	One risk factor but not diabetes
Hemodynamic changes or ECG changes with pain	Probably not angina in diabetic or in nondiabetic patients with two or more other risk factors[a]	T wave flat or inverted <1 mm in leads with dominant R waves
Variant angina	Extracardiac vascular disease	Normal ECG
ST increase or decrease ≥1 mm	ST depression 0.05 to 1 mm	
Marked symmetric T-wave inversion in multiple precordial leads	T-wave inversion ≥1 mm in leads with dominant R waves	

Source: Braunwald et al.[68]
[a]CAD risk factors include diabetes, smoking, hypertension, and elevated cholesterol.
CAD = coronary artery disease; ECG = electrocardiograph.

TABLE 12.4. Short-term risk of death or nonfatal myocardial infarction in
patients with symptoms suggesting unstable angina

High risk	Intermediate risk	Low risk
At least one of the following features must be present:	*No high-risk feature but must have any of the following:*	*No high- or intermediate-risk feature but may have any of the following:*
Prolonged ongoing (>20 min) rest pain	Rest angina now resolved but now low likelihood of CAD	Increased angina frequency, severity, or duration
Pulmonary edema	Rest angina (>20 min or relieved with rest or nitroglycerin)	Angina provoked at a lower threshold
Angina with new or worsening mitral regurgitation murmurs	Angina with dynamic T-wave changes	New-onset angina within 2 weeks to 2 months
Rest angina with dynamic ST changes ≥1 mm	Nocturnal angina	Normal or unchanged ECG
Angina with S_3 or rales	New-onset CCSC III or IV angina in past 2 weeks but not low likelihood of CAD	
Angina with hypotension	Q waves or ST depression ≥1 mm in multiple leads	
	Age >65 years	

Source: Braunwald et al.[68]
CAD = coronary artery disease; ECG = electrocardiograph.

Antiplatelet Therapy

Antiplatelet therapy is an important addition for patients with unstable angina. Several studies have demonstrated that often the cause of crescendo angina is the occurrence of platelet aggregation and thrombus formation on the surface of an ulcerated plaque.[69] In the Veterans Administration Cooperative Study, men with unstable angina who received aspirin (325 mg/day) had a 50% reduction in subsequent death from MI.[70]

Percutaneous Transluminal Coronary Angioplasty

There has been a marked increase in the use of angioplasty, and in 1990, more than 300,000 such procedures were performed.[71] The American College of Cardiology and the American Heart Association Task Force have published guidelines for the selection of patients for coronary angioplasty.[72] Among patients with unstable angina, PTCA is recommended for those who do not show an adequate response to medical treatment (continued chest pain or evidence of ongoing ischemia during ECG monitoring) or who are intolerant to medical therapy because of uncontrollable side effects.

The long-term outcome after successful angioplasty has been reported to be excellent even when compared with patients undergoing bypass surgery.[73] Further research is important in the areas of long-term outcome for multiple lesions, extensive disease, and avoidance of complications. Technologies such as stents, laser angioplasty, and atherectomy await clinical evaluation.

Coronary Artery Bypass Graft

Large randomized trials have shown that surgical revascularization is more effective than medical therapy in relieving angina and improving exercise tolerance for at least several years. Development of atherosclerosis in the coronary artery bypass graft resulting in angina generally occurs within 5 to 10 years. Improved survival with surgical versus medical therapy is seen only in the subset of patients with severe CAD or left ventricular dysfunction.[74]

Silent Ischemia

Many investigations have established that most ischemic episodes in patients with stable angina are not accompanied by chest pain (silent ischemia). It remains unclear the precise nature of events that accompany ischemic events that do or do not produce pain. Patients with predominantly silent ischemia may be hyposensitive to pain in general; denial may play a role, or they may experience pain but attribute the symptoms to a less significant event. It is well documented that personality-related, emotional, and social factors can modulate the perception of pain. It is not surprising that the symptoms among cardiac patients with the same degree of disease vary greatly.[75] Personality inventory studies have shown that patients with reproducible angina have higher scores on indices of nervousness and excitability than do those who are free of symptoms.[76] Patients with clinical depression are also more likely to experience angina than control subjects.[77] Many studies have shown that stress of various types can influence the frequency and duration of ischemic episodes in patients with angina.[78-80] Silent ischemia is prevalent.

Seventy percent of ischemic episodes in patients with IHD are estimated to be asymptomatic. Among patients with stable angina who undergo 24-hour Holter monitoring, 40% to 72% of the episodes are painless. Among patients with unstable angina, more than half manifest painless ST segment depression. In 1988, Cohn[81] proposed classifying silent ischemia into three clinical types to help clarify the prevalence, detection, prognosis, and management of this syndrome. Type 1 includes persons with ischemia who are asymptomatic, never having had any signs or symptoms of cardiovascular disease. Type 2 includes persons who are asymptomatic after an MI but still show painless ischemia. Type 3 includes patients with both angina and silent ischemia. From Cohn's data, 2.5% to 10.0% of middle-aged men have type 1, 18% have type 2, and 40% have type 3.

Methods of Detection

Certain tests can be used to assess the presence of silent ischemia: ETT, ambulatory ECG for ST segment changes (Holter monitor), and radionuclide tests including thallium scintigraphy and gated pooled (MUGA) scan. Of these tests, the most commonly considered are ETT and Holter monitoring.[82] For Holter monitoring when ST segment changes that meet strict criteria are seen in a patient with known IHD, it is generally accepted that they represent episodes of myocardial ischemia. Ischemic criteria include at least 1 mm or horizontal or downsloping ST segment depression that lasts for at least 1 minute and is separated from other discrete episodes by at least 1 minute of a normal baseline. The methodology has limitations, including difficulty reading ST segment changes in patients with an abnormal baseline (left ventricular hypertrophy with strain) or in those with a left bundle branch block. It is not thought at this time that any of the methods to detect silent ischemia are useful for screening for the presence of IHD in apparently healthy populations. Although this subject remains controversial, it may be wise to screen those patients at high risk (i.e., diabetic patients or those patients with two or more cardiac risk factors).

Prognostic Implications

The presence of frequent and prolonged ischemic episodes despite medical therapy in patients with stable and unstable angina has been associated with a poor prognosis. Using Cohn's classification system, those patients with type 2 silent ischemia have the worst prognosis, especially those with left ventricular dysfunction and three-vessel disease. Exercise tests performed 2 to 3 weeks after an MI have shown an adverse 1-year prognosis associated with silent ischemia.[83] It is unclear whether those with type 3 have a worse prognosis.

Management

Antiischemic medical and revascularization therapies have been shown to reduce asymptomatic ischemia. It is prudent to consider patients with persistent asymptomatic ischemia to be at higher risk for subsequent events and therefore to be deserving of more aggressive therapy. Patients with type 1 should be advised to modify risk factors and avoid activities known to produce ischemia. Those with strongly positive tests should be considered for angiography. For patients with types 2 or 3, treatment with β-blockers for a cardioprotective effect should be considered. It remains unresolved whether asymptomatic ischemia has a causal relation with subsequent MI and cardiac death or is merely a marker of high risk.[84]

Myocardial Infarction

Clinical Presentation

The classic initial manifestations of an acute MI include prolonged substernal chest pain with dyspnea, diaphoresis, and nausea. The pain may be described as a crushing, pressing, constricting, vise-like, or heavy sensation. There may be radiation of the pain to one or both shoulders and arms, or to the neck, jaw, or interscapular area. Only a few patients have this classic overall picture. Although 80% of patients with an acute MI have chest pain at the time of initial examination, only 20% describe it as crushing, constricting, or vise-like.[85,86] The pain may also be described atypically, such as sharp or stabbing, or it can involve atypical areas such as the epigastrium or the back of the neck. "Atypical" presentations are common in the elderly. Pathy[87] found that the initial manifestations of an acute MI were more likely to include symptoms such as sudden dyspnea, acute confusion, cerebrovascular events (e.g., stroke or syncope), acute congestive heart failure, vomiting, and palpitations. There is strong evidence to demonstrate that a substantial proportion of MIs are asymptomatic. In an update of the Framingham Study, Kannel and Abbott[88] reported that 28% of infarcts were discovered only through the appearance of new

ECG changes (Q waves or loss of R waves) observed on a routine biennial study. These infarctions had been previously unrecognized by both patient and physician.

Physical Examination

For the patient with the "uncomplicated MI," there are few physical examination findings. The main purpose of the examination is to assess the patient for evidence of complications from the MI and to establish a baseline for future comparison. Signs of severe left ventricular dysfunction include hypotension, peripheral vasoconstriction, tachycardia, pulmonary rales, an S_3, and elevated jugular venous pressure. Preexisting murmurs should be verified. A new systolic murmur can result from several causes: papillary muscle dysfunction, mitral regurgitation as a result of ventricular dilation, ventricular septal rupture, and acute severe mitral regurgitation due to papillary muscle rupture.[86]

Electrocardiography

The classic ECG changes of acute ischemia are peaked, hyperacute T waves, T-wave flattening or inversion with or without ST segment depression, horizontal ST segment depression, and ST segment elevation. Changes associated with an infarction are (1) the fresh appearance of Q waves or the increased prominence of preexisting ones; (2) ST segment elevations; and (3) T-wave inversions.[89] It is important to recognize that with acute MI the ECG may be entirely normal or contain only "soft" ECG evidence of infarction. In the past, infarcts were classified as either transmural or subendocardial, depending of the presence of Q waves. This terminology has now been replaced by the terms *Q-wave* or *non-Q-wave* MI. This distinction has more clinical relevance, as several studies have indicated differences in etiology and outcome.[86] The key differences between these two groupings are as follows: (1) Q-wave infarctions account for 60% to 70% of all infarcts and non-Q-wave infarctions for 30% to 40%. (2) ST segment elevation is present in 80% of Q-wave infarctions and 40% of non-Q-wave infarctions. (3) The peak creatine kinase tends to be higher in Q-wave infarctions. (4) Postinfarction ischemia and early reinfarction are more common with non-Q-wave infarctions. (5) In-hospital mortality is greater in Q-wave infarctions (20% versus 8% for non-Q-wave infarctions). In general, it is thought that the non-Q-wave infarction is a more unstable condition because of the higher risk of reinfarction and ischemia.[86]

Laboratory Findings

Elevation of the creatine kinase MB (CK-MB) isoenzyme is essential for the diagnosis of acute MI. In general, acute elevations of this enzyme are accounted for by myocardial necrosis. Detectable CK-MB from noncardiac causes is rare except during trauma or surgery. The peak level appearance of CK-MB is expected within 12 to 24 hours after the onset of symptoms. Therefore, patients should have a CK-MB level determined on admission and every 12 hours thereafter (repeated twice). Reliance on a single CK assay in an emergency department setting to rule out MI is not sensitive and should be discouraged.

In the event that a patient presents for evaluation past the time for a peak CK-MB to be of value, serum lactate dehydrogenase (LDH) levels may be used. LDH is less specific for myocardial necrosis because elevations may be induced by other diseases as well, such as liver and skeletal muscle disorders and trauma. There are five LDH isoenzymes. An increase in LDH I or an increase in the LDH-1/LDH-2 ratio is characteristically found with an acute MI. Concentrations of LDH isoenzymes usually become abnormal within 14 hours of the onset of infarction and can remain diagnostic for as long as 2 weeks after the infarction.[90] The most common definition of abnormal is an LDH-1/LDH-2 ratio greater than 1.0.[91]

Management Guidelines

The main priority for patients with an acute MI is relief of pain. The frequent clinical observation of rapid and complete relief of pain after early reperfusion with thrombolytic therapy has made it clear that the pain of an acute MI is due to continuing ischemia of living jeopardized myocardium rather than to the effects of completed myocardial necrosis. Effective analgesia should be promptly administered at the time of diagnosis.[92] Analgesia can be achieved by the use of sublingual nitroglycerin or intravenous morphine (or both). Sublingual nitroglycerin should be given immediately unless the systolic blood pressure is less than 90 mm Hg. If the systolic blood pressure is less than 90 mm Hg, nitroglycerin may be used after intravenous access has been obtained. Long-acting oral nitrate preparations should be avoided for management of early acute MI. Sublingual or transdermal nitroglycerin can be used, but intravenous infusion of nitroglycerin allows more precise control. The intravenous dose can be titrated by frequently measuring blood pressure and heart rate. Morphine sulfate is also highly effective in the relief of pain associated with an acute MI. In addition to its analgesic properties, morphine exerts favorable hemodynamic effects by increasing venous capacitance and reducing systemic vascular resistance. The result is to decrease myocardial oxygen demand. As with nitroglycerin, hypotension may occur. The hypotension may be treated with intravenous fluids or leg elevation.

Oxygen

Supplemental oxygen should be given to all patients with an acute MI. Hypoxemia in a patient with an uncomplicated infarction is usually caused by ventilation-perfusion abnormalities.[93] When oxygen is used, it should be administered by nasal cannula or mask at a rate of 4 to 10 L/min. In patients with chronic obstructive pulmonary disease, it may be wise to use lower flow rates.

Thrombolytic Therapy

In addition to relieving pain and managing ischemia, thrombolytic therapy must be considered. Thrombosis has a major role in the development of an acute MI. Approximately 66% of patients with MIs have ST segment elevation, making it likely that the process is caused by an occlusive clot. The goal of thrombolytic therapy is reperfusion with a minimum of side effects. The most common thrombolytic agents include streptokinase, anisoylated plasminogen streptokinase activator complex, recombinant tissue-type plasminogen activator (rt-PA), urokinase, and pro-urokinase.

There have been several large international studies comparing the results with various thrombolytic agents. The Second International Study of Infarct Survival reported baseline and outcome data in 17,187 patients with suspected MI. Streptokinase was compared with placebo. A 23% reduction in vascular deaths was noted for patients on streptokinase.[94] Similar results were found in the GISSI[95] trial (18% reduction with streptokinase compared with placebo). Subsequent studies comparing the effectiveness of the various agents [GISSI-II[96] (rt-PA versus streptokinase)] failed to show a significant difference between the agents. Streptokinase is by far the least expensive of the agents ($125 versus $2800 for rt-PA), but it has more severe side effects (allergic reactions with repeat dosing and hypotension). The thrombolytic effect of streptokinase is more time-dependent. It is best used early (within 2 hours) after an acute MI, whereas rt-PA should be strongly considered for those patients in whom 3 hours has elapsed after infarction. To enhance thrombolysis and inhibit new thrombus formation, heparin should be administered immediately as a bolus of 5,000 to 10,000 units and then by infusion of 1000 units/h to maintain an activated partial thromboplastin time at two to three times control for 3 to 5 days. Low-dose aspirin (80 mg/day) should be started immediately.[97]

Complications (Mechanical)

The most common complications of an acute MI are mechanical and electrical. Mechanical complications include those that are quickly reversible and those that are clearly life-threatening. Reversible causes of hypotension include hypovolemia, vasovagal reaction, overzealous therapy with antianginal or antiarrhythmic drugs, and brady- and tachyarrhythmias. Other, more serious etiologies include primary left ventricular failure, cardiac tamponade, rupture of the ventricular septum, acute papillary muscle dysfunction, and mitral regurgitation.

Killip and Kimball[98] developed a classification of patients with acute MI.

Class I: patients with uncomplicated infarction without evidence of heart failure as judged by the absence of rales and an S_3

Class II: patients with mild-to-moderate heart failure as evidenced by pulmonary rales in the lower half of the lung fields and an S_3

Class III: patients with severe left ventricular failure of pulmonary edema

Class IV: patients with cardiogenic shock, defined as systolic blood pressure less than 90 mm Hg with oliguria and other evidence of poor peripheral perfusion

Cardiogenic shock has emerged as the most common cause of in-hospital mortality in patients with an acute MI. Despite advances in medical therapy, cardiogenic shock has a dismal prognosis (80–90% mortality).[99] The management of patients with cardiogenic shock includes adequate oxygenation, reduction in myocardial oxygen demands, protection of ischemic myocardium, and circulatory support. The potential for myocardial salvage with emergency reperfusion should be considered in all cases.[97]

Complications (Electrical)

The past 30 years has seen major developments in the recognition and treatment of arrhythmias. The most common include brady- and tachyarrhythmias, atrioventricular conduction disturbances, and ventricular arrhythmias. Organized treatment protocols have been developed for each of these dysrhythmias.[100]

Post-MI Evaluation

Recommendations for pre- and postdischarge evaluations of patients with an acute MI have been outlined by the American College of Cardiologists, the American Heart Association, and the American College of Physicians.[101,102] They include recommendations for testing exercise tolerance and strategies to determine those who would benefit from medical or surgical intervention. These recommendations include a submaximal ETT at 6 to 10 days and at 3 weeks to determine functional capacity.

Rehabilitation

The goal of cardiac rehabilitation includes maintenance of a desirable level of physical, social, and psychological functioning after the onset of cardiovascular illness.[103] Specific goals of rehabilitation include risk stratification, limitation of adverse psychological and emotional consequences of cardiovascular disease, modification of risk factors, alleviation of symptoms, and improved function.

Risk stratification is accomplished by exercise tolerance testing. Also, high-risk patients include those with congestive heart failure, silent ischemia, and ventricular dysrhythmias. All patients should undergo an evaluation to reduce risk factors (smoking, hyperlipidemia, and hypertension). Risk modification of these factors has been associated with significant reduction in subsequent cardiac events. Enrollment in a cardiac rehabilitation program with particular emphasis on exercise has been shown to reduce cardiovascular mortality.[104]

References

1. Gunby P. Cardiovascular diseases remain nation's leading cause of death (medical news and perspectives). JAMA 1992;267:335–6.
2. Eisenberg MS, Cummings RO, Litwin PE, Hallstrom AP. Out-of-hospital cardiac arrest: significance of symptoms in patients collapsing before and after arrival of paramedics. Am J Emerg Med 1986;4:116–20.
3. Kuller LH. Sudden death—definition and epidemiologic considerations. Prog Cardiovasc Dis 1980;23:1–12.
4. Gordon T, Kannel WB. Premature mortality from coronary heart disease: the Framingham Study. JAMA 1971;215:1617–25.
5. American Heart Association. Advanced cardiac life support in perspective. In: Textbook of advanced life support. Dallas: American Heart Association, 1987:1–10.
6. Klinkman MS, Stevens D, Gorenflo DW. Episodes of care for chest pain: a preliminary report from MIRNET. J Fam Pract 1994;38:345–52.
7. Kemp HG, Vokonas PS, Cohn PF, Gorlin R. The anginal syndrome associated with normal coronary arteriograms: report of a six-year experience. Am J Med 1973;54:735–42.
8. Marchandise B, Bourrassa MG, Chaitman BR, Lesperance J. Angiographic evaluation of the natural history of normal coronary arteries and mild coronary atherosclerosis. Am J Cardiol 1978;41:216–20.
9. Proudfit WL, Shirey EK, Sones FM. Selective cinecoronary arteriography: correlation with clinical findings in 1000 patients. Circulation 1966;33:901–10.
10. Proudfit WL, Bruschke AVG, Sones FM. Clinical course of patients with normal or slightly or moderately abnormal coronary arteriograms: 10-year follow-up of 521 patients. Circulation 1980;62:712–7.
11. Day LJ, Sowton E. Clinical features and follow-up of patients with angina and normal coronary arteries. Lancet 1979;2:334–7.
12. Ockene IS, Shay MJ, Alpert JS, et al. Unexplained chest pain in patient with normal coronary arteriograms: a follow-up study of functional status. N Engl J Med 1980;303:1249–52.
13. Waxler EB, Kimbiris D, Dreifus LS. The fate of women with normal coronary arteriograms and chest pain resembling angina pectoris. Am J Cardiol 1971;28:25–32.
14. Lavey EB, Winkle RA. Continuing disability of patients with chest pain and normal coronary arteriograms. J Chronic Dis 1979;32:191–6.

15. Isner JM, Salem DN, Banas JS, Levire HS. Long-term clinical course of patients with normal coronary arteriography: follow-up study of 121 patients with normal or nearly normal coronary arteriograms. Am Heart J 1981;102:645–53.
16. Kemp HG, Kronmal RA, Vlietstra RE, Frye RL. Seven year survival of patients with normal or near normal coronary arteriograms: a CASS registry study. J Am Coll Cardiol 1986;7:479–83.
17. DeMeester TR, O'Sullivan GC, Bermudez G, et al. Esophageal function in patients with angina-type chest pain and normal coronary angiograms. Ann Surg 1982;196:488–98.
18. Kline M, Chesne R, Studevant RL, McCallum RW. Esophageal disease in patients with angina-like chest pain. Am J Gastroenterol 1981;75:116–23.
19. Davies HA, Jones DB, Rhodes J. Esophageal angina as the cause of chest pain. JAMA 1982;248:2274–8.
20. Richter JE, Bradley LA, Castell DO. Esophageal chest pain: current controversies in pathogenesis, diagnosis and therapy. Ann Intern Med 1989;110: 66–78.
21. Svensson O, Stenport G, Tibbling L, Wranne B. Oesophageal function and coronary angiogram in patients with disabling chest pain. Acta Med Scand 1978;204:173–8.
22. Schofield PM, Bennett DH, Whorwell PJ, et al. Exertional gastro-oesophageal reflux: a mechanism for symptoms in patients with angina pectoris and normal coronary angiograms. BMJ 1987;294:1459–61.
23. Areskog M, Tibbling L, Wranne B. Noninfarction in coronary care unit patients. Acta Med Scand 1981;209:51–57.
24. Davies HA, Jones DB, Rhodes J, Newcombe RJ. Angina-like esophageal pain: differentiation from cardiac pain by history. J Clin Gastroenterol 1985;7:477–81.
25. Pope CE. Chest pain: Heart? Gullet? Both? Neither? [editorial]. JAMA 1982;248:2315.
26. Richter JE, Obrecht WF, Bradley LA, et al. Psychological comparison of patients with nutcracker esophagus and irritable bowel syndrome. Dig Dis Sci 1986;31:131–8.
27. Clouse RE, Lustman PJ. Psychiatric illness and contraction abnormalities of the esophagus. N Engl J Med 1983;309:1337–42.
28. Katon W, Hall ML, Russo J, et al. Chest pain: relationship of psychiatric illness to coronary arteriographic results. Am J Med 1988;84:1–9.
29. Waxler EB, Kimbiris D, Dreifus LS. The fate of women with normal coronary arteries and chest pain resembling stable angina pectoris. Am J Cardiol 1971;28:25–32.
30. Cannon RO, Quyyumi AA, Mincemoyer R, et al. Imipramine in patients with chest pain despite normal coronary angiograms. N Engl J Med 1994; 330:1411–7.
31. Shub C. Stable angina pectoris. 1. Clinical patterns. Mayo Clin Proc 1990; 65:233–42.
32. Prinzmetal M, Kennamer R, Merliss R, et al. Angina pectoris. I. A variant form of angina pectoris: preliminary report. Am J Med 1959;27:375–88.
33. Kemp HG. Left ventricular function in patients with the angina syndrome and normal coronary arteriograms [editorial]. Am J Cardiol 1973;32:375–6.

34. Cannon RO. Angina pectoris with normal coronary angiograms. Cardiol Clin 1991;9:157–66.
35. Colgan SM, Schofield PJ, Whorwell DH, et al. Angina-like chest pain: a joint medical and psychiatric investigation. Postgrad Med J 1988;64:743–6.
36. Lam HG, Dekker W, Kan G, et al. Esophageal dysfunction as a cause of angina pectoris ("linked angina"). Does it exist? Am J Med 1994;96:359–64.
37. Diamond GA, Forrester JS. Analysis of probability as an aid in the clinical diagnosis of coronary-artery disease. N Engl J Med 1979;300:1350–8.
38. Guidelines for exercise testing: a report of the American College of Cardiology/American Heart Association Task Force on Assessment of Cardiovascular Procedures (Subcommittee on Exercise Testing). J Am Coll Cardiol 1986;8:725–38.
39. Ellestad MH. Stress testing: principles and practice. 3d ed. Philadelphia: Davis, 1986.
40. Evans CH, Karunaratne HB. Exercise stress testing for the family physician. Part I. Performing the test. Am Fam Physician 1992;45:121–32.
41. Evans CH, Karunaratne HB. Exercise stress testing for the family physician. Part II. Am Fam Physician 1992;45:679–88.
42. Chaitman B. The changing role of the exercise electrocardiogram as a diagnostic and prognostic test for chronic ischemic heart disease. J Am Coll Cardiol 1986;8:1195–210.
43. Shub C. Stable angina pectoris. 2. Cardiac evaluation and diagnostic testing. Mayo Clin Proc 1990;65:243–55.
44. Horwitz LD, Herman MV, Gorlin R. Clinical response to nitroglycerin as a diagnostic test for coronary artery disease. Am J Cardiol 1972;29:149–53.
45. Frank CW, Weinblatt E, Shapiro S. Angina pectoris in men: prognostic significance of selected medical factors. Circulation 1973;47:509–17.
46. Kannel WB, Feinleib M. Natural history of angina pectoris in the Framingham study: prognosis and survival. Am J Cardiol 1972;29:154–63.
47. Hilton TC, Chaitman BR. The prognosis in stable and unstable angina. Cardiol Clin 1991;9:27–38.
48. Holmes DR, Vliestra RE, Fisher LD, et al. Follow-up of patients from the Coronary Artery Surgery Study (CASS) potentially suitable for percutaneous transluminal coronary angioplasty. Am Heart J 1983;106:981–8.
49. Hlatky MA, Califf RM, Kong Y. Natural history of patients with single-vessel disease suitable for percutaneous transluminal coronary angioplasty. Am J Cardiol 1983;52:225–9.
50. Pryor DB, Shaw L, Harrell FE, et al. Estimating the likelihood of severe coronary artery disease. Am J Med 1991;90:553–62.
51. Mock MB, Rinquist I, Fisher LD, et al. Survival of medically treated patients in the Coronary Artery Surgery Study (CASS) registry. Circulation 1982;66:562–8.
52. Goodman LS, Gilman A. The pharmacologic basis of therapeutics. 8th ed. New York: Macmillan, 1990.
53. Thadani U, Whitsett T, Hamilton SF. Nitrate therapy for myocardial ischemic syndromes: current perspectives including tolerance. Curr Probl Cardiol 1988;13:725–84.

54. Thadani U, Hamilton SF, Olson E, et al. Transdermal nitroglycerin patches in angina pectoris: dose titration, duration of effect, and rapid tolerance. Ann Intern Med 1986;105:485–92.

55. Cowan C, Bourke J, Reid DS, et al. Tolerance to glyceryl trinitrate patches: prevention by intermittent dosing. BMJ 1987;294:544–57.

56. Thadani U. Medical therapy of stable angina pectoris. Cardiol Clin 1991;9:73–87.

57. Prichard BMC. Beta adrenergic receptor blocking drugs in angina pectoris. Drugs 1974;7:55–84.

58. Thadani U, Davidson C, Singleton W, et al. Comparison of the immediate effects of five beta-adrenoceptor blocking drugs with different ancillary properties in angina pectoris. N Engl J Med 1979;300:750–5.

59. Braunwald E. Mechanism of action of calcium channel blocking agents. N Engl J Med 1982;307:1618–26.

60. Opie LH. Calcium channel antagonists. Part II. Use and comparative properties of prototypical calcium antagonists in ischemic heart disease, including recommendations based on analysis of 45 trials. Rev Cardiovasc Drug Ther 1987;1:4461–75.

61. Packer M. Drug therapy: combined beta-adrenergic and calcium entry blockade in angina pectoris. N Engl J Med 1989;320:709–18.

62. Resnekov L, Chediak J, Hirsh J, Levis HD. Antithrombotic agents in coronary disease. Chest 1989;95:52S–72S.

63. Canner PL. Aspirin in coronary heart disease: comparison of six clinical trials. Isr J Med Sci 1983;19:413–23.

64. Hennekens CH, Buring JE, Sandercock P, et al. Aspirin and other antiplatelet agents in the secondary and primary prevention of cardiovascular disease. Circulation 1989;80:749–56.

65. Manson JE, Grobbee DE, Stampfer MJ, et al. Aspirin in the primary prevention of angina pectoris in a randomized trial of United States physicians. Am J Med 1990;89:772–6.

66. Shah PK. Pathophysiology of unstable angina. Cardiol Clin 1991;9:11–26.

67. Gottlieb SO, Weisfeldt ML, Ouyang P, et al. Silent ischemia as a marker for early unfavorable outcomes in patients with unstable angina. N Engl J Med 1986;314:1214–19.

68. Braunwald E, Mark DB, Jones RH, et al. Diagnosing and managing unstable angina. Quick reference guide for clinicians, Number 10. AHCPR Publication No. 94-0603. Rockville, MD: U.S. Department of Health and Human Services, Public Health Service, Agency for Health Care Policy and Research and National Heart, Lung, and Blood Institute. March 1994.

69. Davies MJ, Thomas AC, Knapman PA, Hangartner JR. Intramyocardial platelet aggregation in patients with unstable angina suffering sudden ischemic cardiac death. Circulation 1986;73:418–27.

70. Lewis HD, Davis JW, Archibald DG, et al. Protective effects of aspirin against acute myocardial infarction and death in men with unstable angina: results of a Veterans Administration cooperative study. N Engl J Med 1983;309:396–403.

71. National Center for Health Statistics. 1986 Summary: National Hospital Discharge Survey. Hyattsville, MD: National Center for Health Statistics, 1987. DHHS Publ No. (PHS) 87-1250.

72. Ryan TJ, Faxon DP, Gunnar RM, et al. Guidelines for percutaneous transluminal coronary angioplasty: a report of the American College of Cardiology/American Heart Association Task Force on assessment of diagnostic and therapeutic cardiovascular procedures (subcommittee on percutaneous transluminal angioplasty). Circulation 1988;78:486–502.

73. Faxon DP. Percutaneous coronary angioplasty in stable and unstable angina. Cardiol Clin 1991;9:99–113.

74. Hammermeister KE, Morrison DA. Coronary bypass surgery for stable angina and unstable angina pectoris. Cardiol Clin 1991;9:135–55.

75. Barsky AJ, Hochstrasser B, Coles A, et al. Silent myocardial ischemia: is the person or the event silent? JAMA 1990;264:1132–5.

76. Droste C, Roskamm H. Experimental pain measurement in patients with asymptomatic myocardial ischemia. J Am Coll Cardiol 1983;1:940–5.

77. Sheps DS, Light KC, Bragdon EE, et al. Relationship between chest pain, exercise endorphin response and depression. Circulation 1989;80 Suppl II:591–4.

78. Deanfield JE, Shea M, Kensett M, et al. Silent myocardial ischemia due to mental stress. Lancet 1984;2:1001–4.

79. Freeman LS, Nixon PGF, Sallabank P, et al. Psychologic stress and silent myocardial ischemia. Am Heart J 1987;114:477–82.

80. Rozanski A, Bairey CN, Krantz DS, et al. Mental stress and the induction of silent myocardial ischemia in patients with coronary artery disease. N Engl J Med 1988;318:1005–12.

81. Cohn PF. Silent myocardial ischemia. Ann Intern Med 1988;109:312–17.

82. Mody FV, Nademanee K, Intarachot V, et al. Severity of silent myocardial ischemia on ambulatory electrocardiographic monitoring in patients with stable angina pectoris: relation to prognostic determinants during exercise stress testing and coronary angiography. J Am Coll Cardiol 1988;12:1169–96.

83. Theroux P, Waters DD, Halphen C, et al. Prognostic value of exercise testing soon after myocardial infarction. N Engl J Med 1979;301:341–5.

84. Gottlieb SO. Asymptomatic or silent myocardial ischemia in angina pectoris: pathophysiology and clinical implications. Cardiol Clin 1991;9:49–61.

85. Kinlen LJ. Incidence and presentation of myocardial infarction in an English community. Br Heart J 1973;35:616–22.

86. Lavie CJ, Gersh BJ. Acute myocardial infarction: initial manifestations, management, and prognosis. Mayo Clin Proc 1990;65:531–48.

87. Pathy MS. Clinical presentation of myocardial infarction in the elderly. Br Heart J 1967;29:190–9.

88. Kannel WB, Abbott RD. Incidence and prognosis of unrecognized myocardial infarction: an update on the Framingham study. N Engl J Med 1984;311:1144–7.

89. Marriott HJL. Practical electrocardiography. 6th ed. Baltimore: Williams & Wilkins, 1977.

90. Lee TH, Goldman L. Serum enzyme assays in the diagnosis of acute myocardial infarction: recommendations based on a quantitative analysis. Ann Intern Med 1986;105:221–33.

91. Vasudevan G, Mercer DW, Varat MA. Lactic dehydrogenase isoenzyme determination in the diagnosis of acute myocardial infarction. Circulation 1978;57:1055–7.

92. Gunnar RM, Lambrew CT, Abrams W, et al. Task force IV: pharmacologic interventions. Am J Cardiol 1982;50:393–408.

93. Fillmore SJ, Shapiro M, Killip T. Arterial oxygen tension in acute myocardial infarction: serial analysis of clinical state and blood-gas changes. Am Heart J 1970;79:620–9.

94. ISIS-2 (Second International Study of Infarct Survival) Collaborative Group. Randomised trial of intravenous streptokinase, oral aspirin, both, or neither among 17,187 cases of suspected acute myocardial infarction: ISIS-2. Lancet 1988;2:349–60.

95. Gruppo Italiano per lo Studio della Streptochinasi nell'Infarto Miocardico (GISSI). Effectiveness of intravenous thrombolytic treatment in acute myocardial infarction. Lancet 1986;1:397–401.

96. GISSI-2 Investigators. GISSI-2: a factorial randomized trial of alteplase vs streptokinase and heparin vs no heparin among 12,490 patients with acute myocardial infarction. Lancet 1990;336:65–71.

97. Lavie CJ, Gersh BJ, Chesebro JH. Reperfusion in acute myocardial infarction. Mayo Clin Proc 1990;65:549–64.

98. Killip T, Kimball JT. Treatment of myocardial infarction in a coronary care unit: a two-year experience with 250 patients. Am J Cardiol 1967;20:457–61.

99. Forrester JS, Diamond G, Chatterjee K, et al. Medical therapy of acute myocardial infarction by application of hemodynamic subsets. N Engl J Med 1976;295:1356–62.

100. American Heart Association. Putting it all together. In: Textbook of advanced cardiac life support. Dallas: American Heart Association, 1987:235–48.

101. Subcommittee to Develop Guidelines for the Early Management of Patients with Acute Myocardial Infarction. ACC/AHA Guidelines for the early management of patients with acute myocardial infarction: a report of the American College of Cardiology/American Heart Association Task Force on Assessment of Diagnostic and Therapeutic Cardiovascular Procedures. Circulation 1990;82:664–707.

102. American College of Physicians. Evaluation of patients after recent acute myocardial infarction [position paper]. Ann Intern Med 1989;110:485–8.

103. Squires RW, Gau GT, Miller TD, et al. Cardiovascular rehabilitation: status 1990. Mayo Clin Proc 1990;65:731–55.

104. O'Connor GT, Buring JE, Yusuf S, et al. An overview of randomized trials of rehabilitation with exercise after myocardial infarction. Circulation 1989;80:234–44.

Case Presentation

Subjective

Patient Profile

John McCarthy is a 54-year-old married white male restaurant operator.

Presenting Problem

"Chest pain, getting worse."

Present Illness

This is the second visit to the office for Mr. McCarthy, who is a well-controlled type 2 diabetic with angina pectoris for 1 year. His coronary artery disease has been stable, and he used three to four nitroglycerin tablets per month—especially after exertion and cold exposure—until the past week. He is now using three to five nitroglycerin tablets per day and has angina with mild exertion or when bending over. His pain radiates to the chin and to the left arm, which it seldom did before.

Past Medical History

No change since the past medical history recorded on his initial "get acquainted" office visit 6 months ago (see Chapter 1).

Social History

His restaurant business has been struggling recently; otherwise, no change since his last visit.

Habits

No change since his prior visit.

Family History

He is especially concerned about his son Mark, aged 28, who has been found to be HIV-positive.

REVIEW OF SYMPTOMS

No other pertinent symptoms noted.

- What further information regarding Mr. McCarthy's chest pain would you like to know? Why?
- What more would you like to know about the current status of his diabetes mellitus?
- What might have caused his chest pain to become worse, and how would you inquire about these possibilities?
- What might this change in symptoms mean to the patient, and how would you ask about this?

Objective

GENERAL

The patient appears apprehensive and describes his pain by holding his clenched fist to the midchest.

VITAL SIGNS

Height, 6 ft; weight, 194 lb; blood pressure, 152/100; pulse, 82; respirations, 22; temperature, 37.2°C.

EXAMINATION

The eyes, ears, nose, and throat are normal. The neck and thyroid gland are unremarkable, and there is no cervical bruit. The chest is clear to percussion and auscultation. The heart has a regular sinus rhythm of 82. There is no cardiac enlargement, rub, or murmur.

LABORATORY

An ECG performed in the office today is normal for age.

- What additional data from the physical examination are likely to be pertinent? Explain.
- What—if any—findings on physical examination might increase or ease your concerns regarding the patient's history today?
- What—if any—laboratory tests would you obtain today? Why?
- What other tests—diagnostic imaging, treadmill ECG, or radionuclide scan—might be important in making a diagnosis today? Explain.

Assessment

- Based on the data available and pending further tests, what is your tentative diagnosis? How would you explain this to Mr. McCarthy and his family?
- What are the implications of this diagnosis for the patient?
- The family asks about the long-term prognosis. How would you respond?
- What symptoms or physical findings—if present—would you consider especially worrisome in this clinical setting? Explain.

Plan

- What are your therapeutic recommendations, and how would you explain them to the patient?
- Is a subspecialist consultation needed? Explain your reasoning.
- The patient wishes to know how soon he can return to work. How would you respond?
- If you decide to admit the patient to the hospital, what is your role in hospital care?

13
Obstructive Airway Disease

HOWARD WEINBERG

Obstructive airway disease includes asthma and chronic obstructive pulmonary disease. Although two distinct entities, these problems share many of the same characteristics. Chronic cough, a prominent symptom of both these ailments, is also presented.

Background

Asthma

Asthma is a disorder of the pulmonary airways characterized by reversible obstruction, inflammation, and hyperresponsiveness. Approximately 10 million Americans have this condition with a mortality of 4000 to 5000 per year.[1] Initial onset can be any age and can afflict either sex and every race. Severity of this illness is difficult to predict; some victims experience a rapidly worsening clinical course, whereas others appear to "outgrow" the disease.

The bronchospasm and inflammation can be triggered by allergens, infection, and psychophysiologic stressors. Allergens include inhaled substances, such as molds, pollens, dust, animal danders, industrial pollutants, side stream or direct tobacco smoke, wood stoves, and cosmetics. Oral inducers include food additives (e.g., tartrazine coloring and preservatives containing sulfiting agents) and medications, especially aspirin and β-blockers (including selective agents and optical preparations).

Respiratory, particularly viral, infections are also a major stimulator of asthma attacks. Some viral infections, such as those caused by the respiratory syncytial virus, induce bronchospasm in most patients. An occasional patient has attacks only with infections.

Psychological factors certainly play a role in inducing asthma episodes. These triggers may be difficult to recognize and may manifest as part of a panic attack, as fear of the disease itself, or as a symptom of abuse.

Chronic Obstructive Pulmonary Disease

Chronic obstructive pulmonary disease (COPD) is defined as an ailment characterized by abnormal expiratory flow that does not change significantly over time. This delineation was intended to exclude asthma. Also excluded are specific upper airway diseases, such as cancers, and conditions affecting the lower airways, such as bronchiectasis, sarcoidosis, and cystic fibrosis.[2] Traditionally included in this category are chronic bronchitis and emphysema. In some patients, however, the overlap with asthma is so strong that a significant distinction cannot be made. Indeed, the term *COPD* was developed in recognition of the large overlap of symptomatology among sufferers of this ailment.

Chronic bronchitis has traditionally been defined as a cough that occurs at least 3 months a year for 2 consecutive years and involves excess mucus secretion in the larger airways. A malady of adults, chronic bronchitis affects about 20% of men and is primarily caused by cigarette smoking. Unfortunately, the incidence in women is increasing as the percentage of women smokers increases. Other contributing factors include air pollution, occupational exposure, and infection.[3]

Emphysema has been defined as a permanent enlargement of distal airspaces with destruction of the acinar walls without fibrosis. This entity can be further subdivided into centriacinar, panacinar, and distal acinar types.[4] Like chronic bronchitis, this illness is primarily found in adult cigarette smokers. However, there is a rare type of congenital emphysema and a genetic syndrome associated with the lack of α_1-antitrypsin in the serum.

Chronic Cough

Certainly, cough is an essential component in the presentation of both COPD and asthma. There are, however, other entities that can cause chronic cough. Although most patients have one cause for cough, a significant number of patients may have two or more causes, the four most common being postnasal drip syndrome, COPD, asthma, and gastroesophageal reflux.[5] Other causes include acute and chronic infection, other lung diseases (embolism, cancer), aspiration, psychogenic factors, and cardiac failure. Cough can also be caused by medications, most prominent of which are angiotensin-converting enzyme (ACE) inhibitors, where the incidence may be as high as 13%.[6]

Clinical Presentation

Asthma

The classic presentation of asthma is cough, dyspnea, and wheezing. Wheezing may be audible or may require auscultation. Infrequently, a patient is so "tight" that wheezing can be detected only after initial therapy. The patient may be comfortable or in extreme respiratory distress. At such times, there may be accessory muscle movement (subcostal, intercostal, supraclavicular), nasal flaring (particularly in children), cyanosis, or altered mental status. Auscultation often reveals rhonchi, wheezing, and a reversal of the normal 2:1 inspiratory/expiratory ratio. An increase in respiratory rate, independent of fever, is also a cardinal sign.

Sometimes, especially in children, the only symptom of asthma is a chronic night cough. Another presentation includes wheezing and shortness of breath that occurs after exercise. This condition is known as exercise-induced asthma or bronchospasm (EIA or EIB). Many Olympic-caliber athletes have EIB.

COPD

The early medical books customarily described two distinct clinical presentations of COPD: the blue bloater of chronic bronchitis and the pink puffer of emphysema. Although these stereotypes are seen on occasion, the more typical presentation is a mixed picture, including cough, dyspnea, and often wheezing. In severe situations, tachypnea, accessory muscle movement, breathing through pursed lips, cyanosis, and agitation are present. Longstanding disease may be indicated by a pronounced barrel chest (i.e., an increase in anteroposterior dimension). Copious sputum production is also noted. Chest auscultation may reveal wheezes, rales, or rhonchi in varying intensity, or it can be normal. Heart sounds might be distant, or a gallop indicative of secondary heart disease may be detected. Examination of the extremities might reveal cyanosis of the nailbeds or clubbing of the fingers. Finally, despite obvious distress, these patients may be smoking.

Chronic Cough

Clinical presentation of cough seems self-explanatory: The patient is coughing. It is important to note, however, whether the cough is productive of sputum (thick, thin, purulent, bloody) or dry. The time of day or night often provides a clue to the extensive differential diagnosis, as does evidence of allergy such as rhinitis, allergic shiners, or a transverse nose crease. Of particular note are symptoms related to gastrointestinal reflux (i.e., heartburn, water brash, or increased belching). Finally, these patients may present with signs and symptoms of a multitude of other underlying diseases.

Diagnosis

The diagnosis of asthma or COPD should be fairly evident from the history and physical examination. Laboratory and radiographic data usually cannot by themselves prove the diagnosis of either disease, but they can provide supportive information or assist in the assessment of severity.

Pulmonary Function Tests

Although extensive pulmonary testing is indicated in the occasional patient, the most useful information is obtained from evaluating the forced expiratory volume in 1 second (FEV_1), the forced vital capacity (FVC), the FEV_1/FVC ratio, and the peak expiratory flow rate (PEFR). Obstructive disease is indicated by a reduced FEV_1 in the presence of a normal FVC (which also causes a reduced FEV_1/FVC ratio). Restrictive disease, however, shows a normal FEV_1, decreased FVC, and increased FEV_1/FVC (this pattern would be representative of pure emphysema).

With asthma, a useful test is to observe the change in FEV_1 after treatment with a bronchodilator. An increase of 15% is indicative of reversible airway disease.[2] Three stimulators—exercise, histamine, and methacholine—may be used for provocative testing. A decrease in FEV_1 of 20% is considered positive. PEFR may be obtained by using a peak flowmeter and can be performed easily in the office or at home. This measurement provides an objective indicator of the severity of an episode or of the response to various therapeutic interventions. It is highly recommended that most patients purchase a peak flowmeter.[1] The National Asthma Education Program has excellent materials available to instruct patients in the use of PEFR meters.

With COPD, the spirometric abnormalities may be a mixture of both obstructive and restrictive diseases. In asymptomatic patients, such as cigarette smokers, abnormal results should serve as an indicator of early illness and, it is hoped, as a stimulus to stop smoking. In symptomatic patients, these measurements can serve as a sign of progressive disease. Finally, the FEV_1 can be used to evaluate the degree of responsiveness to bronchodilators in COPD patients, many of whom have an asthmatic component.

Arterial Blood Gases

Evaluation as to the severity of the disease is assisted by measuring the arterial blood gases (ABGs). Severe hypoxemia in the asthmatic or hypercapnia in the chronic lung patient may serve as important factors in the decision to hospitalize a patient. Most outpatients do not need ABG measurements.

Other Laboratory Tests

Useful tests for very sick patients include (1) counting blood leukocytes as a sign of acute infection, or (2) determining the hematocrit value as indicative of an additional reason for hypoxemia (if it is low) or as a sign of long-standing hypoxemia (if polycythemia is noted). Sputum evaluation is useful when looking for acute infection or in the presence of eosinophilia, Curschmann's spirals, or Charcot-Leydon crystals, all indicative of asthma.

Chest Roentgenography

It is not necessary to obtain a chest roentgenogram on every patient with asthma or COPD. A radiograph may be useful in the undiagnosed patient with chronic cough and may help to identify complications in patients with obstructive disease. These complications might involve pneumonia, pneumothorax, pneumomediastinum, or subcutaneous emphysema. A chest film of the COPD patient may be normal, show a mild increase in lung markings, demonstrate the hyperlucency, overinflation, and bullae often seen with emphysema, or show an enlarged heart or the pulmonary congestion seen with heart failure. On rare occasion, a chest film holds the key to differentiating congestive heart failure with wheezing (cardiac asthma) from true asthma.

Other radiologic procedures such as lung scans, computed tomography scans, and angiography have a role only in the management of complications.

Chronic Cough

The diagnosis of chronic cough is often difficult and time-consuming. Irwin and associates[5] have presented a schema for evaluating previously undiagnosed patients. Their evaluation, in decreasing order of usefulness, includes history, physical examination, pulmonary function tests, methacholine inhalation challenge, upper gastrointestinal radiology, measurement of esophageal pH, sinus roentgenogram, chest film, and bronchoscopy. Following this design, diagnoses are possible in 99% of patients.

Management

The management of asthma and COPD is best viewed from a standpoint of both disease complexes. It includes avoidance, immunotherapy, drug treatment, and psychosocial support (Fig. 13.1).

Avoidance

The life style of any patient with pulmonary problems may be drastically affected by environmental factors: climate, outdoor air pollution, and indoor air pollution.

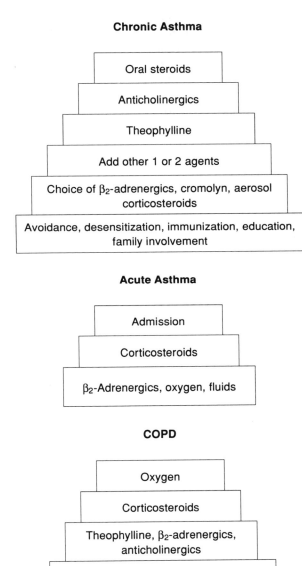

FIGURE 13.1. Recommended stepped treatment plan for asthma and COPD.

Climate

Both asthmatic and COPD sufferers may be affected by changes in wind velocity, humidity, and temperature. Low wind velocity allows accumulation of allergens; high humidity leads to an increase in pollen-producing plants and molds; and sudden temperature drops cause a fall in airway conduction.[7] Barometric pressure changes are also associated with exacerbations of both asthma and COPD. Extremes in climatic events, such as prolonged heat waves or air inversions, often result in increased mortality among COPD patients. Although patients cannot avoid climatic changes, they can stay inside on particularly bad days and can minimize the effects by using filtered air conditioning and heating systems maintained at fairly constant temperature year round.

Outdoor Air Pollution

Potential allergens are either man-made (e.g., smoke and chemical fumes) or natural substances (e.g., pollens, dusts, and molds). Although difficult to avoid, some factors can be minimized by controlling the type of grass, ornamental shrubs, and flowering vegetation around the home.

Indoor Air Pollution

Fortunately, indoor allergens are much more readily controlled. It is of paramount importance to eliminate tobacco smoke. Other potential irritants include building materials, cleaning agents, pest control chemicals, decorative plants, dried flowers, and cosmetics. The bedroom is a particularly important room to allergy-proof. Attention should be directed to pillows, mattresses, carpets, drapes, blankets, shelf ornaments, and stuffed animals (especially stuffed animals in the bed). Wood stoves and kerosene heaters have been shown to aggravate respiratory problems. Sometimes families must make sacrifices concerning pets. This entire aspect of avoidance must be stressed to all patients and may obviate the need for further treatment.[7,8]

Immunotherapy

Desensitization

When avoidance therapy fails, allergic patients should be given trials of antihistamines, nasal steroids, or cromolyn and then be considered for allergy desensitization if needed.

Immunization

Influenza and pneumococcal vaccines should be given to all patients with significant respiratory illness. Influenza vaccine is administered yearly about 2 to 3 months before anticipated outbreaks. October and November are the prime times to immunize in the United States. Pneumococcal vaccine needs to be given only once.

Amantadine

Unvaccinated patients should be treated with amantadine (Symmetrel) during influenza outbreaks. Effective only for influenza A, amantadine is administered in a dosage of 200 mg once a day or 100 mg twice a day (100 mg/day for those older than 65 years of age). The dosage for children, aged 1 to 9 years, is 4.4 to 8.8 mg/kg/day, not to exceed 150 mg/day.[9] Household contacts of patients should also be treated or vaccinated to protect the affected family member.

Drug Treatment

The choice of medication for these illnesses has greatly expanded and is presently undergoing rapid changes in philosophy. This point is especially true for asthma, where most authorities now believe it is essential to treat both the bronchospasm and the inflammation.[1] Unfortunately, those who suffer with COPD have not experienced as great a revolution in drug effect.

Theophylline

Long the cornerstone of asthma treatment, theophylline is no longer the initial drug of choice. A bronchodilator, theophylline is best used for patients needing more than one maintenance drug and for those with pronounced nocturnal symptoms.[10] It is also worth a trial in COPD patients who wheeze.

Theophyllines are available in various formulations: liquid, capsule, tablet, slow-release products, and intravenous solutions. Most patients require several days to reach maximal effectiveness. Once a steady state is reached, it is best to maintain the patient on the same brand-name product, as bioavailability can vary from product to product. Smokers and children tend to metabolize this medication rapidly. Significant interactions are possible with erythromycins, fluoroquinolones, cimetidine (Tagamet), phenytoin (Dilantin), and oral contraceptives. Also, dosages must be monitored closely in patients with liver failure and congestive heart failure. Serum theophylline levels are recommended for all the above situations and in difficult patients in whom "fine tuning" may be needed. Usual therapeutic level is considered to be 10 to 20 μg/ml. Older preparations that contain subtherapeutic doses of theophylline (Marax or Tedral) are no longer considered appropriate therapy (Table 13.1).

TABLE 13.1. Recommended dosages for theophylline, β_2-adrenergic agonists, and corticosteroids

Medication	Age group	Route	Usual dosage
Theophylline	<1 year	PO	Varies considerably
	1–9	PO	24 mg/kg/day
	9–12	PO	20 mg/kg/day
	12–16	PO	18 mg/kg/day
	>16, smoker	PO	18 mg/kg/day
	>16, nonsmoker	PO	13 mg/kg/day
Albuterol	> 2	PO	0.1 mg/kg tid or qid (max. 2–4 mg)
	> 2	MDI	1–2 inhal. q4h
	>12	Nebulizer	2.5 mg q4h
Bitolterol	>12	MDI	2 inhal. q4h or 3 q6h
Metaproterenol	< 6	PO	1.3–2.6 mg/kg/day
	> 6	PO	10–20 mg tid–qid
	> 2	MDI	1–2 inhal. q4h
	>12	Nebulizer	0.2–0.3 ml q4h
Pirbuterol	>12	MDI	1–2 inhal. q4h–q6h
Terbutaline	>12	PO	1.25–5.00 mg tid
	>12	MDI	2 inhal. q4h
Salmeterol	>12	MDI	2 inhal. q12h
Beclomethasone	> 6	MDI	2–4 inhal. bid–qid (max 20/day)
Flunisolide	> 6	MDI	1–2 inhal. bid (max. 8/day)
Triamcinolone	> 6	MDI	1–2 inhal. tid–qid (max. 16/day)
Prednisone	1–12	PO	1–2 mg/kg/day, taper 5–10 days
	>12	PO	40–80 mg/day, taper 5–10 days

Children represent a special group who need close monitoring. With growth, dosage requires constant adjustment. For small children, slow-release capsules (SloBid, Theodur Sprinkles) are particularly useful when sprinkled onto food, thus avoiding the nausea often associated with liquid preparations. Theophylline has come under scrutiny, as have other asthmatic medications, with regard to potential interference with school performance. To date, no significant relation has been established.[11]

In the acute situation, theophylline (as aminophylline) has long been used on an emergency basis. In recent years, it has become clear that intravenous theophylline does not add to the therapeutic regimen but does significantly increase toxicity. This medicine should not, therefore, be used in an emergency situation.[12]

β₂-Adrenergic Agonists

The β-adrenergic agonists now comprise the first step in treating the bronchospasm of asthma. Available as liquids, short- and long-acting tablets, metered-dose inhalers (MDIs), rotohalers, nebulizable solutions, and injectables, they have many potential uses. They are available in the United States as albuterol (Proventil, Ventolin), bitolterol mesylate (Tornalate), metaproterenol sulfate (Alupent, Metaprel), pirbuterol acetate (Maxair), terbutaline sulfate (Brethaire, Brethine), and salmeterol (Serevent) (Table 13.1).

The choice of preparation depends on the patient's age and the acuteness of the situation. MDIs and nebulizers have an almost instantaneous onset of action, and sustained-release tablets offer assistance with nocturnal symptoms. Oral forms have their greatest use in young children. It is rarely necessary to use both the oral route and the inhaled route, a situation that would lead to increase toxicity with little gain in benefit.

β₂-Adrenergic agonists are the treatment of choice for episodic asthmatics and for EIB. Once the need is established for continual usage, some authorities still recommend these agents as solitary treatment, whereas others use them as adjuncts to theophylline or inhaled corticosteroids. Certainly, every patient with significant obstructive disease should always have some form of this medication on hand.

For the treatment of acute situations, β₂-adrenergic agonists are the agents of choice. They can be given by nebulizer (and repeated at 60- to 90-minute intervals if needed[13]) or by MDI using an InspirEase at the rate of one inhalation per minute for 5 minutes. The use of these agents has generally supplanted the need for older agents such as ephedrine, isoproterenol, and epinephrine. Even in the emergency situation, β₂-adrenergic agonists have been found to be equally effective as subcutaneous epinephrine with significantly less toxicity.[14]

Salmeterol, recently released, is a unique new β-agonist for MDI use. It has a longer action (12 hours) than other agents but takes 10 to 20 minutes for onset. It is indicated for maintenance and nocturnal asthma. Other short-acting agents may still be used between the recommended twice-daily dosing.[15]

Some patients experience great trouble in using an MDI. For these situations, there are several spacer devices available: InspirEase, Inhal-aid, Paper tube, and Aerochamber.[16] Home-made alternatives are the inside of a toilet paper roll or a paper lunch bag. These devices greatly increase the use of MDIs and extend their usability for younger and elderly patients. Every patient's technique should be observed to help determine if a spacer device is needed.

In the patient with COPD, these drugs have less application but are still valuable when bronchospasm is prominent. Pulse and blood pressure should be watched carefully. Inhalation is the route of choice.

Cromolyn Sodium

Primarily used as a prophylactic agent for asthma, cromolyn (Intal) has an antiinflammatory action and therefore is of significant advantage. Cromolyn is available for MDI or nebulizer. Onset of action can be as long as 1 to 2 months after the first dose. Dosage is two inhalations four times a day, and tapering can be attempted. This medication has virtually no side effects. Once in usage, cromolyn should be continued throughout an acute episode so as not to lose the prophylaxis. As with inhaled β_2-adrenergic agonists, cromolyn is useful for the prevention of EIB; and along with theophylline and corticosteroids, it is approved for use by the International Olympic Committee.

Nedocromil sodium (Tilade) is a newly released alternative to cromolyn. The recommended dose is two inhalations qid.

Anticholinergic Agents

There are currently two preparations of anticholinergic drugs available: ipratropium bromide (Atrovent) for MDI and atropine for nebulizer. These medicines are most useful in patients with COPD and, due to fewer side effects, may be the agents of choice for the bronchospasm of COPD. Ipratropium is almost devoid of systemic side effects and seems to work much more effectively in COPD patients than in asthma patients. Usual dosage is two inhalations four times a day. Atropine can be tried when more conventional therapy has failed. It is administered in a dosage of 0.01 to 0.025 mg/kg q4h if needed.[17]

Corticosteroids

The usage of steroids for asthma has received considerable attention in recent years. Traditionally thought to be too strong for chronic use, the advent of administration by MDI has minimized side effects and pushed corticosteroids into the forefront of treatment. Also, recognition of the importance of inflammation in the pathophysiology of asthma has made many authorities believe that corticosteroids should be used as first-line treatment in all asthmatics.[18] Unfortunately, the effect of corticosteroids on growth and their potential for adrenal suppression have not been fully addressed, causing many physicians to be reluctant to use these drugs as initial therapy. In the chronic patient, the unstable patient, and the patient in acute crisis, however, there should be no hesitancy.

Aerosol preparations of corticosteroids include beclomethasone dipropionate (Beclovent, Vanceril), flunisolide (AeroBid), and triamcinolone acetonide (Azmacort). The effects of these medications may not be fully seen for up to 4 to 8 weeks, and they are therefore not effective during the acute attack. They also do not protect against adrenal insufficiency. The oral medication must be tapered when attempting to switch to aerosol (Table 13.1).

Oral steroids, usually in the form of prednisone or prednisolone, are essential for use during an acute exacerbation or in an occasional difficult patient, as well in some patients with COPD. When used early in an episode, corticosteroids may prevent a relapse[19] or the need for hospitalization. When steroids are given intravenously, allow 6 to 8 hours before deciding if admission will be necessary.

Some physicians prescribe oral steroids to any patient needing treatment in an emergency setting. Patients with long-standing disease often develop recognizable patterns of deterioration, such as an episode with each upper respiratory infection. In these patients, early or prophylactic treatment often avoids an exacerbation. Dosage varies significantly with weight and age. Also, whereas multiple daily dosing may be best for the acute situation, for chronic treatment it is preferable that the drug be administered every other day.

Corticosteroids are also available for intravenous use. This method is indicated in the acute setting where hospitalization may be necessary. Unfortunately, there is no definitive proof as to the effectiveness of intravenous corticosteroids in preventing the need for hospitalization.

Calcium Channel Blockers

It has been suggested that calcium channel blockers have a mild bronchodilatory effect, but it has not been clinically demonstrated.[20] They are, however, effective medications for the treatment of hypertension in patients with obstructive airways disease, especially compared to β-blockers (can cause bronchospasm) and ACE inhibitors (can cause chronic cough).

Antibiotics

For acute bacterial infections in patients with asthma or COPD, antibiotics are essential. There has been debate concerning when to treat the COPD-afflicted patient. The use of broad-spectrum antibiotics appears to be indicated when COPD sufferers have at least two of the following three symptoms: an increase in dyspnea, an increase in sputum production, or an increase in sputum purulence.[21]

Mucolytics and Expectorants

The value of mucolytics and expectorants has not been demonstrated in objective studies.[22]

Oxygen

Except in the acute situation, oxygen should be reserved for those chronic patients who are in distress when breathing room air. With COPD patients who retain high levels of carbon dioxide, the only functioning respiratory drive may be related to hypoxia. It is therefore critical to adjust the oxygen to a level where the hypoxic drive is not lost.

Pregnancy and Breast-Feeding

Pregnancy is complicated by asthma about 1% of the time. Hypoxia represents a potentially severe risk to a developing fetus, so close control is needed. Theophylline, β_2-adrenergic agonists (terbutaline is considered the safest), cromolyn, and steroids are generally considered safe. Some antibiotics and decongestants, live virus vaccines, and iodides must be avoided.

In lactating mothers, the same medications considered safe during pregnancy are acceptable. Breast-feeding should be encouraged, as studies suggest a delay in the onset of allergies and asthma.[1,10]

Psychosocial Support

Psychosocial support is a critical component in any management program and is addressed in the last section of this chapter.

Prevention

Asthma and COPD are at opposite extremes when it comes to treatment and prevention. Whereas there are several good approaches to the treatment of asthma, management of COPD is at best symptomatic. However, asthma is essentially unpreventable, but COPD should be eliminated.

Smoking cessation is the key to relegating COPD to medical history. Except for a few genetic or occupational cases (which should also be preventable with good industrial hygiene), most cases of COPD are related to cigarette smoking. As a nation, the United States is moving toward an atmosphere of intolerance for smoking, but unfortunately it is a country where the children still have ready access to tobacco. Physicians therefore must remind each and every patient at every encounter to begin the process of smoking cessation. To be successful at quitting, patients must want to stop, as there is no aversion therapy. Once a decision is made to quit, there are literally dozens of methods and programs, although this large number speaks to the relative ineffectiveness of any one method. Perhaps the recently released nicotine patches will prove to be a more effective method.

Smoking cessation is also a key element when treating asthmatic patients, especially when it comes to the prevention of acute attacks. Even side stream smoke has been shown to result in more attacks, more complications, and more frequent need for emergency services.

Prevention of death has always been a priority within the medical profession. It is certainly appropriate when addressing the problems of asthma and COPD.

Asthma is usually viewed as a nonfatal disease, but it does carry the potential for death. Most studies have shown that preventable deaths have been the result of delayed treatment due primarily to two factors: the patient's or family's inability to recognize the severity of an attack, or the physician's poor assessment of the severity of an attack. Suggestions for prevention include frequent use of peak flow meters, establishing effective maintenance therapy, and emphasizing patient and family education. Education is aimed at recognizing an attack, knowing what measures to take at home, and learning to call for help early. The National Asthma Education Program has an excellent teaching packet.[23]

However, COPD is a highly fatal disease, the fifth leading cause of mortality in the United States, with more than 75,000 deaths per annum.[24] Although little can be done to reverse this disease, good management of the environment, appropriate medication, and smoking cessation aid in improving the quality of life for the affected individual.

Family and Community Issues

Family support is an essential factor in the treatment of chronic pulmonary disease. This is true for both asthma, in which victims may be children, and COPD, in which sufferers may be too debilitated to care for themselves.

Asthma

Patient and family attitudes are critical to the acceptance of this disease. Several factors have been identified with regard to poor patient attitude, including the unpredictable nature of asthma leading to a feeling of "beyond my control," a feeling of stigmatization, a false perception that asthma is psychogenic and therefore "in my head," a tendency to deny the disease, and the fear elicited by an experience of being unable to breathe.[25] These attitudes may serve to handicap all attempts at treatment and should be addressed via thorough patient and family education.

Also important is a tendency for families to label their asthmatic member as ill. It is best to view a patient as a person with asthma and not as an asthmatic person. All activities should be continued, especially sports and physical education. It is far better to use an MDI and run than to sit on the sidelines and watch.

COPD

Emotional difficulties are common in COPD sufferers. The dyspnea and fatigue of this disease often leads to depression and fear. Quality of life may be reduced in all areas—social, sexual, vocational, recreational—leading to further loss of self-esteem and isolation.[26] Patients should be encouraged to do as much as possible for themselves and must be given every opportunity to participate in the usual family and community events, even if a wheelchair and oxygen are needed. When the illness becomes terminal, patients should be counseled to keep control of their own lives by participating in the decisions of how and where to die. They can be encouraged to make living wills or execute powers of attorney. If appropriate, patients should be allowed to die at home, and physicians should be willing to make house calls. This decision improves the final quality of life by affording the patient the comfort of dying in a familiar setting, surrounded by family and friends.

References

1. Guidelines for the diagnosis and management of asthma. National asthma education program, expert panel report. Bethesda: National Heart, Lung and Blood Institute; 1991 August, Publ. No. 91–3042.
2. American Thoracic Society. Standards for the diagnosis and care of patients with chronic obstructive pulmonary disease (COPD) and asthma. Am Rev Respir Dis 1987;136:225–44.
3. Ingram RH. Chronic bronchitis, emphysema, and airways obstruction. In: Harrison's principles of internal medicine. New York: McGraw-Hill, 1987:1087–94.
4. Snider GL, Kleinerman J, Thurlbeck WM, Bengali ZH. The definition of emphysema: report of a National Heart, Lung and Blood Institute, Division of Lung Diseases workshop. Am Rev Respir Dis 1985;132:182–5.
5. Irwin RS, Curley FJ, French CL. Chronic cough, the spectrum and frequency of causes, key components of the diagnostic evaluation, and outcome of specific therapy. Am Rev Respir Dis 1990;141:640–7.
6. Goldszer RC, Lilly LS, Solomon HS. Prevalence of cough during angiotensin-converting enzyme inhibitor therapy. Am J Med 1988;85:887.
7. Kemp JP, Meltzer EO. Getting control of the allergic child's environment. Pediatr Ann 1989;18:801–9.
8. Selner JC. Helping asthmatic patients control their environment. J Respir Dis 1986;7:83–104.
9. Physician's desk reference, 42nd ed. Oradell, NJ: Medical Economics, 1992.
10. Weinberg H. Asthma in primary care patients, challenges and controversies. Postgrad Med 1990;88(5):107–14.
11. Gutstadt LB, Gillette JW, Mrazek DA, et al. Determinants of school performance in children with chronic asthma. Am J Dis Child 1989;143:471–5.
12. Seigel D, Sheppard D, Gelb A, Weinberg PF. Aminophylline increases the toxicity but not the efficacy of an inhaled beta-adrenergic agonist in the treatment of acute exacerbations of asthma. Am Rev Respir Dis 1985;132: 283–6.
13. Fanta CH, Israel E, Sheffer AL. Managing—and preventing—severe asthma attacks. J Respir Dis 1992;13:94–108.

14. Becker AB, Nelson NA, Simons FER. Inhaled salbutamol (albuterol) vs. injected epinephrine in the treatment of acute asthma in children. J Pediatr 1983;102:465–9.
15. Med Lett 1994;36(921):37–38.
16. Plaut TF. Holding chambers for aerosol drugs. Pediatr Ann 1989;18:824–6.
17. Gross NJ, Skorodin MS. Anticholinergics: will they be your best option in COPD? J Respir Dis 1986;7(2):38–43.
18. Szefler SJ. A comparison of aerosol glucocorticoids in the treatment of chronic bronchial asthma. Pediatr Asthma Allergy Immunol 1991;5:227–35.
19. Chapman KR, Verbeck PR, White JG, Rebeeck AS. Effect of a short course of prednisone in the prevalence of early relapse after the emergency room treatment of acute asthma. N Engl J Med 1991;324:788–94.
20. Olivier KN, Yankaskas JR. What role for calcium channel blockers in asthma? J Respir Dis 1991;12:703–7.
21. Anthonisen NR, Manfreda J, Warren CPW, et al. Antibiotic therapy in exacerbation of COPD. Ann Intern Med 1987;106:196–204.
22. Brain J. Aerosol and humidity therapy. Am Rev Respir Dis 1980;122 (Suppl):17–21.
23. Teach your patients about asthma: a clinician's guide. Publication 92-2737. Washington, DC: National Institutes of Health, 1992.
24. Rosen MJ. Treatment of exacerbations of COPD. Am Fam Physician 1992;45:693–7.
25. Dirks JF. Patient attitude as a factor in asthma management. Pract Cardiol 1986;12(1):84–98.
26. Dowell AR. Quality of life: how important in managing COPD? J Respir Dis 1991;12:1057–72.

Case Presentation

Subjective

Patient Profile

Samuel Nelson is a 48-year-old single white male farm worker.

Presenting Problem

"My breathing is worse."

Present Illness

For the past 5 years, Mr. Nelson has had gradually progressive cough, shortness of breath on exertion, and occasional wheezing. He has continued to smoke and does not take his medication regularly. When worse, he returns to the physician to refill his β-agonist inhaler for use as needed.

Past Medical History

He had pneumonia 3 years ago that did not require hospitalization.

Social History

Samuel was a high school dropout at age 16. He has never married and lives with his parents. He has no close friends.

Habits

He has smoked two packs of cigarettes daily since age 15. He uses no alcohol or recreational drugs.

Family History

His father, aged 76, has diabetes mellitus and osteoarthritis. His mother, aged 71, has high blood pressure. Three siblings are living and well.

• What additional information would you like about the history of present illness?

• What might be Mr. Nelson's reasons for the visit today? How would you inquire about this?
• What information about Mr. Nelson's work might be useful, and how would you ask about this?
• What more would you like to know about the patient's adaptation to his illness? Why might this be important?

Objective

VITAL SIGNS

Height, 5 ft, 10 in; weight 180 lb; blood pressure, 140/80; pulse, 76; respirations, 22; temperature, 37.2°C.

EXAMINATION

The patient is not in acute distress but has an occasional cough while talking. The head, eyes, ears, nose, and throat are normal. The neck and thyroid gland are normal. The chest has an increased anteroposterior diameter, and there are distant breath sounds throughout. No rales are present, but there are occasional faint wheezes on forced expiration. The heart has a regular sinus rhythm, and no murmurs are present.

• What more—if anything—might be included in the physical examination? Why?
• What—if any—laboratory tests would you order today? Why?
• What—if any—diagnostic imaging would you order today? Why?
• If, in addition to the symptoms described above, Mr. Nelson had lost 12 lb since a previous visit 6 months ago, what might you do differently? Explain.

Assessment

• What is your diagnostic impression today, and how would you explain this to the patient?
• How would you assess the meaning of the illness to Mr. Nelson?
• What is the apparent contribution of smoking to the patient's disease, and how would you describe this to him?
• The patient's employer calls to ask you about how Mr. Nelson is doing? How would you respond?

Plan

- What would be your therapeutic recommendations to the patient regarding medication, activity, and life style? How would you explain this to the patient?
- How might you persuade Mr. Nelson to stop smoking?
- What are the implications of this illness for the family and community?
- What continuing care would you advise? Explain.

14

Gastritis, Esophagitis, and Peptic Ulcer Disease

Alan M. Adelman and James P. Richardson

Dyspepsia and Epigastric Pain

Dyspepsia refers to upper abdominal pain or discomfort and is often associated with fullness, belching, bloating, heartburn, food intolerance, nausea, or vomiting. Dyspepsia is a common problem and can be difficult and expensive to diagnosis specifically. In this chapter, dyspepsia is first discussed in general terms as a symptom that prompts a visit to the physician, after which its common causes are presented.

Epidemiology

Dyspepsia is a common problem with an annual incidence of 1% to 2% among the general population; its prevalence may reach 20% to 40%. The five major causes of dyspepsia are nonulcer dyspepsia (NUD), peptic ulcer disease (PUD), gastroesophageal reflux disease (GERD), gastritis, and cholelithiasis. NUD, PUD, GERD, and gastritis account for more than 90% of all causes of dyspepsia. Other, less common causes of dyspepsia are irritable bowel disease, esophageal or gastric cancer, pancreatitis, pancreatic cancer, Zollinger-Ellison syndrome, and abdominal angina. Patients who seek medical attention for dyspepsia are more likely to be concerned about the seriousness of the symptom, worried about cancer or heart disease, and experiencing more stress than individuals who do not seek medical attention for dyspepsia.[1] The association beween *Helicobacter pylori* and dyspepsia is unclear.

Presentation

No single symptom is helpful for distinguishing the various causes of dyspepsia, but some patient characteristics are predictive of serious disease. Age greater than 50 years, male gender, a history of smoking, and a history of peptic ulcer disease or hiatal hernia are associated with gastric carcinoma, ulcers, and esophageal strictures. In several studies, pain occurring within 1 hour of eating, relief of pain by food or milk, vomiting, and pain lasting more than 6 hours are more commonly reported in patients with an organic cause for their pain. As single symptoms, nocturnal pain, relief of pain by antacids, worsening of pain by food, anorexia, nausea, and food intolerance are not helpful for distinguishing the causes of dyspepsia. One study[2] confirmed the tremendous overlap of symptoms described by patients with and without endoscopically confirmed diagnoses. With the possible exceptions of peptic ulcer disease and duodenitis, there was no association of clinical value between endoscopic findings and dyspeptic symptoms. To summarize, single symptoms are not of great value. Symptom complexes are usually more helpful for guiding patients' evaluations.

General Approach

Three strategies are helpful for management of dyspeptic symptoms. First, the patient who presents with a classic complex of symptoms should be managed for the specific diagnosis. For example, a young smoker with a history of postprandial pain, relieved by food or antacids, is a classic presentation for duodenal ulcer. Second, patients with possible complications of PUD (e.g., gastrointestinal bleeding) or signs of systemic disease (e.g., anemia or significant weight loss) should be evaluated immediately. These first two scenarios occur in few patients. Finally, in the absence of a classic history, complications, or systemic disease, the third strategy is to initiate empiric treatment and workup only if there is treatment failure.

The rationale for empiric treatment is based on four underlying principles. First, because most patients have NUD, PUD, or GERD, the initial treatment is the same. Knowing the exact diagnosis does not alter the initial treatment. Second, approximately 70% of patients with PUD are symptom-free within several weeks regardless of the therapy. Third, the risk of cancer, such as gastric or esophageal, is small, especially in patients younger than 50 years of age. Prompt unrestricted use of endoscopy has not increased the early detection of gastric cancer. Even if a gastric carcinoma is initially treated empirically, a delay in definitive treatment for 4 to 8 weeks has no effect on the outcome. Fourth, the natural history of PUD, NUD, and GERD is marked by periodicity and recurrence. Even if the initial episode is successfully treated, recurrence of the symptoms will prompt further evaluation.

If the pain is persistent or recurrent, further evaluation is required whether by upper endoscopy or upper gastrointestinal (GI) series. Although an upper GI series is less expensive and may be more readily available, it has a false-negative rate that exceeds 18% in some studies and a false-positive rate between 13% and 35%. In addition, the upper GI series is poor for diagnosing GERD and gastritis, two of the most common

TABLE 14.1. Histamine-2 receptor antagonists product information[a]

Generic and brand names	Indications	Maximum daily dosage	Duration of therapy
Cimetidine (Tagamet)	Duodenal ulcer		
	Short-term active	1200 mg	4–8 weeks
	Maintenance	400 mg	6 months
	Active benign gastric ulcer	1200 mg	6 weeks
	GERD	1600 mg	Up to 12 weeks
	Hypersecretory conditions	1200 mg	Clinically indicated
Famotidine (Pepcid)	Duodenal ulcer		
	Short-term active	40 mg	6–8 weeks
	Maintenance	20 mg	
	Active benign gastric ulcer	40 mg	8 weeks
	Hypersecretory conditions	80 mg up to 640 mg/day	Clinically indicated
Nizatidine (Axid)	Duodenal ulcer		
	Short-term active	300 mg	4–8 weeks
	Maintenance	150 mg	1 year
	GERD	300 mg	Up to 12 weeks
Ranitidine (Zantac)	Duodenal ulcer		
	Short-term active	300 mg	4–8 weeks
	Maintenance	150 mg	1 year
	Active benign gastric ulcer	300 mg	6 weeks
	GERD	600 mg	6 weeks
	Hypersecretory conditions	300 mg up to 6 g/day	Clinically indicated

Source: Michocki and Richardson.[6] With permission.
[a]Use all histamine-2 receptor antagonists with caution during pregnancy and lactation. Adjust dosage in the presence of renal failure.
GERD = gastroesophageal reflex disease.

causes of dyspepsia. Upper endoscopy has lower false-positive and false-negative rates, and biopsies can be performed. However, upper endoscopy is more costly, and its availability depends on the availability of an endoscopist. A negative upper GI series does not rule out disease; and if indicated, further evaluation with upper endoscopy should be pursued. The indications for upper endoscopy recommended by the American College of Physicians are (1) persistence of symptoms after 6 to 8 weeks of therapy; (2) no response to therapy after 7 to 10 days; (3) signs of complications of peptic disease; (4) signs of systemic illness; and (5) symptom recurrence.[3]

Empiric treatment for dyspepsia consists of either antacids or histamine 2 receptor antagonists (H2RA). If antacids are tried initially and fail to relieve symptoms, an H2RA should be tried before further workup is undertaken (Table 14.1). At the present time, there is no good evidence that treating patients with dyspepsia for H. pylori improves outcome.[4]

Gastroesophageal Reflux Disease

Gastroesophageal reflux disease is a common problem. About 10% of the general population report heartburn daily, and 15% to 40% experience it monthly. GERD results from exposure of the lower esophagus to gastric acid, pepsin, or bile acids. Several factors may lead to GERD including hiatal hernia, incompetence of the lower esophageal sphincter (LES), inappropriate LES relaxation, impaired esophageal peristalsis and acid clearance, impaired gastric emptying, and repeated vomiting.[5] Exposure to excessive acid or pepsin can produce damage of the esophageal mucosa, leading to inflammation and ultimately scarring and stricture formation.

Presentation

The most reliable symptom of GERD is heartburn, a retrosternal burning sensation that may radiate from the epigastrium to the throat. Patients may also complain of pyrosis or water brash, the regurgitation of bitter tasting material into the mouth. GERD can cause respiratory problems including laryngitis, chronic cough, aspiration pneumonia, and wheezing. Atypical chest pain can also be caused by GERD. Finally, patients may complain of odynophagia (pain with swallowing) or dysphagia.

Diagnosis

A young patient with no evidence of systemic illness requires no further workup and can be treated empirically. Older patients, particularly those with the complaint of odynophagia or dysphagia, require evaluation to rule out tumor or stricture. Upper endoscopy is the evaluation of first choice. Ambulatory 24-hour pH monitoring is the most sensitive test for demonstrating reflux if endoscopy is negative. A barium swallow study or esophageal manometry may be necessary if a motility disorder is suspected, as endoscopy is often normal in patients with this problem.

The presence of hiatal hernia does not equate with a diagnosis of GERD. All patients with hiatal hernia do not have reflux, and all patients with GERD do not have a hiatal hernia. Approximately 50% of the population have a hiatal hernia, but most have no reflux symptoms.

Management

Gastroesophageal reflux disease is treated by both nonpharmacologic and pharmacologic approaches. Treatment of gastroesophageal reflux disease can be divided into three phases. Phase 1 involves life-styles changes. All patients with suspected GERD should be advised to reduce weight, avoid large meals, avoid lying down after meals, avoid exercise after meals, and elevate the head of the bed. Because nicotine lowers LES pressure, smoking cessation should be recommended. Medications that can lower LES pressure and should be avoided include alcohol, theophylline, calcium channel blockers, anticholinergics, β-adrenergic agonists, and α-adrenergic antagonists.

Phase 2 involves pharmacologic agents. Antacids can be used for mild intermittent heartburn; however, if symptoms are persistent or severe, an H_2RA should be substituted for or added. H_2RAs have been available for more than 15 years and are among the most widely prescribed drugs in the world.[6,7] Cimetidine, ranitidine, famotidine, and nizatidine suppress acid secretion by competing with histamine and block its effect on parietal cells of the stomach. H_2RAs are effective when used for 6 to 12 weeks. Daytime and nocturnal acid production needs to be inhibited; therefore, twice-daily dosing is recommended rather than just nocturnal dosing. Sucralfate has also been shown to be efficacious for mild-to-moderate GERD. Sucralfate is a sulfated disaccharide that does not neutralize acid but appears to protect against acid by local effects on the mucosa.

Prokinetic agents, such as bethanecol (25 mg four times daily) or metoclopramide (10 mg four times daily) are also effective for mild-to-moderate GERD. They relieve symptoms by enhancing LES pressure, increasing esophageal contraction amplitude, and accelerating gastric emptying. A new prokinetic agent, cisapride (Propulsid; 10 mg four times daily), does not have the neurologic or psychotropic side effects as does metoclopramide. Combining prokinetic agents with H_2RAs may be better than using either agent alone. Both bethanecol and metoclopramide should be used cautiously in the elderly because of the higher incidence of adverse effects in this group.

For severe or refractory GERD, doubling the standard dose of H_2RAs may be effective. Omeprazole, an H^+/K^+-ATPase inhibitor, decreases gastric acid secretion and is more potent than cimetidine or ranitidine in suppressing both basal and stimulated acid production. Omeprazole has been shown to be effective therapy when H_2RAs have failed.

Phase 3 treatment is surgery. Indications for antireflux surgery include recurrent esophageal strictures; aspiration resulting in recurrent pneumonia, asthma, or laryngitis; bleeding from Barrett's ulcers or gastric erosions in a hiatal hernia; intolerable or difficult-to-treat symptoms.[8] Spechler et al.[9] showed that antireflux surgery was more effective than medical therapy in select patients, although the study was performed before omeprazole was available.

The clinical course of GERD is marked by recurrences and relapses. Maintenance therapy with H_2RAs, even at maximum dosage, has been disappointing. Omeprazole has been shown to decrease the rate of relapse, but there are some concerns regarding prolonged administration. Prolonged omeprazole use causes hypergastrinemia and, in animals only, gastric carcinoid tumor.

Peptic Ulcer Disease

Peptic ulcers may involve any portion of the upper GI tract, but ulcers are most often found in the stomach and duodenum. Duodenal ulcers are approximately three times as common as gastric ulcers; perhaps 10% of the population suffer from duodenal ulcers at some time in their lives.[10] Peptic ulcer disease should be considered a chronic disease, marked by periods of healing and recurrence. Ulcers result when so-called aggressive factors (acid and the proteolytic pepsins) overcome the GI tract's defensive factors (prostaglandins and gastric mucus containing bicarbonate ions). Recently, infection with *H. pylori* has been implicated as a cause of duodenal and peptic ulcer occurrence.[4]

Presentation

Epigastric pain is the most common presenting problem of both duodenal and gastric ulcer disease. The pain may be described as gnawing, burning, boring, aching, or severe hunger pains. Patients with duodenal ulcers typically experience pain within a few hours after meals and have complete or partial relief of pain with ingestion of food or antacids. Pain in gastric ulcer patients is more variable; it may even worsen with eating. Both duodenal and gastric ulcers may occur and recur in the absence of pain. Pain is variable among patients for both kinds of ulceration and correlates poorly with ulcer healing. Physical examination usually reveals epigastric tenderness midway between the xiphoid and umbilicus, but maximal tenderness is sometimes to the right of midline. Other findings may include a succussion splash (due to a mixture of air and fluid in the stomach when gastric outlet obstruction occurs from an ulcer in the duodenum or pyloric channel) or abdominal rigidity in the presence of perforation.

Diagnosis

Duodenal and gastric ulcers can be reliably diagnosed by upper GI contrast studies when a double-contrast technique is used. In addition to the indicators listed earlier in this chapter, endoscopy may be considered in patients with negative radiographic studies, those with deformed duodenal bulbs (thus making radiographic examination difficult), and patients with GI bleeding.[10] Endoscopy is used more often in the presence of gastric ulcers because of the possibility of gastric cancer (see Gastric Cancer, below). Contrast studies that demonstrate gastric ulcers without radiating mucosal folds and those larger than 3 cm in diameter are more likely to be malignant.

Treatment

Relief of pain and healing of the ulceration are the twin goals of therapy for peptic ulcer disease. Many regimens have been found effective. Antacids are effective for healing ulcers and were the mainstay of therapy for years. Combination aluminum hydroxide/magnesium hydroxide antacids (e.g., Maalox, Gelusil) are the most popular. This combination is low in sodium and unlikely to produce constipation (common when aluminum hydroxide alone is used) or diarrhea (common when magnesium hydroxide alone is used). Phosphate depletion may be a problem in malnourished patients, and hypermagnesemia may result when these antacids are given to patients with chronic renal failure. The most popular regimen is 30 ml 1 and 3 hours after meals and at bedtime. However, patient compliance is often poor with this regimen because of the number of doses required.

All H$_2$RAs effectively heal ulcers in equipotent doses (Table 14.1).[7] About 75% to 90% of ulcers are healed after 4 to 6 weeks of therapy. Cimetidine is the most inexpensive but appears to have the highest incidence of side effects and drug interactions.

Omeprazole heals ulcers more quickly than H$_2$RAs, but healing rates at 6 weeks are not significantly improved over those when H$_2$-blockers are given.[11] Omeprazole is approved for short-term therapy of duodenal ulcers only. Because of concern over adverse effects of long-term use, omeprazole should be considered only for patients with severe symptoms, a potential for complications, or refractory disease.

Healing rates with sucralfate are comparable with those with H$_2$RAs. There are no significant side effects, but the size of the tablet and frequency of administration (two to four times daily) are possible drawbacks.

Colloidal bismuth is also as effective as H$_2$RAs for healing ulcers but is not approved by the U.S. Food and Drug Administration for this use. Bismuth compounds may work by eradicating *H. pylori*, an organism implicated in the etiology of ulcer disease. Treatment with antimicrobials effective against *H. pylori* has been recommended for all patients with peptic ulcer disease regardless of whether this is the patient's initial presentation or a recurrence. A regimen of bismuth subsalicylate, tetracycline, and metronidazole has been reported to be 90% effective in eradicating *H. pylori*. Elimination of *H. pylori* markedly reduces the rate of duodenal ulcer recurrence.[4,12]

Although *H. pylori* infection can be reliably diagnosed endoscopically by either biopsy and histologic demonstration of the organism or by the demonstration of urease activity of the specimen, reliable noninvasive tests are not yet commercially available. Until noninvasive tests are available, clinicians must use their best judgment to decide which ulcer patients should have antimicrobial therapy in addition to standard regimens.[13]

Anticholinergic agents reduce acid secretion, but most studies have not found them to be effective in ulcer healing. Because of side effects such as confusion, blurred vision, exacerbation of glaucoma, urinary retention, and delayed gastric emptying, these drugs are no longer recommended for the treatment of peptic ulcers.

Prostaglandins protect the gastric mucosa, possibly by enhancing mucosal blood flow. Misoprostol, a prostaglandin E_1 analog, has been used to prevent ulcers due to nonsteroidal antiinflammatory drugs (NSAIDs). Misoprostol also heals ulcers at approximately the same rate as H_2RAs, but severe diarrhea may limit patient compliance. Stimulation of uterine contractions and induction of abortions are the most serious side effects of misoprostol.

Combination therapy is often used for the treatment of ulcers (e.g., sucralfate and an H_2RA), but the evidence to support the use of these regimens is weak.[11] Dietary therapy is now limited to the elimination of foods that exacerbate symptoms and the avoidance of alcohol and coffee (with or without caffeine) because they increase gastric acid secretion. Cessation of cigarette smoking is also recommended to speed healing and prevent recurrence. NSAIDs should be withheld as well.

Refractory Ulcers and Maintenance Therapy

Most duodenal ulcers heal within 4 to 8 weeks of the start of therapy; and after 12 weeks of therapy, 90% to 95% of ulcers are healed. Higher doses of H_2RAs (e.g., ranitidine 600–1200 mg/day) or omeprazole may be used to heal refractory ulcers. Review of compliance with previous recommendations and a search for the Zollinger-Ellison syndrome should also be considered.

The place of maintenance therapy is still unclear. Patients with severe or recurrent ulcers, ulcer complications, or medical conditions that may worsen with recurrence should be considered for 1 year of maintenance therapy. Elderly patients should also be considered for maintenance therapy because of their increased morbidity and mortality from PUD and its complications.

Gastric Ulcer Therapy

Gastric ulcers heal more slowly than duodenal ulcers, but 90% are healed after 12 weeks of therapy.[11] Gastric ulcers respond to the same treatments as duodenal ulcers, although acid hypersecretion is not associated with gastric ulcers. Gastric cancer should be excluded as a cause of the ulcer (see Gastric Cancer, below).

Gastritis

Gastritis, or inflammation of the gastric mucosa, is a collection of disorders most commonly divided into acute and chronic forms.[10] Acute erosive gastritis is common with severe illnesses such as sepsis, trauma or after surgery, or as a consequence of the administration of certain drugs (NSAIDs, aspirin, alcohol). Symptoms range from hematemesis and melena to anorexia, nausea, and vomiting. Pain is much less common than with peptic ulcer disease. Most patients are asymptomatic unless blood loss is appreciable. Patients may present with signs of massive blood loss (e.g., orthostatic hypotension, tachycardia, and pallor) or evidence of chronic blood loss (e.g., iron deficiency anemia).

Treatment consists of management of the underlying disease and removal of possible gastric irritants. For management and treatment of bleeding due to gastritis, see Upper Gastrointestinal Bleeding, below. Administration of antacids or H_2RAs in sufficient quantities to keep the gastric pH above 4 are effective in reducing the incidence of stress gastritis, but whether these therapies help to stop bleeding is not clear. Surgery is a last resort but may be required if medical therapies fail.

Chronic gastritis has been classified into types A and B. Type A involves the body and fundus of the stomach and may lead to pernicious anemia. Antibodies to parietal cells and to intrinsic factor are common. Type B gastritis is much more common than type A. Stomach involvement ranges from only the antrum to the entire stomach. *H. pylori* is frequently found in patients with type B gastritis, but treatment for *H. pylori* is not advocated.

The development of pernicious anemia, the end result of type A gastritis, is the only reason to treat either type A or B gastritis. Oral or parenteral vitamin B_{12} (cyanocobalamin) is required for the remainder of the patient's life.

Upper Gastrointestinal Bleeding

Upper GI bleeding is defined as GI blood loss above the ligament of Treitz. It may present in one of three ways. (1) It may present as hematemesis, which may be either bright red or coffee-ground-appearing material. Usually hematemesis means active bleeding. (2) It may present as melena. Black, tarry stools signify that the blood has transited through the GI tract, causing the digestion of blood. Melena may also be caused by lower GI bleeding. (3) It may present as hematochezia if bleeding is brisk. Blood can have a cathartic effect on the bowel.

Causes

The four most common causes of upper GI bleeding are (1) peptic ulceration, (2) gastritis, (3) esophageal varices, and (4) esophagogastric mucosal tear (Mallory-Weiss syndrome). Because bleeding due to peptic ulceration may present without pain, the latter should always be considered. The causes of gastritis are described above. Bleeding due to varices is usually abrupt and massive, and chronic blood loss is unusual. Varices may be due to alcohol cirrhosis or any other cause of portal hypertension, such as portal vein thrombosis. Mallory-Weiss syndrome classically presents with retching followed by hematemesis. Other causes of upper GI bleeding include gastric carcinoma, lymphoma, polyps, and diverticula.

Diagnosis/Management

The diagnosis and management of the patient with upper GI bleeding depend on the site and extent of bleeding. Vomitus and stool should be tested to confirm the presence of blood. Initial management for all patients includes assessment of vital signs including orthostatic changes. Patients thought to have significant blood loss should also be typed and cross-matched for blood replacement and a large-bore intravenous line placed for fluid and blood replacement.

A nasogastric tube should be placed to help determine the site and extent of the bleeding. The nasogastric aspirate should be tested for blood. If the aspirate consists of red blood or "coffee-ground" materials, the stomach should be lavaged with saline. Blood products and intravenous fluids may be required. Iced saline has been used to halt bleeding, but the efficacy of this treatment has never been demonstrated. Once the patient is hemodynamically stable and the bleeding has stopped, upper endoscopy can be performed. Upper endoscopy can be both diagnostic and therapeutic: Sclerotherapy or ligation of esophageal varices can be performed through the endoscope, and active bleeding from a peptic ulcer can be treated endoscopically.

If the patient has persistent bleeding, many physicians recommend endoscopy to locate the source of bleeding. Massive hemorrhage from varices can make endoscopy useless.

There are two additional therapies for bleeding varices. Peripherally administered vasopressin is as effective as vasopressin given intraarterially. Balloon tamponade with a Sengstaken-Blakemore tube is an alternative treatment for bleeding varices.

As always, prevention of GI bleeding is more effective than treatment. Maintenance therapy for PUD may decrease subsequent bleeding episodes. β-Adrenergic antagonists can prevent and reduce the mortality rate associated with GI bleeding in patients with cirrhosis, regardless of severity.[14]

Gastric Cancer

The incidence of gastric cancer has declined significantly over the past 60 years,[15] but still causes thousands of deaths each year. Ninety percent of these cancers are adenocarcinomas, and non-Hodgkin's lymphomas and leiomyosarcomas comprise the remainder. Possible etiologic factors are ingestion of high nitrate foods, atrophic gastritis, decreased gastric acidity, and *H. pylori* infection.[4]

Early gastric cancers are usually asymptomatic. As the cancer grows, patients may complain of anorexia or early satiety, vague discomfort, or steady pain. Weight loss, nausea and vomiting, and dysphagia may also be present. Physical examination is usually normal in patients with early disease, but a palpable abdominal mass, enlarged liver, ascites, or enlarged supraclavicular nodes may be present with metastatic disease.

Double-contrast radiographic studies usually can detect gastric cancer. However, if a benign-appearing ulcer is found, further workup may be necessary. Endoscopy with biopsy and brushings is advised by many, but others keep track of the healing of the ulcer by radiography. Benign ulcers are assumed if some degree of healing has been demonstrated by 6 weeks. Complete healing should occur within 12 weeks. Another study should be performed several months later to confirm that no new lesions have appeared. If healing has not occurred by 6 weeks, gastric cancer is suspected, and biopsies and brushings should be obtained. Endoscopy should be repeated at 12 weeks to ensure that the ulcer has healed completely. An alternative approach is to recommend endoscopy with biopsy for all patients with gastric ulcers older than the age of 50, as the incidence of gastric cancer peaks during the sixth decade.

Surgical treatment is the only definite chance for a cure. Unfortunately, only one-third of patients present early enough to achieve a cure through surgery. Five-year survival rates are about 25% for distal tumors and 10% for tumors of the proximal stomach. Surgery with or without radiation therapy may be given for palliation.

Chemotherapy has been successful in reducing tumor size, but responses are transient; hence the role of chemotherapy is still evolving. Adjuvant chemotherapy for patients undergoing complete resection is still investigational.

References

1. Lydeard S, Jones R. Factors affecting the decision to consult with dyspepsia: comparison of consulters and nonconsulters. J R Coll Gen Pract 1989;39:495–8.
2. Johnsen R, Bernersen B, Straume B, et al. Prevalences of endoscopic and histological findings in subjects with and without dyspepsia. BMJ 1991;302:749–52.
3. Health and Public Policy Committee, American College of Physicians. Endoscopy in the evaluation of dyspepsia. Ann Intern Med 1985;102:266–9.
4. NIH Consensus Development Panel on Helicobacter pylori in Peptic Ulcer Disease. JAMA 1994;272:65–69.
5. Altorki NK, Skinner DB. Pathophysiology of gastroesophageal reflux. Am J Med 1989;86:685–9.

6. Michocki RJ, Richardson JP. The clinical use of histamine-2 receptor antagonists. Maryland Med J 1992;41:397–400.

7. Feldman M, Burton ME. Histamine$_2$-receptor antagonists: standard therapy for acid-peptic diseases. N Engl J Med 1990;323:1672–80,1749–55.

8. Richter JE. Surgery for reflux disease—reflections of a gastroenterologist. N Engl J Med 1992;326:825–6.

9. Spechler SJ, Department of Veterans Affairs Gastroesophageal Reflux Disease Study Group. Comparison of medical and surgical therapy for complicated gastroesophageal reflux disease in veterans. N Engl J Med 1992;326:786–92.

10. McGuigan JE. Peptic ulcer and gastritis. In: Wilson JD, Braunwald E, Isselbacher KJ, et al., editors. Harrison's principles of internal medicine. 12th ed. New York: McGraw-Hill, 1991:1229–48.

11. Hixson LJ, Kelley CL, Jones WN, Tuohy CD. Current trends in the pharmacotherapy for peptic ulcer disease. Arch Intern Med 1992;152:726–32.

12. Forbes GM, Glaser ME, Cullen DJE, et al. Duodenal ulcer treated with Helicobacter pylori eradication: seven year follow-up. Lancet 1994;343:258–60.

13. Feldman M. The acid test—making clinical sense of the consensus conference on Helicobacter pylori. JAMA 1994;272:70–71.

14. Poynard T, Cales P, Pasta L, et al. Beta-adrenergic-antagonist drugs in the prevention of gastrointestinal bleeding in patients with cirrhosis and esophageal varices: an analysis of data and prognostic factors in 589 patients from four randomized clinical trials. N Engl J Med 1991;324:1532–8.

15. Mayer RJ. Neoplasms of the esophagus and stomach. In: Wilson JD, Braunwald E, Isselbacher KJ, et al., editors. Harrison's principles of internal medicine. 12th ed. New York: McGraw-Hill, 1991:1248–51.

CASE PRESENTATION

Subjective

PATIENT PROFILE

Ralph Martino is a 45-year-old divorced white male attorney.

PRESENTING PROBLEM

"Heartburn."

PRESENT ILLNESS

For the past 6 weeks, Mr. Martino has had a recurrent burning sensation in the upper abdomen, worse after meals, especially if the food is spicy or "acid." Antacids and milk afford some relief. There has been no nausea, vomiting, constipation, or diarrhea. He notes occasional upper abdominal pain that seems different from the "heartburn." Similar heartburn has occurred several times in the past, especially at the time of his divorce 10 years ago.

PAST MEDICAL HISTORY

The patient had hepatitis and a fractured femur as a teenager.

SOCIAL HISTORY

He is divorced and lives alone with two dogs. He is a partner in a law firm and specializes in labor relations.

HABITS

He smokes one pack of cigarettes daily and takes one to two drinks of vodka each evening. He uses six to eight cups of coffee daily but takes no recreational drugs.

FAMILY HISTORY

His father died at age 66 of colon cancer. His mother, aged 78, has had gallbladder surgery. One sister, aged 47, has Crohn's disease.

REVIEW OF SYSTEMS

He has a long history of recurrent headache and low back pain.

- What additional information regarding the medical history would you like to know? Why?
- What diagnostic possibilities are you considering at this time?
- What questions might you ask to learn more about current stressors in his life?
- What is likely to be the patient's adaptation to his illness? Why might this be pertinent?

Objective

VITAL SIGNS

Height, 5 ft 11 in; weight 186 lb; blood pressure, 138/90; pulse, 70; respirations, 18.

EXAMINATION

The patient appears tense and "worried." The chest is clear to percussion and auscultation. The heart has a regular sinus rhythm, and no murmurs are heard. The abdomen is scaphoid, and active bowel sounds are present. There is mild epigastric tenderness, but no mass is found. On rectal examination, the prostate is normal and no rectal mass is palpable. There is a positive test for occult blood in the feces.

- What more data—if any—might be derived from the physical examination? Why?
- Are there specific diagnostic maneuvers that might be helpful today?
- What—if any—laboratory studies might be useful in making the diagnosis?
- What—if any—diagnostic imaging or endoscopy would you recommend today? Why?

Assessment

- What is your diagnostic assessment at this time? How would you explain this to Mr. Martino?
- What is likely to be the meaning of this illness to Mr. Martino? Explain.

- What is the significance of the positive test for occult blood in feces?
- What are the possible contributions of alcohol and tobacco use to his current illness?

Plan

- Pending the results of further tests, what therapeutic recommendations would you make to Mr. Martino regarding diet, life style, and medication?
- Is consultation likely to be necessary? Under what circumstances? Explain.
- If the patient calls tonight describing the passage of large quantities of dark red blood from the rectum, what would be your concern? What would you do?
- What follow-up would you recommend for this patient?

15
Urinary Tract Infections

LARRY W. JOHNSON

Symptoms of urinary tract infections (UTIs) are common problems presented to the family practitioner[1] and account for 5 million office visits yearly in the United States.[2] UTI is a broad term used to describe microbial colonization of the urine and infection of the structures of the urinary tract extending from the kidney to the urethral meatus, as well as infection of adjacent structures, such as the prostate. In this chapter, definitions and associated concepts of UTIs are given and then traced across the age spectrum from birth to senescence and death. Sexually transmitted diseases are covered only superficially with comments about urethritis.

Most commonly, UTIs are caused by bacteria, although occasionally fungi and viruses are implicated. Organisms need not be detectable in the urine to make the diagnosis of a UTI because their presence may be restricted to localized tissue or an abscess. However, with most UTIs there is bacteriuria, and a positive urine culture can be obtained.

Definitions

Bacteriuria: Presence of bacteria in the urine. Normally, bladder urine is sterile.[3] Urine can become contaminated from urethral or periurethral flora during micturition. Asymptomatic bacteriuria occurs most commonly in diabetic patients, pregnant women, preschool children, and the elderly.

Significant bacteriuria: A term used to differentiate true infection from contamination. Clean-catch midstream urine specimen(s) for culture is the gold standard diagnostic tool for UTIs. The traditional threshold for defining significant bacteriuria is 10^5 or more colony-forming units (CFU) of bacteria per milliliter of voided urine.[4] The method of obtaining the urine specimen and the symptoms of the patient should be used for modifying that traditional guideline. Suprapubic aspiration and bladder catheterization more accurately measure the microbiologic status of the urine, but they are uncomfortable and invasive procedures. With a suprapubic aspiration or properly collected catheterized urine specimen, any growth of bacteria is significant.[2] For the acutely symptomatic female patient, 10^2 CFU of coliform bacteria/ml of urine is a more sensitive indicator while being only slightly less specific.[5] In symptomatic male patients, a threshold of 10^3 CFU reliably suggests infection.[6] In the chronically catheterized patient, a quantitative threshold of 10^2 can be used because invariably, over succeeding days, the subsequent culture reaches 10^5 CFU.[7]

Cystitis: Infection of the urinary bladder usually accompanied by symptoms of dysuria, frequency, or urgency. Cystitis may be mimicked by inflammation of the bladder or urethra in the absence of infection, as well as by vaginitis and sexually transmitted diseases such as those caused by *Neisseria gonorrhoeae, Chlamydia trachomatis,* and herpes simplex.

Acute urethral syndrome: Dysuria, frequency, or urgency in the absence of traditional significant bacteriuria on a voided urine specimen. It usually occurs in young sexually active women. These patients can be divided into two groups.[8] One group includes women with pyuria on urinalysis who appear to be infected with either *Chlamydia trachomatis* or coliform bacteria ($>10^2$ CFU/ml) such as Enterobacteriaceae or *Staphylococcus saprophyticus.* The other group includes women without pyuria for whom no bacterial etiology is found, which in some patients is related to the mechanical irritation or massage of the urethra during intercourse. The diagnosis of acute urethral syndrome does not exclude cystitis because patients may have both conditions.

Acute pyelonephritis: Syndrome that consists of localized flank or back pain combined with systemic symptoms such as fever, chills, and prostration. It is caused by infection of the kidney collecting system and parenchyma and may be complicated by bacteremia.[2]

Chronic pyelonephritis: Defined pathologically rather than clinically. The kidneys show uneven scarring and contraction from progressive inflammation of the renal tubules and interstitium. The pathology is not specific and is found in association with other renal diseases, such as chronic obstruction, analgesic abuse, and uric acid nephropathy.[9]

Intrarenal and perinephric abscesses: Uncommon manifestations that are usually complications of acute pyelonephritis or bacteremic seeding. Intrarenal abscesses may be categorized as cortical or corticomedullary. Most cortical abscesses arise from hematogenous seeding of the kidneys, and most (90%) are caused by *Staphylococcus aureus,* with the source usually being skin, oral cavity, lung, or bone. Corticomedullary abscesses usually are complications of UTI and an abnormality, such as reflux or obstruction.[2]

Acute prostatitis: Acute bacterial infection of the prostate gland usually manifesting as abrupt onset of fever and perineal pain associated with irritation and obstructive voiding dysfunction. Bacteriuria often accompanies acute prostatitis.

Chronic prostatitis: Low-grade, persistent bacterial infection of the prostate gland. Relapsing episodes of cystitis and pyelonephritis may be common. Symptoms may be similar to and generally less intense than patients experience with acute prostatitis.

Urosepsis: Symptomatic bacteremia of urinary tract origin. It is a rare but life-threatening complication of UTIs in healthy persons. Community-acquired urosepsis usually arises from acute pyelonephritis or renal abscess, whereas nosocomial urosepsis most often is associated with urinary tract instrumentation.

Two other terms need definition for optimum treatment of patients. *Reinfection* is recurrence of bacteriuria with an organism different from that originally isolated. *Relapse* is recurrence of bacteriuria with the organism originally isolated. It is possible for reinfection to occur with the same organism, making it impossible to distinguish between reinfection and relapse. True *chronic urinary tract infection* means persistent UTI with the same organism. An alternative definition is to specify chronic infections as either relapses or reinfections.[2]

Asymptomatic Bacteriuria

Screening for asymptomatic bacteriuria is somewhat controversial. The U.S. Preventive Services Task Force (USPSTF) recommends testing asymptomatic patients with diabetes mellitus and pregnant women.[10] The optimum frequency for testing in these groups has not been determined and is left to clinical discretion. The urine specimen should be obtained in a manner that minimizes contamination. In general, dipsticks combining leukocyte esterase (found in granulocytes) and nitrite tests (gram-negative bacteria in urine convert nitrates to nitrites) should be used to detect asymptomatic bacteriuria. The sensitivity and specificity of these dipstick tests vary with spectrum bias (sensitivity, 56–92%; specificity, 42–78%).[11] When the leukocyte esterase and nitrite dipstick are positive in patients with diabetes, a urine culture should be obtained. Patients with diabetes can have asymptomatic bacteriuria and asymptomatic UTIs. During pregnancy, a urine culture (perhaps at about week 16) is a more accurate screening test than dipstick urinalysis. An alternative recommendation for the pregnant patient is to test the urine of all prenatal patients at their first visit and to send to the laboratory for culture only those urine samples with 5 or more white blood cells per high power field (WBCs/hpf) on a centrifuged urine specimen.[12] In pregnant women, bacteriuria is a risk factor for prematurity and low birth weight. About 20% to 40% of untreated pregnant women with asymptomatic bacteriuria develop symptomatic UTI.[13] Several randomized, controlled trials have shown that treatment of asymptomatic bacteriuria during pregnancy can reduce the incidence of symptomatic UTI and premature labor.[13,14]

Also, USPSTF stated that it may be clinically prudent to screen pre-school children and patients age 60 and older. Among children, about 13% to 17% of patients with recurrent bacteriuria develop chronic pyelonephritis, and 23% to 29% have evidence of vesicoureteral reflex.[15] Children with significant structural abnormalities are at increased risk of hypertension, renal insufficiency, renal scarring, and obstructive uropathy.[16] The treatment of bacteriuria in the elderly may be of benefit in the ambulatory setting. Randomized trials in elderly women have shown that treatment can reduce the incidence of subsequent bacteriuria and possible symptomatic UTI.[17]

Diagnostic Considerations

Urine Culture and Urinalysis

Urine culture is performed on midstream clean-catch specimens collected into sterile containers. In women, the external genitalia are washed two or three times with a cleansing agent and water before collecting the specimen. This process does not eliminate urethral contamination. The routine cleansing of the urethral meatus in men before a midstream clean-catch specimen is of questionable value, but this technique is widely used.[18] In newborns and infants, urine collection bags are helpful when proper cleansing and collecting have been done, particularly when no growth on culture is found. The reliability of a bag urine culture is increased with multiple, same single bacterial growth samples. Suprapubic tap for culture is the gold standard.[19]

Prompt handling of a urine specimen for culture is best. Refrigeration of the urine is an acceptable alternative if the specimen cannot be inoculated onto appropriate media expeditiously. Office dip slide culture methods are available and are useful when done properly, particularly when no growth occurs or with growth of bacteria for identification of common pathogens such as *Escherichia coli*. At times, they must be followed by a traditional urine culture.

For identification of bacteria causing prostatitis, a two- to four-glass urine culture can be obtained: After foreskin retraction in the uncircumcised male, the glans is prepared. The patient should have a full bladder. The first voided 10 ml is placed in the first sterile container and represents a urethral culture. Then a midstream urine aliquot of urine is obtained after a 200-ml void and is the bladder culture. The patient stops voiding and prostatic massage, milking the prostate toward the urethra, can result in prostatic secretions for culture. The next voided 10-ml of urine is also a prostatic culture.[20]

On urinalysis, the presence of squamous epithelial cells strongly suggests contamination, and a subsequent clean voided specimen should be obtained. In general, an uncentrifuged drop of urine examined by microscopy with more than 8 WBCs/hpf as the cutoff point can be helpful and is more usable than a cytometer count with 20 WBCs/mm^3 as cutoff for predicting a positive culture.[21] There are many variables for direct quantification of pyuria of urinary sediment from a centrifuged specimen, but most laboratories use 2 to 5 WBCs/hpf as an indication of infection.[8] Direct microscopy for the detection of bacteriuria is a readily available but highly variable method of determining bacteriuria. There is no consistent standard method of specimen preparation or for interpretation with various combinations of centrifuging/not centrifuging and Gram staining/not Gram staining. An uncentrifuged, Gram-stained urine specimen with one organism per oil emersion field correlates best with more than 10^5 CFU/ml of urine on culture.[21] Leukocyte esterase and urine nitrite, briefly discussed under asymptomatic bacteriuria, have equal relevance for symptomatic bacteriuria. A urine culture may be necessary to determine if infection is present.

The antibody-coated bacteria (ACB) test is a research tool that merits brief comment. The ACB test is based on the premise that invasive upper UTIs lead to specific host immune response to the invading bacteria and that mucosal infections such as uncomplicated cystitis do not elicit a significant antibody response. When it was developed, it held the promise of differentiating upper from lower UTIs. It can be falsely negative in the presence of early upper UTI and does not distinguish between prostate and renal infection.[18]

Bacterial and Host Factors

Almost all UTIs are caused by bacteria, although occasionally they are due to viruses or fungi. The severity of the infection is determined by host resistance, the size the inoculum, and the virulence factors of the infecting strain.

Host defenses include the urine itself, colonization of the vaginal introitus by *Lactobacillus,* the bladder, ureteral peristalsis, the competence of the vesicoureteral junction, the kidney, and the immune response, including B and T lymphocytes and phagocytes. Inhibitory factors of urine include high osmolality, urea concentration, organic acids, and low pH. Oligosaccharides and uromucoid, now known to be identical to Tamm-Horsfall protein, are found in normal urine and may competitively inhibit attachment of *E. coli* to the mucosal surface of the urinary tract by aggregating the bacteria in the urine. Micturition empties the bladder of most bacteria, and the bladder mucosa has antibacterial properties.

Predisposing host factors for UTI include being elderly, having diabetes mellitus, pregnancy, urinary calculi, and obstruction. Age-associated UTIs may be related to impaired bladder emptying due to neurologic disease, obstructive uropathy, waning bactericidal secretions from the prostate, and decreased Tamm-Horsfall protein secretion. Clinical mechanisms that contribute to patients with diabetes getting UTIs include autonomic neuropathy with impaired bladder emptying, generalized vascular disease, and glycosuria, which inhibits phagocytosis. Urinary calculi can cause obstruction and irritate the urinary tract mucosa, which promotes bacterial adherence. Stones that form in the presence of a UTI (known as struvite or triple phosphate stones) are caused by urea-producing microorganisms including *Proteus mirabilis* and *Pseudomonas aeruginosa*. Finally, obstruction compromises urinary tract defense mechanisms.[22]

The virulence of bacteria affects the host in the battle of a UTI. The more compromised the natural defense mechanisms (including catheterization), the fewer are the virulence requirements of any bacterial strain or species to induce infection. The K antigen, a polysaccharide of the *E. coli* capsule, restricts access to complement, interfering with phagocytosis. Also, O (lipopolysaccharide) and H (flagellar antigen) factors are important determinants of *E. coli* virulence. Bacterial adherence to uroepithelial cells is a specific process involving bacterial surface structures (adhesions) and complementary components (receptors) on uroepithelial cells. Bacterial fimbria are believed to be the most common surface adhesions responsible for attachment. The most frequent uropathogens are aerobic and facultative anaerobic gram-negative bacilli, primarily *E. coli* and other Enterobacteriaceae such as *Proteus mirabilis*, *Klebsiella pneumoniae*, *Enterobacter*, and *Pseudomonas aeruginosa*. Only about six serotypes of *E. coli* cause about 85% of acute UTIs. Gram-positive cocci, such as *Enterococcus*, are infrequent uropathogens. *Staphylococcus aureus*, *Salmonella*, *Candida*, and *Mycobacterium tuberculosis* are unusual uropathogens, found in special clinical situations. Women with nonsecretor Lewis blood group phenotype are prone to recurrent UTIs and increased adhesiveness of *E. coli* to uroepithelium. Bacterial hemolysins are toxic to polymorphonuclear cells and monocytes. Aerobactin enhances iron uptake in *E. coli* and is another virulence factor for *E. coli*. *Staphylococcus* is an important uropathogen in young adult women, causing cystitis, and it has avid adherence to uroepithelial cells.[23]

Indwelling Catheter

Indwelling catheters are associated with UTIs. Prevention includes not using an indwelling catheter whenever possible, the shortest-term use consistent with the overall needs of the patient, and maintaining a closed drainage system. For incontinent men, a condom catheter is a useful alternative. Patient training, special clothes, and medications can be appropriate alternatives to an indwelling catheter. For patients with urinary retention, intermittent catheterization is a good option. Suprapubic catheterization (as an alternative to urethral catheterization) is best used short term in patients undergoing gynecologic operations. Catheter-associated UTIs (UTIc) remain the most common nosocomial infection. Although usually benign, UTIc causes bacteremia in 2% to 4% of patients and have been associated with a case-fatality rate three times as high as in non-bacteriuria patients.[24]

In patients with long-term catheterization, bacteriuria inevitably develops and the infecting strains change frequently. In this setting, *Proteus* and *Morganella* species produce catheter encrustations and persistent bacteriuria. Sterile catheterization technique is important. Bacteria may enter the bladder at the time of catheterization because the urethra cannot be sterilized. Subsequent routes of bacterial entry have been well defined and differ by gender, with the periurethral route predominant in women and the intraluminal route predominant in men. Growth of bacteria in biofilms on the inner surface of catheters promotes encrustations and may protect bacteria from antimicrobial agents. After bacteriuria develops, the ability to limit its complications is minimal.[25]

Management of Urinary Tract Infections

The life cycle is a useful concept when caring for patients and families. Recommended antibiotic therapy changes frequently enough that checking a drug insert and a yearly updated source such as J. P. Sanford's *Guide to Antimicrobial Therapy* (Antimicrobial Therapy Inc., Dallas, Texas, 1995) is prudent.

Infancy and Childhood

During the neonatal period bacteria reach the urinary tract via the bloodstream or urethra, whereas later in life they ascend the urinary tract from below. UTIs are relatively uncommon during the neonatal period and usually are part of the picture of sepsis, rather than the cause of it. An imaging workup is not generally necessary, but consultation (e.g., with a neonatologist) is appropriate to help make the best decision for the patient. Because sepsis is common in renal infections, including those in infants with obstruction, blood cultures should be performed during febrile UTIs[26] (infancy through senescence). After a first UTI, children require an evaluation with imaging studies to screen for urinary tract abnormalities and for reflux.[27] With an acute febrile infection, renal ultrasonography should be done to rule out hydronephrosis and abscess. Approximately 3 weeks after treatment of the acute infection, all children should have a voiding cystourethrogram to assess reflux. Some physicians restrict these studies to all boys and to girls younger than 5 years of age who have initial infection; older female patients are studied at the time of the second infection. Although reflux is more commonly seen in children younger than age three, 25% of all children younger than age 10 who have had symptomatic or asymptomatic bacteriuria experience reflux. Reflux nephropathy or chronic pyelonephritis is the most common cause of arterial hypertension in children.[27]

Treatment of neonates and children with UTIs should be based on cultures and sensitivity tests on specimens appropriately collected. Decisions about oral or parenteral therapy followed by oral therapy for 7 to 14 days should be based on the clinical severity of the illness. Follow-up culture, for example, 1 week after completion of therapy, is prudent. Trimethoprim/sulfamethoxazole (TMP/SMX: TMP 6 mg/kg and SMX 30 mg/kg bid), amoxicillin (25–50 mg/kg tid), cefaclor (20–40 mg/kg tid), and nitrofurantoin (3–7 mg/kg qid) are appropriate starting agents. Intravenous antimicrobials that may be used while cultures are pending including ampicillin (100–200 mg/kg/day), gentamicin and tobramycin (5.0–7.5 mg/kg/day), or cefotaxime (100–150 mg/kg/day).[28] For the acutely ill patient, checking the package insert for current rate, route, and frequency of administration is wise. Consultation may also be appropriate.

Adults

Lower Urinary Tract Infections

As patients age, UTIs in men become uncommon. Consideration of urologic consultation to rule out obstructions in men with UTIs is appropriate. Appropriate culture and sensitivity tests are important in the adult man for documentation of infection with a follow-up culture to ensure that cure has occurred. Depending on the severity of the illness, oral or parenteral antibiotics can be used. TMP/SMX double strength (160 mg/800 mg bid), amoxicillin (250–500 mg tid), or a fluoroquinolone is appropriate. Abdominal ultrasonography, intravenous pyelography (IVP) cystoscopy, and urine cytology may be necessary, particularly if hematuria is persistent. Split cultures may be helpful to help determine if prostatitis is present. Catheterization to measure residual volume or to obtain urine for culture is rarely indicated.[29]

Lower UTI is a common problem for women and tends to be recurrent. It is not associated with significant long-term morbidity.[30] With an acute lower UTI, empiric short-course therapy (single dose or 3-day therapy) with one of several antibiotics is recommended in the absence of complicating factors. Single-dose regimens for uncomplicated cystitis include TMP/SMX (two double-strength tablets), amoxicillin (3 g), sulfisoxazole (1–2 g), trimethoprim (400 mg), and ciprofloxacin (250 mg).[31] Acceptable drugs for short course (3-day) therapy are many and include TMP/SMX (160/800 mg q12h), sulfisoxazole (500 mg q6h), trimethoprim (100 mg q12h), nitrofurantoin (100 mg q6h), amoxicillin (500 mg q8h), cephalexin (500 mg q6h), ciprofloxacin (250 mg q12h), norfloxacin (400 mg q12h), and amoxicillin/clavulanate (500 mg q8h). This list is presented in order of increasing expense.[32] All fluoroquinolones administered for 3 days are generally effective for treatment of uncomplicated UTIs caused by gram-negative bacilli.[33] When complicating factors are present, the antibiotic susceptibility profile of the infecting organism should be determined and therapy with an appropriate agent provided for 7 days. Ampicillin and related drugs are probably inferior to TMP/SMX for treatment of occult renal infection. The role of posttherapy cultures in the management of UTI in women is not well defined, but cultures can probably be safely omitted for most women with uncomplicated acute cystitis.

Postcoital measures to decrease the chance of recurrent UTI in women include nonantibiotic measures of voiding after intercourse, discontinuing use of a diaphragm and spermicide, and emptying the bladder frequently. Postcoital antibiotic regimens for prevention of recurrent UTIs include TMP/SMX (single-strength tablet), nitrofurantoin (50–100 mg), cephalexin (250 mg), and sulfisoxazole (500 mg). Antibiotic prophylaxis regimens for recurrent UTIs include TMP/SMX (half of a single-strength tablet three times a week), trimethoprim (100 mg hs), and cephalexin (250–500 mg hs).[34] Acceptable drugs for a short course of treatment of bacteriuria include amoxicillin (250 mg tid for 7 days or a 3-g single dose with or without a 3-g follow-up dose in 12 hours), nitrofurantoin (100 mg qid for 3–7 days and 200-mg single dose—avoid with glucose-6-phosphate dehydrogenase [G6PD] deficiency), sulfisoxazole (2 g followed by 1 g qid for 7 days or a 2-g single dose—avoid near term as it can cause hyperbilirubinemia), and cephalexin (3-g single dose and 2-g single dose with 1 g probenecid).

Acute Pyelonephritis

Acute pyelonephritis can be sometimes managed on an outpatient basis. Indications for admission to hospital include severe illness with high fever, severe pain, and marked debility, as well as an inability to maintain oral hydration or take medicines, concern about compliance and the patient's social situation, and uncertainty of diagnosis. When parenteral therapy is needed and if the Gram stain is not suggestive of gram-positive pathogens, empiric therapy such as TMX/SMX, a third generation cephalosporin, or an aminoglycoside is appropriate. Because of its coverage against common bacteria that cause pyelonephritis (*E. coli* 80–95%, *Staphylococcus saprophyticus, Proteus mirabilis, Klebsiella*), ceftriaxone (1–3 g/24 hr) is a good choice. Parenteral therapy can generally be tailored at 48 hours, based on susceptibility data, to the least expensive regimen. Oral therapy can sometimes be used initially and generally can be started at 24 to 48 hours for the hospitalized patient. Urologic consultation and evaluation of the upper urinary tract should be considered if the patient remains febrile for more than 72 hours. Oral agents generally should be used for at least 14 days. TMP/SMX, trimethoprim, amoxicillin, ciprofloxicin, and amoxicillin/clavulanate (in the dose ranges given under short-course therapy) can be used. Susceptibility testing results are critically important in the selection. Posttherapy urine culture for patients with pyelonephritis is recommended to ensure that the patient is cured.[32]

Pregnancy

The pregnant patient with a UTI deserves special attention because symptomatic infections are associated with significant maternal and fetal risks. Because most symptomatic UTIs develop in women with bacteriuria early in pregnancy, treatment of bacteriuria is undertaken to prevent symptomatic infections. Culture-positive bacteriuria pregnant women should be treated with short-course therapy, which is as effective as prolonged therapy. A repeat culture should be performed to be sure the patient is cured. Failure to eliminate bacteriuria with repeated therapy or recurrence with the same organism is indicative of renal parenchymal infection or structural abnormality and requires longer individually tailored therapy (see treatment for pyelonephritis, above). All women with persistent bacteriuria or recurrent infection should have follow-up cultures and a urologic consultation after delivery. Amoxicillin, cephalexin, sulfisoxazole, and nitrofurantoin can be used during pregnancy (in doses listed under short-course therapy). Nitrofurantoin poses a risk in patients with G6PD deficiency. Sulfa drugs can cause hyperbilirubinemia in the fetus, so an alternative drug is better near delivery. Finally, TMP/SMX is not recommended during pregnancy because of questions about its teratogenicity.

Initial therapy for pregnant patients with pyelonephritis should be with intravenous antibiotics, usually ampicillin and an aminoglycoside, with adjustment of the antibiotics based on culture results and the clinical response. A 2-week course of appropriate oral antibiotics is followed by suppressive therapy until delivery. Consultation may be prudent in this high-risk situation.[35]

Prostatitis

Prostatitis seldom affects prepubertal boys but is relatively common in adult men. Several distinct types of prostatitis are recognized. Bacterial prostatitis, caused mainly by coliform bacteria, *Pseudomonas,* and *Enterococcus faecalis,* is often difficult to cure and may require extended therapy (4–16 weeks) with an appropriate antimicrobial agent that achieves therapeutic levels in the prostate. TMP/SMX double strength twice a day is the drug of choice, with carbenicillin, erythromycin, minocycline, doxycycline, and cephalexin as alternatives. About 90% of men with prostatitis have nonbacterial prostatitis or prostatodynia. Nonbacterial prostatitis is an inflammation of the prostate of unknown cause, and therefore treating with antibiotics is unwarranted.[36] The multiglass culture of urine and prostate fluid described earlier is the means of differentiating bacterial from nonbacterial prostatitis.

Elderly Patients

UTI is common in the elderly. Bacteriuria is more common in the geriatric population than in younger adults and is frequently asymptomatic. Asymptomatic bacteriuria in the elderly is a benign condition in most individuals and does not warrant therapy. For some asymtomatic bacteriuric older women, 300 ml of cranberry juice daily reduces the frequency of bacteriuria with pyuria.[37] When symptomatic lower UTI occurs in elderly women, short-course (3-day) therapy with any of several agents is indicated and is usually effective. Several good choices exist, including TMP/SMX (160 mg and 800 mg bid), trimethoprim (100 mg bid), norfloxacin (400 mg bid), ciprofloxacin (500 mg bid) (other fluoroquinolones also look promising), cephalexin (250 or 500 mg qid), and amoxicillin/ clavulanate (250–500 mg tid). Elderly women with frequently recurrent symptomatic UTIs may benefit from estrogen therapy. Men with symptomatic UTIs should have a urine culture to confirm the infection and receive 7 to 10 days of culture–antibiotic matched therapy. The first episode UTI in the elderly man warrants a structural abnormality search, as is indicated for the younger man.

Fourteen days of therapy is indicated for patients with an upper UTI. The typical signs of pyelonephritis may be altered or absent in elderly patients. However, bacteremia and hypotension are more common among the elderly with pyelonephritis. Initial therapy is empiric and should be guided by Gram stain of the urine. When only gram-positive cocci in chains are seen (*Enterococcus*), parenteral ampicillin (6–12 g/day) or a ureidopenicillin (piperacillin, mezlocillin 16–18 g/day) would be appropriate therapy. If gram-negative bacilli are seen, initial parenteral therapy can be a third-generation cephalosporin (e.g., ceftriaxone 3–6 g/day), a ureidopenicillin, aztreonam (3–6 g/day), TMP/SMX (320–480 or 1600–2400 mg/day), or an aminoglycoside (e.g., gentamicin 5 mg/kg/day). Occasionally, parenteral therapy is not necessary, and oral therapy with TMP/SMX or ciprofloxacin (1.0–1.5 g/day) may be appropriate. Hospital- or nursing home-acquired gram-negative bacillary pyelonephritis is more likely to be due to multiple-drug-resistant organisms, such as *Pseudomonas aeruginosa*. Ceftazidime (6 g/day) or piperacillin with or without an aminoglycoside would be appropriate empiric antibiotics with which to start. Elderly patients are at risk for aminoglycoside-induced ototoxicity and nephrotoxicity. Once the infecting organism is identified by culture and susceptibilities are known, therapy can be adjusted to use the safest, least expensive antibiotic to which the organism is susceptible.[38]

References

1. Marsland DW, Wood M, Mayo F. Virginia Study. J Fam Pract 1976;3(4):25–68.
2. Johson CC. Definition and classification and clinical presentation of urinary tract infection. Med Clin North Am 1991;71(2):241–9.
3. Monzan OT, Ory EM, Dobson HL, et al. A comparison of bacterial counts of the urine obtained by needle aspiration of the bladder catheterization and mid-stream voided methods. N Engl J Med 1958;25:64.
4. Kass EH, Finland M. Asymptomatic infections of the urinary tract. Trans Assoc Am Physicians 1956;69:56.
5. Stamm WE, Counts GW, Running KR, et al. Diagnosis of coliform infection in acutely dysuric women. N Engl J Med 1982;307:463.
6. Lipsky BA. Urinary tract infections in men: epidemiology, pathophysiology, diagnosis and treatment. Ann Intern Med 1989;110:138–42.
7. Stark RP, Maki DJ. Bacteriuria in the catheterized patient. What quantitative level of bacteriuria is relevant? N Engl J Med 1984;311:560–6.
8. Stamm WE, Wagner KF, Amsel R, et al. Causes of the acute urethral syndrome in women. N Engl J Med 1980;303:409.
9. Freedman L. Chronic pyelonephritis at autopsy. Ann Intern Med 1967;66:697.
10. U.S. Preventive Services Task Force. Guideline to clinical preventive services report. Baltimore: Williams & Wilkins, 1989.
11. Lachs MS, Nachamkin I, Edelstein PH, et al. Spectrum bias in the evaluation of diagnostic tests: lessons from the rapid dipstick tests for urinary tract infection. Ann Intern Med 1992;117:135–40.
12. Aby AD. A screening for asymptomatic bacteriuria in pregnancy: urinalysis versus urine culture. J Fam Pract 1991;33(5):471–4.
13. Institute of Medicine, Division of Health Promotion and Disease Prevention. Preventing low birth weight. Washington, D.C.: National Academy Press, 1985.
14. Andriole VT, Patterson TF. Epidemiology and natural history and management of urinary tract infections in pregnancy. Med Clin North Am 1991;75(2):365–76.
15. Jodol U. Natural history of bacteriuria in childhood. Infect Dis Clin North Am 1987;1:713.
16. American Academy of Pediatrics, Section of Urology. Screening school children for urologic disease. Pediatrics 1977;60:239–43.
17. Boscia JA, Kobasa WD, Knight RA, et al. Therapy versus no therapy for bacteriuria in elderly ambulatory nonhospitalized women. JAMA 1987;257:1067–71.
18. Pappas PG. Laboratory diagnosis and management of urinary tract infections. Med Clin North Am 1991;75(2):317–29.
19. Sherbotie JR, Cornfeld D. Management of urinary tract infections in children. Med Clin North Am 1991;75(2):327–37.
20. Meares EM. Prostatitis. Med Clin North Am 1991;72:405–22.
21. Ditchburn RK, Ditchburn, JS. A study of microscopical and chemical tests for the rapid diagnosis of urinary tract infection in general practice. Br J Gen Pract 1990;40:406–8.

22. Measley RE, Levison ME. Host defence mechanisms and the pathogenesis of urinary tract infection. Med Clin North Am 1991;75(2):275–82.
23. Sobol JD. Bacterial etiologic agents in the pathogenesis of urinary tract infection. Med Clin North Am 1991;75(2):253–67.
24. Stamm WE. Catheter associated urinary tract infections: epidemiology, pathogenesis and prevention. Am J Med 1991;91:65S–78S.
25. Warren JW. The catheter and urinary tract infection. Med Clin North Am 1991;75:481–8.
26. Nelson's Textbook of pediatrics, 14th ed. Philadelphia: W.B. Saunders, 1992.
27. Coff SA. A practical approach to evaluating urinary tract infection in children. Pediatr Nephrol 1991;5:398–400.
28. Leung AK, Robson WL. Urinary tract infection in infancy and childhood. Adv Pediatr 1991;38:258–73.
29. Gillenwater JY. The role of the urologist in urinary tract infection. Med Clin North Am 1992;75(2):478–86.
30. Nicole LE. The optimal management of urinary tract infections. Infection 1990;18:S50–S56.
31. Johnson JR, Stamm WE. Urinary tract infections in women diagnosis and treatment. Ann Intern Med 1989;111:906.
32. Hooton TM, Stamm WE. Management of acute uncomplicated urinary tract infection in adults. Med Clin North Am 1991;75(2):347–50.
33. Two new fluoroquinolones. Med Lett 1992;34:59.
34. Johnson MA. Urinary tract infections in women. Am Fam Phys 1990;41(2):567–75.
35. Andriole VT, Patterson TF. Epidemiology, natural history, and management of urinary tract infections in pregnancy. Med Clin North Am 1991;75(2):368–71.
36. Mears EM. Prostatitis. Med Clin North Am 1991;75(2):416, 422.
37. Avorn J, Monane M, Gurwitz JH, et al. Reduction of bacteriuria and pyuria after ingestion of cranberry juce. JAMA 1994;271(10):751–4.
38. Baldassarre JS, Kaye D. Special problems of urinary tract infection in the elderly. Med Clin North Am 1991;75(2):384–7.

Case Presentation

Subjective

Patient Profile

Nancy Nelson is a 40-year-old married white female accountant.

Presenting Problem

"It hurts when I pass urine."

Present Illness

For 2 days, Mrs. Nelson has had urinary burning, frequency, urgency, and nocturia. She reports some mild left flank pain. She has felt warm but has not taken her temperature.

Past Medical History

She has had two urinary tract infections over the past 18 months, and both responded promptly to medication.

Social History

She works 3 days a week as a bookkeeper in a large firm. Her husband, Ken, is a home builder, and they have two teenage children.

Habits

She uses no tobacco and takes alcohol occasionally. She drinks six cups of coffee daily.

Family History

Her father, aged 71, is living and well. Her mother died at age 68 of breast cancer. She has no siblings.

REVIEW OF SYSTEMS

She has occasional pain in the joints of her hands and low back pain after lifting and carrying.

- What additional medical history would be helpful? Why?
- What symptoms or past history—if present—would you consider especially worrisome? Explain.
- Might a vulvovaginitis be part of her problem? How would you inquire about this possibility?
- What are Mrs. Nelson's possible concerns about her symptoms? How would you address this issue?

Objective

VITAL SIGNS

Blood pressure, 112/64; pulse, 68; respirations, 18; temperature, 37.4°C.

EXAMINATION

The patient is ambulatory and does not appear acutely ill. There is no mass or organ enlargement in the abdomen. There is moderate suprapubic tenderness without bladder distention. There is equivocal left costovertebral angle tenderness. The examination of the vagina, cervix, fundus, and adnexa are normal except for a thin watery vaginal discharge.

LABORATORY

There is a positive nitrite reaction on urinary dipstick. Red blood cells, bacteria, and many white blood cells are present on microscopic examination of a spun urine specimen.

- What additional data—if any—from the physical examination might be useful, and why?
- What—if any—laboratory tests would you obtain today? Why?
- What—if any—diagnostic imaging would you obtain today?
- If the patient had a thick purulent vaginal discharge, what might you do differently? Explain.

Assessment

- What is the probable diagnosis? What is the likely etiologic cause?
- How would you explain your assessment to the patient and her husband?
- What is the possible significance of the prior urinary tract infections?
- What is the possible meaning of this illness to the patient? To her husband?

Plan

- Describe your therapeutic recommendations for the patient. How would you explain this plan to the patient?
- What is your advice regarding work, household duties, and sexual relations?
- Might this patient benefit from consultation with a urologist? Explain.
- What follow-up would you advise?

16
Vulvovaginitis and Cervicitis

MARY A. WILLARD

Although patients have in the past been indoctrinated that vaginal symptoms are the realm of the subspecialist gynecologist, the range of symptoms and diagnoses covered under this category with the concomitant preventive health and risk management issues is ideally suited to the expertise of the family physician. Excellence in the diagnosis and management of these diseases is the standard of care and can be achieved with minimal equipment, time (1-minute slide examination), and cost to the patient. Patients with vaginal complaints account for an estimated 10% of office visits each year,[1] and many more may be inaccurately diagnosed by telephone. This chapter reviews the systematic approach to the evaluation and treatment of vaginal diseases as well as issues of particular interest to family physicians.

Terminology

To manage these cases well, accuracy and clarity of terms is of paramount importance. A well-defined vocabulary helps the physician be specific with the evaluation in thought and action and assists the patient to understand the disease process. This exactitude of terminology encourages patient and physician to understand that not all vaginal discharge is vaginitis. The following are definitions of the terms used throughout the rest of the chapter.

Cervicitis: Inflammation of the cervix that may be caused by infection, local trauma, or certain medications.

Dysuria: Pain on urination that must be clarified by the physician to delineate painful urination with vulvitis versus cystitis.

Leukorrhea: Although not a commonly used term, this general term indicates excess fluid from the vagina without implying etiology.

Vaginitis: Inflammation or infection of the mucosa of the vagina.

Vulvitis: Inflammation of the vulva and labia.

Vulvodynia: Pain in the vulvar and labial areas not necessarily associated with any inflammation or infection.

Diagnostic Assessment

It is critical for the family physician to remember that few symptoms are more annoying to the female patient than vaginal itching and discharge. Tolerance of low-grade symptoms is the norm for some patients until a flare turns the problem into a midnight emergency. Although the history and physical examination are helpful, the diagnosis can be made only by appropriate testing. Therefore, a detailed discussion of laboratory evaluation is essential here.

Laboratory Equipment and Technique

The equipment needed for accurate diagnosis of vaginal complaints is simple: saline in small containers, nonsterile cotton Q-tips, slides, coverslips, a good microscope with 10X and 40X capacity (i.e., low and high dry power), 10% potassium hydroxide solution (KOH preparation), diagnostic media for *Chlamydia* and gonococci and a small magnifying lens. Vaginal fluid should be examined as soon as possible after it is obtained, as *Trichomonas vaginalis* is fragile and may die quickly.

The technique of examining vaginal fluid is straightforward. After inserting the vaginal speculum, a plain cotton-tipped applicator is swept into the vaginal fluid, withdrawn (preferably with a "clump" of discharge), and placed immediately into a small container with 1 ml of saline. Small pediatric red-topped tubes can store the saline in all rooms where pelvic examinations may be performed so they are immediately available. For maximal results, the smallest amount of saline and the largest sample of vaginal fluid should be used. Once the sample of vaginal fluid is obtained, cervical cultures can be prepared if necessary, the pelvic examination completed, and the saline examined.

Microscopic examination of the vaginal fluid in saline should be performed using gloves as per universal precautions. Take the cotton applicator from the tube and place a drop of fluid on two slides, one for saline examination and one for a KOH preparation. If a diagnosis of yeast infection is being entertained, it is critical to try to get a "clump" of the discharge onto the designated KOH slide. A drop of 10% KOH solution (made by mixing 90 ml distilled water with 10 g KOH) is dropped on it and immediately smelled for a fishy odor. If it is to be further evaluated for hyphae, place a coverslip and allow the slide to sit until the saline slide is examined. The KOH destroys some of the vaginal epithelial and white blood cells (WBCs), leaving only hyphae for inspection.

Next examine the saline slide with coverslip under low power. Search for motion of cells, sheets of epithelial cells compatible with denuding of the mucosa, or "clue cells."[2] The latter are vaginal epithelial cells "studded" with bacteria that adhere for unknown reasons. These epithelial cells

TABLE 16.1. Common vaginal
microorganisms

Lactobacillus
Staphylococcus
Group D *Streptococcus*
Corynebacterium
Group B *Streptococcus*
Escherichia coli
Gardnerella vaginalis
Peptostreptococcus
Bacteroides
Candida sp.

appear dense and tend to "glitter" when focus is varied on them. Although clue cells are present normally in up to 10% of the field, a preponderance of them, especially when combined with a fishy odor on the KOH preparation, supports the diagnosis of bacterial vaginosis.[3]

Once the examination under low power is completed, it is appropriate to scan the field under high dry power to check for *T. vaginalis* and better examine the epithelial cells. Trichomonads appear as motile triangular cells, a little larger than WBCs, with long, moving tails. As can be seen in Table 16.1, many bacteria are part of the normal vaginal ecosystem and are nonpathogenic.[4] For this reason, Gram stains and routine cultures are not first-line tests for diagnosing vaginal diseases. If, however, the high power field has more than 10 WBCs, consider an upper genital tract infection.

If an examination for yeast is necessary, place the KOH preparation under the microscope. Hyphae and spores are best seen on this specimen by focusing under low power to find a "clumped" area, then going immediately to high dry power and focusing on the edges of the clump. The clumped material usually represents epithelial cells and hyphae tissue not desiccated by the KOH preparation, and the edge of the clump is the best place to identify the hyphae. Certainly, if the history so warrants and the cervical os reveals discharge from above, appropriate tests for *Chlamydia* or gonococci should be performed.

When analyzing vaginal complaints, few tests other than those noted above need to be performed except in specific circumstances or in refractory cases (which are discussed in relevant sections). However, one area of testing controversy is the role of vaginal pH tests. Because the premenopausal vaginal ecosystem keeps the pH under 4.5, assessment of change might be of some value. Although sensitive, this test is not specific and can be influenced greatly by fluids from the cervix, semen, or douching. It has therefore limited application in the office. There is also investigation into the use of monoclonal antibodies and DNA analysis. Unfortunately, none of these tests is yet of sufficient reliability to replace the simple slide evaluations.

History

As with any clinical problem, the history is a critical clue to diagnosis and must be obtained methodically from each patient. The ambiguous nature of the problem, however, means that the diagnosis cannot be made solely on historical clues, such as a "cheesy" discharge.

Most women can, with minimal clarification by the physician, reveal a clear history of their complaint. Because there is individual variation in the amount and character of leukorrhea that is "normal," the family physician's role is to help patients distinguish a change from that pattern. Ask about skin lesions, internal or external itching, odor, dyspareunia, and the use (and frequency) of douching, new soaps, or deodorant sprays. Always inquire about previous similar episodes, but ask how these diagnoses were made, especially in the patient treated over the telephone. Many patients who state that they "always get yeast infections" probably have never had an accurate diagnosis, and any vaginal cream has the potential of calming an inflamed mucosa (thereby diminishing the symptoms until the next flare).

One of the most commonly missed presentations of vaginitis is the complaint of dysuria. Treating all patients with dysuria as cystitis results in the inevitable telephone call 48 to 72 hours later from a patient who is no better. Because women with vulvitis complain of pain externally with urination, clarification of the type of dysuria at the initial encounter assists in determining which patients require additional evaluation for vaginitis.

It is also essential for the family physician to obtain a complete sexual history in these patients as well as an assessment of risk for sexually transmitted diseases. If the patient is sexually active, the physician should inquire about any new spermicidal agents or condoms, symptom complaints from a partner(s), a new sexual partner, and types of sexual practice. Moreover, the patient should be educated about sexual practices that minimize risk of disease.

Physical Examination

Although the pelvic examination can be tailored by the history, patients with vaginal complaints must be evaluated systematically. The external genitalia should be thoroughly assessed for clues using a hand-held magnifying lens if necessary. The urethra, labia, and vulvae should be completely checked for ulcerations, warts, tears, cysts, abscesses, erythema, and edema. Also, the vaginal mucosa itself must be inspected for color, lesions, and edema. Normal vaginal mucosa is pink with moist folds. A fiery red color or weepy mucosa is a sign of inflammation. Any plaque-type lesions should be scraped for adherence to vaginal mucosa, a sign of possible candidiasis.

As part of the complete evaluation, observe the cervical os for pus as a cause of leukorrhea. Using a large cotton swab (e.g., one used for proctoscopic examinations), clean the cervix of all discharge, and observe the os for a short time, usually 10 seconds. If purulent fluid appears at the os opening from above, it is an indicator of upper pelvic infection, for which *Chlamydia* and gonococci must be tested. At this point, a bimanual examination should also be performed to assess adnexal tenderness or masses.

Clinical Presentation

It is impossible, given the constraints of space, to discuss all forms of vaginitis or other vaginal diseases. Instead, the focus here is on the more common etiologies and important vaginal skin diseases that may masquerade as "itch." This approach assists in clarifying most vaginal complaints.

Traditional medical training clearly defined the "classic" presentations for vaginitis. Unfortunately, this "eyeball" method correctly diagnoses only one-third of the cases,[5] making thorough clinical evaluation necessary (Fig. 16.1). Nevertheless, an appreciation of the textbook presentations is necessary when teasing apart the significant historical details given by the patient. It is equally important to realize the change in epidemiology of vaginitis since the 1970s. The most common cause of vaginitis is now bacterial vaginosis, followed by mycotic diseases (e.g., *Candida* sp.), with trichomoniasis on the decline.[6] Whatever the reason for this shift, a knowledge of the probabilities is useful.

Contact and Chemical Dermatitides

Contact and chemical dermatitides are much overlooked diagnoses for the patient with vulvitis. Any topical agent used in the genital area (including nonoxynol-9 and rubber in condoms) can be an allergen. Symptoms are characterized by a reddened, swollen vulva or a vaginal mucosa exuding a clear exudate. Equally important is the patient who has been douching repeatedly and with increasing frequency. These patients set up a denuding phenomenon that inflames and strips the mucosa. The appropriate treatment for this category of inflammation is to discontinue the product and consider using a short-term course of topical external steroids for symptomatic relief.[7]

Mycotic Diseases

Although the incidence is rising,[6] contrary to popular belief among patients and physicians, true fungal infections probably account for fewer than one-third of all vaginal infections. The textbook presentation is a

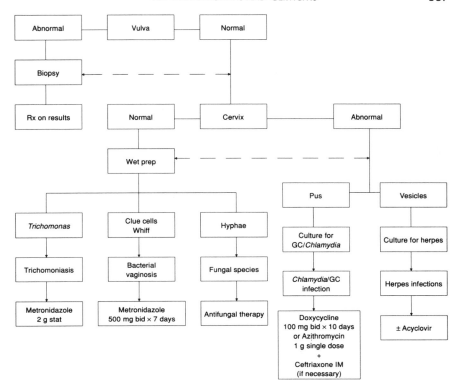

FIGURE 16.1. Diagnostic algorithm for vaginal symptoms. GC = gonococcus; Rx = treatment.

patient complaining of a vaginal itch and cheesy exudate, with white plaques adherent to the vaginal wall and a KOH preparation showing multiple hyphae. Diagnosis should not be made, however, unless hyphae are seen on the slide. Because as many as 20% of asymptomatic women have positive cultures,[8] it is obvious that culture methods are too sensitive and should be reserved for refractory cases,[9] patients with frequent relapses, or when yeast is suspected clinically but the KOH preparation is negative. In this case, suspect *Candida glabrata,* which may present with vaginal burning and, as a spore-former, can be diagnosed only on Gram stain. This infection is often refractory to the standard length of treatment and may need protracted therapy.[7]

Yeast infections typified by *Candida albicans* have been erroneously ascribed to many causes. For example, yeast infections probably do not occur any more frequently in diabetic women but may be more difficult to eradicate.[7] Therefore, consider diabetes in the patient with "chronic" infections, not frequent ones. There is also little proved association between

TABLE 16.2. Drugs for vaginal candidiasis

Generic drug and examples	Formulation	Dose	Cost to patient[a]
Teranazole			
Terazol	Cream 4%	5 g hs × 7 days	$30.79
Terazole	Vag. supp. 80 mg	1 hs × 3	31.69
Nystatin	Vag. tab. 100,000 units	1 hs × 14 days	12.00
Tioconazole			
Vagistat	Ointment 6.5%	4.6 g hs × 1	33.89
Butoconazole			
Femstat	Cream 2%	5 g hs × 3 days	25.00
Clotrimazole			
Gyne-Lotrimin[b]	Vag. tab. 100 mg	1 hs × 7 days	17.59[b]
	Cream 1%	5 g hs × 7–14 days	13.99[b]
Mycelex	Vag. tab. 100 mg[b]	1 hs × 7 days	12.99[b]
	Vag. tab. 500 mg	1 tab. once	18.69
Miconazole			
Monistat 7[b]	Cream 2%	5 g hs × 7 days	15.90[b]
	Vag. supp. 100 mg	1 hs × 7 days	14.99[b]
Monistat 3	Vag. supp. 200 mg	1 hs × 3 days	30.59

[a]Example of over-the-counter or prescription cost at various chain pharmacies in 1994 (not including generic discount drugs).
[b]Available over the counter in 1994.

yeast infection and use of birth control pills.[10] For frequent relapses, consider treating the sexual partner(s) to achieve full eradication and changing the patient's diet since high calories and crude fiber have been associated with susceptibility to infection.[11] Remember, too, that women with human immunodeficiency virus (HIV) disease may manifest persistent or diffuse candidiasis as a presenting symptom.

Treatment is straightforward and consists in topical application of one of several groups of medication (Table 16.2). There has been no proved superiority of one drug over another or of creams over tablets.[12] However, a cream may be used internally and externally if the patient is symptomatic. Several forms of these medications are now available over the counter, but they may be more costly than the one-dose suppository. Physician and patient preferences dictate the specific drug as well as whether vaginal tablets or creams are used, and there is no risk of treating during pregnancy. Truly refractory cases may require longer treatment courses, and the patient with frequent relapses may benefit from oral ketoconazole (Nizoral) 100 mg/day for months except during pregnancy.[13]

Trichomoniasis

Trichomonas vaginalis may cause severe itching or pain often accompanied by frequency of urination because of concomitant cystitis from the organism. On examination, the vulva and vaginal mucosa are fiery red with cervical petechiae ("strawberry cervix"). Typical discharge is yellow-green and bubbly in nature, but any range of color and texture may be seen, making slide examination critical. As noted above, the diagnosis is made by finding motile trichomonads on a saline smear. Because of the low positive predictive value of *Trichomonas* reported on Papanicolaou smears,[8] all these results should be confirmed by a wet preparation before therapy is initiated. Although culture methodology for *T. vaginalis* may have better sensitivity and specificity in theory, there is still debate over the ideal medium and methods, so this technique is not useful.[14]

The drug of choice is metronidazole (Flagyl, Prostat) with the best response noted by a 2-g immediate dose.[15] An alternative regimen of 250 mg tid for 7 days is best used in refractory cases only, as it produces no higher initial cure than the one-time dose. Metronidazole has a significant Antabuse-type reaction, so patients must be cautioned to ingest no alcohol, including cough medicine, during the treatment. As a sexually transmitted disease, it is critically important for the patient's sexual partner(s) to be treated concurrently to prevent reinfection; and although there are some resistant cases, resistance is not an all-or-none phenomenon. Rather, resistance may range from mild (where treatment is effective) to severe, necessitating a treatment dose of 2.5 g/day in divided doses for 7 to 10 days.[16] At this time, no other medication available in the United States can provide better therapeutic results.

Trichomoniasis during pregnancy is difficult to treat. Although the literature is scant, metronidazole may be teratogenic during the first trimester and is therefore contraindicated until the second trimester and then is reserved for severe infections. Clotrimazole (Gyne-Lotrimin, Mycelex-G) may be effective in this situation for controlling symptoms, although it rarely produces eradication.[17]

Bacterial Vaginosis

Formerly known as *Gardnerella,* or nonspecific, vaginitis, bacterial vaginosis has been credited with as many as 50% of all diagnoses of vaginitis.[18] It represents an overgrowth in the vagina of anaerobic organisms typified by *Gardnerella vaginalis.* It produces no vulvar symptoms, no change in vaginal mucosa, little itching, and no pain, unless the discharge is so profuse that the vulvae are simply macerated. Because its course is usually indolent, it is not a cause of an acute change in symptoms. The patient may note only a slight change in normal discharge and an odor that may be more pronounced after intercourse. Patients are frequently inured to the symptoms until treatment is finished and the discharge gone. There may not be an odor immediately on examination, but KOH releases the amines in the epithelial cells and produces the classic fishy odor, which as noted previously is diagnostic when clue cells are present. Because *Gardnerella* bacteria may be a normal inhabitant of the vagina, culture of the organism for a diagnosis has poor specificity and so has not been recommended.[8]

Treatment for this syndrome is metronidazole (Flagyl) 500 mg PO bid for 7 days.[15] Unfortunately, the one-time dose used to treat *Trichomonas* is insufficient for vaginosis, and again the patient must be warned about previously noted side effects. In 1992, the FDA approved usage of a 0.75% vaginal gel formulation of metronidazole (Metrogel-Vaginal) and a 2% vaginal cream formulation of clindamycin phosphate (Cleocin) for this disorder. Preliminary data indicate that both have the same efficacy as oral therapy with side effect profiles similar to but less than their oral forms.[17] Because some association has been noted between bacterial vaginosis and premature rupture of membranes, therapy should be considered during pregnancy after the first trimester. The recommended drug during pregnancy is clindamycin 300 mg bid for 7 days.[18]

At this time, the role of sexual transmission in this disorder is unclear. Studies can be found to support either opinion, and partner therapy has not produced an improved cure rate at least at conventional dosage.[19] Equally unclear is the role of treatment in the asymptomatic patient, but it may be considered in someone undergoing vaginal surgery because of a potential role in pelvic inflammation.[20]

Atrophic Vaginitis

A common cause of vaginal symptoms in the postmenopausal woman, atrophic vaginitis should be considered concomitantly with the evaluation for other etiologies. Lack of estrogen produces thin vaginal epithelium and cells deficient in the acids that provide the premenopausal woman with a balanced vaginal ecosystem. Therefore, the mucosa easily denudes and becomes traumatized. Thus, presenting symptoms may include lack of vaginal lubrication with coitus, pruritus, and dyspareunia, with or without discharge.

On examination the vaginal folds are flattened, and the mucosa is pale pink and shows a lack of lubrication. The cervix is usually atrophic and frequently friable, and the wet preparation is negative. Hormone replacement therapy is the treatment of choice, but vaginal estrogen creams used nightly can provide short-term relief.[21] The patient must be reminded that a vaginal "discharge" may recur as the cells mature back to a premenopausal pattern.

Sexually Transmitted Diseases

Several sexually transmitted diseases (STDs) may present with predominantly vaginal symptoms.

Chlamydia Infection

Even though *Chlamydia* does not produce a vaginitis, it does cause mucopurulent cervicitis.[22] On examination, the cervix may be eroded and present a mucopurulent discharge that when wiped quickly re-forms at the os. When this discharge is seen, the alert clinician should do appropriate testing and examine wet preparations for concomitant vaginal infections, as patients with one STD are at high risk of having more.

Once a diagnosis of chlamydial infection is suspected, empiric treatment is warranted, especially in a high-risk patient (defined as sexually active, nonmonogamous, young). The standard treatment is doxycycline (Vibramycin) 100 mg PO bid for 10 days.[22] Azithromycin as a 1-gram single dose is a reasonable but expensive alternative. If the patient is allergic to tetracycline (rare) or pregnancy is suspected, an appropriate alternative is erythromycin 500 mg PO qid for 7 days. Partners should be treated aggressively, but a test of patient cure is considered unnecessary.

Herpesvirus Infection

Especially in cases of recurrence, patients with herpesvirus infection may present only with symptoms of external burning and minimal liquid discharge. Without ulcerations externally or on the cervix, this diagnosis should not be entertained unless there is a known history of a positive culture.

Human Papillomavirus Infection

Current trends indicate that most human papillomavirus (HPV) disease presents as warts,[23] either externally or internally. Therefore, HPV is unlikely to be a cause of any symptoms unless the growth is large enough to cause an exudative process.

Leukorrhea Secondary to Birth Control Pills

On some occasions, the only cause of leukorrhea is an eroded cervix secondary to the use of birth control pills. The hormones in birth control pills cause more endocervix to be exposed to the environment of the vagina, producing irritation and weeping of the mucosa. It is always asymptomatic. If a patient is having any symptoms, this diagnosis is excluded.

Vulvar Diseases

It is critical to remember that many skin diseases can manifest with vaginal symptoms. Most, such as seborrheic dermatitis, psoriasis, tinea, and pediculosis, have unique characteristics that are obvious. Without these characteristics present, the physician must perform a biopsy with a simple punch instrument for diagnosis and appropriate therapy. All patients must be educated that treatment effects may take months to realize. Also, any pigmented lesion should be biopsied and the patient referred based on biopsy results.

Vestibulitis

With vestibulitis, there is variable redness and edema of the vestibular glands, frequently with a lesion. The number of glands involved can range from 1 to 100, and the symptoms are vulvar pain with dyspareunia. The etiology is still hotly debated but probably HPV is involved. Treatment results are best with vestibular resection or intralesional interferon, but no therapy is 100% effective.[24]

Lichen Sclerosis

Lichen sclerosis produces a white-appearing lesion that is seen predominantly in women older than age 50. There is a typical "keyhole" pattern on both sides of the vulva. The lesion may eventually cover the entire vulva with adhesion and eventual obliteration of the labia minora to the majora. Treatment is a topical testosterone ointment (30 ml of testosterone in oil with 120 g petrolatum) twice a day for 4 to 6 months, then one or two times a week for life.[21] If the patient cannot tolerate the side effects, alternative therapy of progesterone cream can be used. There is a high recurrence rate, even with surgery or laser, so dramatic treatment is best avoided.

Lichen Simplex Chronicus

Caused by chronic itching or irritation, lichen simplex chronicus is a thick scaly condition with localized vulvar lesions without adhesions. Treatment is symptomatic with topical steroids for 1 to 2 months. Because the only recurrences are seen in patients treated by surgery, this intervention is no longer acceptable.[25]

Lichen Planus

Lichen planus may involve mucous membranes in other organ systems. There is vulvar burning, leukorrhea, and redness of the inner labia. Patients may have violaceous papules externally and small, lacy, gray, reticular patterns on the inner labia. Without these identifying marks, this lesion may appear similar to that of atrophic vaginitis; it should be entertained as a diagnosis whenever therapy for atrophic vaginitis fails. Treatment is topical with either a potent fluorinated steroid or a medium potency steroid under occlusion.[25] The patient must be reminded that this condition flares and remits over long periods.

When the Tests Are Negative

A real dilemma ensues when, despite the best efforts of the clinician, the examination and tests reveal no reason for the patient's symptoms. Mentally review the history, the adequacy of the specimen collection, the performance of the laboratory tests, and the possibility of *Chlamydia*. Obtain any history previously overlooked, and consider the diagnosis of an acid-base change in the vaginal environment known as cytolytic vaginosis. Although not easily diagnosed, some patients develop an overgrowth of acidophilic Döderlein's lactobacilli, which produces an increase in enzymes that degrade intracellular glycogen to lactic acid. This action causes massive desquamation and cytolysis and a watery discharge. Because the luteal phase epithelial cells are richer in lactic acid, this syndrome may be cyclic in nature. The hallmark for diagnosis is epithelial cells that have a motheaten appearance, often called pseudo-clue cells, and few WBCs on the wet preparation. Also, because this process is driven by an acidic environment, the symptoms worsen with douching using conventional acidic agents. Instead, these patients can be treated with a douching mixture of sodium bicarbonate and water (1–2 tablespoons in 500 ml water) used three times a week while symptomatic.[5]

If the workup was adequate, resist the urge to perform "shotgun" or even empiric treatment, as such treatment perpetuates old myths. Be supportive and understanding, and encourage the patient to be checked with subsequent recurrences.

Special Considerations for the Family Physician

Much of the success of therapy depends on the unique relationship between the family physician and the patient.

Compliance

The trusting relationship between the patient and the family physician enhances compliance with often distasteful regimens. The patient should be encouraged to finish the full course of therapy despite symptom resolution; and when the therapy demands partner compliance, the patient must be instructed to abstain from intercourse until therapy is completed. Role-playing this discussion with the partner may help allay anxiety in some patients. Choose the shortest regimen possible, and make sure the patient understands the side effects (including local irritation), route of usage, and use of medication during menses. Negotiate with the patient the best time to begin treatment, and inform her of the possibility of recurrence or treatment failure. Also, it is critical to assess the patients' attribution of disease in this condition. Clarity about sexual transmission is important, and if possible, use printed information for the patient to read and to give to her partner(s).

Issues of self-support and control of symptoms can be critical to compliance as well. These issues can be reinforced through good patient education. Sources of self-help for the patient can be found in women's health literature, such as *Our Bodies, Our Selves.*[26] These references may provide the patient with more detailed information on hygiene, as well as alternative remedies. The physician, however, should first read the relevant sections to be sure the information is consonant with good care and to explain areas of disagreement. (For example, there is scant scientific evidence for the use of intravaginal yogurt.) Some patients work best with a combination of conventional medical therapy and time-honored suggestions.

Recurrent or Persistent Vaginitis

Nothing is more frustrating to the patient or physician than recurrence (defined as symptoms recurring after a 1-month disease-free interval) or persistence of symptoms. In this situation, the physician should start over with the history, emphasizing compliance with previous therapy and focusing attention on details of diet, clothing, and irritants. Question the patient about high dairy intake, increased simple sugars, and use of new deodorant tampons, pads, or other topical agents such as perfumes or home remedies. Explore the relation to tight clothing, exercise gear, the use of dildos or vibrators, and the use of hot tubs or pools.

The examination and basic tests should be repeated, but if the history reveals no further clues, culture the cervix for *Chlamydia* and the vaginal vault for bacteria and *Candida,* and perform any necessary vulvar biopsies. In the diabetic patient, the blood glucose must be concomitantly controlled while reinstituting therapy.

Results of these tests dictate therapy. Persistent *Candida* or *Trichomonas* infection may need prolonged (*Candida*) or increased (*Trichomonas*) therapy. Consider treating according to the results of the bacterial culture using an antibiotic[7] targeted to the dominant organism.

If tests are negative, emphasize your support and sympathy, educate the patient about good hygiene and sexual behaviors that minimize risk, and proscribe anything that might exacerbate symptoms. Encourage the patient to return to be examined when symptoms recur.

Management of the HIV-Positive Patient

Other than the fact that patients who are HIV-seropositive may have more problems with HPV, treatment of vaginal disorders follows the same recommendations as for nonpositive patients. Although refractory candidiasis may be a clue for the physician to check a patient for HIV status, a normal vaginal infection should not be of concern. Flares of venereal warts can be treated conventionally, but at least one author suggests that such flares may be a sign to check the patient's CD4 count.[27]

Role of Colposcopy

The role of colposcopy is not well defined for vaginal symptoms. Although it may be a useful tool in the future, its current usage is for evaluating a patient with an abnormal Papanicolaou smear or cervix. Therefore, use it in a patient with persistent cervicitis only to screen for abnormal areas to biopsy. Also, conventional wisdom dictates that patients with HPV should undergo colposcopy to detect a precancerous state of the cervix.

Prevention of Vaginitis

When an STD has caused the vaginitis, the family physician must educate the patient about the difference between a disease that can arise de novo and then be propagated between partners and one acquired *from* someone else. Patients are understandably concerned about *where* they got the disease, but you can help focus the patient on treatment, give basic relevant information, and plan a subsequent visit to continue pursuing their concerns. Clarity about sexual transmission is important, as the patient may also need to be concerned about hepatitis and HIV risk. Acquisition of an STD is certainly threatening to partners who thought of themselves as mutually monogamous, and relationship issues are frequently topics for subsequent visits.

In addition to concerns about sexual transmission, the physician should educate the patient about the causative or associative factors found to be significant in the history. Use of local irritants, clothing, and other offending behaviors must be prevented. Above all, encouraging the patient to come in for evaluation of subsequent infections is critical, as the etiology may differ from the current one.

References

1. Paavonen J, Stamm WE. Lower genital tract infections in women. Infect Dis Clin North Am 1987;1179–98.
2. Fischer PM, Addison LA, Curtis P, Mitchell JM. The office laboratory. Norwalk, CT: Appleton-Century-Crofts, 1983.
3. Bump RC, Zuspan FP, Buesching WJ, et al. The prevalence, six-month persistence and predictive values of laboratory indicators of bacterial vaginosis (nonspecific vaginitis). Am J Obstet Gynecol 1984;150:917–23.
4. Faro S. Bacterial vaginitis. Obstet Gynecol 1991;34:582–6.
5. Cibley LJ, Cibley LJ. Cytolytic vaginosis. Am J Obstet Gynecol 1991;165: 1245–8.
6. Kent HL. Epidemiology of vaginitis. Am J Obstet Gynecol 1991; 165:1168–76.
7. Horowitz BJ, Mardh PA, editors. Vaginitis and vaginosis. New York: Wiley Liss, 1991.
8. Eschenbach DA, Hiller SL. Advances in diagnostic testing for vaginitis and cervicitis. J Reprod Med 1989;34(Suppl18):555–64.
9. Horowitz BJ. Mycotic vulvovaginitis: a broad overview. Am J Obstet Gynecol 1991;165:1188–92.
10. Roy S. Vulvovaginitis: causes and therapies: nonbarrier contraceptives and vaginitis and vaginosis. Am J Obstet Gynecol 1991;165:1240–4.
11. Reed B, Slatery M, French T. Diet and vaginitis. J Fam Pract 1989;29:509–15.
12. Topical drugs for vaginal candidiasis. Med Lett Drugs Ther 1991;33(851): 81.
13. Soble JD. Recurrent vulvovaginal candidiasis: a prospective study of the efficacy of maintenance ketoconazole therapy. N Engl J Med 1986;315: 1455–8.
14. Lossick JG. The diagnosis of trichomoniasis [editorial]. JAMA 1988;259: 1230–2.
15. Drugs for sexually transmitted disease. Med Lett Drugs Ther 1994;36(913):1–8.
16. Lossick JG, Kent HL. Trichomoniasis: trends in diagnosis and management. Am J Obstet Gynecol 1991;165:1217–22.
17. Topical treatment for bacterial vaginosis. Med Lett Drugs Ther 1992; 34(884): 109.
18. Erratum: 1989 sexually transmitted disease treatment guidelines. MMWR 1989;38:664.
19. Eschenbach DA, Hiller S, Critchlow C, et al. Diagnosis and clinical manifestations of bacterial vaginosis. Am J Obstet Gynecol 1988; 158:819–23.
20. Thomason JL, Geebart SM, Scaglione NJ. Bacterial vaginosis: current review with indications for asymptomatic therapy. Am J Obstet Gynecol 1991;165: 1210–6.
21. Byyny RL, Speroff L. A clinical guide for the care of older women. Baltimore: Williams & Wilkins, 1990.

22. Recommendations for the prevention and management of *Chlamydia trachomatis*. MMWR 1993;42(RR12):27.
23. Reid R, Greenberg MD. Human papillomavirus-related diseases of the vulva. Clin Obstet Gynecol 1991;3:630–50.
24. McKay M, Frankman O, Horovitz BJ, et al. Vulvar vestibulitis and vestibular papillomatoses: report of the ISSVD committee on vulvodynia. J Reprod Med 1991;36:413–5.
25. McKay M. Vulvar dermatoses. Clin Obstet Gynecol 1991;34:614–29.
26. Boston Women's Health Book Collective. The new our bodies, ourselves. New York: Simon & Schuster, 1984.
27. Hammill HA, Murtagh CP. Gynecologic care of the human immunodeficiency virus-positive woman. Clin Obstet Gynecol 1991;34:1599–1604.

CASE PRESENTATION

Subjective

PATIENT PROFILE

Ellen McCarthy Harris is a 26-year-old married white female secretary.

PRESENTING PROBLEM

Vaginal discharge.

PRESENT ILLNESS

There is a 10-day history of vaginal discharge with intense itching that began after her last menstrual period. The symptoms have not responded to an over-the-counter vaginal cream.

PAST MEDICAL HISTORY

No serious illnesses or hospitalizations.

SOCIAL HISTORY

She has worked at her secretarial job for 4 years. She and her husband, Andrew, have two children.

HABITS

She does not use tobacco, coffee, or recreational drugs.

FAMILY HISTORY

Her father has diabetes mellitus and coronary artery disease. Her mother is living and well. Her brother, aged 28, is HIV-positive.

REVIEW OF SYSTEMS

No symptoms in other areas.

- What additional information regarding the history of present illness might be important? Explain.
- Why might the over-the-counter medication not have worked?
- Over the past 10 days, what might the patient be doing differently because of her illness? Why might this be pertinent?
- Is it possible that the patient has a sexually transmitted disease? If so, how might you approach this issue?

Objective

VITAL SIGNS

Blood pressure, 112/64; pulse, 68; temperature, 37.0°C.

EXAMINATION

The abdomen is scaphoid with no mass, tenderness, or organ enlargement. The vaginal introitus is moderately inflamed. There is a frothy vaginal discharge. The cervix is mildly injected, and there are a few punctate hyperemic areas. The fundus and adnexa are normal. The rectal examination is normal, and the test for occult blood in the feces is negative.

- What other data—if any—regarding the physical examination might be important?
- What office diagnostic test(s) might you perform, and what are you likely to find?
- What specimens—if any—might you send to the laboratory?
- If the vaginal discharge were thick and purulent, what might you do differently? Explain.

Assessment

- What is the probable etiologic diagnosis? How will you explain this to the patient?
- What—if any—is the likely relationship to her menses?
- What are some concerns that the patient might like to address? How would you give "permission" to address these issues?
- What are the possible family issues in this case? How might you address these?

Plan

- What are your specific therapeutic recommendations? How will you explain these to Mrs. Harris?
- What is your advice regarding her activities, including sexual intercourse?
- Mrs. Harris asks what she can do to prevent recurrence. How would you reply?
- What follow-up would you advise?

17
Disorders of the Back and Neck

WALTER L. CALMBACH

Disorders of the Back

Low back pain occurs in almost 80% of adults at some point in their lives.[1] It is estimated that 1400 workdays per 1000 workers are lost each year in the United States because of low back pain.[2] In many large industrial settings, low back pain is second only to upper respiratory infections as a cause for absence from work.[3] Among chronic conditions, back problems are the most frequent cause for limitation of activity (work, housekeeping, school) among patients younger than 45 years of age.[4] Although low back pain is usually a self-limited problem, it still costs approximately $51 billion per year in lost productivity and compensation.[5] Fortunately, low back pain can be treated simply with a conservative regimen coupled with timely surgical intervention for a few patients plus aggressive rehabilitation for patients with chronic low back pain.[6]

Background

Epidemiology

Estimates of the lifetime prevalence of low back pain range from 60% to 90%, and the incidence has been estimated at 5% per year.[5,7] At any given point in time (point prevalence), 15% to 20% of the population state that they are having back symptoms.[5] Risk factors for low back pain include age, occupation, and multiparity, although these factors are minimally significant for the usual benign and self-limiting back symptoms.[7] When more severe back pain is considered, occupational determinants become much more evident, including repetitive heavy lifting, pulling, or pushing, and exposures to industrial and vehicular vibrations.[8,9] If even temporary work loss occurs, additional important risk factors include job dissatisfaction, supervisor ratings, and job environment (i.e., boring, repetitive tasks).[5] Some factors that are predictive of recurrence of low back pain include traumatic origin of first attack, sciatic pain, radiographic changes, alcohol abuse, specific job situations, and psychosocial stigmata.[10]

Although only 1% of patients with low back pain develop sciatica, the lifetime prevalence of sciatica is estimated to be 40%. Deyo and Tsui-Wu[11] found a 1.5% point prevalence of sciatica, although 11% of patients with low back pain for more than 2 weeks reported sciatica. Most patients with sciatica, even those with significant neurologic abnormalities, recover without surgery.[12,13] Kelsey et al.[14–16] noted a clear association of sciatica with long-distance driving, truck driving, cigarette smoking, and repeated lifting in a twisted posture. Sciatica is most common during the fourth and fifth decades of life, and it peaks during the fourth decade.[17] The rate of laminectomy for low pain back pain and sciatica is much higher in the United States than in European countries or Canada.[10]

Despite the incidence and prevalence of low back pain and sciatica, the major factor responsible for its societal impact relates to disability.[5] At the present time, the National Center for Health Statistics estimates that 5.2 million Americans are disabled with low back pain; and of these individuals, 2.6 million are estimated to be permanently disabled.[18] Between 70% and 90% of the total costs due to low back pain are incurred by the 4% to 5% of patients with temporary or permanent disability.[5] Risk factors for disability due to low back pain include poor health habits, job dissatisfaction, less appealing work environments, poor ratings by supervisors, psychological disturbances, compensatory injuries, and a history of prior disability.[5] These same factors are associated with a high rate of failure for treatment of all types.

Grazier and coworkers[19] performed a comprehensive analysis of the total costs of low back pain in 1984. Frymoyer and Cats-Baril[5] updated this analysis in 1990, estimating that the total direct cost of low back pain exceeded $24 billion annually; they also reported that the total indirect cost exceeds $27 billion annually (workers' lost income, homemakers' lost income, worker's compensation, legal compensation).

Natural History of Low Back Pain

Low back pain is usually a benign, self-limited condition.[5,20] It has been estimated that approximately 60% of the population experience low back pain during any one year, yet most people do not present for medical treatment.[21] Of those who do, 90% recover within 6 weeks with or without therapy.[1,22] Even in industrial settings, 75% of patients with symptoms of acute low back pain return to work within 1 month.[3] Only 2% to 3% of patients continue to have symptoms at 6 months, and only 1% at 1 year. However, there is a 60% rate of recurrence of low back symptoms over the next 2 years.[23] Currently, there is no convincing evidence that age, gender, race, or ethnicity influences the natural history of low back pain.[20] Body habitus, including height and weight, influences the natural history of acute low back pain.[20] Deyo and Tsui-Wu[11] demonstrated that adults in the upper fifth quintile of height and weight showed a greater prevalence of low back pain lasting more than 2 weeks. Cigarette smoking may unfavorably influence the natural history of recovery from acute low back pain, although the cause of this negative influence is not clear. It may be a direct effect of smoking on the nutrition of the lumbar intervertebral disc; it may be due to an indirect mechanical effect of coughing; or smoking may simply be a marker for differences in the behavior and physical fitness of smokers.[20,24] Occupational risk factors also influence the natural history of acute low back pain, and heavier job requirements do prolong recovery. Also, the natural history of low back pain is negatively influenced if the worker views his or her job as dissatisfying, repetitious, or boring; if the employer views the worker as less competent and evaluates the worker poorly; if the interaction between the worker and employer is poor; or if the work environment is perceived as unpleasant and noisy.[20] Finally, psychosocial factors play an important role in the natural history of low back pain, modulating response to pain and promoting illness behavior.[23]

The generally favorable natural history of acute low back pain is significantly influenced by a variety of factors, and the practicing physician must be familiar with this information to counsel patients about expectations and treatment options.

Evaluation

History

Low back pain has many causes and therefore many presentations (Table 17.1). The onset of symptoms can be sudden or insidious. The Canadian Back Institute, for example, found that 70% of patients with noncompensation injuries were unable to identify the specific injury that initiated their back pain.[25] Useful historical items include age, fever, weight loss, adenopathy, steroid use, and previous history of tuberculosis or cancer. Patients should be questioned regarding any aggravating or alleviating factors that affect their back pain. Nonmechanical back pain is usually continuous, whereas mechanical back pain is aggravated by motion and relieved by rest. Low back pain that worsens with cough has traditionally been associated with disc herniation, although studies have now shown that mechanical low back pain also worsens with cough.[25] A history should be elicited regarding leg weakness or leg paresthesias; it is especially important to determine if they are in a dermatomal distribution. Patients should be questioned about bowel or bladder incontinence, the presence of which may indicate a surgical emergency. Patients should be questioned regarding hip pain. Hip pain is often referred to the groin, the anterior thigh, and the knee and is worsened with ambulation. Patients with osteoarthritis or degenerative joint disease complain of morning stiffness that improves as the day progresses. Patients with spinal stenosis may

Table 17.1. Differential diagnosis of low back pain

Mechanical etiology
  Low back "strain"
  Acute disc herniation
  Spondylolisthesis
  Spondylolysis
  Spinal stenosis

Neoplasm
  Multiple myeloma
  Metastases from breast, lung, thyroid, renal, or GI primary cancers
  Hodgkin's or non-Hodgkin's lymphomas

Infectious etiology
  Diskitis
  Osteomyelitis
  Epidural abscess

Spondyloarthropathies
  Osteoarthritis
    Vertebral body
    Posterior facet syndrome
  Rheumatoid arthritis
  Ankylosing spondylitis

Metabolic etiology
  Osteoporosis

Extrinsic disease
  Aortic aneurysm
  Intraabdominal pathology

Psychological etiology
  Hysteria
  Malingering

report symptoms suggestive of spinal claudication, that is, neurologic symptoms in the legs that are worsened with ambulation. Spinal claudication may be differentiated from vascular claudication in that spinal claudication symptoms have a slower onset and slower resolution. A history of pain at rest, pain in the recumbent position, or pain at night suggests infection or tumor as a cause. Osteoporosis may be suspected in women who are postmenopausal or who have undergone oophorectomy. These patients may report unrelenting pain after even "minor" trauma. For patients who present writhing in pain, the presence of an intraabdominal process or vascular cause for the pain, such as abdominal aortic aneurysm, is suggested.

Some investigators have found the McGill pain questionnaire to be useful when interviewing patients with low back pain because it offers precise descriptive terms for common low back symptoms.[26] For example, a crampy or achy type of pain may be due to referred pain or vascular pain, whereas numbness, tingling, or burning sensations may be due to radicular pain.

Physical Examination

The initial examination should be fairly detailed. The patient should be examined in a gown, and the examination should begin with the patient standing. The physician should note the stance and gait of the patient, as well as the presence or absence of the normal curvatures of the spine (e.g., thoracic kyphosis, lumbar lordosis, splinting to one side, scoliosis). The range of motion of the back is examined, including flexion, lateral bending, and rotation. Strength of dorsiflexion and plantar flexion of the foot is examined by asking the patient to heel-walk and toe-walk. The strength of the quadriceps is examined by asking the patient to squat and rise while keeping the back straight.

With the patient seated, the straight-leg-raising test is applied. With the hip flexed to 90 degrees, the flexed knee is brought to full extension. The straight-leg-raising test is positive if the test reproduces the patient's paresthesias in the distribution of a nerve root at less than 60 degrees of knee extension. Sensation to light touch and pinprick is examined. The motor strength of hip and knee flexors is tested. The ankle jerk (S1) and knee jerk (L4) are elicited. Long tract signs are elicited by applying Babinski's maneuver.

With the patient in the supine position, the straight-leg-raising test is applied. With the knee in extension, the leg is raised (i.e., the hip is flexed). A positive test reproduces the patient's reports of leg paresthesias in the distribution of a nerve root. Back pain does not indicate a positive straight-leg-raising test. The crossed straight-leg-raising test (i.e., reproduction of the patient's symptoms by straight-leg-raising of the contralateral leg) is specific for acute disc herniation and suggests a large central disc herniation. Also in the supine position, the hip is examined to test the range of motion and to document pain radiation (hip pathology causes pain radiation to the groin and anteromedial thigh).

With the patient in the prone position, the femoral stretch test is applied. With the hip and knee in extension, the hip is further extended, placing increased stretch on the femoral nerve, which includes elements from the L2, L3, and L4 nerve roots. The hamstring reflex is tested by striking the semitendinosus and semimembranosus tendons at the medial aspect of the popliteal fossa. The hamstring reflex involves both the L5 and S1 nerve roots. Thus an absent or decreased hamstring reflex in the presence of a normal ankle jerk response (S1) implies involvement of the L5 nerve root (Table 17.2). Sensation in the area between the upper buttocks is tested, as is the anal reflex and anal sphincter tone (S2, S3, S4).

TABLE 17.2. Motor, sensory, and deep tendon reflex patterns associated with commonly affected nerve roots

Nerve root	Motor reflexes	Sensory reflexes	Deep tendon reflexes
C5	Deltoid	Lateral arm	Biceps jerk (C5, C6)
C6	Biceps, brachioradialis, wrist extensors	Lateral forearm	Brachioradialis
C7	Triceps, wrist flexors, MCP extensors	Middle of hand, middle finger	Triceps jerk
C8	MCP flexors	Medial forearm	—
T1	Abductors and adductors of fingers	Medial arm	—
L4	Quadriceps	Anterior thigh	Knee jerk
L5	Dorsiflex foot and great toe	Dorsum of foot	Hamstring reflex (L5, S1)
S1	Plantarflex foot	Lateral foot, posterior calf	Ankle jerk

The clinical diagnosis of acute disc herniation requires repeated physical examination demonstrating pain localized to a specific nerve root, with reproduction of pain on straight-leg-raising tests and the appropriate muscle weakness in the nerve root distribution. A positive crossed straight-leg-raising test is helpful for making the diagnosis as well.

Diagnostic Imaging

Plain Radiographs

Plain radiographs are rarely useful for diagnosing low back pain.[1] They cannot demonstrate an acute herniated disc and are used mostly to rule out such diagnoses as vertebral fracture, tumor, infection, spondylolisthesis, spondylolysis, or inflammatory spondyloarthropathies.[27] In the absence of neurologic deficits, plain radiographs for evaluating low back pain should be reserved for patients older than 50 years of age and those with a history of trauma, previous cancer, pain at rest, unexplained weight loss, drug or alcohol abuse, steroid use, any other reason for immunosuppression, or temperature greater than 38°C.[28] Some investigators believe that initial plain radiographs of the spine during early evaluation of acute low back pain should not include routine oblique views, which add little to the diagnosis but double the patient's exposure to radiation.[1] Others, however, believe that the oblique views aid in the diagnosis, especially when evaluating spondylolysis, a point that is particularly true when evaluating young patients active in gymnastics and football.[29] It is important to remember that roentgenographic findings are nonspecific and are observed equally in patients with and without symptoms of low back pain.[30] It is vital to connect patient's complaints of pain with a specific nerve root distribution and not assume that these observed radiographic findings are the cause of the patient's pain.

Computed Tomography, Magnetic Resonance Imaging, Myelography

Computed tomography (CT), myelography, and magnetic resonance imaging (MRI) add to the diagnostic acumen when managing patients with low back pain. A common mistake is to undertake these special imaging studies early in the clinical course for a patient with low back pain but no neurologic findings. The difficulty is that many asymptomatic patients demonstrate bulging or even herniated discs.[1] For example, it has been estimated that 30% to 40% of CT scans show abnormalities of disc bulging in asymptomatic patients.[6] These special imaging studies should probably be reserved for patients with neurologic findings who do not respond to conservative therapy for 3 to 4 weeks.[1] Earlier imaging should be considered if the patient demonstrates the cauda equina syndrome or a progressive neurologic deficit, or if tumor or infection is suspected.[1,6] Few studies have been done directly comparing the three most commonly used modalities for investigating the spine. The CT scan is probably best at noting bony abnormalities, such as fracture or spinal stenosis, as well as a bulging disc. Myelography is especially useful for differentiating significant disc herniation from incidental disc bulging that is not responsible for the patient's signs or symptoms. MRI is a promising technique that is particularly useful for examining the soft tissues of the central nervous system, but limited data are available comparing it with CT scans or the myelogram.[1] A greater potential for MRI in identifying trauma, infection, and neoplasia has been documented. MRI is especially valuable for assessing the postoperative spine and delineating postoperative scarring, recurrent disc disease, and fusion stability.[31] Some believe MRI has become the procedure of choice for lumbar spine imaging, whereas others recommend judicious use of CT and myelography as well.[27,32]

Differential Diagnosis

For most patients with acute low back pain, a definitive diagnosis is not possible.[10] Most of these cases are probably due to strain of the muscles supporting the vertebral spine (Table 17.1). Acute disc herniation has changed little from its description in the classic article of Mixter and Barr,[33] wherein degeneration of the annulus fibrosus leads to partial or complete herniation of the nucleus pulposus. Usually, this herniation is in the posterolateral position, producing unilateral symptoms. Occasionally, the disc herniates in the midline, and a large herniation in such a position can lead to bilateral symptoms.

Posterior Facet Syndrome

The posterior facet syndrome is caused by degenerative changes in the posterior facets, which are true diarthrodial joints and can develop degenerative joint changes visible on roentgenography. Pain caused by degenerative changes in the posterior facet joints radiates to the groin, hip, or thigh, causing a dull achy pain that is difficult to localize.[34] The low back pain typically associated with posterior facet syndrome can be worsened with hyperextension of the spine or with twisting. Steroid injections into the posterior facet joints to relieve presumed posterior facet joint pain have gained popularity. Well-designed studies have demonstrated the dramatic placebo effect of any injection in this area but fail to demonstrate any benefit from steroid injection into the posterior facet joint.[35,36] The presence of degenerative changes in the facet joints on roentgenograms does not necessarily imply that the posterior facets are the true cause of the patient's pain. Caution must be used when ascribing the patient's pain to these degenerative changes. Historically, the posterior facet syndrome has been diagnosed by demonstrating pain relief after injection of local anesthetic into the posterior facet joints,[6] but more recent studies have cast doubt on the validity of this procedure.[34]

Osteoarthritis

Osteoarthritis of the vertebral spine is common during later life (see Chapter 18). It is especially prevalent in the cervical and lumbar spine. Typically, the pain of osteoarthritis of the spine is worse in the morning, increases with motion, and is relieved by rest. It is associated with morning stiffness and decreased range of motion of the spine in the absence of systemic symptoms. The severity of symptoms does not correlate well with roentgenographic findings; that is, patients who have severe degenerative changes seen on radiographs may be asymptomatic, whereas patients with symptoms suggestive of osteoarthritis of the spine may have minimal radiographic findings. Exuberant osteophytic changes may lead to compression of lumbar nerve roots or may even cause cauda equina syndrome.[37]

Ankylosing Spondylitis

Ankylosing spondylitis is a spondyloarthropathy that most commonly affects young men, who present with mild-to-moderate low back pain centered in the back and radiating to the posterior thighs. During its initial presentation, the symptoms are vague, and the diagnosis is often overlooked. The pain is intermittent, but the decrease in range of motion of the back is constant. Early signs of ankylosing spondylitis include limitation of chest expansion, tenderness of the sternum, and decreased range of motion and flexion contractures at the hip. The radiologic hallmarks of ankylosing spondylitis include periarticular destructive changes, obliteration of the sacroiliac joints, development of syndesmophytes on the margins of the vertebral bodies, and bridging of these osteophytes by bone between vertebral bodies, the so-called bamboo spine. Laboratory analysis shows a negative test for rheumatoid factor, an elevated erythrocyte sedimentation rate (ESR), and a positive test for HLA-B27 antigen.[37]

Neoplasia

Multiple myeloma is the most common primary malignancy of the vertebral spine. However, metastatic lesions are the most common cause of cancers of the spine, arising from breast, lung, prostate, thyroid, renal, or gastrointestinal tract primary tumors. Hodgkin's and non-Hodgkin's lymphomas also frequently involve the vertebral spine. The primary site of the tumor is often overlooked, and so back pain is frequently the presenting complaint for many cancers. In an unselected population, fewer than 1% of patients who present with low back pain have cancer as the cause.[38] Findings significantly associated with cancer as a cause of low back pain include age older than 50 years, previous history of cancer, pain lasting more than 1 month, failure to improve with conservative therapy, elevated ESR, and anemia.[38] These patients complain of a dull constant pain that is worse at night and not relieved by rest or the recumbent position. Typical radiographic changes may be absent early in the course of this illness. A bone scan is usually positive owing to increased blood flow and reactive bone formation. However, with multiple myeloma and metastatic thyroid cancer, the bone scan may be negative.[39] Symptomatic spinal cancer is an ominous sign, with a potential for devastating morbidity, which underscores the importance of early recognition and treatment.[40]

Osteoporosis

Osteoporosis is a common problem among elderly patients, affecting up to 25% of women older than 65. It leads to an increased risk for spinal compression fractures.[6] Patients with osteoporosis develop low back pain due to compression fractures, the pain of which is worse after prolonged sitting or standing. The pain may resolve over 3 to 4 months as these compression fractures heal. These patients usually have no neurologic complaints and suffer no neural compression. Laboratory tests are normal with primary osteoporosis. Any abnormalities should prompt an exploration for secondary causes of osteoporosis. On radiography, a loss of height is seen that is due to compression fractures. The diagnosis of primary osteoporosis is made on clinical grounds, i.e., diffuse osteopenia, compression fractures, and normal laboratory findings.[41,42]

Spinal Stenosis

Spinal stenosis can occur at a single level or at multiple spinal levels. In these cases, low back pain is aggravated by standing; the pain increases during the day and is relieved by rest. Over time, the posture may become progressively flexed forward. Symptoms usually begin during the sixth decade. Plain radiographs often show osteophytes at many levels, but as mentioned before, caution must be used when ascribing back pain to these degenerative changes. The "spinal claudication" of spinal stenosis can be differentiated from vascular claudication in that vascular claudication has a faster onset and faster relief of symptoms.[6]

Abdominal Aortic Aneurysm

Abdominal aortic aneurysm can cause low back pain due to compression of surrounding tissues or to extension or rupture of the aneurysm. Most patients complain of dull steady back pain that is unrelated to activity and that may radiate to the hips or thighs. Patients with an acute rupture or extension of the aneurysm complain of severe tearing pain, diaphoresis, syncope, or circulatory shock.[41]

Psychosocial Factors

Psychological factors are frequently associated with complaints of low back pain, influencing both pain symptoms and therapeutic outcome.[43] The Minnesota Multi-phasic Personality Index (MMPI) demonstrates elevated scales for depression, anxiety, and hypochondriasis among these patients. Such findings on MMPI testing are associated with unfavorable outcomes after surgery.

When examining patient outcomes after surgery, psychological factors seem to influence outcomes more strongly than do the initial physical examination or surgical findings. Therefore, patients should be evaluated with standard pain indices, activities of daily living scales, and psychometric testing before surgery. Results of surgery for treating lumbar disc herniation are excellent in well-selected patients.[44]

Management

Most physicians would agree that almost all patients with low back pain, except those with cauda equina syndrome, require a trial of conservative therapy.[4] Such a 4- to 6-week trial should be pursued if there is no evidence of cauda equina syndrome and if there is no rapidly progressive neurologic deficit.

Bed Rest

One of the mainstays for treatment of low back pain is bed rest, although the optimal duration has not been clearly elucidated.[45] However, the value of bed rest for patients with typical findings of a herniated disc are not disputed. At least one well-designed study has demonstrated that 2 days of bed rest are as effective and may be superior to 7 days of bed rest.[4] It is clear that prolonged immobilization can lead to muscle weakness, cardiovascular deconditioning, and bone mineral loss. Therefore, whereas the literature may support the prescription of bed rest for 3 days to 2 weeks, current thinking leans toward a short course of bed rest—on the order of 2 to 3 days. Sitting in bed should be avoided because the sitting position increases intradiskal pressures.[1]

Medications

Antiinflammatory Drugs

Several well-designed clinical trials have shown that nonsteroidal antiinflammatory drugs (NSAIDs) are effective in treating low back pain. In particular, naproxen has been shown to be effective.[46] Therapy is titrated to provide pain relief at a minimal dose and is continued for 4 to 6 weeks. Use of NSAIDs should not be continued indefinitely.[4]

Narcotics

Narcotic pain medications are useful, especially for acute disc herniations with sciatica. However, they should be used for only a brief period, with a time-limited prescription (i.e., narcotics should not be prescribed in a symptom-limited fashion).

Muscle Relaxants

Muscle relaxants should also be prescribed in a time-limited fashion, although evidence for the effectiveness of muscle relaxants is scant. Diazepam (Valium), cyclobenzaprine (Flexeril), and methocarbamol (Robaxin) are commonly used muscle relaxants. Carisoprodol (Soma) has been demonstrated to be effective.[4] The main value of muscle relaxants is less for their relaxant effect than for their sedative effect. Finally, it should be emphasized that muscle relaxants and narcotics should not be used in patients who present with complaints of chronic low back pain (i.e., low back pain of more than 3 months' duration).

Unproved Treatments

Some commonly used treatments for low back pain, such as traction, corsets, or braces, have never been demonstrated to be effective.[1,3,6] To date, there are no convincing data to support benefit from lumbar corsets or braces in the treatment of most low back complaints. Transcutaneous electrical nerve stimulation (TENS) has been shown to be ineffective treatment for low back pain.[47]

Exercise

Exercise is a commonly used and often misunderstood therapy for treatment of acute low back pain. Even in the setting of acute herniation, patients should avoid prolonged inactivity and the debilitation that results from prolonged bed rest.[1] Patients should be prescribed a short 2- to 3-day course of bed rest followed by standing and walking by the third day of treatment. Within the first week of therapy, the patient should be advised to walk 20 minutes for every 3 hours in the supine position. A moderate exercise program can increase activity and decrease pain scores and pain frequency.[47]

Flexion Exercises

Many types of exercise have been recommended for the treatment of acute low back pain and prevention of recurrences.[4] Kendall and Jenkins[48] first demonstrated the effectiveness of isometric flexion exercises. These flexion exercises are probably the most commonly used exercise program, although Williams' flexion exercises have undergone many changes.[49] The rationale for flexion exercises is that strong abdominal muscles protect the lumbar disc from excessive loads. Williams' flexion exercises are contraindicated in the setting of acute disc herniation, immediately after a prolonged period of rest (the disc is hyperhydrated and prone to injury), in cases of postural low back pain (where flexion should be relieved), and in cases of a lateral trunk shift or lift.

Extension Exercises

The less commonly prescribed extension exercises are also useful. McKenzie[50] described a set of hyperextension exercises for the spine as a means of treating chronic back pain. Another study documented the safety and efficacy of these maneuvers.[51] Extension-to-neutral exercises, with the patient in the prone position, have been shown to strengthen the perivertebral muscles that support the spine and promote endurance and full function.[52]

Aerobic Fitness

Cady and Bischoff[53] demonstrated that aerobic fitness training is an effective means of preventing low back injury and rehabilitating patients in whom low back pain has developed. Evidence supports use of exercises that increase fitness in patients with low back pain. For example, in patients with acute low back pain, bed rest for 2 to 3 days can be prescribed. After a pain-free interval of 2 weeks, the patient can begin aerobic training, gradually increasing its duration, frequency, and intensity. A typical prescription would include 30 to 40 minutes of aerobic exercise three to five times a week, including warm-up and cool-down. Exercises should be aerobic in nature, involving large muscle groups. Typical exercises include walking and jogging with good shoes on a level surface; swimming and aerobic dance are useful exercises as well. Cycling can be problematic in that the sitting position increases the workload on the lower back. Jumping rope should be avoided because it places a high compression load on the spine and requires a high level of intensity before aerobic benefit is achieved.[52]

Back School

Another therapeutic modality that has received much attention is the enrollment of patients in "low back school." In these classes, patients receive education in proper sitting, standing, and lifting techniques. Some studies have shown that patients receiving such education return to work 1 week earlier than patients who do not receive such education[54]; it can even lead to decreased incidence of low back injuries in the workplace.[55] Other investigators have found that "back school" is less effective than McKenzie extension exercises.[56] Even in cases of low back pain that has persisted for more than 6 months, enrollment in a "back school" can lead to improvement in both function and pain profile.[57] A structured educational program promoting effective back "hygiene" is probably of benefit to most patients with low back pain.[8]

Surgery

The rate of lumbar surgery in the United States is three to eight times higher than in most European countries.[1] The presence of a bulging disc on imaging procedures or isolated low back pain without neurologic complaints is not an adequate indication for surgery. Surgery in the presence of an acute herniated disc is indicated when there is a combination of definite herniation documented by imaging techniques, a corresponding pain syndrome, a corresponding neurologic deficit, and failure to respond to 4 to 6 weeks of conservative management.[1] Frymoyer and Cats-Baril[5] estimated that 2% to 3% of patients with low back pain may be surgical candidates on the basis of sciatica alone. Overall, the lifetime prevalence of lumbar spine surgery ranges between 1% and 3%.[5]

The major benefit of surgery is relief of sciatica. Among well-selected patients, 75% have complete relief of sciatic symptoms and an additional 15% have partial relief. Patients with clear symptoms of radicular pain have the best surgical outcome, whereas those with the least evidence of radiculopathy have the poorest surgical outcome.[58] Relief of back pain itself is less consistent. Complications of surgery include death (0.2%), thromboembolism (1.7%), and infection (2.9%).

Diskectomy

The most common surgical procedure for treating an acute herniated disc is diskectomy. The sole objective of diskectomy is to decompress the nerve root. This procedure is effective in 60% to 80% of patients. Microscopic diskectomy permits a small incision and less postoperative pain among patients, but there is an increased rate of recurrent symptoms and missed disc fragments. Conventional diskectomy has a short-term success rate of 90%, but over the 10 years after surgery, this success rate decreases to 70%. Five to fifteen percent of patients later require another operation, usually because of recurrent disc herniation or failure to recognize spinal stenosis. The most common cause of failure of lumbar disc surgery is poor patient selection; that is, the cause of pain is not certain, patients are referred for surgery to treat isolated low back pain in the absence of neurologic abnormalities, or the patient has a psychological state that is associated with poor results.[6] To be considered for diskectomy, all patients should demonstrate persistent, unremitting radiculopathy, failure of conservative therapy, neurologic abnormalities on examination, or correlative electromyographic findings and correlative imaging studies.[59]

Chymopapain

Chymopapain injections have been demonstrated to be better than placebo for treating patients with acute disc herniations. However, subsequent trials have demonstrated that surgery is much better than chymopapain therapy for treating these conditions.[60] Surgical therapy is significantly better than chymopapain injection for relieving back and leg pain, and recurrent low back pain is much more common among patients treated with chymopapain.[61] Chymopapain injection was initially considered a "noninvasive" procedure, but the complications and morbidity associated with these injections was found to equal or exceed those of standard surgical therapy. Enthusiasm for this procedure has waned owing to the incidence and severity of complications, including transverse myelitis, allergic reactions (0.5%), and persisting muscle spasms (20%).[6] Therefore, it is much less commonly used now.[1]

Therapeutic Goals and Expectations

When treating patients with low back pain, the physician's goal is to keep the patient as active as reasonable with return to work as soon as possible. It is obviously important to be sure there is no significant pathology causing the patient's low back pain, but in most cases, the patient can be reassured that the back pain is due to a simple muscular strain. Patients should be reassured that they will improve with time, usually quickly. Patients may require a brief period of bed rest during the acute phase, usually 1 to 2 days, and adequate pain relief is necessary during the acute stage as well. Physicians should encourage early mobilization, usually within a few days and always by 2 weeks at the latest. Patients should be encouraged to return to work, usually within 1 to 2 weeks and almost always by 6 weeks. Work activities may be modified at first, but it is important to avoid iatrogenic disability.[21]

Chronic Low Back Pain

Chronic low back pain (i.e., pain persisting >3 months) is a special problem and deserves special consideration. Patients presenting with a history of chronic low back pain require an extensive diagnostic workup on at least one occasion, including an in-depth history, physical examination, and the appropriate imaging techniques (plain radiography, CT scanning, myelography, or MRI). Therapy is directed at strengthening the musculature that supports the spine, including aerobic fitness, flexion and extension exercises, and an educational program on proper sitting, standing, and working techniques.[6] Decompressive laminectomy is reserved for patients with persistent spinal claudication, important myelographic blocks at the spinal level of involvement, or progressive loss of bowel or bladder control. In patients with no surgically correctable lesions, conservative therapy is the mainstay of treatment, complemented by the appropriate use of antidepressants (desipramine, imipramine, doxepin).[4,6]

Prevention of low back injury and consequent disability has received a great deal of attention. Attempts at patient education and preemployment physical examination have not been shown to decrease the occurrence of job-related low back pain, but measuring strength and prescribing general fitness exercises have been beneficial.[6] Similarly, job design, modification of the workplace, cessation of smoking, correction of obesity, and aerobic fitness training are effective ways to decrease the occurrence of low back pain.[10,24,53]

Disorders of the Neck

Cervical Radiculopathy

One of the most common causes of neck pain is cervical radiculopathy, which is defined as pain in the distribution of a particular cervical nerve root. Cervical radiculopathy can be caused by compressive pathology, a herniated cervical disc, spur formation, or a hypermobile state of the cervical spine. Studies have shown that as many as 51% of the adult population experience neck and arm pain at some time in their lives.[62] Risk factors that have been identified to cause neck pain include heavy lifting, smoking, diving, working with vibrating heavy equipment, and possibly riding in cars.[63] Cervical radiculopathy rarely progresses to myelopathy, although as many as two-thirds of patients who are treated with conservative therapy without surgery report persistent symptoms. In severe cases of cervical radiculopathy, where motor function has been compromised, 98% of patients recover full motor function after decompressive laminectomy.[64]

The symptoms of cervical radiculopathy can be single or multiple, unilateral or bilateral, symmetric or asymmetric.[65] There are three main types: (1) The *acute* form is commonly due to a tear of the annulus fibrosus, leading to prolapse of the nucleus pulposus. It is usually the result of some mild-to-moderate trauma. (2) Another type is *subacute* in nature and is usually due to long-standing spondylosis accompanied by mild trauma or overuse. Most of these patients experience resolution of their symptoms within 6 weeks with rest and analgesics. (3) The last type is *chronic* radiculopathy, which occurs during middle or old age. It presents with complaints of neck or arm pain due to heavy labor or atypical activity.[65]

Cervical nerve roots exit the spine above the corresponding vertebral body (i.e., the C5 nerve root exits above C5). Therefore, disc herniation at the C4–C5 interspace causes symptoms in the distribution of C5. Radicular symptoms may be caused by a "soft disc" (i.e., disc herniation) or by a "hard disc" (i.e., osteophyte formation and foraminal encroachment).[66] The most commonly involved interspaces are C5–C6, C6–C7, C4–C5, C3–C4, and C7–T1.[63]

Evaluation

With cervical radiculopathy, sensory symptoms are much more prominent than motor changes. Typically, patients report proximal pain and distal paresthesias.[66] The fifth, sixth, and seventh nerve roots are most commonly affected. Pain may be referred. Referred pain is often vague, diffuse, and lacking in the sharp quality of radicular pain. For example, pain referred from a herniated disc may present as pain in the neck, pain at the top of the shoulders, or pain around the scapulas.[65]

On physical examination, radicular pain increases with certain maneuvers, such as neck range of motion, Valsalva maneuver, cough, or sneeze. Active and passive neck range of motion is tested, examining flexion, extension, and lateral tilt in detail.

Diagnosis

The differential diagnosis of cervical nerve root pain includes cervical disc herniation, spinal canal tumor, trauma, degenerative changes, inflammatory disorders, congenital abnormalities, toxic and allergic conditions, hemorrhage, and musculoskeletal syndromes (thoracic outlet syndrome, shoulder pain).

In cases of cervical radiculopathy unresponsive to conservative therapy but without evidence of a progressive motor deficit, investigation of other pathologic processes is indicated. Plain radiographs are usually not helpful because abnormal findings are equally common among symptomatic and asymptomatic patients. CT scans, myelography, and MRI have a role to play in the diagnosis of cervical radiculopathy.

Management

Conservative Therapy

Immobilization

The purpose of immobilizing the cervical spine is to reduce the intervertebral motion that may cause compression, mechanical irritation, or stretching of the cervical nerve roots.[67] Immobilization is easily achieved by use of the soft cervical collar or the more rigid Philadelphia collar, both of which help hold the neck in slight flexion. The collar is useful in the acute setting, but prolonged use can lead to deconditioning of the paracervical musculature. Therefore, the collar should be prescribed in a time-limited manner, and the patient should be instructed in the use of isometric neck exercises.

Bed Rest

Bed rest is another form of immobilization, serving to help modify the patient's activities and eliminate the axial compression forces of gravity.[67] It is important to hold the neck in slight flexion, which can be accomplished by arranging two standard pillows in a V with the apex pointed cranially, then placing a third pillow across the apex. This arrangement provides mild cervical flexion and internally rotates the shoulder girdle, thereby relieving some traction on the cervical nerve roots.

Medication

Analgesics such as codeine are useful in the acute setting but should be prescribed in a strictly time-limited manner.[67] The physician should be alert to the possibility of addiction or abuse.

Muscle relaxants are helpful for relieving muscle spasm, and several authors have recommended carisoprodol (Soma). Methocarbamol (Robaxin) and diazepam (Valium) are useful alternatives.

The NSAIDs are particularly beneficial, although patient intolerance is high. Often, two or three of these medications must be tried before benefit results without unacceptable side effects.

Physical Therapy

Moist heat, ice packs, ultrasound therapy, and patient education have a role to play in the conservative management of patients with cervical disc disease.[67]

Surgery

Surgical intervention is reserved for patients with radicular signs and symptoms who have failed conservative therapy and who have positive neuroradiologic studies that correspond to their clinical signs and symptoms.[66]

Cervical Myelopathy

The mechanism of pain production in cases of cervical myelopathy is not clearly understood but is presumed to be multifactorial, including vascular changes, cord hypoxia, changes in spinal canal diameter, and hypertrophic facets. Therefore, these patients may present with a variable clinical picture. The usual course is one of increasing disability over the course of several months. Changes usually begin with dysesthesia in the hands, leading to weakness or clumsiness, eventually leading to weakness in the lower extremities.[65]

Evaluation

In cases of cervical myelopathy secondary to cervical spondylosis, symptoms are usually insidious in onset, often with short periods of worsening followed by long periods of relative stability. Acute onset of symptoms or rapid deterioration suggests a vascular etiology.[66] Unlike cases of radicular pain, patients with cervical myelopathy rarely present with neck pain but complain of headache, usually occipital, with pain radiating anteriorly to the frontal area. These patients report that the headache is worse on waking but improves throughout the day.[65] Patients complain of deep aching pain and burning sensations, as well as loss of hand dexterity.[66] Other symptoms include vertebrobasilar insufficiency, presumably due to osteophytic changes in the cervical spine.[65]

On physical examination, these patients are often found to have motor weakness and muscle wasting, particularly of interossei muscles of the hand. Lhermitte's sign is present in approximately 25% of patients[66]; that is, rapid flexion or extension of the neck causes a shock-like sensation in the trunk or limbs. Deep tendon reflexes can be variable. For example, involvement of the anterior horn cell causes a decrease in deep tendon reflexes, whereas involvement of the corticospinal tracts leads to an increase in deep tendon reflexes. The triceps jerk is the reflex most commonly lost owing to frequent involvement of the sixth nerve root. Almost all patients with cervical myelopathy show signs of muscular spasticity.[66]

Diagnosis

The intrathecal contrast-enhanced CT scan is a highly specific test that allows evaluation of the intradural contents and the disc margins. It helps differentiate an extradural defect due to disc herniation from that due to osteophytic changes.[68] MRI has multiplanar capabilities, allowing visualization in both the sagittal and axial planes. Resolution with MRI is sharp enough to allow visualization of the effects of disc herniation or spinal stenosis. MRI is especially helpful for evaluating lesions of the spinal cord.[68]

The CT scan is preferred when evaluating osteophytes, foraminal encroachment, and other bony changes, whereas MRI is superior for demonstrating disc changes and abnormalities of the spinal cord. CT scanning and MRI complement one another, and their use should be individualized to the patient.[69]

It is important to correlate positive radiologic findings with the clinical examination. Degenerative changes of the cervical spine and cervical disc are common, and several studies have demonstrated significant radiologic changes among asymptomatic patients.[68,69]

Management

Conservative Therapy

Most patients with cervical myelopathy present with minor symptoms and demonstrate long periods of nonprogressive disability. Therefore, these patients should be treated conservatively and observed over time.[70] Patients may be treated with a soft cervical collar, physical therapy to promote range of motion, and judicious use of NSAIDs. It must be remembered that only 30% to 50% of patients demonstrate improvement with conservative treatment.

Surgery

Early surgical decompression may be appropriate when patients with cervical myelopathy present with moderate or severe disability or when rapid deterioration is present.[70] Anterior decompression with fusion, posterior decompression, laminectomy, and laminoplasty are each appropriate to particular clinical situations.[71]

The best surgical prognosis can be achieved through careful patient selection. Obviously, accurate diagnosis is essential. Patients with a relatively short duration of symptoms have the best prognosis.[66] If surgery is to be performed, it should be done early in the course of the disease, before irreversible cord damage has occurred.

Cervical Whiplash

Cervical whiplash should be considered a valid clinical syndrome, with symptoms consistent with anatomic sites of injury and a potential for significant impairment.[72] Symptoms associated with cervical whiplash injuries are due to soft tissue trauma, particularly musculoligamentous sprains and strains to the cervical region of the spine. After a rear-end impact in a motor vehicle accident, the driver and passenger are accelerated forward; and owing to inertia, the head is thrown into hyperextension. This hyperextension usually centers on the C5–C6 area and is followed by flexion of the neck, which is limited by the chin striking the chest.

Hyperextension commonly causes an injury to the anterior longitudinal ligament of the cervical spine and other soft tissue injuries of the anterior neck, including muscle tears, muscle hemorrhage, esophageal hemorrhage, and disc disruption. Muscles most commonly injured include the sterno-cleidomastoid, scalenus, and longus colli muscles. Patients may also develop visual disturbances, possibly due to vertebral, basilar, or other vascular injury, or injury to the cervical sympathetic chain.

Evaluation

The patient usually describes a typical rear-end-impact motor vehicle accident that caused hyperextension of the neck followed by hyperflexion; the neck pain that results either appears immediately or is delayed hours or even days after the accident. This pain, usually felt at the base of the neck, increases over time. The patient complains of decreased range of motion and neck pain that is worse with motion or activity. The patient may also complain of paresthesias, weakness, dysphagia, or hoarseness.

The physical examination may be negative if the patient is seen within hours of the accident. Over time, however, the patient develops tenderness in the cervical spine area, decreased range of motion, and muscle spasm. Neurologic examination of the upper extremity should include assessment of motor function, sensory changes, adequacy of deep tendon reflexes, range of motion (especially of the shoulder), and grip strength.

Diagnosis

Radiographic findings are usually minimal. Five views of the cervical spine should be obtained: anteroposterior, lateral, two obliques, and odontoid. Films should be examined for soft tissue swelling anterior to the C3 vertebral body. Straightening of the cervical spine or loss of normal cervical lordosis may be due to positioning during radiologic studies, muscle spasm, or derangement of the skeletal alignment of the cervical spine. Films should be examined for the presence of previous changes to the cervical spine, including osteophytes, disc space narrowing, and narrowing of the foramina on oblique views. Electromyography and nerve conduction velocity tests should be considered if the patient complains of paresthesias or radicular pain. Some believe that MRI is superior to CT scanning for evaluating patients with cervical radiculopathy. The bone scan is highly sensitive for detecting occult injuries. It should be remembered that whiplash injuries often cause soft tissue lesions, which are not seen on most of these studies.

Management

Rest

Initially, the patient should be treated with rest and protection of the cervical spine, usually with a soft cervical collar. The collar helps hold the neck in slight flexion, so the widest part of the cervical collar should be worn posteriorly. The cervical collar is especially useful for decreasing pain if worn at night or when driving. If worn during the day, it should be kept on for 1 to 2 hours and then removed for 1 to 2 hours. The cervical collar should be prescribed for a specific period, usually a few weeks.

Medications

NSAIDs are helpful for treating the muscle spasm and pain associated with whiplash injuries. Muscle relaxants are a useful adjunct, especially when used nightly, and should be prescribed in a time-limited manner. Narcotics are usually not indicated for treatment of whiplash injuries.

Physical Therapy

Physical modalities can help alleviate symptoms of pain and muscle spasm. Early in the course of whiplash injuries, heat for 20 to 25 minutes, no more often than every 3 hours, is useful. However, excessive use of heat can actually prolong healing. Later in the course of whiplash injury, cold therapy is useful for decreasing muscle spasm and pain. Isometric exercises for the neck and range of motion exercises can be initiated early in the therapy of whiplash injuries, even immediately after injury. Patients should receive specific directives regarding exercises and daily activities. Patients may benefit from specific programmed instruction regarding exercises, daily activities, body mechanics, and the use of heat and cold.

Prognosis

Most patients who sustain whiplash injuries have negative investigative studies and do improve, although slowly and irregularly; they benefit from a program of rest, immobilization, exercises, and return to function. Some patients do more poorly, and many factors contribute to a poor prognosis, including chronic symptoms for more than 12 months, loss of employment, persistent neurologic symptoms (e.g., pain radiation, paresthesias, altered reflexes, and muscle weakness or atrophy), osteophytic radiographic changes, or abnormalities on CT scans or MRI.

References

1. Deyo RA, Loeser JD, Vigos SJ. Herniated lumbar inter-vertebral disc. Ann Intern Med 1990;112:598–603.

2. Jackson CP, Brown MD. Is there a role for exercise in treatment of patients with low back pain? Clin Orthop 1983;179:39–45.

3. Spitzer WO, LeBlanc FE, Dupuis M, et al. Scientific approach to the assessment and management of activity related spinal disorders: a monograph for clinicians; report of the Quebec Task Force on Spinal Disorders. Spine 1987; 12(Suppl1):S1–59.

4. Deyo RA. Conservative therapy for low back pain. JAMA 1983;250:1057–62.

5. Frymoyer JW, Cats-Baril WL. An overview of the incidences and costs of low back pain. Orthop Clin North Am 1991;22:263–71.

6. Frymoyer JW. Back pain and sciatica. N Engl J Med 1988;318:291–300.

7. Frymoyer JW, Pope MH, Clements JH, et al. Risk factors in low back pain: an epidemiological survey. J Bone Joint Surg [Am] 1983;65:213–8.

8. Nachemson A. Work for all: for those with low back pain as well. Clin Orthop 1983;179:77–85.

9. Waddell G. A new clinical model for the treatment of low back pain. Spine 1987;12:632–44.

10. White AA III, Gordon SL. Synopsis: workshop on idiopathic low back pain. Spine 1982;7:141–9.

11. Deyo RA, Tsui-Wu YJ. Descriptive epidemiology of low back pain and its related medical care in the United States. Spine 1987;12:264–8.

12. Hazard RG, Fenwick JW, Kalisch SM, et al. Functional restoration with behavioral support: a one-year prospective study of patients with chronic low back pain. Spine 1989;14:157–69.

13. Weber H. Lumbar disc herniation: a controlled prospective study with ten years of observation. Spine 1983;8:131–40.

14. Kelsey JL. Epidemiology of radiculopathies. Adv Neurol 1978;19:385–9.

15. Kelsey JL, Githens PB, O'Conner T, et al. Acute prolapsed lumbar inter-vertebral disc: an epidemiologic study with special reference to driving automobiles and cigarette smoking. Spine 1984;9:608–11.

16. Kelsey JL, Githens PD, White AA, et al. An epidemiologic study of lifting and twisting on the job and risk for acute prolapsed lumbar inter-vertebral disc. J Orthop Res 1984;2:61–69.

17. Spangfort EV. The lumbar disc herniation: a computer-aided analysis of 2,504 operations. Acta Orthop Scand Suppl 1972;142:5–95.

18. National Center for Health Statistics. Prevalence of selected impairments, U.S., 1977, Series 10, No. 132. DHHS Publ. (PHS) 81-1562. Hyattsville, MD: NCHS, 1981.

19. Holbrook TL, Grazier KL, Kelsey JL, Stauffer RN. The frequency of occurrence, impact, and cost of musculoskeletal conditions in the United States. Chicago: American Academy of Orthopaedic Surgeons; 1984.

20. Frymoyer JW, Nachemson A. Natural history of low back disorders. In: Frymoyer JW, editor. The adult spine: principles and practice. New York: Raven Press, 1991:1537–50.

21. Waddell G. A new clinical model for the treatment of low back pain. In: Weinstein JN, Wiesel SW, editors. The lumbar spine. Philadelphia: Saunders, 1990:38–56.

22. Nachemson A. Newest knowledge of low back pain: a critical look. Clin Orthop 1992;279:8–20.

23. Cassidy JD, Wedge JH. The epidemiology and natural history of low back pain and spinal degeneration. In: Kirkaldy-Willis WH, editor. Managing low back pain. 2nd ed. New York: Churchill Livingstone, 1988:3–14.
24. Deyo RA, Bass JE. Lifestyles and low back pain: the influence of smoking and obesity. Spine 1989;14:501–6.
25. Fairbank JCT, Hall H. History taking and physical examination: identification of syndromes of back pain. In: Weinstein JN, Wiesel SW, editors. The lumbar spine. Philadelphia: Saunders, 1990:88–106.
26. Melzack R. The McGill Pain Questionnaire: major properties and scoring mechanisms. Pain 1975;1:277–99.
27. Modic MT, Ross JS. Magnetic resonance imaging in the evaluation of low back pain. Orthop Clin North Am 1991;22:283–301.
28. Deyo RA, Diehl AK. Lumbar spine films in primary care: current use and effects of selective ordering criteria. J Gen Intern Med 1986;1:20–25.
29. Hensinger RN. Spondylolysis and spondylolisthesis in children and adolescents. J Bone Joint Surg [Am] 1989;71:1098–107.
30. Frymoyer JW, Newberg A, Pope MH, et al. Spine radiographs in patients with low back pain: an epidemiological study in men. J Bone Joint Surg [Am] 1984;66:1048–55.
31. Ross JS, Masaryk TJ, Modic MT. Lumbar spine. In: Stark DD, Bradley WG Jr, editors. Magnetic resonance imaging. 2nd ed. St. Louis: Mosby, 1992: 1339–69.
32. Modic MT, Masaryk T, Boumphrey F, et al. Lumbar herniated disc disease and canal stenosis: prospective evaluation by surface coil MR, CT, and myelography. AJR 1986;147:757–65.
33. Mixter WJ, Barr JS. Rupture of inter-vertebral disc with involvement of the spinal canal. N Engl J Med 1934;211:210–5.
34. Jackson RP. The facet syndrome: myth or reality? Spine 1992;279:110–21.
35. Carette S, Marcoux S, Truchon R, et al. A controlled trial of corticosteroid injections into facet joints for chronic low back pain. N Engl J Med 1991; 325:1002–7.
36. Lilius G, Laasonen EM, Myllynen P, et al. Lumbar facet joint syndrome: a randomized clinical trial. J Bone Joint Surg [Br] 1989;71:681–4.
37. Camins MB, O'Leary PF, editors. The lumbar spine. New York: Raven Press, 1987.
38. Deyo RA, Diehl AK. Cancer as a cause of back pain: frequency, clinical presentation, and diagnostic strategies. J Gen Intern Med 1988;3:230–8.
39. Bates DW, Reuler JB. Back pain and epidural spinal cord compression. J Gen Intern Med 1988;3:191–7.
40. Perrin RG. Symptomatic spinal metastases. Am Fam Physician 1989;39: 165–72.
41. McCowin PR, Borenstein D, Wiesel SW. The current approach to the medical diagnosis of low back pain. Orthop Clin North Am 1991;22:315–25.
42. Barth RW, Lane JM. Osteoporosis. Orthop Clin North Am 1988;19:845–58.
43. Frymoyer JW, Rosen JC, Clements J, Pope MH. Psychologic factors in low back pain disability. Clin Orthop 1985;195:178–84.
44. Hurme M, Alaranta H. Factors predicting the results of surgery for lumbar inter-vertebral disc herniation. Spine 1987;12:933–8.

45. Deyo RA, Diehl AK, Rosenthal M. How many days of bedrest for acute low back pain? A randomized clinical trial. N Engl J Med 1986;315:1064–70.

46. Berry H, Bloom B, Hamilton EBD, et al. Naproxen sodium, diflunisal and placebo in the treatment of chronic back pain. Ann Rheum Dis 1982;41: 122–32.

47. Deyo RA, Walsh NE, Martin DC, et al. A controlled trial of transcutaneous electrical nerve stimulation (TENS) and exercise for chronic low back pain. N Engl J Med 1990;322:1627–34.

48. Kendall PH, Jenkins JM. Exercises for backache: a double blind controlled trial. Physiotherapy 1968;54:154–9.

49. Williams PC. Lesions of lumbo-sacral spine. Part 2. J Bone Joint Surg 1937; 19:690–703.

50. McKenzie RA. Prophylaxis in recurrent low back pain. N Z Med J 1979; 89:22–23.

51. Elnaggar IM, Nordin M, Sheikhzadeh A, et al. Effects of spinal flexion and extension exercises on low back pain and spinal mobility in chronic mechanical low-back pain patients. Spine 1991;16:967–72.

52. Jackson CP, Brown MD. Analysis of current approaches a practical guide to prescription of exercise. Clin Orthop 1983;179:46–54.

53. Cady LD, Bischoff DP. Strength and fitness and subsequent back injuries in firefighters. J Occup Med 1979;21:269–73.

54. Berquist-Ullman M, Larsson U. Acute low back pain in industry: a controlled prospective study with special reference to therapy and confounding factors. Acta Orthop Scand Suppl 1977;170:1–117.

55. Hall H, Iceton JA. Back school: an overview with specific reference to the Canadian back education units. Clin Orthop 1983;179:10–17.

56. Stankovic R, Johnell O. Conservative treatment of acute low back pain. Spine 1990;15:120–3.

57. Klaber-Moffett JA, Chase SM, Portek I, Ennis JR. A controlled prospective study to evaluate the effectiveness of a back school in the relief of chronic low back pain. Spine 1986;11:120–2.

58. Abramovitz JN, Neff SR. Lumbar disc surgery: results of the prospective lumbar discectomy study. Neurosurgery 1991;29:301–8.

59. Kambin P, Schaffer JL. Percutaneous lumbar discectomy: review of 100 patients in current practice. Clin Orthop 1989;238:24–34.

60. Muralikuttan KP, Hamilton A, Kernohan WS, et al. A prospective randomized trial of chemonucleolysis and conventional disc surgery. Spine 1992;17: 381–7.

61. Herkowitz HN. Current status of percutaneous discectomy and chemonucleolysis. Orthop Clin North Am 1991;22:327–32.

62. Hult L. The Munkfors investigation. Acta Orthop Scand Suppl 1959;16:1–16.

63. Kelsey JL, Githens PB, Walter SD, et al. An epidemiological study of acute prolapsed cervical intervertebral disc. J Bone Joint Surg [Am] 1984;66:907–14.

64. Dillin W, Booth R, Cuckler J, et al. Cervical radiculopathy: a review. Spine 1986;11:988–91.

65. Lestini WF, Wiesel SW. The pathogenesis of cervical spondylosis. Clin Orthop 1989;239:69–93.

66. Clark CR. Degenerative conditions of the spine. In: Frymoyer JW, editor. The adult spine: principles and practice. New York: Raven Press, 1991:1145–64.
67. Murphy MJ, Lieponis JV. Non-operative treatment of cervical spine pain. In: Sherk HH, editor. The cervical spine. Philadelphia: Lippincott, 1989:670–7.
68. Jahnke RW, Hart BL. Cervical stenosis, spondylosis, and herniated disc disease. Radiol Clin North Am 1991;29:777–91.
69. Russell EJ. Cervical disk disease. Radiology 1990;177:313–25.
70. La Rocca H. Cervical spondylotic myelopathy: natural history. Spine 1988;13:854–5.
71. White AA III, Panjabi MM. Biomechanical considerations in the surgical management of cervical spondylotic myelopathy. Spine 1988;13:856–69.
72. Hirsch SA, Hirsch PJ, Hiramoto H, Weiss A. Whiplash syndrome: fact or fiction? Orthop Clin North Am 1988;19:791–5.

CASE PRESENTATION

Subjective

PATIENT PROFILE

Andrew Harris is a 27-year-old white male married truck driver.

PRESENTING PROBLEM

"Back strain."

PRESENT ILLNESS

Mr. Harris describes a 4-day history of low back pain that began when he lifted a heavy box while unloading his truck. The pain occasionally radiates to the right leg and foot. He has difficulty walking and is unable to work despite 3 days of rest.

PAST MEDICAL HISTORY

He has had several episodes of back strain over the past 5 years, but none as severe as the current illness.

SOCIAL HISTORY

Mr. Harris has been employed by a national freight line for 8 years. He lives with his wife and their two young children.

HABITS

He uses no alcohol, tobacco, or recreational drugs. He drinks four cups of coffee daily.

FAMILY HISTORY

His father had surgery for prostate enlargement 2 years ago and is now living and well at age 61. His mother died at age 60 of a stroke. There is one 32-year-old brother who has had lumbar disc surgery.

REVIEW OF SYSTEMS

Andrew has an occasional tension headache and some pain in his shoulders and knees during cold damp weather.

- Discuss the possible reasons for Mr. Harris' visit today.
- What additional historical information might be useful? Why?
- What more would you like to know about the previous instances of back strain?
- What further information about the patient's job might be useful? Explain.

Objective

VITAL SIGNS

Height, 5 ft 10 in; weight, 232 lb; blood pressure, 140/84; pulse, 74.

EXAMINATION

The patient is ambulatory but moves carefully owing to low back pain. He has difficulty climbing onto the examination table. There is mild tenderness of the lumbosacral spine with adjacent right paraspinal muscle tenderness. Straight leg raising is positive on the right but not on the left. Deep tendon reflexes are +2 and symmetrical. There is decreased perception of pinprick on the lateral right lower leg and foot.

- What further information obtained from the physical examination might be helpful? Why?
- What is the relationship of the patient's weight to his ideal weight and height?
- What—if any—diagnostic maneuvers might help clarify the problem?
- What—if any—diagnostic imaging would you obtain today?

Assessment

- Describe your diagnosis. What is the likely anatomical cause?
- How will you explain your assessment to Mr. Harris?
- What might be the meaning of this illness to the patient? How would you ask about this concern?

- What is the potential economic impact of this illness on the family? How would you address this issue?

Plan

- What would be your therapeutic recommendation? How would you explain this to the patient?
- What would you advise regarding Mr. Harris's weight? How might you persuade him to lose weight?
- Is a subspecialist consultation appropriate at this time? If so, how would you explain this to the patient?
- What follow-up would you plan for Mr. Harris?

18
Osteoarthritis

JOHN B. MURPHY AND ELISE M. COLETTA

Osteoarthritis (OA) is a condition that is best defined by its characteristics. A definition that is widely accepted was developed at a National Institutes of Health workshop on the etiopathogenesis of OA.[1]

OA (osteoarthrosis, degenerative joint disease) is a degenerative disease of the cartilage of joints. It is of diverse etiology and obscure pathogenesis. *Clinically,* the disease is characterized by joint pain, tenderness, limitations of movement, crepitus, occasional effusion, and variable degrees of local inflammation, but without systemic effects. *Pathologically,* the disease is characterized by irregularly distributed loss of cartilage, more frequent in the areas of increased load, sclerosis of subchondral bone, subchondral cysts, marginal osteophytes, increased metaphyseal blood flow, and variable synovial inflammation. *Histologically,* the disease is characterized early by fragmentation of the cartilage surface, cloning of chondrocytes, vertical clefts in the cartilage, variable crystal deposition, remodeling, and eventual violation of the tidemark of blood vessels. It is also characterized by evidence of repair, particularly in osteophytes and later by total loss of cartilage, sclerosis, and focal osteonecrosis of the subchondral bone. *Biomechanically,* the disease is characterized by alterations of the tensile, compressive, and shear properties and hydraulic permeability of the cartilage; increased water; and excessive swelling. These cartilage changes are accompanied by increased stiffness of the subchondral bone. *Biochemically,* the disease is characterized by reduction in the proteoglycan concentration, possible alterations in the size and aggregation of the proteoglycans, alterations in collagen fibril size and weave, and increase synthesis and degradation of matrix macromolecules. *Therapeutically,* the disease is characterized by a lack of a specific healing agent.

Epidemiology

OA is the most common joint condition affecting humans.[2] It is the third most common principal diagnosis recorded by family practitioners for office visits made by older patients, and it is in the top 20 primary diagnoses for office visits to family physicians made by patients of all ages.[3]

Population-based studies of OA demonstrate that the prevalence of radiographic OA is much higher than is symptomatic OA and that there is a progressive increase in the prevalence of OA with advancing age.[4,5] The prevalence of symptomatic OA is about 2% for women younger than age 45, 30% for women age 45 to 64, and 68% for women 65 and older.[6] In general, the figures are similar for men, although slightly lower in the upper two age groups.

It has been estimated that OA is second only to ischemic heart disease as a cause of work-related disability among persons older than 50 years of age and that 80% of individuals with OA report some limitation of activity, with 25% of these individuals being unable to perform a major daily activity.[7] OA results in more hospitalizations and longer hospital stays than does rheumatoid arthritis, and it is the major contributor to the estimated $4 billion spent annually in the United States for total joint replacements.[8]

Beyond age, there are only a few well-documented risk factors for OA. They include major trauma, chronic excess body weight, and heredity with certain forms of OA.[9–12] There is also a growing body of evidence that certain occupational groups (e.g., older men and women in laboring professions) are at increased risk of OA. The role of more subtle forms of trauma and the evidence that participation in certain sports increases the risk of developing OA is much less clear. Further research is needed to clarify these associations.[2]

Pathophysiology

Normal articular cartilage serves two essential mechanical functions. The first is to provide a smooth weight-bearing surface that allows bones to articulate with a minimum of friction. The second is to efficiently transmit load to subchondral bone. Articular cartilage is made up of water (70%), cells (chondrocytes), and a matrix composed of primarily two macromolecules: proteoglycans and collagen. Proteoglycans provide elasticity and stiffness on compression, whereas collagen (primarily type II collagen) provides tensile strength. The integrity of this cartilage matrix is maintained by the chondrocytes.

The pathologic and biochemical changes found in OA cartilage appear to be mediated by complex remodeling interactions between chondrocytes, the matrix, cytokines, growth factors, other inflammatory mediators, the synovium, and mechanical factors. The precise mechanism of these interactions is not fully understood, but the net result includes increasing water content and disorganization of the cartilage matrix. As the disease advances, disorganization gives way to erosion and ulceration. During the later stages of the disease, degradation exceeds repair, and cartilage is irreversibly destroyed. As the cartilage degenerates, joint stresses are increasingly transmitted to the underlying bone, thereby initiating the bony remodeling process consisting of subchondral sclerosis, subchondral cysts, and marginal osteophytes.

Although age is highly associated with OA, it is not thought that OA is an inevitable consequence of aging. OA is much more common with advancing age, but the changes seen in OA cartilage are clearly distinct from those seen with normal aging.[13]

Classification

There is increasing consensus that OA is not a single disease entity but that the observed clinical pattern represents a "final common pathway" for several conditions of diverse etiologies.[14] Until further research elucidates these etiologies, OA has been and will continue to be classified in two major categories: primary (idiopathic) and secondary.[15] Interested readers are referred to the classification scheme developed by the American College of Rheumatology.[15]

Clinical Presentation and Diagnosis

Symptoms

OA is generally a monarticular or oligoarticular disease. Commonly affected joints and joints that are usually spared are listed in Table 18.1.

Early in the symptomatic phase of OA, pain occurs with motion, particularly with weight-bearing, and is relieved by rest. As the disease progresses, pain can occur with minimal motion and even at rest. The pain is often described as a deep aching discomfort, that except in the case of hip OA is localized to the joint. Pain associated with OA of the *hip* is often localized to the anterior inguinal region or to the medial or lateral thigh regions. The pain of hip OA may also radiate, or present in, the buttock, the anterior aspect of the thigh just above the knee, or the knee itself. The pain associated with OA of the *spine* is usually localized, but radicular symptoms may also occur. The discomfort of cervical spine OA may radiate to the supraclavicular and upper trapezius regions as well as to the occiput and the distal upper extremity. In addition to radicular pain, nerve root compression (caused by osteophytic spurs or degeneration of intervertebral discs with protrusion of the nucleus pulposus) may cause paresthesias and muscle weakness. Rarely, large anterior osteophytes in the cervical region can cause dysphagia.

TABLE 18.1. Clinical features of osteoarthritis

Monarticular or oligoarticular joints involved
DIP, PIP, first CMC (thumb)
Knee, hip, first MTP
Lumbosacral and cervical spine
Acromioclavicular, subtalar
Sacroiliac, temporomandibular

Joints spared
MCP, wrist, elbow, shoulder

Symptoms
Pain (primarily with weight-bearing and motion; rest pain is a
　late finding)
Stiffness of <30 minutes' duration after rest
Paresthesias and weakness (secondary to nerve root
　impingement in OA of spine)

Signs
Heberden's/Bouchard's nodes
Gelatinous cysts (dorsal aspect or DIP joint)
Marginal bony overgrowth (knees)
Decreased joint range of motion
Joint crepitance
Joint effusion
Varus joint angulation (knee)
Motor weakness (spinal OA)
Diminished reflexes (spinal OA)
Antalgic gait
Joint instability
Muscle atrophy

CMC = carpometacarpal; MTP = metatarsophalangeal; MCP =
metacarpophalangeal; DIP = distal interphalangeal; PIP = proximal
interphalangeal.

Although *joint* stiffness can occur, it is usually of short duration
(<30 minutes). There is also an absence of systemic symptoms such as
fatigue, weight loss, and fever.

It is not unusual for the symptoms of OA to go unmentioned by an older
patient. Patients and families frequently and incorrectly accept pain, stiffness, and disability as normal consequences of aging. Functional assessment can serve as a valuable aid to diagnosis in that it may detect
functional impairment (i.e., disability) caused by previously unrecognized
OA. A standard functional assessment should include activities of daily
living (ADLs), instrumental activities of daily living (IADLs), and some
measure of mobility.[16,17] ADLs are self-care skills necessary to remain safely
in the home: bathing, dressing, toileting, transferring, feeding, and continence (bowel and bladder). IADLs are higher level skills required for

successful living in the community: shopping, transportation, doing laundry and housework, preparing a light meal, managing finances, using a telephone, and taking medications.

Signs

Physical examination of an affected joint may show decreased range of motion, joint deformity, bony hypertrophy, and occasionally an intra-articular effusion. Crepitance, pain on passive and active movement, and mild tenderness may be found. Evidence of inflammatory changes are usually absent. During late stages, there may be demonstrable joint instability. Table 18.1 lists the physical findings associated with OA.

Heberden's nodes represent cartilaginous and bony enlargement of the dorsolateral and dorsomedial aspects of the distal interphalangeal (DIP) joints. Bouchard's nodes are similar findings at the proximal interphalangeal joints. Heberden's nodes may have a soft consistency and can present acutely with signs of inflammation. However, they more often develop gradually with little or no pain or inflammatory signs. Gelatinous cysts sometimes develop over the dorsal aspect of the DIP joints. These cysts, which are often attached to tendon sheaths, may resolve spontaneously or persist indefinitely.

Quadriceps muscle atrophy, marginal bony overgrowth, joint crepitance, effusion, and mediolateral joint instability (in late stages) are all possible physical findings in OA of the knee. Limitation of joint motion, initially with extension, may be found with active and passive motion. Varus angulation can also develop as a result of degenerative cartilage changes, which are more prominent in the medial compartment of the knee.

The patient with OA of the hip often holds the hip adducted, flexed, and internally rotated, which may result in functional shortening of the leg and the characteristic limp (antalgic gait). Invariably, some degree of limitation in motion can be found with OA of the hip, usually with loss of full extension and internal rotation.

OA of the spine may be associated with limited range of motion and muscle spasm. Nerve root compression can result in motor weakness as well as diminution of reflexes in the distribution of the involved root.

Laboratory Findings

There are no specific laboratory tests for OA. Unlike the inflammatory arthritides (e.g., rheumatoid arthritis), the erythrocyte sedimentation rate and hemogram are normal, and autoantibodies are not present. If there is a joint effusion, the synovial fluid is noninflammatory, with fewer than 2000/mm^3 white blood cells (WBCs), a predominance of mononuclear WBCs, and a good mucin clot. The diagnosis of OA is usually based on

TABLE 18.2. Laboratory and
radiologic assessment of OA

Laboratory tests
Normal erythrocyte sedimentation rate
Normal hemogram
Negative rheumatoid factor
Negative antinuclear antibody
Radiologic findings
Narrowing of joint space
Subchondral bony sclerosis
Subchondral cysts
Marginal osteophyte formation

clinical and radiologic features, with the laboratory assessment being use-ful for excluding other arthritic conditions or secondary causes of OA.

Radiographic Features

During the early stages of OA, radiographs may be normal. Joint space narrowing becomes evident as articular cartilage is lost. Subchondral bony sclerosis (eburnation) appears radiographically as increased bone density. Subchondral bone cysts develop and vary in size from several millimeters to several centimeters; they appear as translucent areas in periarticular bone. Bony deformity and joint subluxation, as well as loose bodies, may be seen in advanced cases. Marginal osteophyte formation is seen as a result of bone proliferation. Although the presence of osteophytes is seen with OA, this feature alone is not thought to be sufficient for the diagnosis of OA, as osteophytes can occur with aging alone (in the absence of OA).

The newer imaging modalities—computed tomography, magnetic reso-nance imaging, and ultrasonography—are potentially powerful tools for the assessment of OA; however, diagnosis rarely requires such expensive modalities. Tables 18.1 and 18.2 outline the clinical, laboratory, and radiologic characteristics of OA.

Management

The management of OA should focus on pain relief, prevention of progressive joint damage, and maximization of functional ability. Nonpharmacologic, pharmacologic, and surgical interventions play important roles in the man-agement of patients with OA. Ongoing functional assessment—using one of the many tools developed specifically for monitoring OA or the standard components of functional assessment—is important to the care of the patient with OA.[18] Such a functional approach is particularly important when assessing the effectiveness of treatment interventions and for monitoring the progress of the disease.

Nonpharmacologic Management

Nonpharmacologic management strategies for OA include limited periods (1–2 hours) of rest when symptoms are at their worst, avoidance of repetitive movements or static body positions that aggravate symptoms, joint preservation techniques, heat (or cold) for the control of pain, weight loss if the patient is obese, adaptive mobility aids to diminish the mechanical load on joints, adaptive equipment to assist in ADL skills, range of motion exercises, strengthening exercises, and endurance exercises.[19–21] Immobilization should be avoided because of the deleterious effects on muscle strength, exercise capacity, and joint range of motion with the associated risk of contracture development.

The use of adaptive mobility aids (e.g., canes, walkers) is an important strategy, but care should be taken to ensure that the mobility aid is the correct device, appropriately sized, and in good repair. In addition, the patient should be instructed in the correct use of the adaptive mobility aid. For OA of the hip, when a cane is used it should be carried in the contralateral hand and advanced at the same time as the affected extremity. The heel of the hand, resting on the top of the cane, should be at the level of the greater trochanter, resulting in elbow flexion of roughly 25 degrees. When an adaptive mobility aid is not properly sized and appropriately used, it can increase joint stress and pain as well as become a hazard that precipitates a fall.

Pharmacologic Management

Pharmacologic approaches to the treatment of OA (Table 18.3) include acetaminophen, salicylates, nonsteroidal antiinflammatory drugs (NSAIDs), and intraarticular steroids. Acetaminophen is advocated for use as a first-line therapy by some authors based on clinical experience and short-term intervention studies.[22] Salicylates and NSAIDs are, however, still the most commonly used first-line medications for the relief of pain related to OA. Intraarticular steroids are generally reserved for the occasional instance when there is a single painful joint or a large effusion in a single joint, and the pain is unresponsive to other modalities. Systemic steroids and narcotics should be avoided if possible.

Salicylates and NSAIDs have analgesic and antiinflammatory effects, probably because they act to inhibit prostaglandin synthesis. Toxic side effects, many of which are thought to be related to inhibition of prostaglandin synthesis, involve several organ systems, are usually reversible after drug withdrawal, and can be severe. The most common adverse effects encountered with salicylates, NSAIDs, and nonacetylated salicylates are listed in Table 18.4. In addition to the adverse effects of salicylates, compliance can be a major problem, given the drugs' short duration of action and the need for frequent dosing, which is one of the reasons NSAIDs are preferred to salicylates.

Many NSAIDs are available, and most are relatively expensive. Because an individual patient's response to one drug is not predictive of the therapeutic response to other agents, it is often necessary to try several drugs before optimal therapy is obtained. With the exception of phenylbutazone (which should be avoided) and perhaps indomethacin (which has a slightly higher incidence of side effects), there is little compelling evidence for choosing one NSAID over another as initial therapy. Misoprostol, a prostaglandin E analog, has been shown to reduce the incidence of gastric ulceration in some patients taking NSAIDs. However, misoprostol is expensive and is not necessary as a routine measure when starting a patient on NSAIDs.

The nonacetylated salicylate preparations are less potent inhibitors of prostaglandins and, as such, are thought to have less gastrointestinal and

TABLE 18.3. Medications for OA

Drug	Dosage range and frequency
Acetaminophen	650 mg q4h *or* 1000 mg q6h
Salicylates	
Aspirin	650 mg q4h
Aspirin, extended release	1600 mg bid
Nonacetylated salicylates	
Choline magnesium trisalicylate (Trilisate)	2–3 g in 1–2 doses/day
Salsalate (Disalcid)	3 g in 2–3 doses/day
NSAIDs	
Acetic acid	
Diclofenac (Voltaren)	75–100 mg bid
Toletin (Tolectin)	200–400 mg tid–qid
Anthranilic acid	
Meclofenamate (Meclomen)	200–400 in 3–4 doses/day
Indoleacetic acid	
Indomethacin (Indocin)	50–200 in 3 doses/day
Sulindac (Clinoril)	300–400 in 2 doses/day
Propionic acid	
Ibuprofen (Motrin)	1.2–3.2 g in 3–4 doses/day
Naproxen (Naprosyn)	500–750 mg in 2 doses/day
Oxicam	
Piroxicam (Feldene)	20 mg in 1–2 doses/day

Table 18.4. Adverse effects of drugs for OA

Drug class	Adverse effects
Salicylates	Dyspepsia, gastrointestinal toxicity Interference with platelet function Tinnitus Hepatitis and renal damage (both rare) Interacts with oral anticoagulants
NSAIDs	Dyspepsia and gastrointestinal toxicity, including bleeding, ulceration, perforation, diarrhea (Meclomen) Interference with platelet function Decreased renal blood flow, fluid retention, renal failure, renal papillary necrosis, interstitial nephritis, nephrotic syndrome Dizziness, anxiety, drowsiness, tinnitus, confusion Mild hepatic dysfunction, rarely hepatitis Aplastic anemia (rare except with phenylbutazone)
Nonacetylated salicylates	Do not affect platelet function Interfere with oral anticoagulants

renal toxicity than do NSAIDs. The nonacetylated salicylates are also thought to have the advantage of not impairing platelet function. Unfortunately, some authorities note that they are not as efficacious in the treatment of OA pain as are salicylates and NSAIDs.[23]

Surgical Management

Arthroscopic lavage and osteotomy are surgical approaches that have been used to decrease the pain of OA of the knee. However, total joint replacement is the primary surgical approach for OA of the knee and hip. Candidates for arthroplasty are individuals with severe pain, impaired joint function, or those who have experienced declines in functional status that do not improve with nonpharmacologic and pharmacologic measures.

The orthopedic surgeon plays the primary role in surgical management of the patient with OA, but the family physician retains a significant role in perioperative management. An important preoperative concern for the patient undergoing hip or knee surgery is the risk of deep vein thrombosis. In this regard, successful prophylactic regimens have included low-dose warfarin, adjusted-dose subcutaneous heparin, and, more recently, low-molecular-weight heparin.[24,25] The latter may prove to be the most efficacious, especially when combined with gradient compression stockings.[25] However, the use of low-molecular-weight heparin does appear to be associated with a small added risk of significant bleeding.[25] Nonpharmacologic methods (compression stockings, external pneumatic compression boots) may be useful in patients who cannot be anticoagulated and may confer additional protection when used as an adjunct to the pharmacologic methods discussed above.[24] Postoperatively, the orthopedic surgeon, family physician, physical therapist, and, as necessary, occupational therapist should work together to develop a rehabilitation program. Physical therapists can also provide valuable assistance in preoperative preparation of the patient with OA through stretching exercises and positioning programs to prevent or reduce contracture and muscle strengthening exercises to prevent or reduce muscle atrophy.

Family Issues

OA should be considered a condition that affects the entire family. The costs of treatment for OA can be substantial, and the direct costs for drug therapy (which can easily exceed $60 per month) are not the only costs to the patient and the family.[23] OA can result in lost income related to time spent on physician and physical therapy visits, disability-related work absences, and absences related to surgery. OA can preclude an individual from performing his or her previous occupation; hence, vocational rehabilitation should be considered an important component of OA management. Not uncommonly, the pain and functional disability associated with OA can contribute to social isolation and depression, which affects the family as well as the patient and obviously requires appropriate treatment.

Sexual intercourse can become difficult and painful, thereby adding to family stress. Sexuality is an often neglected aspect of care and should be dealt with openly. Suggestions for adaptive measures to improve sexual function include exercise to increase mobility, use of heat (e.g., shower or tub) before sexual activity, avoidance of positions that prolong pressure on involved joints, experimentation with adaptive positions, premedication with analgesic/antiinflammatory medications, use of a water bed, a period of rest before sexual activity, and alternatives to intercourse such as masturbation and oral sex.[26]

A valuable resource for patients and families is the Arthritis Foundation, which has local chapters throughout the United States. This foundation not only conducts research on the prevention and treatment of arthritis but, more important, provides services and education for patients and families with arthritis. Emphasis should be placed on educating the patient and family with OA.

Prevention

Attempts at primary prevention of OA appear feasible with our current knowledge base.[27] Potentially modifiable risk factors include obesity, mechanical stress/repetitive joint usage, and joint trauma.[10] Weight reduction, avoidance of traumatic injury, prompt treatment of injury, and work site programs designed to minimize work-related mechanical joint stress may be effective interventions for preventing OA. Early treatment of congenital and developmental disorders known to be associated with the development of secondary OA have the potential of preventing OA. Another approach to primary prevention is prescription of an appropriate exercise program, performed regularly, to maintain joint range of motion and muscle strength, thereby minimizing abnormal joint stresses.

For secondary prevention, screening for decrements in physical functional status using historical screening data such as ADLs, IADLs, and mobility questionnaires as well as using physical performance measures such as the "get up and go test" has the potential for identifying undiagnosed, but treatable, conditions such as OA.[16,17,28,29] The "get up and go test" is a simple maneuver in which a patient rises from a chair, walks 3 meters, turns, walks back to the chair and sits down.[30] Tertiary prevention includes the prescription of appropriate adaptive equipment and mobility aids to reduce disability in the patient with known osteoarthritis.

References

1. Mankin HJ, Brandt KD, Shulman LE. Workshop on etiopathogenesis of osteoarthritis. J Rheumatol 1986;13:1130–60.
2. Felson D. Epidemiology of rheumatic disease: osteoarthritis. Rheum Dis Clin North Am 1990;16:499–512.
3. Facts about family practice. Kansas City, MO: American Academy of Family Physicians, 1987:30–37.
4. Lawrence RC, Hochberg MC, Kelsey JL, et al. Estimates of the prevalence of selected arthritic and musculoskeletal diseases in the United States. J Rheumatol 1989;16:427–41.
5. Croft P. Review of UK data on the rheumatic diseases: osteoarthritis. Br J Rheumatol 1990;29:391–5.
6. Brandt KD. Osteoarthritis. Clin Geriatr Med 1988;4:279–93.
7. Wilson MG, Michet CJ Jr, Ilstrup DM, Melton LJ III. Idiopathic symptomatic osteoarthritis of the hip and knee: a population based study. Mayo Clin Proc 1990;65:1214–21.
8. Felts W, Yellin E. The economic impact of the rheumatic diseases in the United States. J Rheumatol 1989;16:867–84.
9. Hartz AJ, Fischer ME, Bril G, et al. The association of obesity with joint pain and osteoarthritis in the HANES data. J Chronic Dis 1986;39:311–9.
10. Felson DT, Anderson JJ, Naimark A, et al. Obesity and knee osteoarthritis: the Framingham study. Ann Intern Med 1988;109:18–24.
11. Mankin HJ. Clinical features of osteoarthritis. In: Kelley WN, Harris ED Jr, Ruddy S, Sledge C, editors. Textbook of rheumatology. 3rd ed. Philadelphia: Saunders, 1989:1480–500.
12. Hochberg MC. Epidemiology of osteoarthritis: current concepts and new insights. J Rheumatol 1991;27(Suppl):4–6.

13. Hamerman D. The biology of osteoarthritis. N Engl J Med 1989;320:1322–30.
14. Ettinger WH, Maradee AD. Osteoarthritis. In: Hazzard WR, Andres R, Bierman EL, Blass JP, editors. Principles of geriatric medicine and gerontology, 2nd ed. New York: McGraw-Hill, 1990:880–8.
15. Altman RD. Classification of disease: osteoarthritis. Semin Arthritis Rheum 1991;20(Suppl):40–47.
16. Katz S, Ford AB, Moskowitz RW, Jackson BA, Jaffe MW. Studies of illness in the aged; the index of ADL: a standardized measure of biological and psychosocial function. JAMA 1963;185:914–9.
17. Lawton MP, Brody EM. Assessment of older people: self-maintaining and instrumental activities of daily living. Gerontologist 1969;9:179–86.
18. Laquesne M. Indices of severity and disease activity for osteoarthritis. Semin Arthritis Rheum 1991;20:48–54.
19. Dunning RD, Materson RS. A rational program of exercise for patients with osteoarthritis. Semin Arthritis Rheum 1991;21(Suppl2):33–43.
20. Kovar PA, Allegrante JP, MacKenzie CR, et al. Supervised fitness walking in patients with osteoarthritis of the knee: a randomized controlled trial. Ann Intern Med 1992;116:529–34.
21. Puett DW, Griffin MR. Published trials of nonmedicinal and noninvasive therapies for hip and knee osteoarthritis. Ann Intern Med 1994;121:133–40.
22. Bradley J, Brandt K, Katz B, et al. Comparison of an inflammatory dose of ibuprofen, an analgesic dose of ibuprofen and acetaminophen in the treatment of patients with osteoarthritis. N Engl J Med 1991;325:87–91.
23. Drugs for rheumatoid arthritis. Med Lett 1991;33:65–70.
24. King MS. Preventing deep venous thrombosis in hospitalized patients. Am Fam Pract 1994;49(6):1389–96.
25. Imperiale TF, Speroff T. A meta-analysis of methods to prevent venous thrombolism following total hip replacement. JAMA 1994;271(22):1780–5.
26. Laflin M. Sexuality and the elderly. In: Lewis CB, editor. Aging: the health care challenge. Philadelphia: Davis, 1985:293–309.
27. Peyron JG. Is osteoarthritis a preventable disease? J Rheumatol 1991;18 (Suppl27):2–3.
28. Tinetti ME, Ginter SF. Identifying mobility dysfunction in elderly patients. JAMA 1988;259:1190–3.
29. Lachs M, Feinstein A, Cooney L, et al. A simple procedure for general screening for functional disability in elderly patients. Ann Intern Med 1990;112:699–706.
30. Mathias S, Nayak USL, Isaacs B. Balance in the elderly: the "get-up and go" test. Arch Phys Med Rehabil 1986;67:387–9.

CASE PRESENTATION

Subjective

PATIENT PROFILE

Harold Nelson is a 76-year-old married white male retired welder.

PRESENTING PROBLEM

"My knees and hands hurt."

PRESENT ILLNESS

Mr. Nelson has a 20-year history of "arthritis" involving multiple joints, especially the hands and knees. The symptoms seem worse for the past 6 to 8 weeks, especially since the weather turned cold and snowy. He currently takes six to eight aspirin a day but is afraid to use other medication because of his diabetes, especially since he had an episode of incontinence after taking an over-the-counter cold remedy in the past.

PAST MEDICAL HISTORY, SOCIAL HISTORY, HABITS, AND FAMILY HISTORY

These are all unchanged since his previous visit 7 months ago (see Chapter 5).

REVIEW OF SYSTEMS

Mild constipation present for the past 4 to 6 weeks.

- What additional historical data might be useful? Why?
- What might be causing the increasing joint pain, and how would you inquire about these possibilities?
- What more would you like to know about his constipation? Why might this be significant?
- What might Mr. Nelson be doing differently because of his joint pain? How would you address this issue?

Objective

VITAL SIGNS

Height 5 ft 7 in; weight, 166 lb (This is a 10-lb weight gain in the past 7 months); blood pressure, 152/82; pulse, 72; temperature, 37.2°C.

EXAMINATION

There are Heberden's nodes of the distal joints of the fingers. There is a knobby deformity of multiple joints of the hands, wrists, and knees. The involved joints are not hot, but grip strength is decreased and the knees lack about 10 degrees of flexion and extension. The low back is not tender, and no muscle spasm is present. He lacks about 20 degrees of flexion at the waist.

LABORATORY

A blood glucose test performed in the office reveals a level of 110 mg/dl.

- What—if any—additional information might be derived from the physical examination? Why?
- What other areas of the body should be examined? Why?
- What—if any—laboratory determinations should be ordered today?
- What—if any—diagnostic imaging should be obtained?

Assessment

- What is your diagnostic assessment? How would you describe this to the patient?
- What might be the significance of the weight gain over the past 7 months?
- What might be the meaning of the joint pain to the patient? How would you ask about this?
- What would be your thoughts if the patient developed warm swollen tender joints? What would you do differently?

Plan

- What would be your therapeutic recommendation today? How would you explain this to Mr. Nelson?
- How would you approach the patient's concern about medication use?
- What life-style and activity recommendations would you make today?
- What continuing care would you advise?

19
Common Dermatoses

DANIEL J. VAN DURME

Acne

Acne is the most common dermatologic condition presenting to the family physician's office. It is usually found in patients between the ages of 12 and 25, with about 85% of teenagers affected.[1] It can present with a wide range of severity and may be the source of significant emotional, psychological, and physical scars. As teenagers develop their self-image, the physical appearance of the skin can be critically important. Despite excellent medical treatments for this disorder, many patients (and their parents) view acne as a normal part of development and do not seek treatment. The importance of early treatment to prevent the physical and emotional scars cannot be overemphasized.

It is important to understand the pathogenesis of acne as most treatments are not curative but, rather, are directed at disrupting selected aspects of development. Acne begins with abnormalities in the pilosebaceous unit. There are four key elements involved in its development: (1) keratinization abnormalities; (2) increased sebum production; (3) bacterial proliferation; and (4) inflammation. Each may play a greater or lesser role, depending on the type of acne. Initially, there is an abnormality of keratinization. Cohesive hyperkeratosis causes blocking of the follicular canal and the development of a microcomedo. This blocked canal leads to a buildup of sebum behind the plug. Sebum production can be increased by androgens and other factors as well.

This plugged pilosebaceous unit is seen as a closed comedone ("whitehead") or as an open comedone ("blackhead") when the pore dilates and the fatty acids in the sebaceous plug become oxidized. The normal bacterial flora of the skin, especially *Proprionibacterium acnes,* proliferate in this plug and release chemotactic factors, drawing in leukocytes. The plug may cause rupture of the unit under the skin, also causing an influx of leukocytes. The resulting inflammation leads to the development of papulopustular acne. This process can be marked and accompanied by hypertrophy of the entire pilosebaceous unit leading to nodules and cyst formation.

Diagnosis

Diagnosis is straightforward and is based on the finding of comedones, papules, pustules, nodules, and cysts primarily on the face, back, shoulders, and chest. The presence of comedones is considered necessary for the diagnosis of acne vulgaris. Without comedones, one must consider rosacea, steroid acne, or other acneiform dermatoses. It is important for both choice of therapy and long-term follow-up to describe and classify the patients appropriately. One should note the quantity *and* the type of lesions. The number of lesions indicate whether the acne is mild, moderate, severe, or very severe (sometimes referred to as grades I–IV). The predominant type of lesion should also be noted (i.e., comedonal, papular, pustular, nodular, cystic). Thus a patient with hundreds of comedones on the face may have "very severe comedonal acne," and another patient may have only a few nodules and cysts and have "mild nodulocystic acne."[2]

Management

Before pharmacologic management, it is important to review and dispel some of the misperceptions about acne held by many patients. For example, acne is not due to poor hygiene, and aggressive and frequent scrubbing of the skin may actually aggravate the condition. Mild soaps should be used regularly, and the face should be washed gently and dried well before the application of topical medication. Several studies have also failed to implicate diet as a significant contributor to acne,[3,4] and fatty foods and chocolates are not causative agents.

All patients should be taught that acne can be suppressed or controlled when medicines are used regularly but that initial therapy takes several weeks to show its effects. As the current lesions heal, the medications work to prevent the eruption of further lesions. Response to medication is typically seen in about 6 weeks.

The treatment options for acne should be based on the patient and the classification of the acne. Benzoyl peroxide serves as the foundation of most acne therapy. This bacteriostatic agent is available as cleansing liquids and bars and as gels or creams, with strengths ranging from 2.5% to 10.0%. The increase in strength increases the drying (and often irritation) of the skin; it does not provide additional antibacterial activity. This medication is used once or twice daily as basic therapy in most patients.

As all acne starts with some degree of keratinization abnormalities and microcomedone formation, it is also prudent to start with a comedolytic agent. Currently, the most effective agent is tretinoin (Retin-A). It should be started at the lowest dose possible (0.025% cream) and applied nightly. Mild erythema and irritation are common at first; if this reaction is severe, the frequency of application can be decreased to three times per week. The strength can be gradually increased as needed and as tolerated over several months. Patients should be warned about photosensitivity. If benzoyl peroxide is also used, it is crucial to separate the application of these compounds by several hours. When applied together, they can greatly increase the amount of irritation to the skin while inactivating each other, rendering treatment ineffective.

Antibiotics are recommended for papulopustular acne. They act by decreasing the proliferation of *P. acnes* and particularly by inactivating the neutrophil chemotactic factors released during the inflammatory process.[5] Topical agents include erythromycin, clindamycin, tetracycline, and meclocycline. These agents are available in a variety of delivery vehicles and are applied once (sometimes twice) a day in conjunction with benzoyl peroxide. Oral antibiotics are indicated in patients with severe or widespread papulopustular acne and in patients with difficulty reaching the affected areas on their body (i.e., on the back). Tetracycline and erythromycin are the most common agents used and should be started at 1 g/day in divided doses. Tetracycline patients must be warned of photosensitivity and are advised to take the medicine on an empty stomach, without dairy products. Erythromycin patients should be warned of potential gastrointestinal upset. Other options include minocycline, doxycycline, and occasionally trimethoprim-sulfamethoxazole. As the acne improves, the dose of the oral medications can often be gradually decreased to about one-half the original dose for long-term maintenance therapy.

Severe nodulocystic acne requires initial therapy with benzoyl peroxide, tretinoin, and antibiotics. If these agents fail to adequately control the acne, 13-*cis*-retinoic acid (Accutane) may be used. This agent has been highly effective in shrinking the hypertrophied sebaceous glands of nodulocystic acne. In most patients, it induces a "remission" for many months or may cure the condition. If lesions remain, they are more susceptible to conventional therapy. Treatment is a 16- to 20-week course at 0.5 to 2.0 mg/kg/day. There are many side effects, including xerosis, epistaxis, myalgias, arthralgias, and elevated liver enzymes. Liver function tests, triglyceride level, and the complete blood count should be frequently monitored. The medicine is also highly teratogenic and must be used with extreme caution in all women with childbearing potential. Patient selection guidelines for women have been proposed that include serum pregnancy tests before starting, maintenance of highly effective contraception, and written informed consent.[6]

Atopic Dermatitis

Atopic dermatitis (AD) is a common, chronic, relapsing skin condition with an estimated incidence of 10% in the United States. It usually arises during childhood, with about 85% of cases developing during the first 5 years of life.[7]

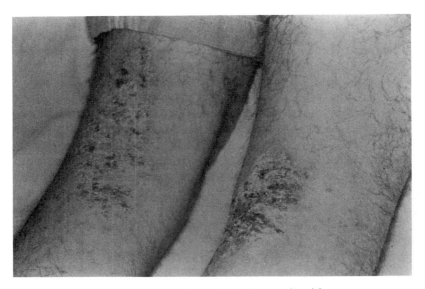

FIGURE 19.1. Atopic dermatitis in the popliteal fossae.

The disease presents with severe pruritus and various morphologic features. It has been described as "the itch that rashes." Although AD is found as an isolated illness in some individuals, it is often a manifestation of the multisystemic process of atopy, which includes asthma, allergic rhinitis, and AD. A family or personal history of atopy is a key element in making the diagnosis.

The eruption is eczematous and usually symmetric. It is erythematous, with papules and plaques, and often has secondary changes of excoriations and lichenification. The persistent excoriations can lead to secondary bacterial infection, which may be noted by the presence of more exudative and crusting lesions. In infants, AD is commonly seen on the face and the extensor areas, whereas in older children and adults it is seen in flexural areas of the popliteal and antecubital fossae as well as the neck and wrists (Fig. 19.1). Patients with AD often have generalized xerosis and some decreased cell-mediated immunity (especially to herpes simplex and wart viruses) and are frequently sensitive to wool and lipid solvents (e.g., lanolin).[8]

Treatment of AD should begin with attempts at decreasing the dryness of the skin. Bathing should be done with cool or tepid water and a mild soap (e.g., Dove or Purpose) or a soap substitute (e.g., Cetaphil). Immediately after bathing and gently patting the skin dry, an emollient should be applied to the skin to help seal in the moisture. This emollient should have no fragrances, no alcohol, and no lanolin (e.g., Eucerin or Aquaphor) and should be used daily to maintain well-lubricated skin. If some areas are particularly severely affected during an acute outbreak, wet dressings with aluminum acetate solution (Burow's solution) can be applied two or three times daily.[8] If the affected area has dry noninflamed skin, a moisturizer with lactic acid (e.g., Lac-hydrin) can be of such help that steroids can be avoided.

Controlling the intense pruritus is important. Keeping the nails trimmed short and using mittens at night can decrease the excoriations in children. Topical steroids can control the inflammatory process, always using the lowest possible dose. In infants and children, one can often maintain good control with 0.25% to 2.5% hydrocortisone cream or ointment two or three times a day. For more severe cases and in adults, 0.1% triamcinolone cream or ointment (or an equivalent-strength steroid) may be needed. Only rarely should fluorinated steroid preparations be used. The intense pruritus can be controlled with the use of antihistamines such as diphenhydramine (Benadryl) or hydroxyzine (Atarax, Vistaril). If sedation is a problem, daytime use of terfenadine (Seldane) or astemizole (Hismanal) may be helpful. If the affected area becomes secondarily infected, antibiotics directed at *Staphylococcus aureus* should be used. Dicloxacillin, erythromycin, and topical mupirocin (Bactroban) are good choices. When these measures fail to provide adequate control, it may be reasonable to pursue specific provocative factors such as foods, dust mites, and psychological stressors.[9]

This condition can produce a great deal of anxiety in both patients and parents, and stress can further aggravate the condition. It is crucial to provide psychological support to the family involved. Although affected children may appear "fragile," they are not and may desperately need some affectionate handling to help ease their own anxieties about the condition.[10]

Miliaria

Miliaria (heat rash) is a common condition resulting from the blockage of eccrine sweat glands. There is an inflammatory response to the sweat that leaks through the ruptured duct, and papular or vesicular lesions result.

One of the most common forms of miliaria is miliaria crystallina, in which blockage occurs near the skin surface and sweat collects below the stratum corneum. A thin-walled vesicle results, and there is little to no erythema. This condition is often seen in infants or bedridden patients and can be treated with cool compresses and ventilation to control perspiration.

Miliaria rubra (prickly heat) is commonly seen in susceptible patients of any age group when exposed to sufficient heat. The occlusion in this case is at the intraepidermal section of the sweat duct. As a result, there is more erythema, sometimes a red halo, or just diffuse erythema with papules and vesicles. There is usually more of a mild stinging or "prickly" sensation than real pruritus. This condition is self-limited but can be alleviated by a low- to medium-dose steroid lotion (e.g., 0.1% triamcinolone lotion) and by keeping the patient cool.[8]

Pityriasis Rosea

Pityriasis rosea (PR) is a benign self-limited condition primarily found between the ages of 10 and 35; it is slightly more common in women (1.5:1.0). The cause is unknown, but a viral etiology is suspected, as some patients have a prodrome of a virus-like illness with malaise, low-grade fever, cough, and arthralgias.[11]

The disorder usually starts with a single, 2- to 10-cm, oval papulosquamous patch on the trunk or proximal upper extremity. This "herald patch" is followed by a generalized eruption of discrete, small, oval plaques on the trunk and proximal extremities, sparing the palms, soles, and oral cavity. These plaques align their long axis with the skin lines, thus giving the rash a characteristic "Christmas tree" appearance (Fig. 19.2). The plaques often have a fine, tissue-like "collarette" scale at the edges.

The differential diagnosis includes tinea corporis, as the initial herald patch can be confused with "ringworm." The diffuse eruption of PR may

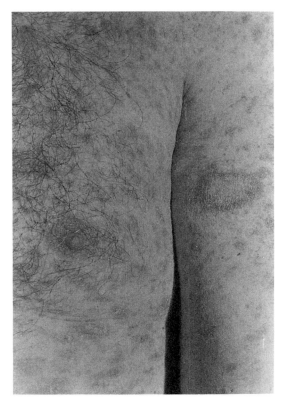

FIGURE 19.2. Pityriasis rosea. (Note herald patch on arm.)

resemble secondary syphilis but can often be distinguished by the sparing of the palms and soles with PR. It may also give the appearance of psoriasis, but it has much finer plaques that are not clustered on the extensor areas. Finally, the eruption may also be confused with tinea versicolor. Skin scrapings for potassium hydroxide preparations should be strongly considered in any patient with apparent PR, as well as serologic testing for syphilis in any sexually active patient.

The management of PR is fairly easy. Pruritus is generally mild and can be controlled with oral antihistamines or topical low-dose steroid preparations. Patients can be reassured that the lesions will fade over about 6 weeks. They should be warned, however, that postinflammatory hypo- or hyperpigmentation (especially in blacks) is possible.[12]

Psoriasis

Diagnosis

Psoriasis, a chronic recurrent disorder, is characterized by an erythematous, scaling, hyperproliferative papulosquamous eruption. Lesions are well-defined plaques with a thick, adherent, silvery-white scale. If the scale is removed, pinpoint bleeding can be seen (Auspitz's sign). Psoriasis occurs in about 1% to 3% of the worldwide population. The etiology is unknown, although some genetic link is suspected, as one-third of patients have an affected first-degree relative.[13] It may start at any age, with the mean age of onset during the late twenties.[14] Lesions most commonly occur on the extensor surfaces of the knees and elbows but are also typically seen on the scalp and sacrum and can affect the palms and soles as well. The nails may show pitting, onycholysis, or brownish macules ("oil spots") under the nail plate. Finally, about 7% of the patients develop psoriatic arthritis, which can be severe and crippling.[13,14]

Although psoriasis is usually not physically disabling and longevity is not affected, the patient's physical appearance can be profoundly affected and may cause significant emotional trauma, including withdrawal from social activities and even depression. Attention to the psychosocial implications of this chronic disease is crucial for every family physician.

The classic presentation, with its erythematous plaques and thick silvery scales on elbows or knees (Fig. 19.3), is usually easy to diagnose, but there are many morphologic variants. Discoid, guttate, erythrodermic, pustular, flexural (intertriginous), light-induced, and palmar-plantar psoriasis are among the many clinical presentations of this condition. The plaques may be confused with seborrheic dermatitis or AD, or the guttate form may resemble PR or secondary syphilis. If the diagnosis is unclear, referral to a dermatologist or performing a biopsy (read by a dermatopathologist, if possible) is in order.

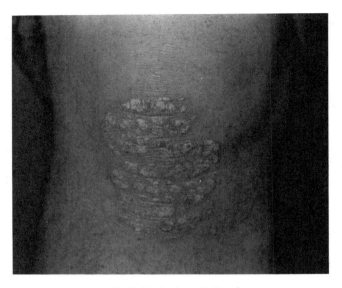

FIGURE 19.3. Typical psoriatic plaque.

The lesions often appear on areas that are subjected to trauma (Koebner phenomenon). Other precipitating factors include infections (particularly upper respiratory infections) and stress. Several drugs, particularly lithium, β-blockers, and antimalarial agents, are well known to exacerbate psoriasis in some patients.[14] The nonsteroidal antiinflammatory drugs (NSAIDs) that are used for psoriatic arthritis may worsen the skin manifestations. Systemic corticosteroids can initially clear the psoriasis, but a "rebound phenomenon" or worsening lesions, even after a slow taper, is common.

Management

There is no cure for psoriasis, and all treatments are designed to control the manifestations and hopefully induce a remission. Although no treatment is necessary, most patients desire some improvement in the cosmetic appearance of their skin. Therapy can start with emollients to keep the skin as moist as possible and attaining exposure to moderate amounts of sunlight while avoiding sunburn. After this basic treatment, modalities are divided into topical agents and systemic therapies. The decision to use systemic agents is often based on the percentage of body surface area involved, with 20% often being used as the cutoff for changing to systemic treatment. In practice, however, the decision to use systemic therapy is based on the severity of the disease, the resistance of the disorder to topical treatments, the availability of other agents, and a complex of social and psychological factors.[15] This decision is usually best made by an experienced dermatologist.

Topical steroid preparations can provide prompt relief, but the relief is often temporary. Tolerance to these agents is common, and one must remain vigilant for the long-term side effects of skin atrophy and telangiectasia. The lowest effective dose should be used (always using caution with higher strengths in the face, groin, and intertriginous areas), and occlusive dressings are often helpful.

Chronic plaques are often best managed using the antimitotic agents anthralin (Dithranol) or coal tar. Anthralin preparations (e.g., Dritho-Creme or Dritho-Scalp) can be applied to thick plaques in the lowest dose possible for about 15 min/day and then showered off. Care must be taken to avoid the face, genitalia, and flexural areas. The duration and strength of the preparation is gradually increased as tolerated until irritation occurs. This preparation is messy and can stain normal skin, clothing, and bathroom fixtures. Coal tar preparations can be used alone or, more successfully, in combination with ultraviolet B (UVB) light therapy (Goeckerman regimen).[13] Coal tar can be found in both crude and refined preparations as bath preparations, gels, ointments, lotions, creams, solutions, soaps, and shampoos. In general, the treatment is similar to that with anthralin: Higher concentrations are used until irritation or improvement results. The preparations are left on overnight, and staining can be a problem. The newest agent for moderate psoriatic plaques is calcipotriene ointment (Dovonex), a synthetic analog of vitamin D_3. It has shown beneficial results without significant systemic side effects; however, it is expensive and may cause skin irritation in about 10% of patients.

When systemic therapy is generally needed, treatment with ultraviolet light can be effective using either UVB (alone or with coal tar or anthralins) or ultraviolet A (UVA) light therapy with psoralens. The psoralen acts as a photosensitizer, and the UVA is administered in carefully measured amounts via a specially designed unit. Phototherapy or photochemotherapy can be expensive and carcinogenic, so they should be administered only by an experienced dermatologist. Other systemic agents include methotrexate, etretinate (Tegison—a retinoid), and cyclosporine.

The psoriatic lesions may disappear with treatment, but residual erythema and hypo- or hyperpigmentation is not uncommon. Patients must be instructed to continue treatment until the induration resolves and not always to expect complete resolution.

Family and Community Issues

Proper patient and family education are crucial for managing the physical and psychosocial manifestations of psoriasis. The patient should be allowed to participate in the decision of which treatment modalities are to be used and must be carefully instructed on the proper use of whichever one is chosen. The ongoing emotional support the family physician provides can help prevent the emotional scars that psoriasis may leave behind. The National Psoriasis Foundation is a nonprofit organization dedicated to supporting research and education in this field. They provide newsletters and other educational material for patients and their families. A written prescription with their address (National Psoriasis Foundation, 6600 SW 92nd, Suite 300, Portland, OR 97223; phone 503-244-7404) can be one of the most effective long-term "treatments" for these patients.

Rhus Allergy

Plant-related contact dermatitis can be triggered by many plant compounds, but the most common allergen is the *Rhus* agent of poison ivy, oak, and sumac. These three plants cause more allergic contact dermatitis than that from all other contact materials combined.[8] The plants are all from the genus *Rhus* and contain the oleoresin urushiol. This resin, which serves as the allergen (and rarely as a primary irritant), is located within all parts of the plant.[16]

The clinical presentation varies with the amount of the allergen and the patient's sensitivity. The eruption is erythematous, with papules, wheals, and often vesicles. With severe cases, large bullae or diffuse urticarial hives can be seen. The distribution is often linear or streak-like on exposed skin from either direct contact with the plant or by inadvertent spreading of the resin by the patient.

A history of exposure to the plant or to any significant activities outside helps in the diagnosis. It must be remembered, however, that the resin adheres to animal hair, clothing, or other objects; and the patient may have no known direct exposure. The thick skin on the hands often prevents eruption on the palms, even though the resin is transferred to another part of the body where an eruption does occur. An outbreak may occur within 8 hours, or the initial exposure may sensitize the patient so the rash occurs after a couple of weeks of exposure to the resin remaining on or in the skin.[16] This ability of the resin to remain on the skin and cause a later eruption has led to the mistaken belief that the fluid of the vesicles can cause spreading of the lesions.

Treatment begins with removal of any remaining allergen by thorough skin cleansing with soap and water as soon after exposure as possible. Any clothing that may have come in contact with the plant should also be washed. If the affected area is small and there is no significant vesicular formation, topical steroids (high dose, e.g., triamcinolone 0.5%) are sufficient. The blisters can be relieved by frequent use of cool compresses of water or of Burow's solution (1 packet of Domeboro in 1 pint of water). Oral antihistamines (e.g., diphenhydramine 25 mg or hydroxyzine 10–25 mg, four times a day) can help relieve the pruritus. If the outbreak is severe or widespread, oral steroids may be needed. Prednisone (0.5–

1.0 mg/kg/day) can be tapered over several days if treating an outbreak that started 1 week or more after exposure; but it should be tapered over a longer time (10–14 days) if treating an outbreak that started within 1 to 2 days of exposure. This regimen treats the lesions that are present and should suppress further development of lesions as the skin is sensitized.[17]

Prevention is best done by avoidance, but there has been some success with barrier creams (e.g., Stokogard). Desensitization attempts have not been successful and are not recommended.

Seborrheic Dermatitis

Seborrheic dermatitis is a common (incidence 3–5%), recurrent scaling eruption. It typically occurs on the face and scalp and on intertriginous areas of the body. It usually occurs in two age groups: infants during the first few months of life (sometimes presenting as "cradle cap") and adults aged 30 to 60 ("dandruff"). It causes mild pruritus and is generally gradual in onset and fairly mild in presentation. An increased incidence (30–80%) has been described in patients with acquired immunodeficiency syndrome, and these patients often present with a sudden severe eruption.[18] The etiology is unknown, but there is thought to be some infectious process with the *Pityrosporum* yeasts, particularly *P. ovale*.

The lesions are scaling macules, papules, and plaques that are sometimes yellowish, thick, and greasy and at other times white, dry, and flaky. Thicker, more chronic lesions occasionally crust, then fissure and weep. Secondary bacterial infection leading to impetigo is not uncommon. The differential diagnosis includes atopic or contact dermatitis, candidiasis, or a dermatophytosis. When the scalp is involved, the plaques are often confused with psoriasis, and in fact the two conditions may overlap, which has led to the term *seboriasis*. When the trunk is involved, the lesions may be confused with PR.

Treatment of hair-bearing areas consists of periodic use of shampoos containing ketoconazole (Nizoral) or over-the-counter products with selenium sulfide (e.g., Selsun Blue), or pyrithione zinc (e.g., Head and Shoulders). Salicylic acid and sulfur combinations (e.g., Sebulex) and other combination agents including tar-based products, and some preparations that include low-dose steroids are also available. These preparations should be left on the skin for several minutes before rinsing and should be used alternating with regular shampoos every other wash. This protocol may prevent the tachyphylaxis that can occur with daily use. Other areas (including the face, groin, and chest) can be treated with ketoconazole cream or a low-potency topical steroid such as 1.0% to 2.5% hydrocortisone cream. Thick scales on an infant's scalp can be gently scrubbed off after application of warm mineral oil or a salicylic acid shampoo. Although in infants the condition can be expected to resolve over several months, adults must be informed that this is a chronic *recurrent* condition.

Rosacea (Acne Rosacea)

Acne rosacea, a chronic facial skin condition, usually starts in patients between ages 30 and 60. It is characterized by acneiform lesions such as papules, pustules, and sometimes nodules (Fig. 19.4). Patients also have facial flushing, generalized erythema, telangiectasias, and mild-to-severe sebaceous gland hyperplasia. Conjunctivitis, blepharitis, and episcleritis are the ocular manifestations of the disease (present in about one-half the patients), and severe involvement of the nose can lead to soft tissue hypertrophy and rhinophyma. Otherwise, most lesions are on the forehead, cheeks, and nose. Pathogenesis is unknown, but increasing evidence sug-

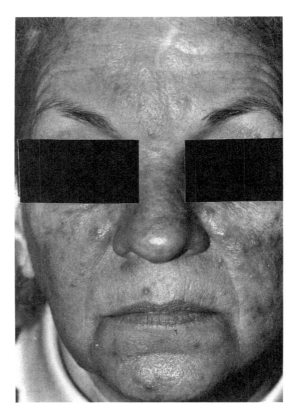

FIGURE 19.4. Acne rosacea.

gests that it is primarily a cutaneous vascular disorder, which leads to lymphatic damage, followed by edema and erythema, and finally papules and pustules develop.[19] Despite popular conception, alcohol is not known to play a causative role, but the vasodilatory effects of alcohol may make the condition appear worse. There is also some vasomotor instability in response to hot liquids and spicy foods, and they should be avoided.[8]

Treatment with oral erythromycin or tetracycline 1 g/day in divided doses can help both the facial and ocular manifestations of the disease. Response is variable, with some patients showing a prompt response followed by weeks or months of remission and others requiring long-term suppression with antibiotics. If long-term treatment is needed, the dose should be titrated downward to the minimal effective amount. Topical metronidazole (Metrogel) can be helpful in mild-to-moderate cases and seems safe for long-term use.[20] Oral metronidazole (Flagyl) may be used with caution in more resistant cases. Isotretinoin (Accutane) can also be used for severe refractory rosacea.[8]

Pompholyx (Dyshidrotic Eczema)

Pompholyx, a recurrent eczematous dermatosis of the fingers, palms, and soles, is more common in a young population (<age 40) and presents with pruritic deep-seated vesicles. The etiology is unknown. Despite the name and the fact that many patients have associated hyperhidrosis, it is not a disorder of sweat retention. Many of these patients have a history of AD, and it is considered a type of hand and foot eczema. Stress is thought to play a role in some cases, as is the ingestion of certain allergens (e.g., nickel).[8]

Onset is typically abrupt, and the disorder lasts a few weeks; it may also be chronic, however, and lead to fissuring and lichenification. Secondary bacterial infection can also occur. The vesicles are usually small but can be bullous and may give the appearance of tapioca. The most common site is the sides of the fingers in a cluster distribution (Fig. 19.5). The nails can also show involvement with dystrophic changes such as ridging, pitting, or thickening.

Treatment is difficult and should be directed at removing the inciting stressor when possible. Further treatment is similar to that for AD: Cool compresses may provide relief, and topical steroids can alleviate the inflammation and pruritus. Pompholyx is one of the dermatoses in which high-potency fluorinated or halogenated steroids (in a gel or ointment formulation) are often needed to penetrate the thick stratum corneum of the hands. If secondary infection is present, erythromycin may be helpful. Severe cases may require oral steroids, but these agents should be reserved for the worst cases.

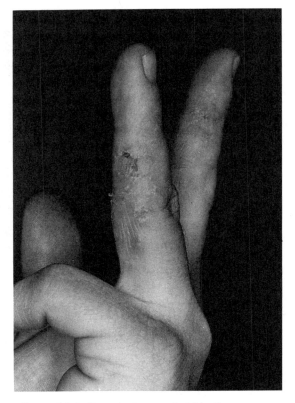

FIGURE 19.5. Pompholyx, or dyshidrotic eczema.

Drug Eruptions

Various types of rash are common reactions to medications. The dermatologic manifestations include maculopapular (or morbilliform) eruptions; urticaria; fixed hyperpigmented lesions; photosensitivity reactions; vesicles and bullae; acneiform lesions; and generalized pruritus. Patients frequently take several medications, they may also have other coexisting illnesses, and the drug-induced eruption may not manifest until the patient has been taking the drug for several days (sometimes weeks). All these factors combine to make it difficult to definitively attribute a particular eruption to a single agent. Only when the eruption (1) follows administration of a particular agent, (2) resolves with removal of that agent, and (3) recurs with its readministration—and other causes have been excluded—can one say that the eruption is definitely due to a specific drug. Obviously, caution must be exercised before any rechallenge with an agent; thus, readministration is often not undertaken. Subsequently, many patients mistakenly believe they have dermatologic reactions to certain medications.

TABLE 19.1. Adverse reactions to common drugs

Anaphylaxis	*Maculopapular (morbilliform)*	*Urticaria*
Aspirin	Barbiturates	Antibiotics
NSAIDs	Gentamicin	NSAIDs
Penicillins	Isoniazid	Opiates
Sulfonamides	Penicillin compounds	Radiocontrast agents
Serum (animal derived)	Phenothiazines	
	Phenytoin	*Vesicular eruption*
Fixed drug eruptions	Quinidine	Barbiturates
Aspirin	Sulfonamides	Captopril
Barbiturates	Thiazides	Clonidine
NSAIDs		Nalidixic acid
Phenolphthalein	*Photosensitivity*	Penicillin
Sulfonamides	Furosemide	Piroxicam
Tetracyclines	Griseofulvin	Sulfonamides
	Methotrexate	
Lupus-like eruptions	Phenothiazines	
Hydralazine	Quinidine	
Hydrochlorothiazide	Sulfonamides	
Isoniazid	Sulfonylureas	
Methyldopa	Tetracyclines	
Procainamide	Thiazides	
Quinidine		

Table 19.1 is a listing of several of the typical reactions to some of the more common drugs used in clinical practice.[8,10,17,21,22] Treatment obviously consists of stopping the offending (or suspected) agent. Topical low-potency steroids or antihistamines can relieve the pruritus that accompanies certain eruptions.

Contact Dermatitis

Contact dermatitis is the clinical response of the skin to an external stimulant. It is a common condition, with chemically caused dermatitis being responsible for 30% of all occupational illness.[21] This condition is such a problem with a wide variety of pathogenetic mechanisms and potential products involved that there is an international journal titled *Contact Dermatitis* devoted to this topic. By suspecting virtually everything and anything and obtaining a thorough history, the family physician nevertheless should be able to diagnose and manage most of these problems.

There are a few subtypes of contact dermatitis, with the most common being irritant contact dermatitis (accounting for 70–80% of cases of contact dermatitis).[23] It is the result of a break in the skin's integrity and subsequent local absorption of an irritant. No allergen is demonstrable. A single exposure can induce an inflammatory response if the agent is caustic enough or if the exposure is striking. Often the response is the result of prolonged exposure with repeated minor damage to the skin, such as in those who must wash their hands frequently. Common offending agents include soaps, industrial solvents, and topical medications (e.g., benzoyl peroxide, tretinoin, lindane, benzyl benzoate, anthralin).[23–25]

The second most common type is allergic contact dermatitis, which is a delayed hypersensitivity reaction that occurs after the body is sensitized to the offending agent. The reaction is thus often delayed somewhat from the time of exposure. The response varies depending on the individual's sensitivity, the amount and concentration of the allergen, and the amount of penetration.[24] Poison ivy (or *Rhus*) dermatitis is perhaps the most common form of allergic contact dermatitis (see above). Other common offenders include nickel, fragrances, rubber chemicals, neomycin, parabens (found in sunscreens and lotions), and benzocaine (topical anesthetic).[26,27] Even topical steroid preparations have been reported to cause allergic contact dermatitis in some patients.[26]

Physical findings vary somewhat with the different forms of contact dermatitis. The irritant type causes an erythematous scaling eruption with a typically indistinct margin (Fig. 19.6). The allergic type usually causes

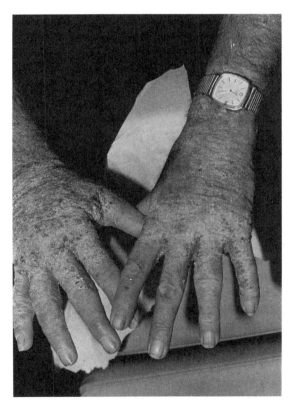

FIGURE 19.6. Contact dermatitis, irritant type.

more erythema, edema, and with vesicular formation, weeping. These eruptions are more sharply defined and may correspond to the shape of the offending agent (e.g., a watchband or the elastic band of some clothing).

Treatment is symptomatic after removal of the irritant or allergen. Cool compresses can provide relief from the pruritus, particularly if there is any weeping. Oral antihistamines may be needed along with topical steroids. Ointment compounds should be used, as they are less irritating and sensitizing. The patient should avoid any topical preparations with benzocaine or other "-caines," as they may aggravate the condition. With severe cases, a tapering course of oral steroids (prednisone) over 1 to 2 weeks is necessary. Subacute and chronic cases may also be colonized with *Staphylococcus aureus,* and an oral antibiotic may speed resolution.[27]

Avoidance of the irritant or allergen is sometimes difficult for patients. Their job may require some exposure, or it may be difficult to verify the agent. Patch testing may be a reasonable solution for determining the likely offending agent(s) and thus assist in a long-term plan of avoidance.

Urticaria

Urticaria is a common skin condition affecting about 20% of the population and is characterized by transient wheals or hives.[28] It is typically a type I immunologic reaction (mediated by immunoglobulin E) but may be due to physical or environmental exposure (pressure- or cold-induced). Urticaria can be acute, lasting less than 6 weeks, or chronic. Perhaps the most frustrating issue for both the patient and the physician faced with urticaria is that the underlying cause is difficult to ascertain. In only 20% of cases of chronic urticaria can the specific etiology be determined.[28]

Diagnosis is relatively easy. A generalized eruption of pruritic wheals with erythema and localized edema and the presence of lesions lasting less than 24 hours establish the diagnosis. Angioedema is a closely related process in which deeper tissues may be involved, particularly mucous membranes. Severe generalized urticaria can be a systemic illness leading to cardiac problems and even death.

One should search carefully to determine the underlying etiology by obtaining a careful and comprehensive history and performing a thorough physical examination. Common causes include medications (antibiotics, NSAIDs, narcotics, radiocontrast dyes), illnesses (viral hepatitis, parasitic), physical agents (pressure, cold, heat, exercise), contacts (chemicals, fragrances, dyes, soaps, lotions, feathers, animal dander), insect bites and bee stings, foods (chocolates, shellfish, strawberries, nuts), and stress.[8,10,29,30] The question of how much laboratory work and other testing are necessary to elucidate the etiology is variable. In general, an extensive workup is not advised during the early weeks and is begun only when the patient seems otherwise ill, is pressing hard for an etiology, or other signs and symptoms point to another cause.[29]

Treatment consists of avoidance of any known or suspected precipitant plus symptomatic treatment to provide comfort. H_1 blockers such as hydroxyzine, astemizole (Hismanal), clemastine (Tavist), chlorpheniramine, or diphenhydramine can be used alone or in combination with an H_2 blocker such as cimetidine (Tagamet). For severe acute urticaria, a dose of prednisone tapered over 2 weeks can be helpful. Chronic urticaria may require a great deal of maintenance emotional support, as the condition can make normal activities difficult. Patients need to be reassured, and medications may have to be given on a long-term, daily basis.

The author gratefully acknowledges the contribution of Stephen J. Brozena, M.D.

References

1. Winston MH, Shalita AR. Acne vulgaris: pathogenesis and treatment. Pediatr Clin North Am 1991;38:889–903.
2. Pochi PE, Shalita AR, Strauss JS, et al. Report on the Consensus Conference on Acne Classification: Washington, DC, March 24 and 25, 1990. J Am Acad Dermatol 1991;24:495–500.
3. Rosenberg EW. Acne diet reconsidered. Arch Dermatol 1981;117:193–5.
4. Rasmussen JE. Diet and acne. Int J Dermatol 1977;16:488–92.
5. Leyden JT, Shalita AR. Rational therapy for acne vulgaris: an update on topical therapy. J Am Acad Dermatol 1986;15:907–14.
6. American Academy of Dermatology, Guidelines of care for acne vulgaris. J Am Acad Dermatol 1990;22:676–80.
7. Hanifin JM. Atopic dermatitis in infants and children. Pediatr Clin North Am 1991;38:763–89.
8. Habif TB. Clinical dermatology: a color guide to diagnosis and therapy. 2nd ed. St. Louis: CV Mosby, 1990.
9. Przybilla B, Eberlein-Konig B, Rueff F. Practical management of atopic eczema. Lancet 1994;343:1342–6.
10. Goldstein BG, Goldstein AO. Practical dermatology. St. Louis: Mosby-Year Book, 1992.
11. Parsons JM. Pityriasis rosea update. J Am Acad Dermatol 1986;15:159–67.
12. Bjornberg A. Pityriasis rosea. In: Fitzpatrick TB, Eisen AZ, Wolff K, et al., editors. Dermatology in general medicine. 4th ed. New York: McGraw-Hill, 1993:1117–23.
13. Gibson LE, Peary HD. Papulosquamous eruptions and exfoliative dermatitis. In: Moschella SL, Hurley HJ, editors. Dermatology. 3rd ed. Philadelphia: WB Saunders, 1992:607–51.
14. Christophers E, Sterry W. Psoriasis. In: Fitzpatrick TB, Eisen AZ, Wolff K, et al., editors. Dermatology in general medicine. 4th ed. New York: McGraw-Hill, 1993:489–514.
15. Guidelines for the management of patients with psoriasis. Workshop of the research unit of the Royal College of Physicians of London; Department of

Dermatology, University of Glasgow; British Association of Dermatologists. BMJ 1991;303:829–35.

16. Baer RL. Poison ivy dermatitis. Cutis 1990;40:34–36.

17. Pariser RJ. Allergic and reactive dermatoses. Postgrad Med 1991;89:75–85.

18. Frioschl M, Land HG, Landthaler M. Seborrheic dermatitis and atopic eczema in human immunodeficiency virus infection. Semin Dermatol 1990;9:230–2.

19. Wilkin JK. Rosacea. Pathophysiology and treatment. Arch Dermatol 1994;130:359–62.

20. Schmadel LK, McEvoy GK. Topical metronidazole: a new therapy for rosacea. Clin Pharm 1990;9:94–101.

21. Kalish RS. Drug eruptions: a review of clinical and immunologic features. Adv Dermatol 1991;6:221–37.

22. Bigby M, Stern RS, Arndt KA. Allergic cutaneous reactions to drugs. Prim Care 1989;16:713–27.

23. Contact dermatitis and urticaria from environmental exposures. Agency for Toxic Substances and Disease Registry. Am Fam Physician 1993;48:773–80.

24. Oxholm A, Maibach MI. Causes, diagnosis, and management of contact dermatitis. Compr Therapy 1990;16:18–24.

25. Hogan DJ. Review of contact dermatitis for non-dermatologists. J Fl Med Assoc 1990;77:663–6.

26. Adams RM. Recent advances in contact dermatitis. Ann Allergy 1991;67:552–66.

27. Whittington C. Clinical aspects of contact dermatitis. Prim Care 1989;16:729–38.

28. Huston DP, Bressler RB. Urticaria and angioedema. Med Clin North Am 1992;76:805–40.

29. Cooper KD. Urticaria and angioedema: diagnosis and evaluation. J Am Acad Dermatol 1991;25:166–74.

30. Soter NA. Urticaria and angioedema. In: Fitzpatrick TB, Eisen AZ, Wolff K, et al., editors. Dermatology in general medicine. 4th ed. New York: McGraw-Hill, 1993:1483–95.

CASE PRESENTATION

Subjective

PATIENT PROFILE

Ruth Nelson McCarthy is a 51-year-old married white female restaurant operator.

PRESENTING PROBLEM

"Rash on hands."

PRESENT ILLNESS

For 8 to 10 months, the patient has noticed a rash on her hands. It occurs especially between the fingers and, when present, is red, irritated, and scaling. The itching of the rash prompts scratching, especially during her sleep at night.

PAST MEDICAL HISTORY

She has been taking cyclic estrogen and progesterone tablets since her previous visit 8 months ago (see Chapter 2).

FAMILY HISTORY, SOCIAL HISTORY, AND HABITS

All are unchanged since her previous visit.

- What additional information would you like regarding the history of present illness? Explain.
- What more would you like to know about her work?
- What might the patient be doing to treat her rash? Why might this be important?
- What are possible reasons for the patient's visit today? How would you address this issue?

Objective

VITAL SIGNS

Blood pressure, 136/88; pulse, 72; respirations, 18; temperature, 37°C.

EXAMINATION

There is dermatitis of both hands, worse on the right. The rash especially involves the fingers and the interdigital folds. The skin is cracked and bleeding in places, and there is evidence of excoriation.

- What additional data about the examination of the hands might be useful?
- Are there additional areas of the body that you might examine? Why?
- What—if any—laboratory tests might be useful? Why?
- What physical findings might suggest that the problem is other than a localized dermatitis? Explain.

Assessment

- What is the probable diagnosis and its cause? How will you explain this to the patient?
- How might this relate to activities in her life?
- What are some implications of the diagnosis for Mrs. McCarthy and her family?
- If a similar rash were also present on other areas of the body, what diagnostic possibilities would you consider?

Plan

- What specific therapy would you recommend? How would you explain this to Mrs. McCarthy?
- How might this problem be prevented in the future? What changes in her work would you advise?
- If the rash became infected, with purulent drainage and crusting, what might you do differently?
- What continuing care would you recommend?

20
Diabetes Mellitus

CHARLES KENT SMITH, JOHN P. SHEEHAN, AND
MARGARET M. ULCHAKER

Diabetes mellitus (DM) affects 12 million to 15 million individuals in the
United States, incurring an immense cost in terms of morbidity and
premature death. The most common form is type II, or adult-onset, DM,
which has racial preponderances, female predilection, and strong associations with obesity. There was a revolution in DM management during the
1980s with the advent of home blood glucose monitoring devices, human
insulin, and reliable laboratory markers of long-term glycemic control.
Also, published national and international standards of care have been
disseminated directly to patients and physicians, heightening the importance of adequate care and glycemic control to minimize devastating long-
term complications.[1,2] Table 20.1 describes diagnostic criteria for diabetes
mellitus, impaired glucose tolerance, and gestational diabetes.

Heightened clinical awareness of the genetics and predisposing factors
should foster early diagnosis and adequate metabolic control of the type II
patient. By contrast, the type I DM patient generally presents with a more
precipitous clinical picture of ketoacidosis. Declining islet cell secretory
function is more gradual, however, and can evolve over a 10-year period.
Understanding the autoimmune nature of islet destruction has led to
experimental protocols attempting to interrupt this process. Occasionally,
there is diagnostic confusion owing to a lack of a family history, the absence
of significant ketosis, and the absence of significant obesity and other
diagnostic hallmarks. The measurement of C-peptide levels and islet cell
antibodies provides useful diagnostic clarification.[3] Careful clinical follow-
up can clarify evolving absolute insulin deficiency even in the absence of
these laboratory markers.

Pathophysiology

Previously, type I DM was considered to be an acute event. Viral associations were invoked with regard to the seasonal trends in its incidence.
However, patients can have markers of islet destruction in the form of islet

Table 20.1. Diagnostic criteria for diabetes mellitus,
impaired glucose tolerance, and gestational diabetes

Nonpregnant adults

Criteria for diabetes mellitus: Diagnosis of diabetes mellitus in nonpregnant adults
should be restricted to those who have one of the following:
Random plasma glucose level of 200 mg/dl or more plus classic signs and symptoms
of diabetes mellitus including polydipsia, polyuria, polyphagia, and weight loss.
Fasting plasma glucose level of 140 mg/dl or more on at least two occasions, *or*
Fasting plasma glucose level less than 140 mg/dl with the 2-hour sample *and* the
sample at one previous interval being 200 mg/dl or more after a 1.75 g/kg (up to
75 g) glucose load.

Criteria for impaired glucose tolerance: Diagnosis of impaired glucose tolerance in
nonpregnant adults should be restricted to those who have *all* the following:
Fasting plasma glucose of less than 140 mg/dl
Two-hour oral glucose tolerance test plasma glucose level between 140 and
200 mg/dl
Intervening oral glucose tolerance test plasma glucose level of 200 mg/dl or more

Pregnant women

Criteria for gestational diabetes: After an oral glucose load of 100 g, gestational diabetes
may be diagnosed if two plasma glucose values equal or exceed:

Fasting:	105 mg/dl
1 Hour:	190 mg/dl
2 Hour:	165 mg/dl
3 Hour:	145 mg/dl

Source: Physician's Guide to Non-Insulin-Dependent (Type II) Diabetes: Diagnosis and Treatment.
2nd ed. Alexandria, VA: American Diabetes Association, 1988:4. With permission.

cell antibodies for up to 10 years before the development of overt DM. Islet and insulin autoantibodies along with the loss of first-phase insulin secretion in response to an intravenous glucose tolerance test are highly predictive of evolving type I DM.[4] Attempts to interrupt this autoimmune process with immunosuppressive agents have been tried with some encouraging results, but toxicity remains a concern. Clinical trials are ongoing in this area, as are trials with early insulin replacement therapy. Insulin has been given to experimental animals that have autoimmune islet destruction without overt DM in an attempt to suppress the autoimmune process. A recent pilot study of 12 patients holds exciting promise for clinical applicability of this approach in humans.[5] From the clinical perspective, only patients who have newly diagnosed DM can be offered early aggressive insulin replacement treatment unless they are willing to participate in research protocols at specialized centers.

Type II DM is associated with genetic predispositions, advancing age, obesity, and lack of physical exercise. The importance of caloric intake and energy expenditure has been clearly established.[6] Although type II DM is a syndrome of insulin resistance and islet secretory defects, in any given individual it is not possible to define the degree of insulin resistance versus secretory defects with any precision. The earliest metabolic defect found in first-degree relatives of individuals with type II DM is defective skeletal muscle glucose uptake with later increased insulin resistance at the level of the liver and resultant uncontrolled hepatic glucose output. The ensuing hyperglycemia can have a toxic effect called glucotoxicity on the islets, resulting in secondary secretory defects with declining insulin secretion and self-perpetuating hyperglycemia. Hyperglycemia may also down-regulate glucose transporters. It is unclear whether secretory defects or insulin resistance is the primary defect even in type II DM; they appear to coexist in patients with established disease. Patients may exhibit many abnormalities, including loss of first-phase insulin secretion and loss of the pulsatility of insulin secretion.[7-10] Also, both men and women tend to have abdominal obesity, which is associated with hyperinsulinemia and insulin resistance.[11] Type II DM is a syndrome not only of disordered glucose metabolism but also of lipid metabolism; many patients have a concurrent dyslipidemia manifesting elevations in serum triglycerides, depressions in high-density lipoprotein-cholesterol, and marginal increases in total cholesterol. This dyslipidemia results from uncontrolled hepatic very low-density lipoprotein secretion and defective clearance of lipoprotein molecules. The associations of hyperinsulinemia and insulin resistance with essential hypertension have been documented[12] along with the marked tendency for patients with essential hypertension to develop DM and the converse: patients with type II DM developing essential hypertension. A central unifying hypothesis focuses on hyperinsulinemia and insulin resistance being primary metabolic aberrations that result not only in hyperglycemia but also hypertension and dyslipidemia. Thus, our current understanding of type II DM and the more recently described syndrome X[13] (hyperinsulinemia, dyslipidemia, hypertension, and hyperglycemia) highlight the important issue not only of primary prevention of type II DM but also secondary prevention.

Importance of Glycemic Control

The relationship between microvascular complications of DM and glycemic control has been debated for decades. Many studies suggest an association between poor long-term glycemic control and retinopathy, neuropathy, and nephropathy. Unfortunately, many of these studies were not randomized, and the role of genetic factors was unclear. However, positive trends with glycemic control have been described. Smaller human studies and several animal studies link sustained metabolic control to the prevention of complications. One study showed, however, that early poor control despite later good control results in diabetic complications.[14] The results of the Diabetes Control and Complications

Trial were published in 1993.[15] This study conclusively demonstrated the benefit of tight control with blood glucose maintained as close to the normal range as possible. In the primary prevention group, intensive therapy reduced the risk for developing retinopathy by 76% and in the secondary intervention group slowed the progression of retinopathy by 54%. Microalbuminuria and neuropathy were also very favorably affected.

Decades of questions about the glucose hypothesis are therefore finally answered, with the obvious recommendation that most individuals with type I DM be treated with intensive therapy. The major negative aspect of attempts to achieve optimum glycemic control in intensive insulin therapy is the potential for severe hypoglycemia. Careful screening of individuals with a history of severe unconscious reactions is necessary to redefine realistic treatment goals. Many individuals, though, can safely achieve excellent metabolic control as defined by normal glycohemoglobin levels without significant hypoglycemia.

Defining Control

The definition of DM control has varied. During the era of urine testing, predominantly negative urine tests were indicative of good glycemic control. However, because blood glucose can be twice normal in the absence of glycosuria, urine glucose monitoring is now outmoded. Home blood glucose monitoring (HBGM) provides positive feedback of daily glycemic control to patients and physicians. Patients engaged in intensive insulin therapy can monitor themselves four to seven times per day and make adjustments in their regimen to optimize blood glucose control. The precision and accuracy of the home units has improved considerably, as has the simplicity and duration of the test (Table 20.2). Each system has its inherent weaknesses and limitations in such areas as blood volume, timing, hematocrit, temperature, and humidity. It is important that patients adhere strictly to the manufacturers' guidelines because attention to proper calibrations, strip handling, and ongoing maintenance are critical.[16] Noninvasive HBGM with infrared technology may be the wave of the future. Markers of long-term control such as the glycohemoglobin assays are also available. These tests measure the degree of glycosylation of hemoglobin either as total glycosylated hemoglobin (TGH) or glycosylation of subfractions such as the A_1 or A_1c. Hemoglobinopathies can affect all of these tests except the TGH. Glycohemoglobins reflect the average blood glucose over the previous 60 to 90 days. They are useful not only for confirming the degree of glycemic control but also for identifying possible falsification or errors in HBGM results. Glycohemoglobins are useful motivating tools for the patient; it often becomes a perceived challenge to reduce the result within the constraints of hypoglycemia. It is recommended that this test be

TABLE 20.2. Home blood glucose monitoring units

Meter	Manufacturer	Test time (seconds)	Blot/wipe required	Telephone no.
Medisense 2	MediSense	20	No	800-537-3575
Exactech Companion/Pen	MediSense	30	No	800-537-3575
Accu-Chek Advantage	Boerhinger-Mannheim	40	No	317-845-7169
Accuchek III	Boerhinger-Mannheim	120	Yes	317-845-7169
Tracer II	Boerhinger-Mannheim	120	Yes	317-845-7169
Accuchek Easy	Boerhinger-Mannheim	*	No	317-845-7169
Glucometer Elite	Ames	60	No	800-348-8100
Glucometer III	Ames	60	Yes	800-348-8100
One Touch II	Lifescan	45	No	800-227-8862
Checkmate	Wampole	90	No	800-525-6718
Diascan Ultra	HDI	90	No	800-342-7226

* Test time dependent on blood glucose level.

performed at least two to four times per year in all patients. In addition to markers of glycemic control, it is critical to monitor other clinical parameters. Annual lipid profiles are an integral part of overall DM care in view of the high prevalence of dyslipidemia, especially in the patient with type II DM. In type I DM patients, lipid disturbances are uncommon unless patients are in poor glycemic control, have a familial dyslipidemia, or have renal insufficiency. Markers of nephropathy are also important to measure. The earliest marker, microalbuminuria, is not only a forerunner of overt clinical nephropathy but also a marker for greatly increased cardiovascular risk in both type I and type II patients.[17,18] Microalbuminuria can be conveniently measured in either spot urine specimens or by overnight albumin excretion rates.[19]

Patient Education

Patient attention to management principles decidedly affects short-term metabolic control and ultimately has an impact on long-term complications. The interactions of nurse educators and dietitians are important. The presence of family members and significant others during the educational sessions is vital to a successful outcome. Education must encompass a comprehensive understanding of the pathophysiology of DM and its complications and the importance of attaining and sustaining metabolic control. Accurate HBGM is critical; after initial instruction, periodic reassessment of performance technique helps to ensure continued accuracy.

Education should also focus on dietary principles. For individuals with diabetes, the current dietary recommendations are a diet containing at least

50% carbohydrate, less than 30% fat, and 20% or less protein. Caloric requirements are based on ideal body weight (IBW)—*not* actual body weight. We calculate IBW by the Hamwi formula.[20]

Women
  100 pounds for 5 feet
  5 pounds for every additional inch
  Example: Woman 5'3" = 115 pounds IBW

Men
  106 pounds for 5 feet
  6 pounds for every additional inch
  Example: Man 5'8" = 154 pounds IBW

Based on anthropometric measures, 10% may be subtracted or added based on small body frame or large body frame, respectively.

Basal caloric requirements then are as follows.

Woman 5'3": IBW = 115 pounds
115 × 10 kcal = 1150 kcal/day

Add 300 to 400 kcal/day for moderate to strenuous activity.
Subtract 500 kcal/day for 1 pound per week weight loss.

As individuals with DM type II are generally hyperinsulinemic, diet prescriptions for weight loss and maintenance require a lower caloric level than previously mentioned. The activity factor in kilocalories (300–400 kcal/day) can be modified in these individuals. For the type II DM patient, caloric restriction is of major importance. By contrast, diet for the type I DM patient should involve careful consistency of carbohydrate intake. Achieving this degree of dietary education generally requires several sessions with a nutrition specialist. Dietary principles are an ongoing exercise, and eradication of myths and misconceptions is a major task. Unfortunately, many patients still perceive that "sugar-free" implies carbohydrate-free and that "sugar-free" foods cannot affect blood glucose control. This belief, of course, fails to recognize the monomer/polymer concept and the fact that most carbohydrates are ultimately digested into glucose. In addition to maintaining carbohydrate consistency, patients must learn carbohydrate augmentation for physical activity in the absence of insulin reduction. Patients also need instruction on carbohydrate strategies for dealing with intercurrent illness during which the usual complex carbohydrate may be substituted with simple carbohydrate. Although it has long been said that diet is the cornerstone of DM management,[21] effective DM dietary education is still problematic owing to time constraints and reimbursement problems.

Insulin-requiring patients must be aware of the many facets of insulin therapy. Accurate drawing-up and mixing of insulin is an assumption that is often not founded in reality. Site selection, consistency, and rotation are crucial. Insulin absorption is most rapid from the abdomen; the arms, legs, and buttocks, respectively, are next. We find that administering the pre-meal insulin in the abdomen optimizes postmeal control (assuming the use of Regular insulin). By contrast, the buttocks, as the slowest absorption site, is not a good choice for premeal injections. However, the lower buttocks is an ideal site for bedtime injections to minimize nocturnal hypoglycemia. Haphazard site selection and rotation can lead to erratic glycemic control. Because of the variability in absorption among sites, we suggest site consistency, i.e., using the same site at the same time of day (all breakfast injections in the abdomen, all dinner injections in the arms, all bedtime injections in the lower buttocks). Broad rotation *within* the sites is important to eliminate local lipohypertrophy.[22] Careful premeal timing of insulin injections (generally 30 minutes) is also required for optimal postprandial glycemic control. Patients need a comprehensive perspective on insulin adjustments[23] for hyperglycemia, altered physical activity, illness management, travel, and alcohol consumption.

Patients need education on the pathophysiology, prevention, and treatment of microvascular complications. Education on macrovascular risk factors and their modification for prevention of cardiovascular, cerebrovascular, and peripheral vascular disease is also critical. Patients can have a considerable impact on decreasing foot problems and amputations with simple attention to hygiene (avoidance of foot soaks), daily foot inspection, and the use of appropriate footwear. These measures can greatly reduce the incidence of trauma, sepsis, and ultimately amputations.[24]

Diabetic Complications

Complications of DM include those that are specific to DM and those that are nonspecific but are accelerated by the presence of DM. The specific complications of DM are microvascular, the triad of retinopathy, neuropathy, and nephropathy. Atherosclerosis, a common complication in patients with DM, is not specific to DM but is greatly accelerated by its presence. A major misconception among patients and even physicians is that the complications of DM tend to be less severe in patients with type II DM. In terms of macrovascular disease, patients with type II DM or impaired glucose tolerance have greatly accelerated macrovascular disease; patients with type II also suffer significant morbidity from microvascular complications.

Retinopathy

Retinopathy is the commonest cause of new-onset blindness during middle life. Retinopathy is classified as background, preproliferative,

Table 20.3. Classification of diabetic neuropathy

Type	Signs and symptoms
Sensory peripheral polyneuropathy	Pain and dysesthesia Glove and stocking sensory loss Loss of reflexes Muscle weakness/wasting
Autonomic	Orthostatic hypotension Gastroparesis, diarrhea, atonic bladder, impotence, anhidrosis, gustatory sweating, cardiac denervation on ECG
Mononeuropathy	Cranial nerve palsy Carpal tunnel syndrome Ulnar nerve palsy
Amyotrophy	Acute anterior thigh pain Weakness of hip flexion Muscle wasting
Radiculopathy	Pain and sensory loss in a dermatomal distribution

and proliferative. Early diagnosis and treatment with laser cannot be overemphasized for the preservation of vision. Several studies clearly document the importance of annual examinations by an ophthalmologist for all patients.[25] Good visual acuity does not exclude significant retinal pathology; unfortunately, many patients believe good visual acuity implies an absence of significant retinal disease.

Neuropathy

The clinical spectrum of diabetic neuropathy is outlined in Table 20.3.

Nephropathy

Diabetic nephropathy may first manifest as microalbuminuria, either detected on a spot urine determination or by timed overnight albumin excretion rate. The presence of microalbuminuria should alert the patient and physician to the need for stringent glycemic control; such control has been shown to decrease the progression from microalbuminuria to clinical proteinuria and attendant evolution of hypertension.[26] Hypertension increases the rate of deterioration of renal function in patients with DM, and aggressive treatment is mandatory. We favor the use of angiotensin-converting enzyme inhibitors and calcium channel blockers in the light of data that show decreasing proteinuria with many of these agents over and above that achievable with conventional antihypertensive therapy. In 1993, results from a randomized, controlled trial using captopril in patients with insulin-dependent DM (IDDM) who had a urine protein excretion of more than 500 mg/day and a serum creatinine concentration of less than 2.5 ng/dl showed clearly that captopril protected against deterioration in renal function and was significantly more helpful than blood pressure control alone. This was thought to slow the progression by a mechanism independent of its antihypertensive properties.[27] Also, α-blockers have a favorable metabolic and side effect profile. Avoidance of excessive dietary protein intake is also important, as excessive dietary protein may be involved in renal hypertrophy and glomerular hyperfiltration. Strict glycemic control even over a 3-week period can decrease renal size (as seen on ultrasonography) and decrease the hyperfiltration associated with amino acid infusions to levels comparable with those of normal non-DM individuals.[28]

Patients with DM in general are salt-sensitive, having diminished ability to excrete a sodium load with attendant rise in blood pressure; therefore, avoidance of excessive dietary sodium intake is important. Hyperinsulinemia and insulin resistance are also important in the genesis of hypertension, with insulin-resistant patients having higher circulating insulin levels to maintain normal glucose levels. Associated with this insulin resistance and hyperinsulinemia is the occurrence of elevated blood pressures even in nondiabetic individuals. Insulin is antinatriuretic and stimulates the sympathetic nervous system; both mechanisms may be important in the genesis of hypertension.

Macrovascular Disease

Macrovascular disease is the major cause of premature death and considerable morbidity in individuals with DM, especially those with type II DM. Conventional risk factors for macrovascular disease deserve special attention in DM; they include smoking, lack of physical activity, dietary fat intake, obesity, hypertension, and hyperlipidemia. Correction and control of hyperlipidemia through improved metabolic control and the use of diet or pharmacotherapy is mandatory for the DM patient. The National Cholesterol Education Program guidelines[29] are of special importance to the diabetic, as are the American Diabetes Association guidelines[30] for the treatment of hypertriglyceridemia, with pharmacotherapy now being indicated for patients with persistent elevation in triglycerides greater than 250 mg/dl. DM is one of the few diseases in which women have greater morbidity and mortality than men, especially in terms of macrovascular disease, with the black woman bearing the greatest load.

Foot Problems

Foot problems in the diabetic patient are a major cause of hospitalization and amputations. They generally constitute a combination of sepsis, ischemia, and neuropathy. The presence of significant neuropathy facilitates repetitive trauma without appropriate pain and ultimately nonhealing. Also, neuropathy may mask manifestations of peripheral vascular disease (PVD), such as claudication and rest pain such that patients may have critical ischemia with minimal symptoms. Therefore, PVD may be difficult to diagnose on usual clinical grounds alone. Not only may neuropathy mask clinical symptoms, the clinical signs may be somewhat confusing. Patients with less severe neuropathy may exhibit cold feet related to arteriovenous shunting, and patients with more severe neuropathy may exhibit cutaneous hyperemia related to autosympathectomy. Noninvasive vascular testing along with clinical evaluation is helpful for the diagnosis and management of PVD. Calcific medial arterial disease is common and can cause erroneously high blood pressure recordings in the extremities, confusing the assessment of the severity of PVD. Severe ischemia with symptoms and nonhealing wounds generally require surgical intervention. Milder symptoms and disease may respond favorably to enhanced physical activity and the use of the hemorrheologic agent pentoxifylline. Appropriate podiatric footwear and management are important to both ulcer healing and prevention of repetitive trauma.[24–31]

Achieving Glycemic Control

Type I DM

Optimal management of type I DM requires an educated, motivated patient and a physiologic insulin regimen. The major challenge is physiologic insulin replacement matched to dietary carbohydrate with appropriate compensation for variables such as exercise. Physiologic insulin replacement involves intensive insulin therapy with multiple injections (three or more per day) or the use of continuous subcutaneous insulin infusion (CSII) pumps. Several regimens have been used to achieve glycemic control and are outlined in Table 20.4. The conventional split-mix regimen combining regular and an intermediate-acting insulin in the morning before breakfast and in the evening before dinner has the major limitation of nocturnal hypoglycemia from the predinner intermediate-acting insulin when stringent control of the fasting blood glucose is sought. Dividing the evening insulin dose—delivering Regular insulin before dinner and the intermediate-acting insulin at bedtime—can afford a significant reduction in the risk of nighttime hypoglycemia.[32] Most patients require 0.5 to 0.8 units/kg body weight to achieve acceptable glycemic control. It is generally distributed as two-thirds in the morning and one-third in the evening, with (1) one-third of the morning dose being Regular and two-thirds being intermediate-acting insulin; (2) 50% of the

TABLE 20.4. Multiple injection regimens

Breakfast	Lunch	Dinner	Bed (10 p.m.–1 a. m.)
R + N or L	0	R	N or L
R + U	R	R + U	0
R	R	R	N or L

R = Regular; N = NPH; L = Lente; U = Ultralente.

evening insulin as Regular insulin before dinner; and (3) the remaining 50% as intermediate-acting insulin at bedtime (10 p.m. to 1 a.m.). These doses are modified according to individual dietary preferences and carbohydrate distribution.

Also, patients need algorithms to adjust their insulin for hyperglycemia, varying physical activity, and intercurrent illnesses. Many episodes of severe hypoglycemia occur in the context of unplanned physical activity and dietary errors; likewise, many episodes of ketoacidosis occur during episodes of intercurrent illness. For physical activity, a reduction in insulin dosage of 1 to 2 units per 20 to 30 minutes of activity generally suffices pending the intensity of the activity. The other option is to augment carbohydrate intake (i.e., 15 g carbohydrate before every 20 to 30 minutes of activity). During illness, it is important that patients appreciate the fact that illness is a situation of insulin resistance and that all the routine insulin should be administered. Carbohydrate from meals and snacks may be substituted as simple carbohydrate in the form of liquids such as juices and regular ginger ale. It is important that all treatment regimens be individualized and that therapeutic options for insulin administration are discussed. In this way, patients' life styles can be accommodated and appropriate insulin regimens tailored.[23] For example, using a basal-bolus regimen with Ultralente, it is possible to delay the lunchtime injection pending the patient's time constraints; furthermore, the insulin dose can be adjusted depending on carbohydrate intake and physical activity. In some individuals, a noontime injection is not feasible. A schoolchild or a person engaged in construction work might find it difficult to accommodate a prelunch insulin injection and might be better off with a morning intermediate-acting insulin to cover the lunchtime carbohydrate intake, with Regular insulin being taken to cover the breakfast carbohydrate intake as a combined prebreakfast dose.

Severe hypoglycemia in the well-educated, adherent, motivated patient on a physiologic insulin regimen is uncommon. Most severe hypoglycemic episodes are explained on the basis of diet or exercise and insulin-adjustment errors.[33] The individual who is attempting to achieve true euglycemia, however, is at risk for periodic easily self-treated hypoglycemia. See Table 20.5 for management strategies. For the individual with type I DM

TABLE 20.5. Hypoglycemia management strategies

Causes	Signs and symptoms	Treatment
Insulin/OHA overdose	Sympathomimetic	Conscious—15-G
Carbohydrate omission	Coldness	Simple carbohydrate
Missed/late meal	Clamminess	Juice 4 oz
Missed/late snack	Shaking	Regular soda 6 oz
	Diaphoresis	3 B-D glucose tabs
	Headaches	7 Lifesavers
Uncompensated	Neuroglycopenic	Unconscious
activity/exercise	Confusion	Glucagon S.C.[a]
	Disorientation	D_{50} 50 cc
	Loss of consciousness	

[a]We do not recommend the use of gel products (e.g., Monojel) for treatment of unconscious hypoglycemia, as aspiration is a potential hazard.
OHA = oral hypoglycemic agent.

who has been educated thoroughly, is on a physiologic insulin regimen with an agreed diet plan, and has algorithms for illness and physical activity, failure to attain the desired degree of glycemic control is largely related to psychosocial variables.

Type II DM

In most instances, type II DM is a syndrome of insulin resistance coupled with variable secretory defects, both of which can be compounded by glucotoxicity. As insulin resistance is related to genetic factors, obesity, and sedentary life style, the mainstay of treatment for the type II diabetic patient should be correction of insulin resistance through diet and exercise and reversal of glucotoxicity acutely through reestablishment of euglycemia. Many patients still perceive themselves to be more absolutely insulin-deficient than insulin-resistant and are willing to accept insulin therapy as a compromise in the context of failed weight loss efforts. Also, many patients perceive pharmacotherapy to be equivalent to a diet and exercise regimen alone, assuming the desired degree of glycemic control is achieved. Chronic nonadherence to a diet regimen with resultant failure of weight loss or progressive obesity frequently leads to mislabeling the patient as a "brittle diabetic." It is important to avoid premature and unnecessary insulin therapy in these individuals and to stress to them the importance of diet and exercise as the most physiologic approach to controlling their metabolic disorder.

Oral hypoglycemic agents (OHAs) are useful adjuncts to attaining glycemic control for the type II patient through their enhancement of insulin secretion and insulin action. The second-generation agents, glyburide and glipizide, are preferred in view of their side effect profile, short duration of action, and high potency. Some differences exist between these agents in terms of degree of enhancement of insulin secretion versus control of hepatic glucose output, with glyburide exhibiting increased effects in control of hepatic glucose output.[34,35] Suggested starting doses for a 70-kg individual younger than age 65 with normal renal function are 2.5 mg glyburide or 5.0 mg glipizide. The availability of a sustained-release glipizide preparation allows for once daily dosing of this agent with comparable glucose control and the potential for enhanced patient compliance with OHA treatment. The first-generation OHAs tend to have more prolonged durations of action, lower potencies, and a more significant side effect profile compared with the second-generation OHAs. Concern about possible cardiotoxicity of OHAs related to the University Group Diabetes Program study has largely disappeared, given the emergence of data to support the safety of these agents from the cardiovascular perspective. Indeed, the current literature is largely focusing on the atherogenicity of insulin and the impact of hyperinsulinemia and insulin resistance on hypertension and dyslipidemia, thus making OHAs a relatively attractive alternative to insulin therapy.[36,37]

Insulin therapy in type II diabetic patients is indicated in situations in which patients are acutely decompensated and are more insulin-resistant due to intercurrent illnesses. Clearly, short-term insulin therapy can reestablish glycemic control acutely in many individuals. However, reevaluation of endogenous insulin production with C-peptide determinations is important. Most obese patients with type II DM have considerable elevation in their C-peptide levels, assuming they are not glucotoxic from antecedent chronic hyperglycemia. The initiation of insulin therapy in a type II patient remains controversial in terms of indications and optimum insulin regimen. The dilemma revolves around the obese C-peptide-positive patient who was achieving good glycemic control in the short term with insulin. This individual often suffers progressive obesity and worsening glycemic control owing to worsening insulin resistance, thereby increasing requirements for exogenous insulin. Thus, frequently insulin therapy in an obese C-peptide-positive patient fails to achieve its primary goal of sustained improved glycemic control. Also, perpetuation of the obese state, or indeed worsening thereof, in conjunction with progressive hyperinsulinemia raises concerns about the impact of this worsened metabolic milieu on hypertension, dyslipidemia, and the atherosclerotic process. Initiation of insulin therapy should therefore be undertaken cautiously in most patients, and their progress should be carefully monitored in terms not only of glycemic control but also of hypertension, dyslipidemia, and obesity.

Many insulin regimens have been used to treat individuals with type II DM with insulin, many being similar to those used in the type I setting. Recent trends have focused on the use of bedtime insulin therapy in these individuals on the grounds that it can maximally affect the dawn hepatic glucose output/disposal and peak insulin resistance, thereby achieving the best possible fasting blood glucose and minimizing glucotoxicity. Minimizing glucotoxicity facilitates daytime islet secretory function and minimizes the need for daytime insulin therapy.[38] Combination therapy with insulin and OHAs seems theoretically sound, with OHAs presumably enhancing insulin sensitivity and reducing the need for exogenous insulin. The data, however, support only modest improvements in glycemic control and modest reduction in insulin requirements at best. One such regimen has been the use of an intermediate-acting insulin at bedtime at a dose of 0.2 U/kg coupled with a daytime second-generation OHA. Unlike the situation in the type I diabetic patient, hypoglycemia tends to be uncommon in type II patients owing to their fundamental insulin resistance. Metformin, available in 1995, will add a new dimension to the management of type II DM. It is a biguanide and a true insulin sensitizer that can be used alone or in combination with sulfonylureas or insulin. It also facilitates weight loss and improvement in the lipid profile.

In 1994, the American Diabetes Association published a paper with significant implications for family physicians. This was entitled "The Standards of Medical Care for Patients with Diabetes Mellitus."[39] Goals were set for IDDM and non-insulin-dependent diabetes (NIDDM), the latter having particular implications for family physicians. The paper acknowledged that there were no randomized clinical trial results similar to those of the DCCT that proved the benefits of near-normalization of blood glucose in NIDDM. However, the authors thought that it was likely that there would be benefits of close control and that this should be taken into consideration and, in fact, that it was reasonable to use the same glycohemoglobin and blood glucose goals detailed as for IDDM. Several controlled trials are looking at this question.

Several studies are now appearing confirming that euglycemia and tight control of diabetes by primary care physicians are very difficult to achieve in real life despite a desire to do so on the part of patients and physicians.[40]

Gestational Diabetes Mellitus

Gestational DM (GDM) is an important entity in terms of maternal morbidity, fetal macrosomia, associated obstetric complications, and neonatal hypoglycemia. GDM should be screened for in all patients using current screening and diagnostic guidelines (Table 20.1). Early and aggressive management can significantly improve outcome. The initial strategy for the patient with GDM is dietary control; however, when the goals of pregnancy are not being achieved (i.e., premeal and bedtime glucose <90 mg/dl and 1 hour postprandial glucose <120 mg/dl), insulin therapy should be initiated. Given the data linking postprandial blood glucose levels to macrosomia, it is important that postprandial glucose levels are controlled adequately and that target glucose levels are achieved.[41,42] In our center, this goal is most readily and predictably reached with premeal Regular insulin and overnight intermediate-acting insulin. Most women with GDM have reestablishment of euglycemia immediately postpartum. These individuals, however, should be counseled on the long-term risks of prior GDM for developing overt type II DM, which may occur in as many as 70% of these individuals.[43] Also, the hazards of uncorrected obesity, associated insulin resistance, dyslipidemia, hypertension, and potential for premature cardiovascular death must be addressed.[44]

Individuals with type I DM who are contemplating pregnancy should be in optimal glycemic control before conception to decrease the risk of congenital malformations and the incidence of maternal/fetal complications. The achievement of two consecutive glycosylated hemoglobin levels in the nondiabetic range is recommended before conception. A regimen of premeal Regular insulin and overnight intermediate-acting insulin (alternatively, CSII) may readily achieve these goals. Careful follow-up by a skilled management team is essential to an optimum outcome.[42]

Contraception and DM

The use of oral contraceptives (OCs) in women with either type I or type II DM has been an area of controversy,[42] with many believing that significant elevations occur in blood glucose along with an increased risk of vascular complications. In our experience, the incidence of such problems is minimal given a woman who is normotensive and has an absence of vascular disease; therefore, we believe OCs can be safely used. Even for a woman in poor glycemic control, OCs are still the most effective form of contraception.

Diabetic Ketoacidosis

Diabetic ketoacidosis (DKA) is the ultimate expression of absolute insulin deficiency resulting in uncontrolled lipolysis, free fatty acid delivery to the liver, and ultimately accelerated ketone body production. Insulin deficiency at the level of the liver results in uncontrolled hepatic glucose output via gluconeogenesis and glycogenolysis; and with insulin-mediated skeletal muscle glucose uptake being inhibited, hyperglycemia rapidly ensues. The attendant osmotic diuresis due to hyperglycemia results in progressive dehydration and a decreasing glomerular filtration rate. Dehydration may be further compounded by gastrointestinal fluid losses (e.g., emesis from ketones or a primary gastrointestinal illness with concurrent diarrhea). Insensible fluid losses from febrile illness may further compound the dehydration.

Diagnosis of DKA is fairly characteristic in the newly presenting or established type I diabetic patient. The history of polydipsia, polyuria, weight loss, and Kussmaul's respirations are virtually pathognomonic. Physical examination should be directed at assessing the level of hydration (e.g., orthostasis) and possible underlying and precipitating illness. Measurement of urine ketone, urine glucose, and blood glucose levels can rapidly confirm the clinical suspicion, with arterial pH, serum bicarbonate, and ketones validating the diagnosis. A thorough search for an underlying precipitating illness remains axiomatic (e.g., urosepsis, respiratory tract infection, or silent myocardial infarction). Treatment should be directed at correcting (1) the dehydration/hypotension; (2) ketonemia/acidosis; (3) uncontrolled hepatic glucose output/hyperglycemia; (4) insulin resistance of DKA/underlying illness; and, of course, (5) specific treatment of any defined underlying illnesses.

Dehydration and hypotension require urgent treatment with a 5- to 6-liter deficit to be anticipated in most individuals. Initial treatment should be with 0.9% NaCl with 1 to 2 L/hr being given for the first 2 hours and flow rates thereafter being titrated to the individual's clinical status. Use of a Swan-Ganz catheter is prudent in the individual with cardiac compromise. Potassium replacement at a concentration of 10 to 40 mEq/L is critical to replace the usual deficits of more than 5 mEq/kg once the patient's initial serum potassium level is known and urine output is documented. Giving 50% of the potassium as KCl and 50% as KPO$_4$ appears theoretically sound, but phosphate replacement has not been shown to alter the clinical outcome. Bicarbonate therapy is generally reserved for patients with a pH of less than 7.0, plasma bicarbonate less than 5.0 mEq/L, severe hyperkalemia, or a deep coma. Bicarbonate should be administered by slow infusion 50 to 100 mEq over 1 to 2 hours with the therapeutic endpoint being a pH higher than 7.1 rather than normalization of the pH. Overzealous use of bicarbonate can result in severe hypokalemia with attendant cardiac arrhythmogenicity, paradoxical central nervous system acidosis, and possible lactic acidosis due to tissue hypoxia. Intravenous insulin therapy should be initiated at the starting dose of 0.1 U/kg/hr with rapid titration every 1 to 2 hours should a 75 to 100 mg/dl/hr decrease in glucose not be achieved. Insulin therapy at this relatively high dose is needed to combat the insulin resistance of the hormonal milieu of DKA (i.e., high levels of glucagon, cortisol, growth hormone, and catecholamines). Given that hepatic glucose output is more rapidly controlled than ketogenesis, the insulin infusion rate can be maintained by switching the intravenous infusion to dextrose 5% to 10% when blood glucose is less than 250 mg/dl. The insulin infusion should be continued until the patient is ketone-free, clinically well, and able to resume oral feeding. It is of paramount importance that subcutaneous insulin be instituted promptly at the time of refeeding.

Flow sheets should be generated documenting the following.

1. Patient admission weight relative to previous weights with serial weights every 6 to 12 hours, urine ketones, and fluid balance
2. Vital signs and mental status every 1 to 2 hours
3. Bedside glucose monitoring every 1 to 2 hours
4. Urine ketones every 1 to 2 hours
5. Fluid balance
6. Blood gases and arterial pH on admission, repeating until pH is over 7.1
7. Serum potassium on admission and then every 2 to 4 hours
8. Serum ketones on admission and then every 2 to 4 hours
9. Complete blood count, serum chemistries, chest roentgenogram, electrocardiogram, and appropriate cultures on admission
10. Abnormal chemistries other than potassium repeated every 4 hours until normal.[45,46]

References

1. Clinical practice recommendations: 1990–1991. Diabetes Care 1991;14 (Suppl2): 1–81.
2. The European patient's charter. Diabetic Med 1991;8:782–3.
3. Landin-Olsson M, Nilsson KO, Lernmark A, Sunkvist G. Islet cell antibodies and fasting C-peptide predict insulin requirement at diagnosis of diabetes mellitus. Diabetalogia 1990;33:561–8.
4. Zeigler AG, Herskowitz RD, Jackson RA, et al. Predicting type I diabetes. Diabetes Care 1990;13:762–75.
5. Keller RJ, Eisenbarth GS, Jackson RA. Insulin prophylaxis in individuals at high risk of type I diabetes. N Engl J Med 1993;341:8850:927–8.
6. Helmrich SP, Ragland DR, Leung RW, Paffenbarger RS. Physical activity and reduced occurrence of non-insulin-dependent diabetes mellitus. N Engl J Med 1991;325:147–52.
7. DeFronzo RA. The triumverate: B-cell, muscle, and liver: a collusion responsible for NIDDM. Diabetes 1988;37:667–87.
8. Erikkson J, Franssila-Kallunki A, Ekstrand A. Early metabolic defects in persons at increased risk for non-insulin-dependent diabetes mellitus. N Engl J Med 1989;321:337–43.
9. DeFronzo RA, Bonadonna RC, Ferrannini E. Pathogenesis of NIDDM. Diabetes Care 1992;15:318–68.
10. Clark PM, Hales CN. Measurement of insulin secretion in type 2 diabetes: problems and pitfalls. Diabetic Med 1992;9:503–12.
11. Bjornstorp P. Metabolic implications of body fat distribution. Diabetes Care 1991;14:1132–43.
12. Ferrannini E, Buzzigoli G, Bonadonna B, et al. Insulin resistance in essential hypertension. N Engl J Med 1987;317:350–7.
13. Zavaroni I, Bonora E, Pagliara M, et al. Risk factors for coronary artery disease in healthy persons with hyperinsulinemia and normal glucose tolerance. N Engl J Med 1989;320:703–6.

14. Kern TS, Engerman RL. Arrest of glomerulonephropathy in diabetic dogs by improved glycemic control. Diabetalogia 1990;33:522–5.
15. Diabetes Control and Complications Trial Research Group. The effect of intensive treatment of diabetes on the development and progression of long-term complications in insulin-dependent diabetes mellitus. N Engl J Med 1993;329:977–86.
16. Self-monitoring of blood glucose: American Diabetes Association Consensus Statement. Diabetes Care 1992;15:56–61.
17. Viberti GC. Etiology and prognostic significance of albuminuria in diabetes. Diabetes Care 1988;11:840–8.
18. Deckert T, Feldt-Rasmussen B, Borch-Johnson K, et al. Albuminuria reflects widespread vascular damage: the Steno hypothesis. Diabetologia 1989;32:219–26.
19. Marshall SM. Screening for microalbuminuria: which measurement? Diabetic Med 1991;8:706–11.
20. Hamwi GL. Changing dietary concepts in therapy. In: Danowski TS, editor. Diabetes mellitus: diagnosis and treatment. New York: American Diabetes Association, 1964:73–78.
21. Wood FC, Bierman EL. Is diet the cornerstone in management of diabetes? N Engl J Med 1986:1244–7.
22. Zehrer C, Hansen R, Bantl J. Reducing blood glucose variability by use of abdominal injection sites. Diabetes Educator 1990;16:474–7.
23. Skyler JS, Skyler DL, Seigler DE, O'Sullivan M. Algorithms for adjustment of insulin dosage by patients who monitor blood glucose. Diabetes Care 1981;4:311–8.
24. Frykberg RG. Management of diabetic foot problems (Joslin Clinic). Philadelphia: Saunders, 1984.
25. Singerman LJ. Early-treatment diabetic retinopathy study: good news for diabetic patients and health care professionals [editorial]. Diabetes Care 1986;9:426–9.
26. Feldt-Rasmussen B, Mathiesen ER, Deckert T. Effect of two years of strict metabolic control on the progression of incipient nephropathy in insulin-dependent diabetes. Lancet 1986;2:1300–4.
27. Lewis EJ, Hunsicker LG, Bain RP, Rohde RD for the Collaborative Study Group. The effect of angiotensin-converting-enzyme inhibition on diabetic nephropathy. N Engl J Med 1993;329:1456–62.
28. Tuttle KR, Bruton JL, Perusek MC, et al. Effect of strict glycemic control on renal enlargement in insulin-dependent diabetes mellitus. N Engl J Med 1991;324:1626–32.
29. Report of the National Cholesterol Education Program expert panel on detection, evaluation, and treatment of high blood cholesterol in adults. Arch Intern Med 1988;148:36–69.
30. Role of cardiovascular risk factors in prevention and treatment of macrovascular disease in diabetes. Diabetes Care 1992;15:68–74.
31. Flynn MD, Tooke JE. Aetiology of diabetic foot ulceration: a role for the microcirculation? Diabetic Med 1992;9:320–9.
32. Skyler JS. Insulin treatment: therapy for diabetes mellitus and related disorders. Alexandria, VA: American Diabetes Association, 1991:127–37.

33. Bhatia V, Wolfsdorf JI. Severe hypoglycemia in youth with insulin-dependent diabetes mellitus: frequency and causative factors. Pediatrics 1991;88: 1187–93.
34. Groop L, Luzi L, Melander A, et al. Different effects of glyburide and glipizide on insulin secretion and hepatic glucose production in normal and NIDDM subjects. Diabetes 1987;36:1320–8.
35. Halter JB, Ward WK, Best JD, Pfeifer MA. Glucose regulation in non-insulin-dependent diabetes mellitus: interaction between pancreatic islets and the liver. Am J Med 1985;79(Suppl):6–12.
36. Stout RW. Insulin and atheroma: 20-yr perspective. Diabetes Care 1990;13: 631–54.
37. Fontbonne AM, Eschwege EM. Insulin and cardiovascular disease: Paris Prospective Study. Diabetes Care 1991;14:461–9.
38. Groop LC, Widèn E, Ekstrand A, et al. Morning or bedtime NPH insulin combined with sulfonylureas in treatment of NIDDM. Diabetes Care 1992; 15:831–4.
39. American Diabetes Association. The standards of medical care for patients with diabetes mellitus. Diabetes Care 1994;17:616–23.
40. Peterson KA. Diabetes care by primary care physicians in Minnesota and Wisconsin. J Fam Pract 1994;38:361–7.
41. Proceedings of the Third International Workshop-Conference on Gestational Diabetes Mellitus. Diabetes 1991;40(Suppl2):1–201.
42. Jovanovic-Peterson L, Peterson CM. Pregnancy in the diabetic woman: guidelines for a successful outcome. Endocrinol Metab Clin North Am 1992; 33:433–56.
43. Kaufmann RC, Amankwah KS, Woodrum J. Development of diabetes in previous gestational diabetic [abstract]. Diabetes 1991;40:137A.
44. Kaufmann RC, Amankwah KS, Woodrum J. Serum lipids in former gestational diabetics [abstract]. Diabetes 1991;40:192A.
45. Kozak GP, Rolla AR. Diabetic comas. In: Kozak GP, editor. Clinical diabetes mellitus. Philadelphia: Saunders, 1982:109–45.
46. Siperstein MD. Diabetic ketoacidosis and hyperosmolar coma. Endocrinol Metab Clin North Am 1992;33:415–32.

Case Presentation

Subjective

Patient Profile

Harold Nelson is a 76-year-old married white man.

Presenting Problem

"Blood sugar going up and down."

Present Illness

Mr. Nelson has been diabetic for 24 years. He was initially diet-controlled but now takes glyburide, 5 mg daily in the morning for the past 3 years. For about 2 months, he has noted wide swings in his blood sugar levels from 60 to more than 300 mg/dl on HBGM. He has had no shakiness or sweating at times of low blood sugar, although sometimes he feels inappropriately weak and sleeps more than usual. His appetite is fair, and he has lost some weight in the past few weeks.

Past Medical History, Social History, and Family History

All are unchanged since his previous visits 2 and 9 months ago (see Chapters 5 and 18).

Habits

Unchanged except that he reports drinking alcoholic beverages "a little more than usual."

Review of Systems

Occasional constipation. Sometimes he has lower leg pain after walking.

- What additional medical history might be important? Why?
- What questions about his diet might be important? Explain.
- What might you ask to clarify his alcohol use?
- What might you ask to further evaluate the leg pain?

Objective

Vital Signs

Height, 5 ft 7 in; weight, 160 lb (a decrease of 6 lb in 2 months); blood pressure, 162/84; pulse, 74; respirations, 20; temperature, 37.0°C.

EXAMINATION

The patient is ambulatory and alert. The eyes, ears, nose, and throat—including a funduscopic examination—are normal. The chest is clear to percussion and auscultation. The heart has a regular sinus rhythm, and no murmurs are present. On the abdominal examination, there is no mass or tenderness, and the liver is palpable about 1 cm below the right costal margin. There are Heberden's nodes of both hands and osteoarthritic swelling of other joints, especially the knees. The deep tendon reflexes are normal, and there is no decreased perception of pinprick in the lower extremities.

LABORATORY

An office determination reveals a blood sugar of 270 mg/dl approximately 2 hours after breakfast.

- What more data could you obtain from the physical examination, and why?
- What might you do to help clarify the patient's lower leg pain?
- What—if any—laboratory tests would you order today? Explain.
- What—if any—diagnostic imaging would you order today? Why?

Assessment

- What are possible causes of Mr. Nelson's problems with blood sugar control? How would you explain this to the patient?
- Could the presenting complaint be related to problems in the family? How might you assess this possibility?
- What are possible causes of the weight loss? Of the leg pain?
- What might be the meaning of these problems to the patient? How might you address this issue?

Plan

- Describe your therapeutic recommendations for the patient. How would you explain this to Mr. Nelson?
- Describe your advice regarding diet, alcohol use, and exercise.
- How might you involve other family members in dealing with the problem?
- What continuing care would you advise?

21
Human Immunodeficiency Virus Infection and Acquired Immunodeficiency Syndrome

RONALD H. GOLDSCHMIDT

Care for patients with human immunodeficiency virus (HIV) infection requires excellence in all aspects of family practice. The family physician's roles are many: providing patient education to prevent uninfected persons from becoming infected; identifying and instituting early intervention for infected persons; delivering comprehensive care of symptomatic disease including the acquired immunodeficiency syndrome (AIDS); and providing support and care for the family. This broad scope of clinical responsibilities is in an area of clinical medicine where the knowledge base and management strategies are evolving rapidly. New manifestations of HIV disease, diagnostic protocols, and drug recommendations (Table 21.2)[1] change on a regular basis. Epidemiologic, social, and community trends also continue to have important effects on clinical care. This chapter provides an overview of important clinical aspects of HIV disease for the family physician.

Acute HIV infection is followed by an asymptomatic phase, usually lasting more than 5 years. Immunodeficiency, the hallmark of which is progressive destruction of CD4+ (T-helper) lymphocytes, then results in susceptibility to opportunistic infections and malignancies. Early symptomatic disease (with manifestations such as oral candidiasis, oral hairy leukoplakia, and lymphadenopathy) is followed by the opportunistic infections and malignancies that characterize AIDS.[2] The average time from infection to AIDS-defining illnesses appears to be about 8 to 11 years.

Risk Factors, Risk Reduction, and Patient Education

The virus is usually transmitted from person to person by the passage of blood or body fluids such as semen and vaginal secretions. Urine, sweat, and saliva are not considered to be infectious. Persons engaging in unsafe sexual activity and intravenous drug use with needle sharing account for most cases of HIV infection. Transfusion-related infection now occurs in only about 1 of every 40,000 units of donated blood. Without treatment, vertical transmission (from mother to child) occurs in 25% of children of infected mothers. Casual transmission (in the absence of sexual contact or passage of blood) from person to person does not seem to occur. Transmission from infected patients to health care workers occurs at a rate of 0.3% to 0.4% (one seroconversion for every 250 to 333 needlestick or similar injuries) and constitutes an uncommon but important transmission category. Universal blood and body fluid precautions are essential to minimize health care worker risk.[3,4]

The family physician's role in educating patients to prevent HIV transmission by reduction or elimination of at-risk behaviors is important. Physicians should assess their patients' risk for HIV infection by obtaining a sexual and drug history. Education about the use of condoms or non-insertive sex can be life-saving for persons who do not remain celibate or in a mutually monogamous relationship. Intravenous drug users can be encouraged to enter a drug treatment program. Those who do not abstain from intravenous drug use must be educated about safer needle use by cleaning their injection equipment with bleach. Physicians' offices should have health education materials about HIV and sexually transmitted disease openly available for patients and families to read and take with them.

Counseling and Testing

Counseling about HIV is the beginning of a critical medical intervention.[5,6] During the pretest counseling session(s), the physician and patient need to discuss the patient's risk of being infected, ongoing activities that put the patient or others at risk, and methods of future risk reduction. Before offering testing, the physician should assess whether the patient appears psychologically and socially prepared to undergo it. An assessment of the availability of support from friends and family is a key part of the decision to offer testing. Persons with risk factors (and patients who request HIV testing even if they do not admit to risk factors) can then be offered HIV antibody testing. A discussion of the risks of testing (including false-positive results, false-negative results, the possible loss of confidentiality, and family and social disruption) precedes obtaining informed consent for testing.

The difference between confidential and anonymous testing needs to be discussed. Confidential testing can be performed in the physician's office but results in charted documentation that can reveal HIV status to health care workers and others who process medical records. To avoid possible breaches of confidentiality, referral to an anonymous test site or special procedures within the office to ensure anonymity must be arranged.

Testing for HIV generally requires an enzyme-linked immunosorbent assay (ELISA) screening test followed by either a Western blot or immunofluorescent antibody confirmatory test. Other tests that approach the sensitivity of the ELISA and specificity of the confirmatory tests are in development. A "window period" exists between the time of infection and seroconversion. During that time, patients can be infected but have not had a sufficient antibody response to result in positive serologic testing. In most cases, this "window period" lasts about 6 weeks to 3 months. For patients with recent at-risk activities, retesting in 3 to 6 months is advised. In a few patients, serologic evidence of HIV infection may not occur for 6 months to 2 years or, rarely, not at all.

Posttest counseling for HIV-negative patients should include discussions about future risk reduction as well as a reassessment of risk factors to ensure that the patient is not in the "window period." Posttest counseling for the HIV-positive patient is likely a turning point in his or her life. The patient should be told clearly that the test is positive and that he or she is infected with the HIV virus. It is important to reassure the patient that HIV positivity does not mean he or she has AIDS. Because there is a long asymptomatic phase of HIV infection and rapid advances in treatment of HIV infection and opportunistic infections occur, it may be many years before problems arise. On hearing an HIV-positive result, however, most patients are in some degree of psychological shock and may not be able to assimilate much information. Perhaps the most important intervention the family physician can make is to reassure the patient that the physician will remain his or her personal physician while assembling a multidisciplinary team to meet problems should they arise. Offering to meet with the family and members of the patient's social network can be helpful. In general, a commitment to ongoing care should be the focus of the first posttest counseling session. A more detailed patient care plan can be developed at subsequent visits.

Early Intervention for Asymptomatic Seropositive Patients

The seropositive patient requires both routine health care maintenance and special attention to specific signs, symptoms, and laboratory markers for HIV disease progression. Routine health care maintenance includes a comprehensive history and physical examination with special attention to a history of sexually transmitted diseases and physical findings of skin and oral conditions. Laboratory evaluation includes a routine complete blood count including platelet count, chemistry panel, syphilis serology, and urinalysis. A chest roentgenogram is required for persons with a history of cardiopulmonary problems but is not required for all HIV-infected persons. A tuberculin skin test (intermediate-strength purified protein derivative [PPD]) should be performed with the recognition that in HIV-infected persons a 5-mm (rather than the usual 10-mm) reaction to an intermediate-strength PPD is considered indicative of tuberculous infection.[7,8] For HIV-infected persons known to be at high risk for tuberculosis, such as injection drug users, homeless persons, and persons from countries with a high incidence of tuberculosis, even a negative tuberculin skin test cannot eliminate the possibility of co-infection with tuberculosis. These patients should probably be given prophylactic (INH) therapy regardless of their PPD status. Patients with positive tuberculin skin tests and patients with high risk of tuberculosis require a chest roentgenogram to exclude active tuberculosis. Immunizations, including annual influenza vaccination and one-time pneumococcal vaccination, should be current. Hepatitis B vaccine is recommended if there is an ongoing risk of exposure to hepatitis B.

The most widely used surrogate marker for HIV disease progression is the CD4+ lymphocyte count. The normal range for CD4+ lymphocyte counts is broad and variable, so multiple measurements are required to detect trends. In general, CD4+ lymphocyte counts decrease by about 85 cells/mm³/year from an average baseline level of about 1000 cells/mm³. CD4+ cell counts should be obtained annually until the count is fewer than 500 cells/mm³. Thereafter, CD4+ cell counts can be performed every 3 to 6 months to help guide decisions about initiating antiretroviral therapy and *Pneumocystis carinii* pneumonia (PCP) prophylaxis.

Antiretroviral Therapy

The optimal time to initiate antiretroviral therapy is not established.[9] The most extensive studies of the clinical effects of zidovudine (AZT, Retrovir)[10,11] indicate that zidovudine therapy delays disease progression, but this effect is time-limited, probably to less than 1 year. Therefore, the timing of antiretroviral therapy is a decision that should be made jointly by the patient and provider. Some patients and providers will initiate therapy when the CD4+ lymphocyte counts are as high as 500 cells/mm³; most initiate therapy at lower CD4+ levels. Some choose not to initiate therapy until symptomatic disease occurs. The recommendations[9] that are generally followed are that all symptomatic patients and patients with fewer than 200 CD4+ lymphocytes/mm³ receive therapy and that asymptomatic patients with 200 to 500 CD4+ lymphocytes/mm³ be offered therapy.

Zidovudine is the agent most frequently used. Standard treatment with 500 to 600 mg/day in divided doses is recommended, but dosages as low as 300 mg/day have been shown to be effective. Didanosine (ddI, Videx) and zalcitabine (ddC, Hivid) are alternatives to zidovudine for patients intolerant to side effects of zidovudine, patients with clinical progression despite zidovudine therapy, or in combination with zidovudine for patients selecting combination therapy.[12,13] Changing or adding agents is often instituted when disease progression occurs or the CD4$^+$ lymphocyte counts decrease to (arbitrary) low levels, such as 50% of baseline level at time of initial treatment, or 100 CD4$^+$ cells/mm^3.

Prophylaxis Against *Pneumocystis carinii* Pneumonia and *Mycobacterium avium* Complex

When CD4$^+$ lymphocyte counts fall to fewer than 200 cells/mm^3 and when patients develop symptoms of advanced HIV disease, prophylaxis against PCP should be initiated.[14] Prophylaxis has been shown to delay or prevent the development of PCP and improve the survival and health of HIV-infected persons. Trimethoprim/sulfamethoxazole (TMP/SMX), one double-strength tablet daily, is the drug of choice. For patients unable to tolerate TMP/SMX, dapsone or aerosolized pentamidine are alternate prophylactic agents.

Rifabutin prophylaxis against *Mycobacterium avium* complex (MAC) disease has been recommended for all patients with fewer than 100 CD4$^+$ lymphocytes/mm^3.[15] However, MAC disease is a very late-stage disease, so many providers are withholding prophylaxis and treating those patients who develop symptomatic disease.

Clinical Presentations of HIV Disease

The clinical manifestations of HIV disease are widespread and varied. Virtually every organ system can be affected by a broad range of opportunistic infections and malignancies.[16–18] The Centers for Disease Control 1993 surveillance case definition for AIDS includes the identifier diseases listed in Table 21.1 as well as a CD4$^+$ lymphocyte count less than 200 cells/mm^3. Some guidelines for treatment of the most common syndromes, along with recommendations for early intervention, are listed in Table 21.2.

Nonspecific Symptoms and Signs

Nearly all patients with HIV disease develop weight loss, weakness, malaise, and anorexia. Unexplained fevers are also common with advanced HIV disease. Investigation for specific organ system disease and opportunistic infections and malignancies is the first step in evaluating these symptoms and signs. The most common causes are pulmonary disease including PCP, central nervous system (CNS) disease, and disseminated MAC infection. Multidrug treatment of symptomatic MAC disease is

TABLE 21.1. Identifier diseases for AIDS surveillance case definition

Candidiasis of bronchi, trachea, or lungs
Candidiasis, esophageal
Cervical cancer, invasive
Coccidioidomycosis, disseminated or extrapulmonary
Cryptococcosis, extrapulmonary
Cryptosporidiosis, chronic intestinal (>1 month duration)
Cytomegalovirus disease (other than liver, spleen, or nodes)
Cytomegalovirus retinitis
HIV encephalopathy
Herpes simplex: chronic ulcer (>1 month duration); or bronchitis, pneumonitis, or
  esophagitis
Histoplasmosis, disseminated or extrapulmonary
Isosporiasis, chronic intestinal (>1 month duration)
Kaposi's sarcoma
Lymphoma, Burkitt's
Lymphoma, immunoblastic
Lymphoma, primary in brain
Mycobacterium-avium intracellularae complex or *M. kansasii* infection, disseminated or
  extrapulmonary
Mycobacterium tuberculosis infection, any site (pulmonary or extrapulmonary)
Mycobacterial disease, other species or unidentified species, disseminated or
  extrapulmonary
Pneumocystis carinii pneumonia
Pneumonia, recurrent
Progressive multifocal leukoencephalopathy
Salmonella septicemia, recurrent
Toxoplasmosis of brain
Wasting syndrome due to HIV

Source: Adapted from Centers for Disease Control. 1993 revised classification system for HIV infection and expanded case definition for AIDS among adolescents and adults. MMWR 1992;41(RR-17):1–19.

generally administered to patients able to tolerate the drugs.[17] Treatable sepsis caused by bacteria and fungi (including cryptococcal sepsis) can also be identified. Frequently, however, no specific pathogenic process can be found, so the nonspecific symptoms and signs are attributed to HIV infection itself. Fevers can be treated with nonsteroidal antiinflammatory drugs (NSAIDs), but these drugs appear to be especially nephrotoxic in AIDS patients and should be used only for persistent symptomatic fevers. Vigorous nutritional programs, including hyperalimentation, can increase the daily caloric intake but have not been shown to alter the course of advanced HIV disease.

Skin and Oral Cavity

Skin and oral cavity lesions are the most frequent first manifestation of HIV disease.[19] A form of seborrheic dermatitis is the most common skin condition found in HIV-infected persons. This condition is readily treated with a combination of low-strength hydrocortisone cream plus ketoconazole cream. Drug rashes can be bothersome and serious. Careful investigation to identify and discontinue the offending drug, including nonprescription drugs the patient may be taking without the physician's knowledge, is essential.

Kaposi's sarcoma (KS) is an AIDS-defining condition. The violaceous to brown lesions can occur anywhere on the body. A biopsy is required to establish the diagnosis of AIDS (when KS is the initial manifestation) and when bacillary hemangiomatosis (a bacterial condition that can produce lesions similar to those of KS) or other conditions are possible. KS does not require treatment unless the lesions are cosmetically bothersome, bulky, or painful, or the patient wishes the lesions to be treated. Localized lesions can be treated successfully with radiation therapy, cryotherapy, or with intralesional injections of chemotherapeutic agents or interferon. Extensive KS sometimes can be treated with systemic chemotherapeutic agents. Other skin conditions include bacterial folliculitis, fungal rashes, and molluscum contagiosum. Herpes zoster infections (shingles) can antedate the diagnosis of AIDS or can occur during the course of AIDS. Intravenous acyclovir (Zovirax) is usually required, although oral acyclovir is sometimes effective.

Herpes simplex infections of the perioral and perirectal areas can be extensive and persistent. Treatment with oral acyclovir is usually effective, but extensive lesions sometimes require intravenous acyclovir. Apparent bacterial infections of the perioral and perirectal areas should prompt investigation (by viral culture) for underlying herpes infections. Disseminated herpes simplex and zoster infections usually require intravenous acyclovir treatment.

Oral candidiasis (thrush) can be identified in most HIV-infected patients at some time. Oral candidiasis is not an AIDS-defining condition and occurs in patients without HIV infection as well. Candidiasis usually takes the form of white removable plaques on the tongue or other areas of the oral mucosa but at times can be erythematous and atrophic. Treatment with topical or systemic antifungal agents is usually effective. Oral hairy leukoplakia is a viral lesion that usually appears on the lateral borders of the tongue. Because this condition is asymptomatic and recedes spontaneously, no treatment is required. Other oral conditions include KS, angular cheilitis, and periodontal disease.

Eyes

Cytomegalovirus (CMV) retinitis usually occurs late in the course of AIDS, when CD4$^+$ lymphocyte counts are fewer that 50 cells/mm^3 in most cases. Hemorrhages, perivascular exudates, and white, gray, or yellow discoloration of the peripheral retina are characteristic. When CMV retinitis is

TABLE 21.2. Treatment regimens for HIV disease

Problem	Drug	Comments
Antiretroviral therapy	Zidovudine (AZT; Retrovir) 500–600 mg PO daily in divided doses	Hematologic toxicity. Give 300–400 mg daily in divided doses for patients unable to tolerate higher dosages
	and/or	
	Didanosine (ddI; Videx) 200 mg PO bid; 125 mg PO bid for patients <60 kg	Can be used in patients who fail or are intolerant to zidovudine, or in combination with zidovudine
	and/or	
	Zalcitabine (ddC; Hivid) 0.75 mg PO tid	Can be used in patients who fail or are intolerant to zidovudine, or in combination with zidovudine
Mycobacterium avium complex (MAC)	Use two or three of the following drugs in combination	Treatment indicated for patients with signs, symptoms, and laboratory abnormalities consistent with MAC disease who can tolerate multidrug regimen. Use ethambutol and clarithromycin whenever possible. Azithromycin appears effective and can substitute for clarithromycin
	Ethambutol 15 mg/kg PO qd	
	plus	
	Clarithromycin (Claricid) 500 mg PO qid or 1 g PO bid	
	plus	
	Rifampin 10 mg/kg PO qd	
	or	
	Clofazimine (Lamprene) 100 mg PO qd	
	or	
	Ciprofloxacin (Cipro) 500–750 mg PO bid	
Prophylaxis against MAC disease	Rifabutin (mycobutin) 300 mg PO qd	Reduce dosage in combination with fluconazole
Cytomegalovirus (CMV) retinitis	Ganciclovir (Cytovene)	Neutropenia, dosage modification in renal failure
	Induction: 5 mg/kg IV q12h	
	Maintenance: 5 mg/kg IV as 1 hr infusion 5–7 times/week	
	or	
	Foscarnet (Foscavir)	Nephrotoxicity common
	Induction: 60–90 mg/kg/dose IV q8h for 2 weeks as 2-hr infusion	
	Maintenance: 90–120 mg/kg IV qd as 2-hr infusion	
Mucocutaneous herpes simplex (localized)	Acyclovir (Zovirax) 200–400 mg PO 5 times/day	Chronic maintenance therapy (200–400 mg PO 3–5 times/day) may be necessary when repeated episodes occur

Condition	Treatment	Comments
Disseminated, extensive, or persistent herpes simplex	Acyclovir 5 mg/kg/dose IV q8h	Chronic maintenance therapy (200–400 mg PO 3–5 times/day) may be necessary
Herpes zoster: shingles, disseminated, extensive, or persistent infection	Acyclovir 10 mg/kg/dose IV q8h; oral acyclovir 800 mg PO 5 times/day sometimes effective	Chronic maintenance therapy may be necessary
Acute *Pneumocystis carinii* pneumonia (PCP)	TMP/SMX (Septra, Bactrim) 15 mg TMP/kg daily given in 3–4 divided doses PO or IV	TMP/SMX first-line therapy
	or	
	Pentamidine isethionate (Pentam) IV, dapsone plus trimethoprim PO, clindamycin plus primaquine IV and PO, or trimetrexate plus leucovorin IV and PO	Second-line therapies
Prophylaxis or suppression of PCP for patients with CD4+ <200 cells/mm³ or prior episode of PCP	TMP/SMX 1 DS tablet PO qd or bid or 3 times weekly	TMP/SMX considered most effective for prophylaxis or suppression
	or	
	Inhaled pentamidine (Aeropent) 300 mg q4wk	Less effective than TMP/SMX
	or	
	Dapsone 50–100 mg PO daily	Less effective than TMP/SMX
	or	
	Clindamycin 450–600 mg PO bid–tid plus primaquine 15 mg PO qd	Less effective than TMP/SMX
Toxoplasma gondii	Sulfadiazine 1 g PO q6h or clindamycin 600–900 mg PO or IV qid	Maintenance required
	plus	
	Pyrimethamine 75–100 mg PO as loading dose, then 25–50 mg PO qd–qod	
	plus	
	Leucovorin calcium (folinic acid) 10–25 mg PO qd	
Cryptococcus neoformans	Amphotericin B 0.7–1.0 mg/kg/day IV over 4–6 hours	Fluconazole maintenance required
	or	
	Fluconazole	
	Acute: 400–800 mg PO qd	
	Maintenance: 200–400 mg PO qd	Maintenance required

Source: Adapted from Goldschmidt RH, Dong BJ. Treatment of AIDS and HIV-related conditions: 1994. J Am Board Fam Pract 1994;7:155–78.

identified, treatment with gancyclovir (Cytovene) or foscarnet (Foscavir) should be instituted,[16,20] as progression to blindness can occur rapidly and without warning symptoms. Cotton-wool spots are nonspecific signs of ischemia that are frequently noted on funduscopic examination of many AIDS patients. These small white lesions with indistinct margins can come and go and do not threaten vision.

Lymph Nodes and Hematopoietic Systems

Generalized lymphadenopathy caused by HIV-induced nodal hyperplasia is common and does not require biopsy or specific treatment. Treatable causes of lymphadenopathy, including lymphoma, tuberculosis, fungal infections, and KS, should be considered when suspicious clinical syndromes are present, lymphadenopathy is asymmetric, or prominent hard lymph nodes are present. Biopsy may be required in these instances.

All blood cell lines can be affected by HIV infection. Neutropenia is common, with reductions in the absolute neutrophil count to fewer than 300 to 500 neutrophils/mm^3. Careful observation, blood cultures, and consideration of empiric antibiotic treatment are required for severe neutropenia. Granulocyte-macrophage stimulating factors can help raise the neutrophil count to noncritical levels. Anemia caused by HIV disease can require transfusions or erythropoietin therapy. Macrocytosis is a normal hematologic response to zidovudine therapy. Zidovudine-induced macrocytosis does not require or respond to treatment. However, some patients receiving zidovudine develop a severe anemia with or without macrocytosis, requiring discontinuation of the drug or blood transfusion. Thrombocytopenia can occur early in the course of HIV infection and does not appear to constitute a major prognostic risk factor, nor is it a condition that requires treatment. Thrombocytopenia late in the course of HIV disease does not require treatment unless bleeding is present.

Heart and Pericardium

Congestive cardiomyopathy has been described in patients with AIDS but is infrequent. More common is fluid overload and congestive heart failure caused by large-volume intravenous fluid administration required for the treatment of opportunistic infections and other AIDS-associated problems. Fungal, bacterial, and tuberculous infections of the heart and pericardium can occur in AIDS patients and require standard therapy.

Lungs

Pulmonary disease is the most common cause of morbidity and mortality in HIV-infected persons. Pulmonary symptoms and signs can vary from only minimal shortness of breath or nonproductive cough to severe respiratory distress. The physical examination usually reveals tachypnea. Rales and cough with purulent sputum are not usually present unless bacterial pneumonia or pulmonary tuberculosis is present. Evaluation focuses on the findings of the chest radiograph and arterial blood gas measurements. The chest film of PCP and many other pulmonary processes in AIDS typically shows diffuse interstitial infiltrates or alveolar infiltrates. Thoracic and mediastinal lymphadenopathy and pleural effusions, when present, usually indicate fungal disease, *M. tuberculosis* infection, lymphoma, or pulmonary KS. Pleural effusions are not seen with PCP alone. The chest film is normal in 5% of patients with PCP. Arterial blood gas measurements usually show substantial hypoxemia with hypocarbia. Lactic dehydrogenase levels are frequently elevated in AIDS pulmonary disease but do not provide sufficient information on which to base differential diagnostic decisions. Abnormalities of chest radiographs or arterial blood gases require further investigation to establish the pathologic diagnosis.

The most common pulmonary disease in HIV-infected persons is PCP.[21,22] Therefore, evaluation focuses on establishing whether PCP is present. Examination of pulmonary specimens for *P. carinii* requires sputum induction or bronchoscopy, as patients with PCP do not expectorate sputum containing *P. carinii* organisms. Purulent sputum (e.g., from bacterial pneumonias) usually cannot be evaluated for PCP. *P. carinii* cysts can be detected for at least 3 weeks after initiation of therapy. Therefore patients seriously ill with presumptive PCP should be treated empirically, with diagnostic procedures performed at a later point in time. First-line treatment of PCP is with intravenous or oral TMP/SMX. The duration of therapy is 3 weeks. Shorter courses of therapy have been used, but anecdotal reports of failures are of concern. TMP/SMX has the added advantage of treating possible concurrent bacterial pneumonia. TMP/SMX therapy has substantial toxicity, but most toxicity can be managed successfully to permit a full treatment course. Patients with PaO$_2$ less than 70 mm Hg should also receive concurrent corticosteroids.[23] Patients with acute PCP can have clinical deterioration during the first 4 to 5 days of treatment. Careful intravenous fluid monitoring can help avoid fluid overload that can contribute to such deterioration. Marked clinical worsening after 1 week or failure to respond after 2 weeks of therapy are reasonable indications for changing to an alternative agent. PCP recurrences can be treated with the same agent that was successful on previous episodes.

Patients with moderate to severe PCP, those with first episodes of PCP, and those with their first AIDS-defining diagnosis are usually hospitalized to provide monitoring, adequate medication administration, and psychological support. Patients with mild PCP who have adequate home support services can be treated with oral medications as outpatients. Oral treatment of PCP is with TMP/SMX or with dapsone plus trimethoprim.

Other pathogenic processes to be excluded include bacterial pneumonia (most commonly pneumonia caused by *Haemophilus influenzae* and *Streptococcus pneumoniae*), tuberculosis,[18] KS, and disease caused by *Legionella pneumophila, Mycoplasma pneumoniae,* and MAC.

Gastrointestinal Tract

Esophagitis with dysphasia, odynophagia, and retrosternal pain can be caused by *Candida albicans,* CMV, or herpes simplex virus. Candidal esophagitis is most common. In patients with coexisting oral candidiasis, systemic treatment with ketoconazole or fluconazole should be initiated as an empiric trial. However, if the patient does not have oral candidiasis or a previous case diagnosis of AIDS, esophagoscopy with biopsies and cultures is advised to establish the diagnosis of candidal esophagitis (which is an AIDS-defining disease) and to direct therapy. Other causes of esophageal symptoms include CMV esophagitis and herpes esophagitis. Treatment of CMV esophagitis with gancyclovir or foscarnet and herpes esophagitis with acyclovir is usually effective.

Diarrhea and weight loss are common. Bacterial cultures and parasite determination should be performed to identify treatable causes. HIV infection itself can cause diarrhea but is a diagnosis of exclusion.

Perianal disease, most commonly caused by herpes simplex virus infections, often requires prolonged therapy with oral acyclovir. Extensive perianal disease may require intravenous therapy.

Liver disease can be the result of drug toxicity, hepatitis, or other infections and malignancies. Patients with laboratory findings suggesting a predominantly obstructive pattern (as indicated by a disproportionately elevated alkaline phosphatase) should undergo ultrasound examination to identify hepatic masses or biliary tract obstruction. An AIDS-associated cholangiopathy[24] with strictures and papillary stenosis can be identified by upper endoscopy with retrograde cholangiography. Sphincterotomy can effectively palliate symptoms of a biliary tract obstruction. When the ultrasound examination is negative, MAC disease, tuberculosis, fungal diseases, or other infiltrative hepatic processes should be considered.

Gynecologic Problems

Women with HIV infection can have severe, persistent vaginal candidiasis. Prolonged or repeated antifungal treatment is often necessary. Cervical dysplasia and cancer are also reported to be more frequent and more aggressive than in women not infected with HIV.[25] Papanicolaou smears should be performed every 6 months; dysplasia should be evaluated by colposcopy.

Renal and Adrenal Disease

The most common renal problem is drug toxicity. Special attention is required when patients are taking TMP/SMX, NSAIDs, or other drugs known to cause nephrotoxicity. Adrenal insufficiency, especially with hypotension and inadequate response to stress, occurs in some patients with HIV disease, requiring formal evaluation to establish the need for acute (stress) and maintenance therapies.

Musculoskeletal System

Polyarthralgias, Reiter syndrome, and other arthritis syndromes have been described in HIV-infected persons. A myopathy caused by zidovudine can be overlooked. Patients can be asymptomatic or can present with weakness and pain. The diagnosis is established by noting marked elevation of muscle enzymes in serum chemistry determinations. Discontinuation of zidovudine is required.

Neurologic Problems

Neurologic problems include peripheral neuropathies, myelopathies, and CNS disorders. Most common are the CNS disorders, including dementia caused by HIV encephalopathy and other pathogenic processes.

The AIDS dementia complex is usually a late manifestation of HIV disease. It can present with cognitive impairment, motor disturbances, or behavioral dysfunction. The most typical presentation is confusion, forgetfulness, and lethargy. At times, predominant features include ataxia and clumsiness. Behavioral changes are dominated by apathy, listlessness, and withdrawal. The major cause of the AIDS dementia complex is HIV infection of the brain, also termed HIV encephalopathy. The diagnosis is one of exclusion of other treatable causes of CNS disease. Treatment with high dose (1000–1200 mg/day) zidovudine has been reported to be successful in some cases.

The differential diagnosis of CNS disorders includes two common and treatable AIDS complications: cryptococcal meningitis and toxoplasmic encephalitis. Cryptococcal meningitis can present with the AIDS dementia complex, fever, photophobia, headache, or stiff neck.[26] Serum and cerebrospinal fluid cryptococcal antigen tests are positive more than 90% of the time. Treatment with amphotericin B, fluconazole, or both is usually effective. Toxoplasmic encephalitis can present as the AIDS dementia complex but also can cause seizures and focal neurologic signs. Empiric treatment is usually given when suspicious lesions on computed tomography or magnetic resonance imaging scans are noted. Failure to respond within 3 weeks can be an indication for a brain biopsy to rule out lymphoma and other CNS problems.

Kaposi's Sarcoma and Lymphomas

Multisystem involvement by KS can present with mass lesions or disseminated disease. Most patients with systemic KS also have involvement of the skin or oral mucosa. Involvement of the lungs, pleura, and gastrointestinal tract can be associated with bleeding and other problems. Obstruction of lymphatic flow caused by regional lymph node involvement is best treated with local radiation therapy. Systemic chemotherapy has been used for widespread KS but with variable results. Non-Hodgkin's lymphoma can occur in the brain, thoracic and abdominal lymph nodes, gastrointestinal tract, bone marrow, and elsewhere. Mass lesions can be treated with radiation therapy. Systemic disease can be treated with combination chemotherapy, although the drug toxicities limit the effective use of chemotherapy.

HIV Disease in Children

Without treatment, 25% of children born to mothers with HIV infection are also infected. Infection can occur transplacentally, at the time of delivery, and at breast-feeding. With zidovudine treatment of the mother during pregnancy (PO), intrapartum (IV), and to the child (PO), transmission can be reduced to 8.3%[27] Cesarean section is not recommended on a routine basis. Establishing the diagnosis of HIV infection in infants is problematic, because testing for antibodies measures maternal antibodies until approximately 15 months of age. Therefore, the diagnosis is made by viral culture or clinical syndromes. The polymerase chain reaction test can be helpful but is associated with false-positive test results. Maternal antibody is lost by 15 to 18 months of age, so diagnosis of infection is more readily made at that time.

Children infected with HIV should receive routine DPT, Hib, MMR, and inactivated (intramuscular) poliovirus vaccine. Oral poliovirus vaccine should not be given to HIV-infected children or to children living with immunocompromised persons. Influenza and one-time pneumococcal vaccines are recommended for children with symptomatic HIV infection.

In children,[28] AIDS usually presents with constitutional symptoms (e.g., fever and failure to thrive), oral candidiasis, lymphadenopathy, hepatosplenomegaly, and persistent or recurrent bacterial infections. Viral infections can also be severe and persistent. Pulmonary manifestations include PCP and lymphocytic interstitial pneumonitis. Gastrointestinal complications include diarrheal syndromes and candidial esophagitis. Neurologic problems also occur and must be evaluated thoroughly. The prognosis for children with AIDS is generally poor. Antiretroviral treatment with zidovudine and prophylaxis against PCP with TMP/SMX have shown to improve outcomes, and these measures are routinely recommended.

References

1. Goldschmidt RH, Dong BJ. Treatment of AIDS and HIV-related conditions: 1994. J Am Board Fam Pract 1994;7:155–78.
2. Centers for Disease Control; Council of State and Territorial Epidemiologists; AIDS Program, Center for Infectious Diseases. Revision of the CDC surveillance case definition for acquired immunodeficiency syndrome. MMWR 1987;36(Suppl1):1S–15S.
3. Guidelines for prevention of transmission of human immunodeficiency virus and hepatitis B virus to health-care and public-safety workers. MMWR 1989;38(Suppl6):1–37.
4. Public Health Service statement on management of occupational exposure to human immunodeficiency virus, including considerations regarding zidovudine postexposure use. MMWR 1990;39(No. RR-1):1–14.
5. Public Health Service guidelines for counseling and antibody testing to prevent HIV infection and AIDS. MMWR 1987;36:509–15.
6. Goldschmidt RH, Legg JJ. Counseling patients about HIV test results. J Am Board Fam Pract 1991;4:361–3.
7. Centers for Disease Control. Tuberculosis and human immunodeficiency virus infection: recommendations of the Advisory Committee for the Elimination of Tuberculosis (ACET). MMWR 1989;38:236–8, 243–50.
8. Purified protein derivative (PPD)-tuberculin anergy and HIV infection: guidelines for anergy testing and management of anergic persons at risk of tuberculosis. MMWR 1991;40(No. RR-5):27–33.
9. Sande MA, Carpenter CC, Cobbs CG, et al. Antiretroviral therapy for adult HIV-infected patients. Recommendations from a state-of-the-art conference. National Institute of Allergy and Infectious Diseases State-of-the-Art Panel on Anti-Retroviral Therapy for Adult HIV-Infected Patients. JAMA 1993; 270:2583–9.
10. Volberding PA, Lagakos SW, Koch MA, et al. Zidovudine in asymptomatic human immunodeficiency virus infection: a controlled trial in persons with fewer than 500 CD4-positive cells per cubic millimeter. N Engl J Med 1990; 322:941–9.
11 Concorde: MCR/ANRS randomised double-blind controlled trial of immediate and deferred zidovudine in symptom-free HIV infection. Concorde Coordinating Committee. Lancet 1994;343:871–81.
12. Caliendo AM, Hirsch MS. Combination therapy for infection due to human immunodeficiency virus type I. Clin Infect Dis 1994;18:516–24.
13. Hirsch MS, D'Aquila RT. Therapy for human immunodeficiency virus infection. N Engl J Med 1993;328:1686–95.
14. Centers for Disease Control. Recommendations for prophylaxis against Pneumocystis carinii pneumonia for adults and adolescents infected with human immunodeficiency virus. MMWR 1992;41(No. RR-4):1–11.
15. Recommendations on prophylaxis and therapy for disseminated Mycobacterium avium complex for adults and adolescents infected with human immunodeficiency virus. U.S. Public Health Service Task Force on Prophylaxis and Therapy for Mycobacterium Avium Complex. MMWR 1993;42(RR-9):14–20.

16. Jacobson MA, Mills J. Serious cytomegalovirus disease in the acquired immunodeficiency syndrome (AIDS): clinical findings, diagnosis, and treatment. Ann Intern Med 1988;108:585–94.
17. Horsburgh Jr CR. Mycobacterium avium complex infection in the acquired immunodeficiency syndrome. N Engl J Med 1991;324:1332–8.
18. Barnes PF, Bloch AB, Davidson PT, Snider DE Jr. Tuberculosis in patients with human immunodeficiency virus infection. N Engl J Med 1991;324:1644–50.
19. Berger TG, Obuch ML, Goldschmidt RH. Dermatologic manifestations of HIV infection. Am Fam Physician 1990;41:1729–42.
20. Palestine AG, Polis MA, De Smet MD, et al. A randomized, controlled trial of foscarnet in the treatment of cytomegalovirus retinitis in patients with AIDS. Ann Intern Med 1991;115:665–73.
21. Murray JF, Mills J. Pulmonary infectious complications of human immunodeficiency virus infection. Am Rev Respir Dis 1990;141:1356–72, 1582–98.
22. Goldschmidt RH. Recommendations for the treatment of acute Pneumocystis carinii pneumonia. J Am Board Fam Pract 1991;4:58–60.
23. National Institutes of Health—University of California Expert Panel for Corticosteroids as Adjunctive Therapy for Pneumocystis Carinii Pneumonia. Consensus statement on the use of corticosteroids as adjunctive therapy for Pneumocystis carinii pneumonia in the acquired immunodeficiency syndrome. N Engl J Med 1990;323:1500–4.
24. Cello JP. Acquired immunodeficiency syndrome cholangiopathy: spectrum of disease. Am J Med 1989;86:539–46.
25. Spence MR, Reboli AC. Human immunodeficiency virus infection in women. Ann Intern Med 1991;115:827–9.
26. Saag MS, Powderly WG, Cloud GA, et al. Comparison of amphotericin B with fluconazole in treatment of acute AIDS-associated cryptococcal meningitis. N Engl J Med 1992;326:83–89.
27. Centers for Disease Control and Prevention. Recommendations for the use of zidovudine to reduce perinatal transmission of human immunodeficiency virus. MMWR 1994;43(RR-11):1–20.
28. Falloon J, Eddy J, Wiener L, Pizzo PA. Human immunodeficiency virus infection in children. J Pediatr 1989;114:1–30.

CASE PRESENTATION

Subjective

PATIENT PROFILE

Mark McCarthy is a 28-year-old single white male waiter.

PRESENTING PROBLEM

"Cough and HIV-positive."

PRESENT ILLNESS

Mark has had a cough for 3 weeks with a recurrent low-grade fever. His cough has been productive of gray-yellow sputum with an occasional fleck of blood. He was found 10 months ago to be HIV-positive when he requested the test after several worrisome sexual contacts.

PAST MEDICAL HISTORY

Unremarkable since tonsillectomy, age 5.

SOCIAL HISTORY

The patient dropped out of college to organize a rock group that disbanded 2 years ago. He now works as a waiter in his parents' restaurant.

HABITS

Smokes one and a half packs of cigarettes daily. He uses no alcohol. He drinks four cups of coffee a day and occasionally smokes marijuana.

FAMILY HISTORY

His father, aged 54, is diabetic and has coronary artery disease. His mother, aged 51, and sister are living and in good health.

REVIEW OF SYSTEMS

Over the past month, he has had a poor appetite and believes that he has lost 3 to 5 pounds.

- What additional information about the history of present illness would be pertinent?
- What additional information about his HIV history might be pertinent? How would you elicit this information?
- What information about his current life style and work might be important? How would you frame this inquiry?
- What might be Mr. McCarthy's unstated reasons for the visit today? Why might this be important?

Objective

VITAL SIGNS

Height, 5 ft 9 in; weight, 145 lb; blood pressure, 110/72; pulse, 78; respirations, 24; temperature, 38.2°C.

EXAMINATION

The patient is a thin white man who does not appear acutely ill but coughs from time to time while speaking. The eyes, ears, nose, and throat are unremarkable except for mild pharyngeal injection. There are a few enlarged cervical nodes bilaterally. The chest has scattered rhonchi at both bases. The heart has a normal sinus rhythm with no murmurs. The skin has a few dark, slightly elevated areas of pigmentation on the dorsum of the hands.

- What other information obtained from the physical examination might be important? Why?
- Are there other areas of the body that you might examine? Why?
- What—if any—laboratory tests should be ordered today?
- What—if any—diagnostic imaging should be ordered today?

Assessment

- Pending the outcome of the tests you have ordered, what is your diagnostic assessment? How would you explain this to the patient?
- How would you assess Mr. McCarthy's knowledge of his health status and prognosis?

- What might be the meaning of the current illness to the patient? How would you address this issue?
- Describe the family implications of the illness?

Plan

- What are your specific recommendations for this patient? How would you explain this to the patient?
- What—if any—changes would you advise in his future work responsibilities?
- Mr. McCarthy's parents ask for an explanation of their son's illness. How would you respond?
- What are your recommendations for continuing care?

22
Anxiety Disorders

David A. Katerndahl

The lifetime prevalence of any anxiety disorder in the general population is 14.6%.[1] Not only are anxiety disorders important for the distress they cause, they are also associated with "excessive" suicide-related mortality.[2] Patients suffering from anxiety disorders tend to present to primary care settings. It is estimated that about 20% of family practice patients suffer with significant anxiety. Although recognition of anxiety disorders by private practitioners results in a shorter duration of illness and a greater frequency of mental health treatment, only 50% of patients with anxiety disorders are recognized by their physician.[3] Yet recognition of the presence of a disorder is only part of the problem. Once the presence of an anxiety disorder is recognized, primary care physicians are accurate in determining which disorder is present only 49% of the time.[4]

This chapter deals with the following "high impact" anxiety disorders: (1) panic disorder with agoraphobia; (2) generalized anxiety disorder; (3) obsessive compulsive disorder; and (4) posttraumatic stress disorder. These four disorders are associated with considerable morbidity to the patient and family, and they frequently overlap.

Panic Disorder and Agoraphobia

Panic attacks typically begin with cardiopulmonary symptoms and peak rapidly, finally dissipating within 1 to 2 hours. When unexpected attacks recur and leave the sufferer with a 1-month period of concern or dread of another attack, the condition is termed panic disorder (PD). Although patients frequently use multiple health care sites, more than 40% of panic attack patients seek care for their symptoms from their personal physician.[5] As many as 20% of family practice patients have a history of panic attacks.[6] Because PD patients believe they have a physical disorder causing their symptoms, they preferentially use general health providers instead of mental health providers. Consequently, emergency department usage is frequent in PD patients. Although anxiety is not a frequent presenting complaint in patients with PD, panic-related symptoms (Table 22.1) often

Table 22.1. Criteria for panic attack

Note: A panic attack is not a codable disorder. Code the specific diagnosis in which the panic attack occurs (e.g., 300.21 Panic Disorder with Agoraphobia).

A discrete period of intense fear or discomfort, in which four (or more) of the following symptoms developed abruptly and reached a peak within 10 minutes:
1. palpitations, pounding heart, or accelerated heart rate
2. sweating
3. trembling or shaking
4. sensations of shortness of breath or smothering
5. feeling of choking
6. chest pain or discomfort
7. nausea or abdominal distress
8. feeling dizzy, unsteady, lightheaded, or faint
9. derealization (feelings of unreality) or depersonalization (being detached from oneself)
10. fear of losing control or going crazy
11. fear of dying
12. paresthesias (numbness or tingling sensations)
13. chills or hot flushes

Source: American Psychiatric Association. Diagnostic and statistical manual of mental disorders. 4th ed. Washington, DC: APA, 1994. With permission.

induce help-seeking. Patients with chest pain present to their personal physician or the emergency department, whereas those with dizziness more frequently use the paramedics.[5]

Consequences and Complications

The longitudinal course of PD is one of persistent or recurring disability, with the quality of life frequently being impaired. As many as 90% of PD patients have a history of major depression, and 20% of PD patients report previous suicide attempts, irrespective of the presence of depression. As patients try to self-medicate their anxiety, the risk of substance abuse increases, such that up to 20% of PD patients abuse alcohol.

When patients associate their panic attacks with the situations in which they occurred, fear and avoidance of those situations may develop as the patient attempts to prevent another panic attack. When this phobic avoidance becomes severe enough that it restricts the patient's life, agoraphobia has developed. Up to two-thirds of PD patients have some degree of phobic avoidance.[7]

Diagnosis

Diagnosis of PD is based on the clinical history and the application of DSM-IV criteria (Table 22.2). Evaluation should consist of a thorough

TABLE 22.2. Diagnostic criteria for 300.21 panic disorder with agoraphobia

A. Both (1) and (2):
  1. recurrent unexpected panic attacks
  2. at least one of the attacks has been followed by 1 month (or more) of one (or more) of the following:
    a. persistent concern about having additional attacks
    b. worry about the implications of the attack or its consequences (e.g., losing control, having a heart attack, "going crazy")
    c. a significant change in behavior related to the attacks
B. The presence of agoraphobia
C. The panic attacks are not due to the direct physiological effects of a substance (e.g., a drug of abuse, a medication) or a general medical condition (e.g., hyperthyroidism).
D. The panic attacks are not better accounted for by another mental disorder, such as social phobia (e.g., occurring on exposure to feared social situations), specific phobia (e.g., on exposure to a specific phobic situation), obsessive-compulsive disorder (e.g., on exposure to dirt in someone with an obsession about contamination), post-traumatic stress disorder (e.g., in response to stimuli associated with a severe stressor), or separation anxiety disorder (e.g., in response to being away from home or close relatives).

Source: American Psychiatric Association. Diagnostic and statistical manual of mental disorders. 4th ed. Washington, DC: APA, 1994. With permission.

history and physical examination with assessment of possible complications. Because panic attacks are associated with a variety of organic pathology, patients must be evaluated for hyperthyroidism, cardiac arrhythmias, medication effects (stimulant use, sedative withdrawal), and partial complex epilepsy. However, without supporting evidence in the history or physical examination, routine laboratory screening is probably inappropriate.

Management

Management begins with patient education. This point is especially important when dealing with patients with PD because they frequently believe that a physical disorder is causing their symptoms. An explanation of the role of neurotransmitters in psychiatric disease and "labeling" their symptoms as "panic disorder" frequently reassures these patients.

If an organic cause for the panic attacks is found, management begins with treatment directed at this condition. Dietary measures such as the avoidance of caffeine and other stimulants is important. Also, patients should be encouraged to discontinue use of tobacco and marijuana.[8] The goal of therapy is for the patient to be panic-free. Unfortunately, the relapse rate after successful treatment is high.

Behavioral Therapy

Although based on few studies, behavioral therapy can be successful. Individual psychotherapy and insight therapy are probably not helpful, but applied relaxation and cognitive therapy are appropriate in the PD patient. Also, patients with agoraphobia eventually need some form of behavioral therapy following resolution of their panic attacks. Systematic desensitization in which agoraphobic patients are progressively exposed to their situational fears is effective when coupled with physician and family support. Even if drug therapy is used, exposure to phobic situations should be encouraged in all patients with PD.

Drug Therapy

A variety of medications are successful in preventing recurrent panic attacks in susceptible individuals. No medication is effective in aborting a panic attack once it has begun, however. Tricyclic antidepressants are effective in up to 90% of PD patients. Although imipramine (Tofranil) is used in most studies, other tricyclics such as desipramine (Norpramin) and clomipramine (Anafranil) are also effective. Because patients may respond to subantidepressant dosages and may be highly sensitive to imipramine, the initial starting dose should be low: 25 to 50 mg at bedtime. Patients should be warned that a sense of "jitteriness" may be seen early in the course of imipramine therapy. Maintenance of imipramine dosage usually results in resolution of this symptom. The dosage may be increased at regular intervals up to 300 mg/day. Three weeks of treatment may be necessary before panic suppression is achieved.

Although neuroleptics are contraindicated in PD, certain benzodiazepines are highly effective. The high-potency benzodiazepines—alprazolam (Xanax) and clonazepam (Klonopin)—have efficacy similar to that of the tricyclics. The literature recommends high doses of these benzodiazepines (3–10 mg alprazolam per day and 2–6 mg clonazepam per day), but experience in primary care settings suggests that lower doses are effective in primary care patients. Based on plasma levels and balancing side effect and remission rates, the optimal alprazolam dose may be 2 to 3 mg/day. Although alprazolam is the only medication with U.S. Food and Drug Administration approval for the treatment of PD, clonazepam may produce less sedation and fewer withdrawal side effects.

Monoamine oxidase inhibitors such as phenelzine (Nardil) may be even more effective than the tricyclics. Beginning with a dose of 15 mg at bedtime, the dose can be increased up to 60 mg/day. Due to the dietary restrictions, these drugs are not the first line of therapy. Other medications may also be effective for the management of PD. There is evidence to support the antipanic efficacy of fluoxetine (Prozac), lorazepam (Ativan), sodium valproate (Depakene), clonidine (Catapres), and verapamil (Calan). β-Blockers do not appear effective for management of PD.

Drug selection depends on the patient's age, concurrent medications, and co-morbid states. Elderly patients and those with a history of substance abuse should not be started on benzodiazepines. In the presence of major depression, a tricyclic antidepressant would be appropriate. Treatment should be continued until patients are panic-free for at least 6 to 12 months. Medication should be tapered slowly to avoid withdrawal symptoms.[9]

Point of Referral

Because these patients are frequently seen by family physicians and treated with medications with which most family physicians are familiar, there is no immediate need for referral. Family physicians who make home visits can diagnose and manage agoraphobic patients more readily than other specialists. Referral is appropriate if the physician is uncomfortable with an indicated therapy (e.g., monoamine oxidase inhibitors). Referral is also considered for patients who are potentially suicidal or are actively abusing drugs or alcohol.

Family Issues

Studies have shown a strong familial pattern for both PD and agoraphobia. Children of PD patients frequently have behavioral problems associated with the avoidance behavior in the parents.[10] Family members can be helpful in the management of agoraphobia, providing support at home while patients begin to confront their fears. PD and agoraphobia are stressful on the marital relationship, but the family frequently adapts to the agoraphobic's fears. Successful therapy implies changes in the family situation and dynamics. Hence, successful treatment of agoraphobia generates stress on the family unit.

Generalized Anxiety Disorder

The hallmark of generalized anxiety disorder (GAD) is excessive or unrealistic worry, out of proportion to the problems that exist. More than 85% of patients state that they spend more than half of their day anxious, with 36% of patients claiming that they spend more than 90% of their day in an anxious mood. Although 79% worry excessively about their families, about half of patients worry about finances and work.

Generalized anxiety disorder is frequently associated with other anxiety disorders: social phobia, panic disorder, simple phobia, and obsessive compulsive disorder. More than 70% of patients claim to have had at least one panic attack previously.[11] The lifetime prevalence of major depressive episode is 67%. This relation is particularly important because depression may represent a predisposing factor to GAD, and its presence frequently alters management.[12]

Although patients rarely seek psychiatric help, they do frequently seek help from family physicians, cardiologists, and pulmonologists. They often present to their family physician with multiple nonspecific complaints, usually including fatigue and muscular pain.[13]

Differential Diagnosis

The diagnosis of GAD is based on DSM-IV criteria (Table 22.3). Not only must the patient have experienced excessive anxiety for at least a 6-month period, but they must have at least three symptoms related to motor tension, autonomic hyperactivity, and vigilance and scanning. Because of the association between GAD and other anxiety disorders, GAD can be diagnosed only when the anxiety is unrelated to the focus of the other anxiety disorder, such as panic attacks. If depression is present, the anxiety must be present when the depression is not. Organic factors known to be associated with anxiety must not be responsible for initiating *and* maintaining the anxiety. Hence, hyperthyroidism, drugs such as cocaine and amphetamines, and general stimulants such as caffeine and tyramine must be excluded as the cause of the anxiety. Due to symptomatic similarity, adjustment disorder with

TABLE 22.3. Diagnostic criteria for 300.02 generalized anxiety disorder

A. Excessive anxiety and worry (apprehensive expectation), occurring more days than not for at least 6 months, about a number of events or activities (such as work or school performance).
B. The person finds it difficult to control the worry.
C. The anxiety and worry are associated with three (or more) of the following six symptoms (with at least some symptoms present for more days than not for the past 6 months). *Note:* Only one item is required in children.
   1. restlessness or feeling keyed up or on edge
   2. being easily fatigued
   3. difficulty concentrating or mind going blank
   4. irritability
   5. muscle tension
   6. sleep disturbance (difficulty falling or staying asleep, or restless unsatisfying sleep)
D. The focus of the anxiety and worry is not confined to features of an axis I disorder, e.g., the anxiety or worry is not about having a panic attack (as in panic disorder), being embarassed in public (as in social phobia), being contaminated (as in obsessive-compulsive disorder), being away from home or close relatives (as in separation anxiety disorder), gaining weight (as in anorexia nervosa), having multiple physical complaints (as in somatization disorder), or having a serious illness (as in hypochondriasis), and the anxiety and worry do not occur exclusively during posttraumatic stress disorder.
E. The anxiety, worry, or physical symptoms cause clinically significant distress or impairment in social, occupational, or other important areas of functioning
F. The disturbance is not due to the direct physiological effects of a substance (e.g., a drug of abuse, a medication) or a general medical condition (e.g., hyperthyroidism) and does not occur exclusively during a mood disorder, a psychotic disorder, or a pervasive developmental disorder.

Source: American Psychiatric Association. Diagnostic and statistical manual of mental disorders. 4th ed. Washington, DC: APA, 1994. With permission.

anxious mood must be excluded. This disorder differs from GAD in that a psychosocial stressor is present, the duration of disorder is less than 6 months, and the full symptomatic picture of GAD is usually not present.

Management

Behavioral Therapy

A variety of modalities exist to help the GAD patient cope with stress and anxiety. Progressive relaxation, stress management, and assertiveness training with or without hypnosis are frequently used,[14] as are family and group therapy as well as other forms of supportive psychotherapy. However, studies with cognitive behavioral therapy, during which anxious thoughts are identified and then changed, suggest that such cognitive therapy may be superior to other forms of behavioral therapy.[15]

Drug Therapy

Benzodiazepines

At least 70% of GAD patients respond to benzodiazepines (Table 22.4). Such response is more likely if a precipitating stress exists, significant depression is lacking, patients are aware of the psychological nature of their symptoms, there has been a prior response to benzodiazepines, and the patient expects recovery. Most patients who respond to benzodiazepines note improvement within the first week of therapy. Unfortunately, benzodiazepines frequently decrease alertness and performance. Although it is unusual for GAD patients without prior substance abuse to abuse benzodiazepines, physical dependence frequently develops. Tapering of the benzodiazepine dosage by reducing the dose by 10% per week can be tried after 2 months of therapy. Relapse is not uncommon and requires reinstituting the benzodiazepine or attempting intermittent therapy. Tricyclic antidepressants may reduce the chance of relapse.

TABLE 22.4. Commonly used benzodiazepines

Drug	Rate of onset	Usual daily dosage (mg)	Half-life (hours)
Alprazolam (Xanax)	Intermediate	0.5–4.0	12–15
Chlordiazepoxide (Librium)	Intermediate	15–100	5–30
Clonazepam (Klonopin)	Intermediate	1–10	30–60
Clorazepate (Tranxene)	Rapid	7.5–60.0	30–200
Diazepam (Valium)	Rapid	2–60	20–100
Lorazepam (Ativan)	Intermediate	2–6	10–20
Oxazepam (Serax)	Intermediate	30–120	5–15
Prazepam (Centrax)	Slow	20–60	30–200

Buspirone

Patients with respiratory disease, dementia, prior substance abuse, or on central nervous system (CNS) depressants may benefit from buspirone (BuSpar). Buspirone is helpful in patients in whom psychomotor impairment may be life-threatening. Because of its delayed onset of anxiolytic activity, buspirone is useful only in patients with chronic anxiety. Adequate doses of buspirone may be required for 2 to 3 weeks before patients note a response. Because there is no potential for dependence, buspirone does not need to be tapered once therapy is completed.

Other Medications

Although β-blockers may reduce somatic symptoms, they have no place in the management of GAD. Tricyclic depressants may be of some benefit in patients with GAD.[15] If present, depression should be treated aggressively. Hence, the drug of choice in the management of GAD with major depression is a tricyclic antidepressant. Buspirone is the next alternative. Because benzodiazepines may worsen depression, they should not be first-line agents in patients with GAD and depression.[12]

Point of Referral

Because the management of GAD requires patience and frequent office visits initially, not every physician wishes to manage these patients. Referral should be considered in the presence of co-morbid anxiety or depressive disorders if the physician lacks comfort in management. Patients with current substance abuse or those requiring behavioral techniques unfamiliar to the physician may also be referred to appropriate mental health providers. Because some patients may indeed require chronic benzodiazepine therapy, the recurrence of symptoms or difficulty tapering benzodiazepines does not necessarily indicate the need for referral.

Family Issues

Although there is no reported familial pattern to GAD, family issues may be important. As mentioned before, many patient worries focus around family problems. Involvement of the family in therapy is helpful. Specifically, family and friends should be enlisted to encourage socialization and confrontation of fears.[13] Although not frequently recognized, the presence of GAD within a family has serious implications. Not only can GAD produce functional impairments and affect quality of life, it represents a serious stress for the family. GAD in parents may be a risk factor for the development of autism in children.[16]

Obsessive Compulsive Disorder

The hallmark of obsessive compulsive disorder (OCD) is the presence of recurrent obsessions or compulsions (or both) that markedly distress or significantly interfere with the patient's life. Obsessions—intrusive ideas or thoughts—occur in more than half of OCD patients. Fears of contamination are common, as are thoughts of harming others, counting, praying, and blasphemous or sexual thoughts. *Compulsions*—repetitive intentional behaviors designed to neutralize discomfort—also occur in more than half of these patients. Rituals such as cleaning and hand washing, arranging items, and "checking" are common. Compulsions include acts to control the behavior of others, hoarding behaviors, and hair pulling. Fewer than 10% of patients have both obsessions and compulsions, but the presence of multiple obsessions or multiple compulsions is common.[17] Delusions may occur in as many as 12% of patients, but they are usually transient and their absurdity is realized by the patient.[18] Although patients frequently consider themselves "crazy," they do not always believe that their obsessions are senseless, and their compulsions are not always resisted.[19]

Obsessive compulsive disorder is a continuous disorder in about 85% of patients; in only 5% is it episodic.[20] Although 35% of OCD patients seek mental health care from general health physicians,[17] most of the cases are not recognized by the primary care physician. When such patients do present, they may expect extensive laboratory testing to assess what they consider serious physical problems.[21]

Co-morbidity and Complications

Up to 80% of OCD patients have evidence of depression, anxiety, substance abuse, or work disability.[21] Between 32% and 67% of patients have major depressive disorder, usually beginning after the onset of OCD. Substance abuse is seen in 14% to 24% of patients, again usually beginning after the onset of OCD. Although panic disorder is seen in fewer than 15% of patients,[17,20] almost 40% of patients do report panic attacks; 19% of these patients note panic attacks triggered only by OCD symptoms.[22] Usually beginning before the onset of OCD, phobias are present in almost half the patients.[17] Although more than 50% of patients have at least one personality disorder,[23] fewer than 15% have an obsessive compulsive personality.[24]

With an obsession to body parts, it is not surprising that a high rate of eating disorders are seen in these patients.[20] CNS disease is also common; abnormal scans are frequently seen, and more than 90% of patients have some abnormality on neurologic testing.[25] In addition to a high degree of psychosocial disability, OCD patients frequently have behavioral problems and find it difficult to maintain employment.[24] Their social involvement is usually poor, and half of OCD patients have some marital distress.[26]

TABLE 22.5. Diagnostic criteria for 300.3 obsessive-compulsive disorder

A. Either obsessions or compulsions:
   Obsessions as defined by (1), (2), (3), and (4):
   1. recurrent and persistent thoughts, impulses, or images that are experienced, at some time during the disturbance, as intrusive and inappropriate and that cause marked anxiety or distress
   2. the thoughts, impulses, or images are not simply excessive worries about real-life problems
   3. the person attempts to ignore or suppress such thoughts, impulses, or images, or to neutralize them with some other thought or action
   4. the person recognizes that the obsessional thoughts, impulses, or images are a product of his or her own mind (not imposed from without as in thought insertion)
   Compulsions as defined by (1) and (2):
   1. repetitive behaviors (e.g., hand washing, ordering, checking) or mental acts (e.g., praying, counting, repeating words silently) that the person feels driven to perform in response to an obsession, or according to rules that must be applied rigidly
   2. the behaviors or mental acts are aimed at preventing or reducing distress or preventing some dreaded event or situation; however, these behaviors or mental acts either are not connected in a realistic way with what they are designed to neutralize or prevent or are clearly excessive
B. At some point during the course of the disorder, the person has recognized that the obsessions or compulsions are excessive or unreasonable. *Note:* This does not apply to children.
C. The obsessions or compulsions caused marked distress, are time consuming (take more than 1 hour a day), or significantly interfere with the person's normal routine, occupational (or academic) functioning, or usual social activities or relationships.
D. If another axis I disorder is present, the content of the obsessions or compulsions is not restricted to it (e.g., preoccupation with the food in the presence of an eating disorder; hair pulling in the presence of trichotillomania; concern with appearance in the presence of body dysmorphic disorder; preoccupation with drugs in the presence of a substance use disorder; preoccupation with having a serious illness in the presence of hypochondriasis; preoccupation with sexual urges or fantasies in the presence of a paraphilia; or guilty ruminations in the presence of major depressive disorder).
E. The disturbance is not due to the direct physiological effects of a substance (e.g., a drug of abuse, a medication) or a general medical condition.
Specify if:
   With poor insight: if, for most of the time during the current episode, the person does not recognize that the obsessions and compulsions are excessive or unreasonable

Source: American Psychiatric Association. Diagnostic and statistical manual of mental disorders. 4th ed. Washington, DC: APA, 1994. With permission.

Differential Diagnosis

Patients with OCD frequently use primary care physicians for their mental health care. The physician must therefore have a high index of suspicion because embarrassment usually prevents patients from spontaneously revealing their obsessions or compulsions.[27] The diagnosis of OCD is based on DSM-IV criteria (Table 22.5). Two screening questions can be useful for identifying possible OCD patients:

1. Are you bothered by thoughts coming into your mind that make you anxious and that you are unable to get rid of?
2. Are there certain behaviors you do over and over that may seem silly to you or to others but that you feel you just have to do?

Physical examination can provide clues to the physician. Such clues are important because patients often do not voluntarily describe their obsessions or compulsions. Dermatologic changes may be due to compulsive hand washing or self-mutilations. Similarly, hoarding behaviors may lead to collecting garbage, which can result in poor hygiene or infections. Hair-pulling behaviors—trichotillomania—may be evidenced by areas of alopecia. Similarly, a normal physical examination in the presence of repeated evaluations for somatic symptoms suggests OCD. Evidence of plastic surgery may reflect patients' obsessions with their bodies. Routine laboratory testing is not helpful for differentiating OCD from other disorders unless specifically indicated by the history or physical examination.

Several physical disorders simulate OCD. CNS infections such as encephalitis, head trauma, brain tumors involving the frontal or prefrontal cortex or residing near the basal ganglia, Huntington's chorea, and diabetes insipidus should be considered in the differential diagnosis.[21] A variety of psychiatric disorders may also be suggested. However, the content of the obsessions suggests the true diagnosis. For example, the realization by OCD patients that delusions are not real differentiate them from schizophrenics. Specific personality disorders such as obsessive compulsive and schizotypal personality should also be considered.[27]

Management

Behavioral Therapy

Although flooding therapy—sudden intense exposure to objects of fear until anxiety dissipates—may be helpful for OCD; insight therapy,[27] dynamic psychotherapy, and systematic desensitization are not. Exposure therapy with response prevention is the behavioral technique of choice. Office-based, with homework assignments, exposure therapy involves exposure to stimuli associated with the patient's obsessions until the discomfort diminishes—within about 30 to 35 minutes. This therapy is coupled with response prevention in which patients are asked to refrain from rituals for progressively longer periods until their discomfort diminishes. If performed as directed, this therapy produces a 70% reduction in symptoms for at least 50% of patients. Unfortunately, 25% of patients either refuse or cannot comply.[28] Patients who do comply report improvement in their work and social adjustment, and they experience diminished OCD symptoms and depression. Persistence of benefit is related to the duration of therapy and compliance with homework activities.[29]

Drug Therapy

Drug therapy is helpful in patients who are purely obsessional, have a history of substance abuse, or cannot comply with behavioral therapy.[28] Clomipramine (Anafranil) in doses of up to 250 mg/day is more effective than other tricyclic antidepressants in OCD patients. Although there may be improvement in symptoms and in the ability to function, clomipramine-treated patients are rarely symptom-free. OCD tends to relapse quickly after discontinuance of clomipramine.[30] Although up to 10 weeks of therapy may be required before improvement is seen, once improvement occurs the clomipramine dose can frequently be reduced without exacerbation of obsessive compulsive symptoms.[31] Fluoxetine (Prozac) in doses up to 80 mg/day and fluvoxamine (Luvox) in doses up to 300 mg/day may also be effective in OCD patients.[32] However, monoamine oxidase inhibitors and benzodiazepines are not helpful; and in fact, benzodiazepines may interfere with behavioral therapy.[27] Buspirone (BuSpar) and lithium carbonate (Eskalith, Lithobid) may be useful for augmenting a response to clomipramine or fluoxetine.[32]

The presence of co-morbid conditions affects the choice of therapeutic agents. In the presence of other anxiety disorders or major depressive disorder, the agent of choice is probably clomipramine. Depressed patients may also respond to fluoxetine or fluvoxamine to a lesser extent. Buspirone may also be appropriate in the depressed patient. When using drug therapy, patients should be treated for at least 1 year. Clomipramine and fluoxetine should be tapered every 2 months in decrements of 50 mg and 20 mg, respectively.

In general, patients with purely obsessional disorders should be treated with drug therapy first, followed by a variety of behavioral techniques—cognitive therapy, assertiveness training, flooding—if necessary.[33] Drug therapy causes a reduction in symptoms in 30% to 42% of patients. Although behavioral therapy may reduce symptoms in up to 50% of patients, OCD patients must have some ritual behavior for it to be effective. Although self-exposure techniques are the most potent, therapist-aided techniques are of marginal value but may be necessary. Behavioral therapy is less likely to succeed in patients who are depressed, delusional, or noncompliant because covert rituals may undermine therapy.[34] Although OCD is treatable, a poor response is more likely in patients who have personality disorders (especially schizotypal personality), patients who have overvalued ideas (a strong belief in the value of their rituals), and patients with a family history of psychiatric problems.[33]

Although electroconvulsive therapy has not been shown to be helpful in OCD,[28] patients refractory to behavioral and drug therapy can be improved with surgery. Techniques that interrupt the connections between the frontal cortex and the limbic system result in marked improvement in 28% of patients, with an additional 37% of patients being symptom-free. Only 12% of patients show no improvement. The intelligence of patients receiving such surgery is usually increased after the procedure.[34]

Point of Referral

There is no reason a family physician cannot use the medications or behavioral techniques mentioned.[27] Therefore, referral usually depends on physician comfort with the therapeutic program. Consider referral in patients who do not respond to adequate therapy or in those with complicating medical or psychiatric problems.

Family Issues

The patient's family is important in OCD. Not only is the disorder a familial one,[24] but OCD patients frequently have marital problems. However, behavioral therapy can produce improvement in OCD patients despite these marital problems. Also, the spouse improves as the patient responds, regardless of whether the family has been involved in the treatment.[26] Unfortunately, because of the embarrassing nature of the disorder, evaluation is sometimes viewed as "taboo" by the family, thus presenting an obstacle to the help-seeking of the patient. However, if the family is involved as co-therapist in family-based therapy, OCD patients have lower levels of anxiety, depression, and OCD symptoms, and they increase their social adjustment. If family members are to be involved in such therapy, they must have low levels of anxiety themselves and be able to tolerate the frustrating nature of this therapy.[35]

Posttraumatic Stress Disorder

Posttraumatic stress disorder (PTSD) occurs in people experiencing a stressful event that occurs beyond the range of usual human experience and is particularly distressing to anyone experiencing it. It is associated with persistent reexperiencing of the event, avoidance of stimuli associated with the event, and symptoms of increased arousal. Because of the dissociative nature of some of the symptoms, it has been suggested that PTSD should be classified as a dissociative disorder.

Although the stressful event itself is the precipitant of the disorder, several factors have been identified as important in its development: factors present before the stressful event, characteristics of the stressor, and poststress factors. Patient factors that predispose to the development of

PTSD include poor school performance, a rigid or immature personality, the lack of preparedness for the stressor, a disruptive environment before the stress, and preexisting psychiatric problems such as anxiety or depression.[36] The patient's family of origin may also be important. PTSD is more likely to develop in patients who come from families with low cohesion and expressiveness, early parental separation, familial history of depression, alcoholism, or anxiety, parental neglect, and intrafamilial conflict.[37]

Although the severity of the trauma itself does not predict development of PTSD, its duration and intensity does.[38] If the stress occurs during a vulnerable time in the patient's life or bears a similarity to an earlier traumatic event, PTSD is more likely. In rape victims, PTSD is more likely to develop if the rape is done by a stranger, involves physical force or injury, includes the display of weapons, or is associated with a sense of helplessness in the victim.[39]

After the stress has occurred, the subjective level of distress and weekly alcohol intake predict the development of PTSD.[40] Lack of support during recovery—financial and emotional—is also an important factor.

Symptoms and Course

Although symptoms usually begin immediately after the stressor, there may be a delayed onset. Once established, PTSD frequently persists for years. Symptomatically, 90% of patients note sleep disturbance, loss of interest, emotional detachment, avoidance behavior of situations associated with the stressor, and reexperiencing of the event. Also, a variety of somatic symptoms may develop.

Although patients with PTSD frequently develop depression, generalized anxiety disorder, and violent behavior, criminality without a prior predilection is uncommon.[36] In general, men are at greater risk for developing depression and drug abuse, whereas women are at greater risk of developing panic disorder and phobias. An increased risk of alcoholism and OCD appears similar in both genders.[41]

Diagnosis

Because patients frequently present with vague complaints, diagnosis of PTSD can be challenging. In addition to experiencing a traumatic stressor, DSM-IV criteria (Table 22.6) require evidence that the traumatic event is persistently reexperienced (e.g., flashbacks or nightmares). To be diagnosed with PTSD, a patient must also have persistent avoidance of stimuli associated with the stressor or a generalized numbing of emotions. Finally, patients must have persistent symptoms of increased arousal. Although the DSM-IV requires symptoms of at least 1 month's duration, some authors recommend increasing this criterion to 3 months' duration because of the observation that more than half of rape victims recover within 3 months.[42]

TABLE 22.6. Diagnostic criteria for 309.81 posttraumatic stress disorder

A. The person has been exposed to a traumatic event in which both of the following were present:
1. the person experienced, witnessed, or was confronted with an event or events that involved actual or threatened death or serious injury, or a threat to the physical integrity of self or others
2. the person's response involved intense fear, helplessness, or horror. *Note:* In children, this may be expressed instead by disorganized or agitated behavior.

B. The traumatic event is persistently reexperienced in one (or more) of the following ways:
1. recurrent and intrusive distressing recollections of the event, including images, thoughts, or perceptions. *Note:* In young children, repetitive play may occur in which themes or aspects of the trauma are expressed.
2. recurrent distressing dreams of the event. *Note:* In children, there may be frightening dreams without recognizable content.
3. acting or feeling as if the traumatic event were recurring (includes a sense of reliving the experience, illusions, hallucinations, and dissociative flashback episodes, including those that occur on awakening or when intoxicated). *Note:* In young children, trauma-specific reenactment may occur.
4. intense psychological distress at exposure to internal or external cues that symbolize or resemble an aspect of the traumatic event
5. physiological reactivity on exposure to internal or external cues that symbolize or resemble an aspect of the traumatic event

C. Persistent avoidance of stimuli associated with the trauma and numbing of general responsiveness (not present before the trauma), as indicated by three (or more) of the following:
1. efforts to avoid thoughts, feelings, or conversations associated with the trauma
2. efforts to avoid activities, places, or people that arouse recollections of the trauma
3. inability to recall an important aspect of the trauma
4. markedly diminished interest or participation in significant activities
5. feeling of detachment or estrangement from others
6. restricted range of affect (e.g., unable to have loving feelings)
7. sense of a foreshortened future (e.g., does not expect to have a career, marriage, children, or a normal life-span)

D. Persistent symptoms of increased arousal (not present before the trauma), as indicated by two (or more) of the following:
1. difficulty falling or staying asleep
2. irritability or outbursts of anger
3. difficulty concentrating
4. hypervigilance
5. exaggerated startle response

E. Duration of the disturbance (symptoms in criteria B, C, and D) is more than 1 month.

F. The disturbance causes clinically significant distress or impairment in social, occupational, or other important areas of functioning.

Specify if:
Acute: if duration of symptoms is less than 3 months
Chronic: if duration of symptoms is 3 months or more
Specify if:
With delayed onset: if onset of symptoms is at least 6 months after the stressor

Source: American Psychiatric Association. Diagnostic and statistical manual of mental disorders. 4th ed. Washington, DC: APA, 1994. With permission.

When considering the differential diagnosis, adjustment disorder can usually be ruled out by the lack of severity of symptoms as well as the fact that the stressor is usually not extreme. In the presence of head trauma, either postconcussive disorder or organic aggressive disorder must be considered. The presence of co-morbid conditions such as depression and substance abuse frequently makes the diagnosis difficult. Depression and substance abuse themselves must be considered in the differential diagnosis.[43] Finally, because of the publicity surrounding PTSD and its potential for financial compensation, malingering must be considered.

Certain DSM-IV symptoms appear to be specific for PTSD and may therefore have diagnostic implications. For example, the existence of many triggers for reexperiencing the event suggests the presence of PTSD, as does avoidance of stimuli through the loss of interest, estrangement, or a numbing effect. The presence of a startle response, sleep disturbance, memory disturbance, or disturbed concentration are specific for PTSD. Finally, if patients are either predominantly angry or avoid getting upset, PTSD should be considered.[44]

Management

The disorder is not easily treated. Although two-thirds of PTSD patients completing a 4-week inpatient treatment program were improved, 55% of them required hospitalization within 2 years.[45] Early treatment is important and depends heavily on the attitudes of the family and the physician. Also, the presence of predisposing factors, substance abuse, and subsequent stressors may also impede recovery. Unfortunately, the presence of secondary gain, litigation, and encouragement from others to assume a sick role represent further obstacles to recovery.

Behavioral Therapy

Negative symptoms such as avoidance behavior, loss of interest, and emotional numbing respond better to psychotherapy than to medication.[43] In general terms, the goals of psychotherapy are to encourage the patients to express their emotions and to explore earlier events. Evaluation begins by exploring the stressor itself as well as the patient's status before the stressor. A detailed understanding of the problems experienced and the stressor are also important. A variety of methods have been found to be successful for treating PTSD. Psychodynamic therapy, hypnotherapy, and desensitization to the stressor decrease symptoms.[46] Although flooding therapy has been successful, it has also produced increased depression, the occurrence of panic attacks, and relapse of alcoholism. The use of PTSD groups may be helpful.

Drug Therapy

Although all PTSD patients require psychotherapy, medication frequently has a positive effect on the results of psychotherapy, particularly with hyperarousal and the reexperiencing of the event.[47] Although response to major tranquilizers is poor,[44] both imipramine (Tofranil) in doses sufficient to produce blood levels higher than 150 mg/ml and phenelzine (Nardil) in doses from 15 to 75 mg/day alleviate symptoms over an 8-week period.[48] Also, a variety of other medications may augment medication response.

Two approaches can be applied to the selection of a drug regimen. First, medication can be selected based on co-morbid states. Hence, in the presence of panic disorder or depression, the PTSD patient should be started on a tricyclic antidepressant. In the presence of generalized anxiety disorder, the patient should receive buspirone (BuSpar) or a benzodiazepine. Finally, in the presence of outbursts, the patient should be prescribed propranolol (Inderal).

The second approach to drug therapy is to begin the patient on a tricyclic antidepressant for a 6- to 8-week period. At the end of the 8-week period, the patient is reevaluated for response. In the presence of refractory depression or anger, the tricyclic antidepressant is changed to a monoamine oxidase inhibitor, or lithium (Eskalith, Lithobid) is added. Similarly, symptoms of autonomic arousal such as vigilance or a startle response can be treated with either propranolol in doses of 60 to 640 mg/day or clonidine (Catapres) in doses of 0.2 to 0.6 mg/day. Persistent flashbacks respond to carbamazepine (Tegretol), and distress on reexposure to stimuli responds to propranolol. Finally, persistent aggression can be treated with either propranolol, carbamazepine, or lithium.[43]

Point of Referral

Because most family practitioners are not trained in the psychodynamic techniques used with PTSD patients, most of these patients require referral for co-management. Also, if monoamine oxidase inhibitors or lithium are indicated, some physicians may feel the need to refer those patients to a psychiatrist.

Family Issues

The family is an important factor in the evaluation and treatment of the PTSD patient. The family should be included in the interview process, because patients are often incapable of revealing their own feelings or describing their behavior. Also, the family's attitude is important for treatment. It can help to minimize secondary gain in the patient by discouraging the development of a sick role. Also, through patience and support, the family can provide a positive setting for the patient's recovery.

References

1. Schatzberg AF. Overview of anxiety disorders. J Clin Psychiatry 1991;52 (Suppl):5–9.
2. Allgulander C, Lavori PW. Excess mortality among 3302 patients with "pure" anxiety neurosis. Arch Gen Psychiatry 1991;48:599–602.
3. Ormel J, Koeter MWJ, van den Brink W, van de Willige G. Recognition, management, and course of anxiety and depression in general practice. Arch Gen Psychiatry 1991;48:700–6.
4. Andersen SM, Harthorn BH. Recognition, diagnosis, and treatment of mental disorders by primary care physicians. Med Care 1989;27:869–86.
5. Katerndahl D. Factors associated with persons with panic attacks seeking medical care. Fam Med 1990;22:462–6.
6. Katon W, Vitaliano PP, Russo J, et al. Panic disorder. J Fam Pract 1986;23: 233–9.
7. Noyes R Jr. Comorbidity and mortality of panic disorder. Psychiatr Med 1990;8:41–66.
8. Roy-Byrne PP, Uhde TW. Exogenous factors in panic disorder. J Clin Psychiatry 1988;49:56–61.
9. Roy-Byrne PP. Integrated treatment of panic disorder. Am J Med 1992;92 (Suppl1A):49S–54S.
10. Silverman WK, Cerny JA, Nelles WB, Burke AE. Behavior problems in children of parents with anxiety disorders. J Am Acad Child Adolesc Psychiatry 1988;27:779–84.
11. Sanderson WC, Barlow DH. Description of patients diagnosed with DSM-III-R GAD. J Nerv Ment Dis 1990;178:588–91.
12. Lydiard RB. Coexisting depression and anxiety. J Clin Psychiatry 1991;51 (Suppl):48–54.
13. Dilsaver SC. Generalized anxiety disorder. Am Fam Physician 1989;39:137–44.
14. Dubovsky SL. Generalized anxiety disorder. J Clin Psychiatry 1990;51 (Suppl):3–10.
15. Butler G, Fennell M, Robson P, Gelder M. Comparison of behavior therapy and cognitive behavior therapy in the treatment of GAD. J Consult Clin Psychol 1991;59:167–75.
16. Piven J, Chase GA, Landa R, et al. Psychiatric disorders in the parents of autistic individuals. J Am Acad Child Adolesc Psychiatry 1991;30:471–8.
17. Karno M, Golding JM, Sorenson SB, Burnam A. Epidemiology of OCD in five US communities. Arch Gen Psychiatry 1988;45:1094–9.
18. Insel TR, Akiskal HS. OCD with psychotic features. Am J Psychiatry 1986; 143:1527–33.
19. Lelliott PT, Noshirvani HF, Basoglu M, et al. Obsessive-compulsive beliefs and treatment outcome. Psychol Med 1988;18:697–702.
20. Rasmussen SA, Eisen JL. Clinical and epidemiologic findings of significance to neuropharmacologic trials in OCD. Psychopharmacol Bull 1988;24:466–70.
21. Alarcon RD. How to recognize OCD. Postgrad Med 1991;90:131–43.
22. Austin LS, Lydiard RB, Fossey MD, et al. Panic and phobic disorders in patients with OCD. J Clin Psychiatry 1990;51:456–8.
23. Baer L, Jenike MA, Ricciard JN, et al. Standardized assessment of personality disorders in OCD. Arch Gen Psychiatry 1990;47:826–30.

24. Riddle MA, Scahill L, King R, et al. OCD in children and adolescents. J Am Acad Child Adolesc Psychiatry 1990;29:766–72.
25. Hollander E, Schiffman E, Cohen B, et al. Signs of central nervous system dysfunction in OCD. Arch Gen Psychiatry 1990;47:27–32.
26. Emmelkamp PMG, de Haan E, Hoogduin CAL. Marital adjustment and OCD. Br J Psychiatry 1990;156:55–60.
27. March JS, Johnston H, Greist JH. Obsessive-compulsive disorder. Am Fam Physician 1989;39:175–82.
28. Greist JH. Treating the anxiety. J Clin Psychiatry 1990;51(Suppl):29–34.
29. O'Sullivan G, Noshirvani H, Marks I, et al. Six-year follow-up after exposure and clomipramine therapy for OCD. J Clin Psychiatry 1991;52:150–5.
30. Feinberg M. Clomipramine for obsessive-compulsive disorder. Am Fam Physician 1991;43:1735–8.
31. Pato MT, Hill JL, Murphy DL. Clomipramine dosage reduction study in the course of long-term treatment of OCD patients. Psychopharmacol Bull 1990; 26:211–14.
32. Insel TR. New pharmacologic approaches to OCD. J Clin Psychiatry 1990; 51(Suppl):47–51.
33. Jenike MA. Approaches to the patient with treatment–refractory OCD. J Clin Psychiatry 1990;51(Suppl):15–21.
34. Greist JH. Treatment of OCD. J Clin Psychiatry 1990;51(Suppl):44–50.
35. Mehta M. Comparative study of family-based and patient-based behavioral management in OCD. Br J Psychiatry 1990;157:133–5.
36. Pary R, Lippmann SB, Turns DM, Tobias CR. Post-traumatic stress disorder in Vietnam veterans. Am Fam Physician 1988;37:145–50.
37. Silven SM, Iacono C. Symptom groups and family patterns of Vietnam veterans with PTSD. In: Figley CR, editor. Trauma and its wake. Vol 2. New York: Brunner/Mazel, 1986.
38. Buydens-Branchey L, Noumair D, Branchey M. Duration and intensity of combat exposure and PTSD in Vietnam veterans. J Nerv Ment Dis 1990; 178:582–7.
39. Bownes IT, O'Gorman BC, Sayers A. Assault characteristics and PTSD in rape victims. Acta Psychiatr Scand 1991;83:27–30.
40. Feinstein A, Dolan R. Predictors of PTSD following physical trauma. Psychol Med 1991;21:85–91.
41. Helzer JE, Robins LN, McEvoy L. PTSD in the general population. N Engl J Med 1987;317:1630–4.
42. Davidson JRT, Foa EB. Refining criteria for PTSD. Hosp Community Psychiatry 1991;42:259–61.
43. Silver JM, Sandberg DP, Hales RE. New approaches in the pharmacotherapy of PTSD. J Clin Psychiatry 1990;51(Suppl):33–38.
44. Bleich A, Siegel B, Garb R, Lerer B. Post-traumatic stress disorder following combat exposure. Br J Psychiatry 1986;149:365–9.
45. Perconte ST, Griger ML, Belucci G. Relapse and rehospitalization of veterans two years after treatment for PTSD. Hosp Community Psychiatry 1989;40:1072–3.
46. Brom D, Kleber RJ, Defares PB. Brief psychotherapy for PTSD. J Consult Clin Psychol 1989;57:607–12.
47. Friedman MJ. Toward rational pharmacotherapy for PTSD. Am J Psychiatry 1988;145:281–5.
48. Frank JB, Kosten TR, Giller EL Jr, Dan E. Randomized clinical trial of phenelzine and imipramine for posttraumatic stress disorder. Am J Psychiatry 1988;145:1289–91.

CASE PRESENTATION

Subjective

PATIENT PROFILE

Nancy Nelson is a 40-year-old white female accountant.

PRESENTING PROBLEM

"Feeling nervous."

PRESENT ILLNESS

Mrs. Nelson reports a long history of recurrent anxiety becoming worse over the last 3 years. Her hands are often moist and tremulous, and she has trouble falling asleep at night. Her symptoms are worse with new people and when with clients at work. She is fearful of making mistakes on the job, especially on clients' tax returns. She has trouble relaxing even on weekends and vacations. She feels some relief when she takes a drink of alcohol.

PAST MEDICAL HISTORY

She has had three urinary tract infections over the past year; the last was treated 4 months ago.

SOCIAL HISTORY, HABITS, AND FAMILY HISTORY

Are unchanged since her last visit 4 months ago (see Chapter 15).

REVIEW OF SYSTEMS

She reports occasional urinary frequency and one to two time nocturia.

- What additional medical history would you like to know? Why?
- What is a likely reason for today's visit?
- What more would you like to know about her symptoms at work?
- What adaptations might Mrs. Nelson had made to her symptoms, and why might this be important?

Objective

GENERAL

The patient appears tense and fidgets with her hair and fingers during the interview.

VITAL SIGNS

Blood pressure, 118/60; pulse, 74 and regular; respirations, 18.

EXAMINATION

The eyes, ears, nose, and throat are normal; the neck and thyroid are unremarkable; the hands are cool with slightly moist palms. No tremor is present.

- What additional information—if any—might you include in the physical examination, and why?
- Are there other areas of the body that should be examined today? Why?
- What physical diseases might cause Mrs. Nelson's symptoms? How might you eliminate these as diagnostic possibilities?
- What laboratory tests or diagnostic imaging—if any—would you obtain today? Why?

Assessment

- What is your diagnostic assessment? How would you explain this to Mrs. Nelson?
- Might today's complaint be a "ticket of admission" to discuss other problems? Explain.
- Might her symptoms be related to life events that have not yet been discussed, and how would you elicit this information?
- What might be the impact of this illness on the family? On coworkers?

Plan

- Describe your therapeutic recommendation. How would you explain this to Mrs. Nelson?
- What—if any—life-style changes would you advise?
- Would you recommend consultation or referral? Explain.
- What continuing care would you recommend?

23
Depression

Rupert R. Goetz, Scott A. Fields, and
William L. Toffler

To effectively diagnose and treat patients with depression, physicians need
a clear understanding of the current systems of classification. The *Diagnostic and Statistical Manual of Mental Disorders* (DSM-IV) divides affective
disorders into 10 categories: major depression, bipolar I, bipolar II, dysthymic and cyclothymic disorders, mood disorders due to medical conditions
and due to substance abuse, as well as depressive, bipolar, and mood disorders
not otherwise specified.[1] We first explore diagnostic and therapeutic concepts, highlighting the structure behind current understanding of these
disorders. Then we discuss application of these concepts to the process of
evaluation and treatment of patients, including special populations.

Epidemiology

Almost half of all office visits resulting in a mental disorder diagnosis are
to nonpsychiatrists, mostly physicians in primary care.[2] Patients seen in
this setting may be in an earlier, less organized stage of illness.[3] Table 23.1
summarizes the prevalence of affective disorders. Generally, women are at
higher risk than men, as are patients with other medical or psychiatric
conditions.

Etiology

Mechanisms of depression in three main areas have been investigated: abnormalities in neurotransmission, neurophysiology, and neuroendocrine function.
The ultimate causes of these disorders remain unclear. Clinically, etiologic
differentiation and specific biologic tests remain limited in their usefulness.
The biopsychosocial model described by Engel in 1980[4] underscores the
interrelation of biologic, psychological, and social issues in illness and may be
used to better understand the possible origins of depression.

TABLE 23.1. Epidemiology of affective disorders
in the general population

Disorder	Current prevalence (%)	Lifetime prevalence (%)
Major depression	3–6	10–20
Dysthymia	1	2–3
Bipolar disorder	<0.5	0.5–1.0

Genetic factors may play a role in increased susceptibility. First-degree relatives of a patient with affective disorder have about a 25% to 30% likelihood of major depression or bipolar disorder. Twin studies have shown concordance for major depression of 50% for monozygotic twins and 25% for dizygotic twins.[5] The variation in risk makes unlikely a single gene with predictable penetrance for specific disorders.

Psychological factors have long been considered important in depression. Behavioral theorists[6] argue that impaired social skills lead to dysphoria and that the addition of secondary gain leads to clinical depression. Cognitive-behavioral theory[7] holds that thought distortions, activated by a stressor, lead some individuals to unrealistically negative and demeaning views of themselves, the world, and the future. Some theories of depression place a high value on the patient's function within society: Patients cannot be understood outside their social context.

Diagnosis

Diagnostic Criteria

A major depressive disorder requires the patient to have a major depressive episode (Table 23.2), and there should never have been a manic, hypomanic, or mixed epixode. Either depressed mood or loss of interest or pleasure is required. Once the diagnosis is made, the severity (mild, moderate, severe), result of treatment (partial or full remission), and presence or absence of psychotic features should be noted. These features may be either mood congruent (depressive in character) or incongruent. Catatonic, melancholic, or atypical features, as well a postpartum onset or longitudinal course (seasonal, rapid cycling), can be described.

Dysthymia is used to describe a specific disorder rather than a "milder depression." It is diagnosed when two of six criteria (see Table 23.3) are met over a period of 2 years, uninterrupted by more than a 2-month period, and not initiated by a major depression. *Bipolar disorders* are divided into type I and II, the former characterized by at least one manic (Table 23.4) or mixed episode, the latter by at least one hypomanic episode and major depressive episodes. Mania is distinguished from hypomania by the longer

TABLE 23.2. DSM-IV diagnostic criteria for a
major depressive episode

A. Five of the following nine symptoms present for at least
   2 weeks
   1. Depressed mood
   2. Diminished interest or pleasure
   3. Significant appetite or weight change
   4. Sleep disturbance (insomnia or hypersomnia)
   5. Psychomotor agitation or retardation
   6. Fatigue or loss of energy
   7. Feelings of worthlessness or inappropriate guilt
   8. Diminished ability to think or concentrate
   9. Recurrent thoughts of death or suicide
B. Not a mixed episode
C. Cause significant distress or impair function
D. Not attributable to medical conditions or substance abuse
E. Not attributable to bereavement

A mnemonic may be useful to recall these criteria: *Depression is
worth seriously memorizing extremely gruesome criteria, sorry.*
(DIWS MEGCS). These initials stand for *D*epressed mood,
*I*nterest, *W*eight, *S*leep, *M*otor activity, *E*nergy, *G*uilt,
*C*oncentration, and *S*uicide.[14]

Source: Adapted from American Psychiatric Association.[1] With
permission.

TABLE 23.3. DSM-IV diagnostic criteria for
dysthymic disorder

A. Depressed mood for at least 2 years
B. Two of the following six symptoms
   1. Poor appetite or overeating
   2. Insomnia or hypersomnia
   3. Low energy or fatigue
   4. Low self-esteem
   5. Poor concentration or difficulty making decisions
   6. Feelings of hopelessness
C. Never interrupted for more than 2 months at a time
D. No major depression during the first 2 years
E. Never had a manic episode
F. Not superimposed on psychotic disorder
G. Not attributable to medical conditions or substance abuse
H. Significant distress or impairment

Source: Adapted from American Psychiatric Association.[1] With
permission.

TABLE 23.4. DSM-IV diagnostic criteria for a manic episode

A. Distinct period of elevated, expansive, or irritable mood for
    1 week
B. Three of the following seven symptoms (four if the mood is
    only irritable)
    1. Inflated self-esteem or grandiosity
    2. Decreased need for sleep
    3. More talkative than usual or pressure to keep talking
    4. Flight of ideas or experience of racing thoughts
    5. Distractibility
    6. Increased goal directed activity or psychomotor agitation
    7. Excessive involvement with pleasurable activities with
        potential for painful consequences
C. Not a mixed episode
D. Disturbance sufficiently severe to cause marked impairment
E. Not based on medical conditions or substance abuse

Source: Adapted from American Psychiatric Association.[1] With
permission.

duration and presence of marked impairment in social or occupational
functioning or the need for hospital admission because of danger to self or
others. A mixed episode is defined as fitting criteria for major depressive
and manic episodes together for 1 week. Analogous to dysthymia, *cyclo-thymia* is a disorder characterized by many hypomanic and depressed
episodes over 2 years, never without affective symptoms for longer than
2 months. Mood disorders caused by general medical conditions and sub-stance-induced mood disorders are now included within the group of
affective disorders, and atypical disorders are divided into the three "not
otherwise specified" categories.

In all cases, an organic basis for the disturbance must be ruled out. The
condition should also not be attributable to a primary psychotic disorder.
Depressive disorders can be linked in a diagnostic algorithm (Fig. 23.1).
The important role of early detection of a possible manic episode is
emphasized by its placement near the top of the sequence.

Related Diagnoses

Several other disorders present with dysphoria as the chief complaint or
prominent feature. They should be considered as part of a differential
diagnosis (Fig. 23.2).

Cognitive Disorders

Cognitive disorders may include both depressed and manic presentation
together with indications of an underlying medical disorder in the physi-cal, mental status, or laboratory examinations. In particular, abnormalities

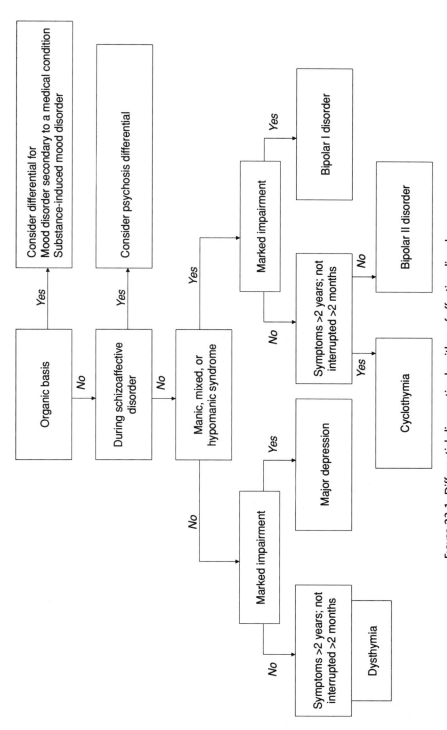

FIGURE 23.1. Differential diagnostic algorithm of affective disorders.

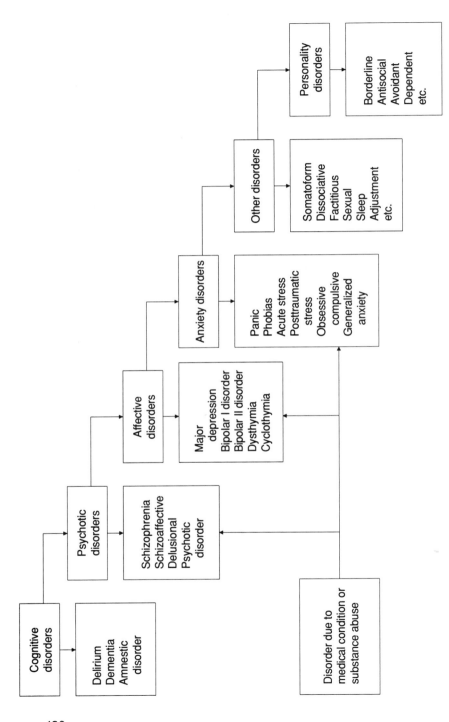

FIGURE 23.2. Implied differential diagnostic cascade of psychiatric disorders.

in cognitive testing, such as disorientation, memory deficits, attention, and concentration difficulties, should raise the concern of such a disorder.

Delirium and dementia may have prominent affective symptoms. *Delirium,* characterized by an inability to sustain attention, is more likely in elderly or medically ill patients. It is often acute in onset and shows fluctuation. *Dementia* begins insidiously. Affective lability, periods of apathy, and concentration and memory problems are prominent. Differentiation from the "pseudodementia of depression" may be difficult, and treatment may have to be directed at an affective disorder to clarify the diagnosis. Alcohol and drug abuse and dependence disorders fall into the category of substance-related mental disorders. The classification of the psychiatric disorders induced by these substances into each category emphasizes the importance of distinguishing them as a first priority.

Psychotic Disorders

Psychotic disorders are characterized by loss of reality contact. When affective symptoms meeting criteria for a major depressive episode or for mania are present as well, a schizoaffective disorder is diagnosed. Differentiation from the affective disorders with psychotic features is possible when there is a 2-week history of psychosis in the absence of affective symptoms. Occasionally, treatment for both disorders over time is required to clarify the underlying diagnosis.

Anxiety Disorders

Anxiety disorders, in particular panic and posttraumatic stress disorder, may have severe dysphoria as the presenting complaint. The prominence of anxiety and vegetative signs characteristic of depression may help define the diagnosis (also see Chapter 22).

Somatoform Disorders

With somatoform disorders, such as chronic pain (somatoform pain disorder) and hypochondriasis, a patient who meets criteria for the affective disorder should be assigned this diagnosis in addition to the somatoform diagnosis.

Personality Disorders

Personality disorders are characterized by long-standing, pervasive, and maladaptive personality traits; they therefore often include significant dysphoria. The presence of a personality disorder should not obviate the diagnosis of a major affective disorder. However, a patient suffering from intense constant depression since adolescence is much less likely to respond to biologic treatments than a patient with major depression alone.

Bereavement

Grief, although intense, needs to be seen within its cultural context. The duration may be variable, although morbid preoccupation with worthlessness, prolonged and marked functional impairment, and marked psychomotor retardation may raise the concern that the patient is suffering from a major depression.

Treatments

Biologic Therapies

Differentiation of unipolar from bipolar affective disorders is crucial because the basic treatment strategies differ. The mainstay of therapy for major depression is the antidepressant, although mood stabilizers and neuroleptics are used adjunctively. Conversely, the main treatment for bipolar disorders is a mood stabilizer, and adjunctive use of neuroleptics and antidepressants may be required.

When major depression is present, treatment with antidepressants should (and, in some cases of dysthymia, may) be offered. The compounds differ little in their antidepressant efficacy, but their side effect profiles are diverse. Choice is dictated by the desire to use or avoid certain side effects. Tables 23.5 and 23.6 outline specifics on the pharmacology and side effects of available preparations. Use of antidepressants in patients with bipolar disorders may increase the number of cycles per year and may provoke a manic episode.

Tricyclic and Related Antidepressants

These classic antidepressants include, for example, amitriptyline, imipramine, nortriptyline, and desipramine. They are well studied, effective, and generally the least expensive.

Once a medication is chosen, the lowest dose indicated is generally initiated. Incremental increases are made until the expected target range is reached, a clinical response is noted, or unacceptable side effects occur. Such dosage increases are often tolerated every 3 or 4 days. The patient should understand that a full therapeutic effect on their mood and energy can be expected after approximately 4 weeks. Sleep may improve within a few days. The patient may experience increased energy before mood and depressive thought patterns are reversed. Thus the early treatment phase is potentially more dangerous for a patient with suicidal thoughts. Because beneficial effects and side effects vary greatly in individual patients, frequent visits, initially weekly or even more often, are required until the depression has improved.

TABLE 23.5. Effects and side effects of common antidepressants

Generic name (trade name)	Chemical type	Mean $T_{1/2}$ (h)	Sedation	Anticholinergic	Orthostasis	Dosage[a] (mg/day)	Other side effects
Amitriptyline (Elavil, Endep)	Tricyclic tertiary amine	21	+++	+++	+++	75–300	
Amoxapine (Asendin)	Dibenzoxapine	8	++	++	++	100–300	Extrapyramidal syndrome
Buproprion (Wellbutrin)	Propiophenone	10	0	0	0	75–450	Seizure, agitation
Clomipramine (Anafranil)	Tricyclic		++	++	++	75–200	
Desipramine (Norpramin, Pertofrane)	Tricyclic secondary amine	21	+	+	+	75–200	
Doxepin (Sinequan, Adapin)	Tricyclic tertiary amine	17	+++	++	+++	75–200	
Fluoxetine (Prozac)	Benzenepropanamine	80	0	0	0	20–60	Insomnia, anxiety
Imipramine (Tofranil, Janimine)	Tricyclic tertiary amine	28	++	++	+++	75–200	
Maprotiline (Ludiomil)	Tetracyclic	43	++	++	++	75–225[b]	Seizure, rash
Nortriptyline (Pamelor, Aventyl)	Tricyclic secondary amine	36	+	+	+	50–150	
Paroxetine (Paxil)	Phenylpiperidine	20	+/–	0	0	20–50	Nausea
Protriptyline (Vivactil)	Tricyclic secondary amine	78	+	+++	+	15–40	
Sertraline (Zoloft)	Hydroxytryptamine	25	+/–	0	0	50–200	
Trazodone (Desyrel)	Triazolopyridine	7	+++	0	+	100–400	Priapism
Trimipramine (Surmontil)	Tricyclic tertiary amine	13	+++	+++	+++	75–200	

[a]Usual daily maintenance dose.   [b]Ceiling dose due to possible seizures.
+++ = marked; ++ = moderate; + = mild; +/– = equivocal; 0 = none. Treat elderly with approximately half the recommended dosage of each of these medications.

483

TABLE 23.6. Preferred use for nontricyclic antidepressants

Targeted symptom	Suggested choices[a]
Insomnia	Amitriptyline, doxepin
Hypersomnia/hyperphagia	Fluoxetine, buproprion, monoamine oxidase inhibitors (MAOIs)
Anergia	Fluoxetine, desipramine, buproprion, protriptyline
Delusions	Amoxapine, neuroleptic plus antidepressant
Weight gain	Fluoxetine, desipramine, buproprion
Obsessions/compulsions	Fluoxetine, clomipramine
Panic	Imipramine, MAOIs, alprazolam
Elderly/frail	Desipramine, nortriptyline, trazodone, buproprion
Cardiovascular disorder	Maprotiline
Chronic pain	Amitriptyline, doxepin, nortriptyline
Peptic ulcer	Amitriptyline, imipramine, doxepin

[a]These suggestions are provisional and meant only as examples; the overall clinical picture guides choices.

When the patient has achieved remission of the depression, the medication is continued for a minimum of 4 to 5 months. In cases of recurring or severe depression, continued medication for longer, possibly years, may be best. Once the decision to stop treatment has been made, dosage should be reduced slowly over several weeks while observing for any signs of relapse for several months.

Serotonin Reuptake Inhibitors

The newest antidepressants (e.g., fluoxetine, sertraline), with almost exclusive serotonin activity, have favorable side effect profiles, which may allow initiation at their regular antidepressant dose. They are activating and should be given during the day. This activation may trigger agitation, anxiety, and restlessness (akathesia), which can be disconcerting to the patient.

Monoamine Oxidase Inhibitors

Monoamine oxidase inhibitors (MAOIs), e.g., phenelzine and tranylcypromine, are often used with psychiatric consultation. The risk of a hypertensive crisis can be avoided with dietary restrictions, excluding foods high in tyramine. Postural hypotension is likely to be the main side effect. MAOIs may be the treatment of choice for "atypical" depression characterized by hypersomnia, hyperphagia, and reverse diurnal variation (energy decreases over the course of the day).[8]

Electroconvulsive Therapy

Electroconvulsive therapy (ECT) remains a useful and effective procedure for treatment of severe depression and mania. Studies have shown it to be as effective or superior to other antidepressant treatments. It is contraindicated in patients with recent strokes, space-occupying intracranial lesions, and recent myocardial infarction. There are no scientifically valid studies showing long-term memory loss or disturbances in the ability to learn new information. Maintenance antidepressant treatment should follow to prevent relapse.[9]

Lithium

Bipolar disorder is most commonly treated with lithium, one of the most effective mood stabilizers. It has antidepressant properties for the bipolar patient with depression as well as antimanic properties for the patient with elevated mood; it works best when used prophylactically.

It is renally excreted, so changes in fluid balance or dietary salt intake can dramatically affect the lithium level and produce toxicity. Dose-dependent side effects include gastrointestinal disturbances such as diarrhea and a fine hand tremor. Hypothyroidism can occur in up to 20% of patients. Thyroid levels should be checked before and every 6 months during treatment. Nephrogenic diabetes insipidus is infrequent, although up to 60% of patients on lithium complain of increased urination. Less frequent side effects seen at higher lithium levels include vomiting and abdominal pain, nystagmus, slurred speech, weakness, dizziness, and ataxia.

After a patient has reached stability, levels should be rechecked every 3 to 6 months. Carbamazepine and valproate may represent alternatives to lithium in nonresponsive patients.[10]

Psychological Therapies

Whereas biologic and, more controversially, psychoanalysis were the main treatments for depression in the past, studies since the 1970s have examined the usefulness of multiple psychotherapeutic modalities. For mild cases of major depression, interpersonal and cognitive-behavioral treatment should be used first. Combination of psychotherapy with antidepressants may be particularly indicated in patients maintained on medications, patients with severe neurotic character problems, and in the context of marital conflicts.[11] There may be significant differences in the usefulness of these therapies for the short-term versus the long-term treatment of depression. Particularly when both biologic and psychological treatments are suggested, clear agreements, possibly contractual, between collaborating providers regarding who is responsible for care are necessary.

Social Treatments

Implications of the depression for marital, family, job, and social functioning must be considered and addressed. The patient's support network must be explored. Expectations regarding length of complete or partial disability should be discussed early. Social work interventions can hasten full recovery, which may otherwise be delayed or even made impossible.

Evaluation and Treatment Process

A clear series of diagnostic and therapeutic steps allows differentiation of disorders and logical treatment choice.

1. *History.* A thorough evaluation should include safety, current history and review of systems, prior episodes of depression (including psychosis and suicide ideations and attempts), treatments, prior medical problems, childhood and developmental difficulties, and family and social histories. The question of suicidal risk is the initial overriding concern. Together with this information, the degree of the patient's competence to participate in treatment planning must be considered.[12] History of a previous manic episode must be investigated. Vegetative signs, including changes in sleep, appetite, weight, and sexual functioning, should be explored owing to their relevance for medication choice.

2. *Mental status examination.* The general appearance of the patient must be noted. Abnormalities in the patient's cognitive function should raise the suspicion of organic etiology. Loose associations, flight of ideas, or loss of reality contact point toward psychosis. Abnormal emotional states are the hallmark of affective disorders. Irritability, as well as euphoria, may speak for mania. Rating scales such as the Mini-Mental Status Examination or the Beck Depression Inventory may be helpful for objectifying this examination.

3. *Laboratory evaluation.* Laboratory workup of depression should include basic chemistries, complete blood count, and thyroid studies. Patients evaluated for depression are at increased risk for physical disorders.

4. *Consultation.* Each family physician must define when to refer a patient. Physician variables regarding consultation may include experience with particular drugs, comfort with psychotherapeutic modalities, and availability of reliable consultants. Patient variables may include trust in the physician, openness to referral, specific diagnostic characteristics such as psychosis, or treatment failure. Admission of a suicidal patient or treatment with ECT generally requires psychiatric consultation.

Treatment Principles

The patient's safety must be established. Voluntary or involuntary hospitalization must be offered when such safety is in doubt. No-harm contracts may be useful when assessing the risk to the patient, but their therapeutic value is unclear. Biologic, psychological, and social interventions must be prioritized. A return visit for more extended evaluation and treatment planning may be necessary.

In the context of depression several basic rules can be formulated to guide treatment.

1. Treat any medical disorders that may underlie the depression first.
2. Address alcohol and drug abuse before attempting other interventions.
3. When a patient meets criteria for major depression, make the diagnosis and provide medical treatment.
4. When a patient does not fully meet these criteria, a treatment trial with antidepressants may be reasonable.
5. A 6-week treatment period, with at least 3 weeks at the highest tolerated safe dose, can be considered an adequate treatment trial.
6. If possible, psychotherapy should be provided in addition to biologic treatments.

Treatment-Resistant Depression

When a patient does not respond to the initial treatment strategy, the history should be reviewed for hidden alcohol or drug abuse, unrecognized underlying medical problems, or subtle psychotic symptoms. Patient compliance and determination of antidepressant blood levels should be considered. The treatment plan should be reviewed and revised as appropriate. Strategies used when there has been no response include changing to another antidepressant, possibly an MAOI, or augmentation with lithium or thyroxine. Finally, ECT or combinations of tricyclic antidepressants, with MAOIs, have been advocated.

Special Populations

Children

Social withdrawal, poor school performance, a phobia, aggression or self-deprecation, and somatic complaints may herald depression, in which case standardized testing of children may be helpful. Biologic treatments are generally considered to be effective for major depression in children and adolescents. The dosage of medications must take into consideration the lower fat/muscle ratio, which leads to a decreased volume for distribution of the drug. The relatively larger liver in children leads to more rapid metabolism of the tricyclic drugs than in adults. Prepubertal children may have more dramatic swings in blood levels; therefore, doses should be divided three times daily, a practice that can likely be discontinued in the adolescent.[13] Psychotherapy is frequently necessary, at times with inclusion of the whole family in treatment.

Elderly Population

Distinction between somatic (vegetative) symptoms of depression and physical problems is a common problem in the elderly. Vague somatic discomforts may herald depression. Psychotic symptoms may be subtle and focus on somatic complaints. When symptoms of cognitive impairment accompany depression, three main disorders must be distinguished: delirium, pseudodementia of depression, and depression with dementia. Delirium is characterized by its course, but the latter two diagnoses may be more difficult to delineate. A family history of affective disorder, concern about the deficits, and inability to try hard at cognitive tasks speak for depression.

A treatment trial with antidepressants to influence the reversible portion of the patient's dysfunction may be helpful. Side effects require particular attention. Of most concern are excess sedation, cardiac arrhythmias, orthostatic hypotension, and anticholinergic syndromes. Medications should usually be begun at half the normal dosages for the average adult patient, and changes should be made less frequently. Side effects should be monitored carefully and blood levels obtained when questions arise. ECT may be useful in elderly patients with refractory depression, psychotic symptoms, medication intolerance, or medical compromise, as rapid progression to severe nutritional depletion is not uncommon.

References

1. American Psychiatric Association. Diagnostic and statistical manual of mental disorders. 4th rev. ed. Washington, DC: APA, 1994.
2. Schurman R, Kramer P, Mitchell J. The hidden mental health network. Arch Gen Psychiatry 1985;42:89–184.
3. Williamson PS, Yates WR. The initial presentation of depression in family practice and psychiatric outpatients. Arch Gen Psychiatry 1989;11:188–93.
4. Engel G. The clinical application of the biopsychosocial model. Am J Psychiatry 1980;137:535–44.
5. Torgersen S. Genetic factors in moderately severe and mild affective disorders. Arch Gen Psychiatry 1986;43:222–6.
6. Lewinsohn PM. A behavioral approach to depression. In: Friedman R, editor. The psychology of depression: contemporary theory and research. New York: Wiley, 1974:157–85.
7. Beck AT. Depression: causes and treatment. Philadelphia: University of Pennsylvania Press, 1972.
8. Stewart JW, McGrath PJ, Quitlein FM, et al. Relevance of DSM III depression subtypes and chronicity of antidepressant efficacy in atypical depression. Arch Gen Psychiatry 1989;46:1080–7.
9. Rose RM. Electroconvulsive therapy—consensus conference. JAMA 1985; 254:2103–8.
10. Janicak PG, Boshes RA. Advances in the treatment of mania and other acute psychotic disorders. Psychiatr Ann 1987;17:145–9.
11. Scott WC. Treatment of depression by primary care physicians: psychotherapeutic treatments for depression. In: Informational report of the Council on Scientific Affairs, American Medical Association. Chicago: AMA, 1991.

12. Gutheil TG, Bursztajn H, Brodsky A. The multidimensional assessment of dangerousness: confidence assessment in patient care and liability prevention. Bull Am Acad Psychiatr Law 1986;14:123–9.
13. Puig-Antich J, Ryan ND, Rabinovitch H. Affective disorders in childhood and adolescence. In: Weiner JM, editor. Diagnosis and psychopharmacology of childhood and adolescent disorders. New York: Wiley, 1985.
14. Andreasen NC, Black DW. Introductory textbook of psychiatry. Washington, DC: American Psychiatric Press, 1990:191.

CASE PRESENTATION

Subjective

PATIENT PROFILE

Mary Nelson is a 71-year-old married white female retired teacher.

PRESENTING PROBLEM

"No energy and sleeping poorly."

PRESENT ILLNESS

For the past 2 months, Mrs. Nelson has noted tiredness and disturbed sleep. She lacks energy all day, yet sleeps for only short periods at night and wakes each morning about 4 a.m. unable to fall asleep again. Her appetite is poor, and she sometimes cries inappropriately. She has had several similar episodes in the past treated with antidepressants. Her last visit, about 8 months ago, focused on management of her hypertension (see Chapter 8).

PAST MEDICAL HISTORY

She is hypertensive on hydrochlorothiazide for 10 years, with a calcium channel blocker added 8 months ago.

SOCIAL HISTORY, HABITS, AND FAMILY HISTORY

All are unchanged since her previous visit.

REVIEW OF SYSTEMS

She occasionally notes flushed skin, especially during the afternoon. She believes she has lost some weight recently.

- What additional medical history might help clarify the problem?
- How might you inquire about life events that could be contributing to Mrs. Nelson's problem?
- What might have prompted the visit today? How would you elicit this information?
- What more might you like to know about the flushed skin?

Objective

VITAL SIGNS

Weight, 119 lb (decrease of 3 lb since her previous visit 8 months ago); blood pressure, 142/76; pulse, 70.

EXAMINATION

The patient has a flat affect, speaks slowly, and becomes tearful several times during the interview. The eyes, ears, nose, and throat are normal. There are no abnormalities of the neck and thyroid. The hands are warm, and there is no tremor.

- What additional data—if any—might you obtain from the physical examination? Why?
- What physical diseases—if any—might account for today's symptoms? How would you examine for these possibilities?
- What—if any—laboratory tests would you obtain today?
- What physical findings—if present—would suggest that the problem is other than a primary affective disorder? Explain.

Assessment

- What is your diagnostic assessment? How would you explain this to the patient?
- How might the family be contributing to the illness?
- How might you assess the possibility of suicidal intent? Describe how you would frame this inquiry.
- What is likely to be the meaning of this illness to the patient? To the family?

Plan

- Describe your specific recommendations. How would you present these to Mrs. Nelson?
- What community resources—if any—might be useful in caring for this patient's problem? How would you gain involvement of these other professionals?
- If Mrs. Nelson indicated that she had thought of suicide, what would you do?
- What continuing care would you advise?

24
Care of Acute Lacerations

GEORGE F. SNELL

Lacerations represent a common clinical problem in both physicians' offices and emergency rooms. Although they are seldom life-threatening, they are usually sustained traumatically and are often associated with a high degree of emotional upset of the patient, parent, or accompanying family member. Calmness and reassurance, coupled with thorough and competent treatment, are essential for optimal handling of both the trauma and the emotional component. Such competence in wound management should be a skill acquired by all family physicians.

It is important for the physician performing the primary wound closure to have a good working knowledge of the anatomy of the skin and underlying tissues. This knowledge provides the key to managing deep lacerations and undermining the skin layers. Figure 24.1 represents a model of the layers of the skin and subcutaneous tissue down to underlying structures such as muscle or bone. An important functional feature of the skin is its lines of cleavage, or Langer's lines. These lines are formed by collagen fibers that lie parallel in the dermis. Incisions that parallel these lines cause little disruption of the collagen bundles, with little new collagen synthesis and therefore little scarring. Incisions that cross these lines disrupt collagen bundles and result in increased amounts of new collagen and, consequently, an increased amount of scar tissue. One should remember that these lines of cleavage, however, are not always consistent with the skin tension lines, which are more obviously indicated by so-called wrinkle lines. When planning débridement, closure, or excision of a lesion, the physician should try to identify the wrinkle lines and follow them closely to minimize scarring and preserve function. Figure 24.2 shows the usual distribution of Langer's lines of cleavage and wrinkle lines on the face.

The goals of primary wound closure are fourfold: (1) stop the bleeding; (2) prevent infection; (3) preserve function; and (4) restore appearance.

Optimal wound healing can be stimulated by the physician who carefully handles tissues and utilizes nature's healing processes. It is helpful for the physician who is managing wounds to know the three phases of skin healing.[1]

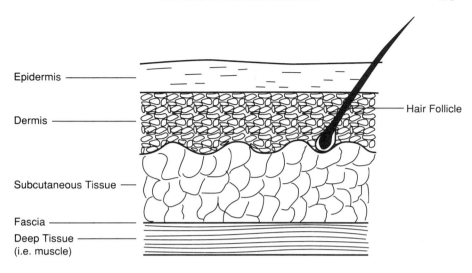

Epidermis

Dermis

Subcutaneous Tissue

Fascia

Deep Tissue
(i.e. muscle)

Hair Follicle

FIGURE 24.1. Model of skin and subcutaneous tissue.

Wound Healing Phases

Substrate (Inflammatory) Phase

The substrate, or inflammatory, phase occurs during the first 5 to 6 days after injury. To neutralize bacteria and foreign bodies, leukocytes, histamines, prostaglandins, and fibrinogen arrive at the wound site through blood and lymph. The amount of inflammation present in the wound is related to the presence of necrotic tissue formed by fluid accumulation in deadspace, or decreased circulation. Specific steps taken during the wound repair that reduce the amount of the inflammatory response include débridement, cleansing and removal of foreign bodies, and control of bleeding by precise ligature or cautery.

Fibroblastic (Collagen) Phase

The fibroblastic, or collagen, phase occupies days 6 through 20 after injury. Fibroblasts enter the wound early, and collagen synthesis occurs, which binds the wound together. As the collagen content rises, wound strength increases, so that supporting sutures can be removed. Sutures placed under too much tension compromise the vascular supply and adversely affect the collagen deposition. The novice may place sutures with too much tension, perhaps thinking it would bind the wound together better. This assumption is false.

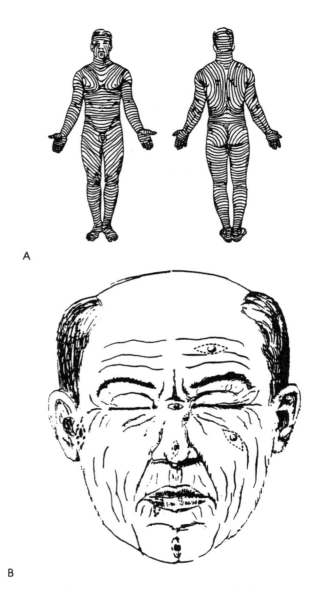

A

B

FIGURE 24.2. (A) Langer's lines on anterior and posterior body surfaces. (B) Wrinkle lines on the face. Sites for elective elliptical excisions also are shown.

Maturation (Remodeling) Phase

The maturation, or remodeling, phase takes many months to complete and consists in collagen restructuring and retraction, which results in a final scar. How much scarring occurs is related to a variety of factors, including genetic tendencies for fibroblastic overproliferation, wound infection, and skin tension at the site of the laceration. Scar revision should not be attempted until 12 months or more after the original repair to see how the mature scar will appear.

Anesthesia

After an initial quick assessment of a wound, it is usually advisable to anesthetize the wound first and then proceed to proper cleansing and inspection. Assessment for neurovascular damage should be performed before anesthesia is accomplished.

Topical Agents

Topical anesthesia can be helpful, particularly in young children, to relieve the pain from injection of the local anesthetic. Sometimes small lacerations, requiring only two or three sutures, can be closed after application of only a topical anesthetic for a few minutes. Topical agents commonly used are the following.

Cocaine

Cocaine is the oldest topical agent known and is the only one with inherent vasoconstrictor properties. Used in a 4% to 10% solution, it is applied by swab or cotton pledget. It is most commonly used in the nasopharynx. It is a stimulant to the cardiovascular system and sometimes causes tachycardia and hypertension.

Tetracaine

Tetracaine (Pontocaine) is commonly used in the eye or on other mucous membranes. It can be obtained in plastic squeeze bottles marketed for ophthalmic use and must be kept in the refrigerator. Cetacaine, a combination of tetracaine and two other chemicals, is an anesthetic frequently used by spraying on mucous membranes before a procedure such as laryngoscopy.

Lidocaine

Lidocaine (Xylocaine) is the most common local anesthetic used but is occasionally used topically in a viscous form or as a 2% to 5% ointment.

Dyclonine

Dyclonine (Dyclone) differs in chemical structure from the other topical agents. It is used in a 0.5 or 1.0% solution that provides an effect lasting 20 minutes.

TAC

Perhaps the most commonly used topical agent for wound repair is a combination called TAC.[2] It consists of 2% tetracaine, aqueous adrenaline 1:1000, and 4.2% cocaine. It is prepared in a volume of 85 ml by mixing 10.5 mg 2% tetracaine, 21 ml 1:1000 aqueous adrenaline, 5 grains cocaine, and sterile water to the total volume of 85 ml. If a child can keep a gauze or cotton pledget saturated with this solution over a laceration for 5 to 10 minutes, the laceration can be repaired sometimes without further anesthesia.

Local and Regional Agents

Local and regional agents are injected to block the nerve supplying the area to be anesthetized.

Lidocaine

Lidocaine (Xylocaine) produces moderate duration of anesthesia and is most often used in a 1% or 2% concentration. It is also mixed with 1:100,000 aqueous epinephrine to prolong the anesthetic action and to provide some local vasoconstriction. Solutions with epinephrine should never be used on the fingers, toes, or penis, thus avoiding necrosis due to ischemia. The usual cause of failure from lidocaine is an impatient doctor. If physicians can wait 5 to 10 minutes after injection, they can then proceed with the repair with better anesthesia. Lidocaine is safe, but systemic toxicity can occur, which usually manifests initially as tinnitus and a feeling of numbness and tingling, sometimes proceeding to mental confusion or coma. Allergies to lidocaine are rare; most so-called allergic reactions to local anesthetics are the result of intravascular injection or autonomic responses on the part of the patient.

Mepivacaine

Mepivacaine (Carbocaine) is a local anesthetic that produces a longer duration of action than lidocaine but cannot be enhanced by the addition of epinephrine. Toxic reactions to mepivacaine are rare and are similar to those mentioned for lidocaine.

Procaine

Procaine (Novocain) is the old standby of local anesthesia. It has a rapid onset of action and a fairly short duration. It has a wide margin of safety, and toxic doses are difficult to achieve. Any procedure should be completed in less than 30 to 45 minutes when this drug is used for anesthesia.

Bupivacaine

Bupivacaine (Marcaine) is the longest acting local anesthetic. Consequently, it is used for therapeutic nerve blocks. It is marketed in 0.25%, 0.50%, and 0.75% solutions.

Field and Infiltration Blocks

Most minor surgical procedures and laceration repairs may be accomplished using the local infiltration technique. Here the physician infiltrates the site of the laceration with multiple injections into the skin and subcutaneous tissue. It is less painful to inject this solution through the open part of the laceration, especially if the physician uses a 27-gauge or smaller needle. The caliber needle decreases the rate at which the solution can be injected and therefore lessens the pain. One should inject as few sites as possible, moving from an area that is already anesthetized or injected to an adjacent unanesthetized area. If possible, a single insertion of the needle should be made and the injecting performed in a fan-like pattern. Longer needles facilitate this technique, in contrast to the short 0.5-inch needle.

Field blocks differ from an infiltration anesthetic in that the area to be repaired is not directly injected but is anesthetized by injecting all around the operating site, thereby blocking the cutaneous nerve supply to the area. Field blocks require more time to produce the anesthesia, but they last longer. Also, no distortion occurs due to swelling in the tissues to be repaired. An intradermal wheal should be made and subsequent injections given through this wheal. One technique that minimizes the discomfort of the anesthetic injections involves injecting a saline wheal and then injecting the anesthetic through that wheal.

Digital Blocks

The common digital nerve at its junction into the dorsal and palmar branches can be anesthetized by infiltrating about 1 ml of local anesthetic just proximal to the webbing between the digits at the metacarpophalangeal joint. It should be done on each side of the finger to anesthetize the entire finger. The site for digital and common digital nerve blocks is shown in Figure 24.3.

Preparing the Wound for Closure

After the initial assessment and local anesthesia has been accomplished, the wound must be reexamined for any damage to deeper structures. Thorough cleansing should take place through (1) mechanical means, including

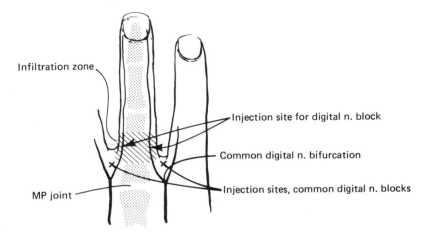

FIGURE 24.3. Digital nerve block.

wiping, brushing, and irrigation; and (2) chemical means, which includes the use of antiseptic soaps such as hexachlorophene (pHisoHex), chlorhexidine gluconate (Hibiclens), or povidone-iodine (Betadine). The most effective irrigating method is to inject saline using a syringe with a 22-gauge needle. This method produces sufficient velocity to facilitate the cleansing process.

After the second inspection and cleansing of the wound are completed, débridement, or removal of devitalized tissue, converts a contaminated or jagged wound into a clean, surgical one. This process is called "freshening the edges." Removal of tissue in certain areas such as the lip or eyelid should be performed with extreme caution. There is no point in increasing the deformity needlessly when a somewhat imperfect scar can provide a much more functional result. If a considerable amount of tissue has been crushed, initial removal of all the crushed tissue may result in undesirable function. A wound over a joint surface is an example of this circumstance. Such wounds should be closed loosely using subcutaneous absorbable sutures, with subsequent revision of the scar if necessary.

For débridement, the sharpest instrument available, a scalpel, should be used to make the initial cut through the skin. The remainder of the tissue can then be excised using sharp tissue scissors for better control. Débridement through a hairy area may need to be done at an angle that parallels the angle of the hair follicles. If it is performed in this manner, fewer follicles are damaged, and there is less likelihood of a hairless area surrounding the scar.

After débridement, skin edges should be held together to see if they can come together with minimum tension. Undermining may be necessary to

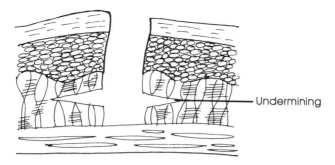

FIGURE 24.4. Undermining in the subdermal layer.

provide more mobility of the skin by releasing some of the subcutaneous attachments that prevent the skin from sliding. Undermining is performed with sharp instruments, such as the scalpel or scissors and is performed in the subcutaneous tissue plane. One should undermine around the entire circumference of the wound so the skin slides together easily. The widest undermining is performed where the skin needs to be moved the farthest, usually in the center portion of the wound (Fig. 24.4).

Hemostasis can be obtained in most cases by applying pressure directly over the wound. If compression is insufficient, vessel ligation or cautery should be performed, taking the precaution to destroy as little tissue as possible within the ligature or cautery. In most cases, absorbable sutures are preferred for the ligature of blood vessels. One precaution should be observed when obtaining hemostasis. Avoid pushing clamps back into the unexposed portion of the wound and grasping for bleeders, as it often unnecessarily damages skin structures. If bleeding cannot be controlled by further exposing the wound, closure may need to be quickly accomplished and a sterile rubber band or other drain mechanism used to decrease hematoma formation. In such cases, a pressure dressing is advisable.

The selection of suture materials for laceration repair depends on physician preference and the purpose for which it is used. Moy et al.[3] have written an excellent article thoroughly covering this topic. Table 24.1 summarizes the advantages and disadvantages of various materials used.

Wound Closure

Previous mention has been made that under ideal circumstances a wound with clean margins is approximated without tension. Two additional goals of the closure process must be emphasized: (1) accurate approximation of tissue layers, and (2) elimination of deadspace. Accurate placement of subdermal sutures in tissue layers that hold the suture well, such as the fat–fascial junction and the dermal–fat junction, are the preferred layers for

TABLE 24.1. Acute care of lacerations: Common suture materials

Suture	Advantages	Disadvantages
Absorbable		
Catgut	Inexpensive	Low tensile strength
		High tissue reactivity
		Absorbed 4–5 days
Chromic catgut	Inexpensive	Moderate tensile strength and tissue reactivity
Polyglycolic acid (Dexon)	Low tissue reactivity	Moderately difficult to handle
	Good tensile strength	
Polyglactic acid (Polysorb, Vicryl)	Easy handling	Absorption delay occasionally results in "spitting"—suture rejected from skin
	Low tissue reactivity	
	Good tensile strength	
Polyglyconate (Maxon)	Easy handling	Expensive
	Good tensile strength	
Nonabsorbable		
Silk	Handles best	Low tensile strength
	Mild skin irritation	High tissue reactivity
		Increased infection rate
Nylon (Ethilon, Dermilon)	High tensile strength	Difficult to handle, has "memory," knots slip—many throws needed
	Minimal tissue reactivity	
	Inexpensive	
Polypropylene (Proline, SurgiPro)	No tissue reaction	Knots slip—many throws needed
	Stretching, accommodating swelling	Expensive
Braided polyester (Ethiflex, Mersilene)	Handles well	Tissue drag high if uncoated
	Knots secure	Expensive
Polybutester (Novafil)	Elasticity—accommodates swelling and retraction	Expensive
	Little drag	

suture placement deep within wounds (Fig. 24.5). For the dermal fat layer, an inverted knot technique should be used or a technique that parallels the tissue plane of the dermal–fat junction instead of placing the suture in a perpendicular fashion through this tissue plane. These deep sutures should provide most of the strength to the wound closure, allowing the skin sutures to just approximate the skin margins.

The skin, or dermal layer, may be closed using a variety of suture techniques. The best results are obtained when the skin edges are everted slightly. The following suture techniques should be within the skill level of all family physicians.

1. *Simple interrupted stitch.* This stitch is placed by passing the needle through the skin surfaces at right angles, placing the suture as wide as

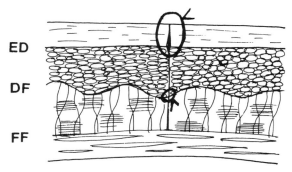

FIGURE 24.5. Proper layered closure. ED = epidermis–dermis junction; DF = dermis–fat junction; FF = fat–fascia junction.

it is deep. The opposite margin is approximated using a mirror image of that placement, as shown in Figure 24.6. A general rule to follow is that the points of entrance and exit from the wound edge should be 2 mm for a so-called plastic closure on the face but can be farther apart for closures in other areas. Using the open-loop knot shown in Figure 24.7 avoids placing the suture under excessive tension. The first throw of the knot with two loops (the so-called surgeon's knot) is placed with just enough tension to approximate the wound margin. The second throw of the knot, a single loop, is then tied, leaving a little space so no additional tension is placed on the first throw. A third and fourth throw can then be tightened snugly down on top of the second throw without causing increased tension on the wound. The knot should be manipulated to one side of the wound after the tying process to allow easier access for suture removal.

2. *Vertical mattress suture and short-hand vertical mattress suture.* This method of closure promotes eversion and can be helpful in circumstances in which considerable skin tension exists or thick layers of the skin (such as on

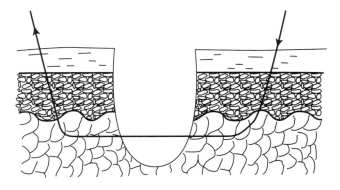

FIGURE 24.6. Simple interrupted suture placement.

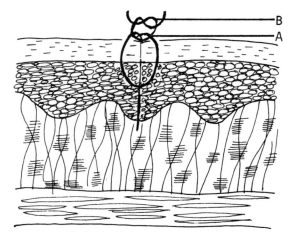

FIGURE 24.7. Open-loop knot. A = first throw, double loop; B = second throw, single loop.

the back) are encountered. This suture can be placed by putting in the more superficial part, then tenting the skin and placing the deeper stitch, which is the short-hand method.[4] The classic method first places the deeper stitch and closes with the superficial portion (Fig. 24.8).

3. *Intracuticular running suture.* This technique is used for closing linear wounds that are not under much tension. It results in minimal scarring and has no suture marks. The principal drawback of the technique is that one is not able to ensure controlled tissue apposition and tension as easily as with the interrupted suture method. The technique, shown in Figure 24.9, is a popular closure method among patients because of cosmetic results. The ends of the suture need not be tied; taping under slight tension preserves approximation.

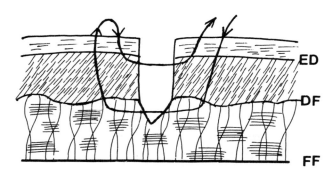

FIGURE 24.8. Vertical mattress suture. ED = epidermis–dermis junction; DF = dermis–fat junction; FF = fat–fascia junction.

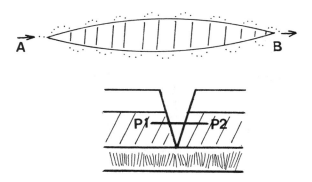

FIGURE 24.9. Intracuticular running suture. A = entrance point of suture; B = exit point of suture; P1, P2 = plane of suture depth.

4. *Three-point, or half-buried, mattress suture.* This technique has been developed to minimize the complication of possible vascular necrosis of the tip of a V-shaped wound. To perform this technique, insert the needle into the skin of the wound edge on one side of the nonflap portion, as shown in Figure 24.10, and bring it out into the wound at the middermis level. The suture is then placed through the tip of the flap transversely at the same mid-dermis level and is returned on the opposite side of the V, paralleling its point of entrance. The suture is then tied, drawing the tip snugly into the concavity without compromising the vascular supply. This suture could also be used to close a stellate laceration that might have several tips, bringing the tips together in a purse-string fashion.

5. *Subcutaneous, or subdermal, suture.* This suture was described in the first paragraph in this section and is an important one to master for cosmetic closures.

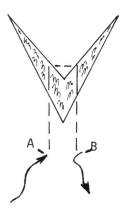

FIGURE 24.10. Three-point, or half-buried, mattress suture. A = entrance point of suture. b = exit point of suture. (Remember: It is an *intradermal* suture.)

Specific Laceration Types

Suggestions for managing specific types of lacerations follow.

1. *Lacerations crossing an obvious landmark.* Lacerations that involve a prominent anatomic feature or landmark, such as the vermilion border of the lip or the eyebrow, require special attention for optimum management. It is common practice to close a laceration from one end to the other. When the wound crosses a landmark, it is advisable to place a marking suture that approximates the wound margins at the landmark accurately. Other portions of the wound can then be closed; and if this marking stitch was placed under considerable tension, it can then be removed and replaced with one that is under less tension when other sutures have closed the wound. An additional caveat with eyebrow lacerations is that the eyebrow should never be shaved.

2. *Beveled laceration* (Fig. 24.11). This wound deserves special mention because one side of the laceration is a thin flap with the edge undercut. This undercut edge will slough because of poor blood supply, resulting in retraction of the scar during the healing process. The margins of this wound should be trimmed and squared as shown, followed by undermining, enabling the squared dermal margins to slide together. The closure should be performed in layers to eliminate the deadspace and to avoid retraction resulting in an unsightly scar.

3. *Lacerations with excess tissue, or "dog ears."* Sometimes after closing a wound, an uneven amount of skin on one side of the laceration bunches up and forms a hump of tissue. This phenomenon also occurs at the ends of a wound of elliptical shape when the mid-portion of the wound has to be brought together and leaves excess tissue at either end. The best way to manage these "dog ears" is to make a linear incision along one side after tenting the skin with a skin hook and then grasp the excess triangle of tissue at the tip and excise the tissue triangle with a second linear incision, as shown in Figure 24.12. This maneuver extends the original wound in a straight line, which can then be closed with additional simple interrupted sutures.

4. *Complex lacerations.* For a wound of unequal length with a dog ear or hump of extra tissue in the middle of one side, the hump of tissue can be excised and the triangular defect thus created then closed after the undermining has taken place (Fig. 24.13). A four-point suture technique can be used to bring the two margins togther, and the wound is then closed, forming a T-shaped incision as shown.

Lacerations can result in skin defects of all shapes and sizes. Defects of circular, rectangular, or square configurations can be closed in a variety of fashions. The physician should not attempt to close these wounds without having had some experience or at least some practice in making additional incisions or creating flaps. Several resources are available to learn these

A

Incisions

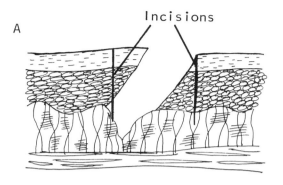

B

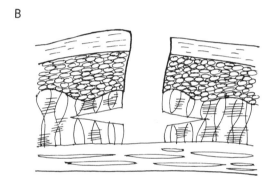

C

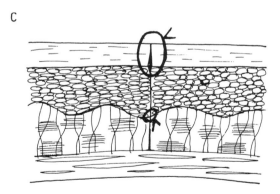

Figure 24.11. Closure of beveled wound. (A) Trimming (squaring) beveled edges. (B) Undermining in the fat layer. (C) Layered closure.

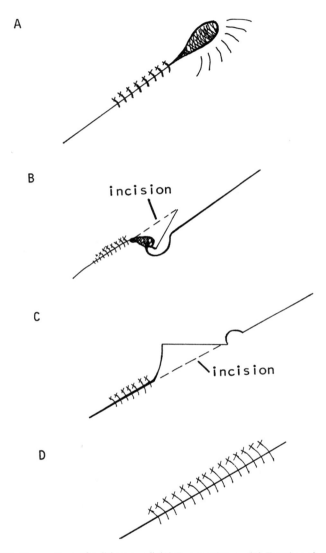

FIGURE 24.12. Correction of a "dog ear." (A) Excess tissue. (B) Tenting the tissue and initial incision. (C) Removing excess after secondary incision. (D) Final closure.

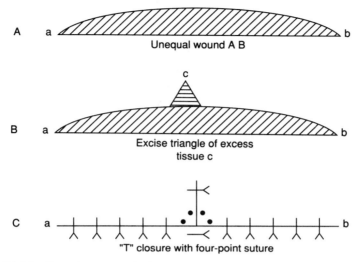

FIGURE 24.13. Complex wound closure. (A) Unequal wound (a–b). (B) Excise triangle of excess tissue (c). (C) T closure with a four-point suture.

methods, including wound closure workshops and other reference material.[5] The detailed management of these complex wounds is beyond the scope of this chapter.

5. *Fingertip wounds.* Because of the commonness of fingertip injuries and the possible complexity and malfunction that may result from these injuries, a brief discussion of management principles is included here.

a. *Amputations of areas of fingertip skin* and subcutaneous tissue less than 1 cm^2 are usually fairly simple and can be managed with thorough cleansing, proper dressing protection, and subsequent healing by secondary intention. Involvement of more of the fingertip in an amputation increases the complexity of treatment. These tip amputations are best described according to the depth and direction of the bevel (Fig. 24.14). The most favorable bevel angle is one in which the defect faces dorsally and distally, and the most unfavorable defect faces volarly. In many cases, the favorably angled amputation can be managed conservatively without suturing or grafting. After proper preparation of the initial wound, the wound is allowed to heal by contraction and epithelialization when the volar skin is preserved. When the volar skin is not preserved, additional coverage is needed to preserve tactile sensation and function. In many cases, the family physician may want to refer these injuries.

b. *Injuries to the nail and nailbed* can be managed by family physicians if they understand the anatomy and follow certain caveats. There are three main rules of treatment: (1) save the nail; (2) reapproximate nail matrix

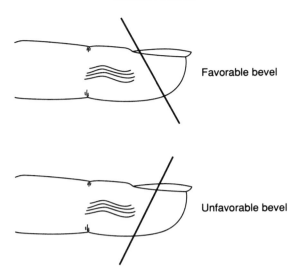

Favorable bevel

Unfavorable bevel

FIGURE 24.14. Fingertip amputations.

lacerations with fine absorbable suture; and (3) use wound contraction and natural epithelialization to advantage. More complex fingertip injuries involving the nail matrices and bone require additional rules: (1) restore the pulp when necessary with rotational flaps of volar tissue (sometimes called a VY closure); (2) replace small, noncrushed skin pulp amputations; (3) use skin grafts to cover exposed areas when needed; and (4) reduce fractures or remove fragmented bone that will not heal. Ditmer[6] excellently covered the management of fingertip and nailbed injuries in a 1989 article.

Postwound Closure Management

Most wounds should be protected during the first 24 to 48 hours after closure. Sometimes a simple Band-Aid will do; but on other occasions, where pressure is needed or continued oozing might be expected, a pressure dressing should be applied. The first layer should be a nonstick type of gauze dressing. (Several such dressings are available and come in convenient packages, e.g., Xeroderm, Adaptic, and Telfa.) Then apply a gauze pad or other mesh and a self-adhering roller gauze such as Kling. Most of these dressings should be left in place for 48 hours and the wound then reexamined for infection and hemostasis. If a wound is repaired under considerable tension, splinting may be necessary to preserve wound approximation. It can be in the form of a bulky dressing or a plaster or fiberglass padded splint. After the initial protective period, many wounds can be left open, and it is certainly permissible to wet them briefly with soap and water. Some simple facial lacerations can be left entirely open if covering with a dressing is impractical.

Follow-up of lacerations to detect infection, continued bleeding, or other undesirable result is important. Additionally, most patients appreciate close attention to detail by their physicians. Removal of sutures should be individualized, depending on the location of the wound, the activity of the individual, and the tension under which the wound was closed. General rules include the following: (1) Remove facial sutures in about 3 to 5 days. (2) In nonstressed areas of the body that are not highly mobile, such as the extremities, remove sutures in 7 to 10 days. (3) On fingers, palms, and soles, where the skin is especially thick or motion occurs, sutures should be left in place for 10 to 14 days or possibly longer. Back wounds and wounds over joints are usually sites where the sutures must be retained for the longest time. Supplemental support of the wounds can be provided by using tape strips after sutures are removed to prevent wound disruption. Table 24.2 is a sample instruction sheet that can be given to patients who have had lacerations sutured.

TABLE 24.2. Care of sutured lacerations: Instructions to patients

1. Keep wound dressing clean. May shower. Do not expose to moisture for prolonged periods.
2. **Dressing wet:** If the dressing gets wet, remove it, blot the wound dry with a sterile gauze, and reapply a clean, dry dressing (e.g., a sterile gauze).
3. **Dressing changes:** Remove the dressing applied in the hospital after 2 days. Reapply a sterile dressing and repeat this procedure every 2 days until the stitches are removed unless instructed otherwise.
4. **Signs of infection:** If any of the following signs of infection appear, contact a physician immediately:
   a. Wound becomes *red, swollen, tender,* or *warm.*
   b. Wound begins to *drain* or *fester.*
   c. *Red streaks* appear up the arm or leg.
   d. *Tender lumps* appear in the groin or under the arm.
   e. *Chills* or *fever* occur.
5. **Infection check:** Because of the nature of the injury, the possibility of infection is increased. Please return to be checked in _____ days.
6. **Stitch removal:** The physician suggests the stitches be removed in about _____ days.
7. **Tetanus immunization:** For your records, you/your child received the following
   a. Tetanus toxoid _____
   b. DT (diphtheria-tetanus) _____
   c. DPT (diphtheria-pertussis-tetanus) _____
   d. Other _____

Concurrent Therapy

Prophylaxis of infection is an important aspect of laceration management that should not be neglected by the family physician. The principal method of infection prevention is thorough cleansing and preparation of the wound before closure or, in some cases, not even closing the wound where contamination is considered likely, such as for wounds that are more than 12 hours old or that are highly contaminated. Antibiotic prophylaxis is probably not helpful in most circumstances unless given in sufficient quantities to obtain good tissue levels while the wound is still open. Where extensive tissue damage and repair is necessary, intravenous antibiotics should be begun during wound closure. The practice of prescribing an oral antibiotic that is started several hours after closure is probably of little value for preventing wound infections. Other wounds that are often considered indications for prophylactic antibiotics include human and animal bites. There is evidence to support an increased incidence of wound infection in human and cat bite wounds.[7] Whether this increased magnitude of infection justifies routine use of antibiotic prophylaxis remains questionable.[8] It is a common practice, however, to administer antibiotics in these circumstances.

Tetanus prophylaxis is indicated from both medical and legal aspects. Table 24.3 is a summary guide to tetanus prophylaxis and routine wound management as published by the Centers for Disease Control in 1991.[9] If passive immunization is needed, human tetanus immune globulin (TIG) is the product of choice. It provides protection longer than antitoxin of animal origin and causes fewer adverse reactions. The current average TIG dose is 250 units IM. There is recent evidence that the TIG dose should be increased to 500 units IM.[10,11] When tetanus

TABLE 24.3. Guide to tetanus prophylaxis during routine wound management

History of adsorbed tetanus toxoid (doses)	Clean, minor wounds		All other wounds[a]	
	Td[b]	TIG	Td[b]	TIG
Unknown or <3	Yes	No	Yes	Yes
≥3[c]	No[d]	No	No[e]	No

[a]Such as, but not limited to, wounds contaminated with dirt, feces, soil, and saliva; puncture wounds; avulsions; and wounds resulting from missiles, crushing, burns, and frostbite.
[b]For children <7 years old; DPT (DT, if pertussis vaccine is contraindicated) is preferred to tetanus toxoid alone. For persons ≥ 7 years of age, Td is preferred to tetanus toxoid alone.
[c]If only three doses of *fluid* toxoid have been received, a fourth dose of toxoid, preferably an adsorbed toxoid, should be given.
[d]Yes, if >10 years since last dose.
[e]Yes, if >5 years since last dose. (More frequent boosters are not needed and can accentuate side effects.)

toxoid and TIG are given concurrently, separate syringes and separate sites should be used for the injections.

References

1. Breitenbach K, Bergera J. Principles and techniques of primary wound closure. Prim Care 1986;13:411–31.
2. Bonadio WA, Wagner V. Efficacy of TAC topical anesthetic for repair of pediatric lacerations. Am J Dis Child 1988;142:203–5.
3. Moy RL, Lee A, Zolka A. Commonly used suture materials in skin therapy. Am Fam Physician 1991;44:2123–8.
4. Moy RL, Lee A, Zolka A. Commonly used suturing techniques in skin surgery. Am Fam Physician 1991;44:1625–34.
5. Warren S, Snell G. Complex wound closure, excisional biopsy, and use of simple flaps. Prim Care 1986;13:433–45.
6. Ditmar DM. Fingertip and nail bed injuries. Occup Med 1989;4:449–61.
7. Phillips L, Heggers J. Layered closure of lacerations. Postgrad Med 1988;83:142–8.
8. Lindsey D, Christopher M, et al. Natural course of the human bite wound: incidence of infection and complications in 434 bites and 803 lacerations in the same group of patients. J Trauma 1987;27:45–48.
9. Centers for Disease Control. MMWR 1991;40(No. Rr-10):1–28.
10. Richardson JP, Knight AL. The management and prevention of tetanus. J Emerg Med 1993;11(6):737–42.
11. Allen T, Audet D. Tetanus prophylaxis: protocols require further change and simplification. J Emerg Med 1993;11(6):757–8.

CASE PRESENTATION

You are called by the hospital emergency department staff at 6 p.m. One of your patients is there with a hand laceration. You go there to meet him.

Subjective

PATIENT PROFILE

Ken Nelson is a 47-year-old married white male home builder.

PRESENTING PROBLEM

"I cut my hand today."

PRESENT ILLNESS

Five hours ago, the patient cut his right hand on sheet metal at work. He finished his work shift and now presents at the end of the day for treatment.

PAST MEDICAL HISTORY

No serious illness or hospitalization.

SOCIAL HISTORY

Ken Nelson is a self-employed building contractor who lives with his wife and 16-year-old daughter.

HABITS

He does not use tobacco or alcohol. He drinks one thermos of coffee per day.

FAMILY HISTORY

Not recorded because of the limited nature of today's problem.

- What more would you like to know about the injury? Why might this information be important?
- What do you need to know about his tetanus immunizations status?
- What are pertinent safety issues that should be elicited?

• What might be the significance of the 5-hour delay in seeking care? How would you inquire about this?

Objective

VITAL SIGNS

Blood pressure, 132/86; pulse, 66.

EXAMINATION

There is a 4-cm-long linear laceration of the lateral right hand; the wound extends into the subcutaneous tissues. The patient has full active and passive motion of the hand and fingers. There is no loss of neurologic function.

• What further information—if any—regarding the physical examination might be important?
• What are some concerns regarding hand injuries, and how would you examine to address these possibilities?
• How can you determine that neurologic function is intact?
• In what circumstances would you obtain laboratory testing or diagnostic imaging?

Assessment

• What are some concerns regarding this injury? How would you describe these concerns to the patient?
• If the patient had lost sensory perception to one of his fingers, what would you do?
• Is this a teachable moment for accident prevention? How would you approach this issue with the patient?
• What are pertinent insurance issues in regard to this injury?

Plan

• How would you prepare the wound for suturing, and what suture material would you use? Describe special considerations in suture technique for hand lacerations.
• What would be your recommendation regarding tetanus prophylaxis?
• Mr. Nelson asks about returning to work. How would you respond?
• What aftercare would you recommend for this injury?

25
Athletic Injuries

M. PATRICE EIFF

Athletic injuries comprise a significant portion of the musculoskeletal problems seen by family physicians. If one accepts the broad definition of an athlete as anyone who engages in physical activity, caring for athletes becomes an even more important part of a family physician's practice.[1] With the increasing popularity of sport and exercise in the United States today, physicians must be prepared to manage an array of acute and chronic athletic injuries. Family physicians are well suited to care for patients with athletic injuries along a spectrum from prevention to injury rehabilitation.

Emergent or Life-Threatening Injuries

Emergent or life-threatening injuries are uncommonly encountered in athletics. As would be expected, they occur most commonly in contact sports such as football, hockey, rugby, and wrestling. Physicians providing fieldside coverage for athletic events must recognize high-risk situations for serious injuries and evaluate the safety of the sports environment. Being prepared for the emergency care and transportation of the seriously injured athlete is essential for the management of these injuries.

Cervical Spine Injury

Cervical spine injuries happen primarily to athletes participating in football, wrestling, and gymnastics.[2] Trauma to the cervical spine may cause a number of clinical syndromes depending on the force of impact. Serious cervical spine injuries include central cord contusion, vertebral subluxation, and cervical fractures and dislocations. The usual mechanism of injury is hyperflexion, such as occurs when a football player attempts a tackle in a head-tucked position. Other mechanisms of injury include axial loading from a fall directly onto the top of the head and hyperextension.

Diagnosis

A significant cervical spine injury should be suspected in any player if, after a collision, there is any loss of consciousness, persistent mental status alterations, abnormalities on neurologic examination, or marked neck pain or stiffness. Extremity numbness, painful paresthesias, weakness, and neck pain in the conscious athlete indicate a possible spinal cord injury. Physicians must maintain a high index of suspicion to differentiate spinal cord injury from routine cervical sprains and strains, as neurologic deficits are not always present after trauma to the spinal cord.

Management

The approach to any athlete with a suspected cervical spine injury starts with the basic principles of emergency care. Checking for the ABCs (airway, breathing, circulation) is essential. Immediately immobilize the head and neck, and then assess the level of consciousness by doing a brief but thorough neurologic function survey. Diagnostic screening for neurologic deficits or symptoms should be performed in a timely manner to ensure that there is no delay in the emergency care of the athlete. If the player is prone, he or she must be moved to a supine position on a rigid backboard using a log roll technique while the head and neck are supported.[3] If a sufficient number of qualified personnel are not available to perform the log roll safely, the head and neck should be immobilized while waiting for emergency medical technicians to arrive. A football player's helmet should be left on and only the face mask removed if necessary for airway management. Once at the hospital, the athlete should have a more complete neurologic examination and radiographic evaluation of the cervical spine. The keys to management of these injuries are a high index of suspicion, early recognition, and proper stabilization to prevent further injury. When in doubt, it is always more prudent to overprotect the athlete and treat the injury as a suspected cervical spine injury until a more complete evaluation can be done.

Concussion

Concussion (defined as immediate but transient posttraumatic impairment of neurologic function) is a common injury in contact and collision sports. An estimated 250,000 concussions occur every year in football alone.[4] Even relatively minor blows to the head can result in a concussion. Confusion and amnesia following a blow to the head are the usual hallmarks of concussion. Concussion may also lead to alteration in coordination, balance, vision, and hearing. Concussion can occur without a definite loss of consciousness. Table 25.1 describes common signs and symptoms of mild, moderate, and severe concussions.

TABLE 25.1. Guide to concussion

Grade	Symptoms	Resolution	Management guidelines[a]
1 Confusion without amnesia No LOC	No loss of consciousness (LOC) Momentary confusion Mild dizziness Headache	Athlete normally recovers quickly but should be watched for changing symptoms.	Remove from contest. Examine immediately and every 5 minutes for amnesia or symptoms. May return after 20 minutes if no amnesia or other symptoms develop.
2 Confusion with amnesia No LOC	Momentary unconsciousness Amnesia Confusion Severe dizziness Blurred or double vision Loss of balance or coordination Nausea Tinnitus	Symptoms usually subside somewhat in 30–60 minutes but usually do not completely disappear for a few days. Some may linger up to 1 week. Athlete should be observed for at least 24 hours for changing symptoms.	Remove from contest and no return to same event. Examine frequently for signs of intracranial pathology. Reexamine within 24 hours. Return to play only after symptom-free for 1 week. Consider CT scan if symptoms persist.
3 LOC	LOC (>1 minute) Prolonged amnesia Severe confusion Loss of balance or coordination Severely altered vision Nausea	Recovery takes several days, and some symptoms can linger for weeks. Athlete should be referred to a neurologist, watched for 48 hours, and checked periodically for several weeks.	Transport to hospital with C-spine immobilization. Thorough neurologic examination essential. CT or MRI scan. Return to play only after symptom-free for 2 weeks. Persistent symptoms indicate a need for additional neurologic evaluation.

[a]Adapted from Kelly et al.[5] With permission.

Diagnosis

Any athlete with a concussion should be examined immediately for signs of neurologic impairment or mental status alternations. Focusing the mental status evaluation on orientation, concentration, and short-term memory can detect the subtle effects of the concussion. Reexamination of the athlete every 5 minutes to assess for amnesia or postconcussive symptoms such as headaches, dizziness, or vision changes aids in determining the severity of the concussion. The development of amnesia during this period of observation precludes the athlete's return to play. Severe head injury such as epidural, subdural, or intracerebral hematomas are distinguished from concussion by the presence of immediate and prolonged loss of consciousness, usually longer than 5 minutes. Brief loss of consciousness followed by severe headache, irritability, vomiting, and lethargy should raise suspicion for an epidural hematoma.

Management

Management decisions for concussion are based on the level of severity. Table 25.1 outlines management guidelines for the three grades of concussion. An athlete with a concussion should not be allowed to return to play if there is any doubt about his or her condition. It has been reported that repeated concussions can predispose the brain to diffuse swelling, which may result in catastrophic outcomes such as cerebrovascular congestion or herniation.[5] Close observation, careful assessment of the head-injured athlete, and adherence to the proposed management guidelines help prevent serious morbidity and mortality associated with concussions.

Traumatic Injuries

Traumatic sports injuries are those resulting from a specific episode of trauma, acute or subacute. Traumatic injury to the bone usually results in a fracture or, less commonly, periosteal injury. Traumatic injury to a joint and its surrounding supporting structures may lead to instability, such as subluxation or dislocation. *Subluxation* is distinguished from *dislocation* in that it is a transient and partial rather than complete displacement of joint surfaces. A *sprain* is a stretch or tear of a ligament, and a *strain* is a stretch or tear of a musculotendinous unit. Sprains and strains are classified according to the following criteria.

Grade 1: Minimal tear of fibers. Mild swelling, pain, and disability. No muscle weakness or joint instability.
Grade 2: Partial tear of fibers. Moderate amount of swelling, pain, and disability. Partial weakness on muscle contraction or partial joint instability.

Grade 3: Complete tear. Severe pain, swelling and disability. Extremely weak
on muscle testing or definite joint instability.

Other traumatic athletic injuries include contusions and hematomas secondary to direct force applied to soft tissues. Traumatic bursitis may also
result from a direct injury to a bursa. Some of the more common traumatic
athletic injuries are discussed below.

Shoulder Dislocation

The glenohumeral joint is a shallow socket; and although it allows a
wide range of shoulder motion, it does little to maintain stability of the
joint. The rotator cuff muscles and the ligamentous structures forming
the capsule provide joint stability. Sufficient impact on the shoulder
stretches or tears the capsule enough to allow the humeral head to slip
out of the glenoid fossa, resulting in a dislocation. The most common
type of shoulder dislocation is an anterior dislocation, usually the result
of forced external rotation and abduction of the shoulder.[6] This injury
may occur as a result of arm tackling in football, when a player's shot is
blocked forcefully in volleyball or basketball, or from a fall on an
abducted arm. Uncommonly, the humerus dislocates posteriorly as a
result of a direct blow to the front of the shoulder or a fall on an
outstretched arm with the shoulder in internal rotation and adduction.
The humerus may also dislocate inferiorly from a blow to the top of the
shoulder with the arm in 90 degrees of abduction.

Diagnosis

The athlete with an anterior shoulder dislocation experiences severe pain,
resists moving the injured arm, and may claim to have heard the shoulder
"pop." On examination, the athlete is unable to rotate the arm or abduct
the arm across the body. On inspection, the dislocated shoulder has a sharp,
square contour compared to the smooth, rounded outline of the uninjured
shoulder. The radiographic evaluation of a clinically suspected anterior
shoulder dislocation should include anteroposterior (AP), lateral, and axil-
lary views of the shoulder. Roentgenograms reveal anterior and slightly
inferior displacement of the humerus out of the glenoid fossa (Fig. 25.1).
Associated injuries may include an avulsion fracture of the greater tuberosity or fracture of the humeral head.

Management

Reducing the dislocation promptly before significant muscle spasm or
joint swelling develops yields a higher reduction success rate. In a prone
position, with a roll under the chest and the arm hanging off the table,
apply downward traction on the arm with the elbow at 90 degrees. An

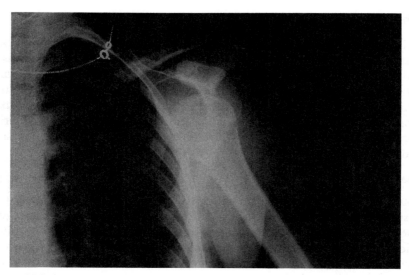

FIGURE 25.1. Anteroposterior view of the shoulder showing anterior and inferior displacement of the humerus after a shoulder dislocation.

assistant rotating the inferior scapula toward the spine during this maneuver can aid in the reduction. If this maneuver is unsuccessful, a countertraction method of reduction may be attempted.[7] The athlete lies supine with the arm held in 30 to 45 degrees of abduction. Apply gentle traction to the arm along its longitudinal axis with countertraction maintained with a sheet around the upper thorax or an unshod foot against the upper chest wall. Use increasing force until the arm slips back into the glenoid fossa. After reduction, the arm is immobilized across the chest and ice applied. If these attempts at early reduction are unsuccessful, reduction using analgesia or anesthesia can be attempted in the emergency department.

The acute management of the athlete with a first-time dislocation is the same as that for the athlete with chronic recurrent dislocations of the shoulder. Prompt relocation is important, but in the athlete with chronic recurrent dislocation immobilization may not be necessary. Shoulder immobilization, with the arm in a sling for 3 to 4 weeks, is necessary for the athlete with a first-time dislocation. Elbow and wrist range of motion as well as internal and external rotation exercises can be started as soon as early pain subsides. Rehabilitation has been shown to reduce the rate of recurrence of anterior shoulder dislocations.[8] Goals of the shoulder rehabilitation include restoration of full shoulder abduction and strengthening of the rotator cuff muscles, especially those involved with internal and external rotation of the shoulder. Athletes with recurrent shoulder dislocations should be referred to an orthopedic surgeon for consideration of surgical repair.

Shoulder Subluxation

Subluxation of the shoulder occurs when the humerus slips out of its socket but then spontaneously relocates. Although subluxation is not as serious as a dislocation, it still results in damage to ligaments or other supporting structures of the joint. Any combination of anterior, posterior, or inferior laxity of the shoulder capsule can lead to a subluxation. Anterior subluxations are fairly common in football, volleyball, and wrestling. Posterior subluxations are more common in athletes who use repetitive overhand motion, such as swimmers and baseball and tennis players.

Diagnosis

The athlete with a shoulder subluxation complains of pain and a feeling of instability in the shoulder joint. He or she may also relate that the arm goes "dead" for a few moments after the subluxation.[9] With a history of subluxation, it is important to examine the shoulder joint for capsular laxity in all directions. Comparison of the amount of joint play of the humerus in the injured shoulder with the uninjured side is a useful guide to evaluation. The *apprehension test* checks for anterior stability of the joint and is performed by standing behind the athlete and externally rotating the arm with the shoulder in 90 degrees of abduction. The athlete who is apprehensive about this test or resists this motion may have anterior subluxation. Another test of shoulder stability is performed by feeling for the amount of humeral movement with upward and downward pressure while the athlete is lying supine on a table with the shoulder hanging just off the edge. Radiographic evaluation of the athlete with recurrent shoulder subluxation may demonstrate a Hill-Sachs lesion, which is a notch defect in the humeral head caused by compression of the head as it passes over the glenoid rim when the humerus subluxes.

Management

During the acute period after a subluxation, rest, ice, and pain medication are required. Rehabilitation begins after the acute discomfort subsides. Exercises aimed at strengthening the shoulder musculature with emphasis on the areas of greatest instability may be needed for 2 to 3 months to properly rehabilitate the shoulder. Usually symptoms are gradually alleviated, and the athlete may return to competition when the apprehension test elicits no pain and no joint laxity is apparent. Athletes who experience recurrent subluxations despite pursuing an aggressive shoulder rehabilitation program for at least 6 months should give serious consideration to discontinuing the sport or consider possible surgical intervention.[6]

Acromioclavicular Separation

Acromioclavicular (AC) separation, also known as shoulder separation, results when the ligaments stabilizing the clavicle, acromion, and coracoid

TABLE 25.2. Acromioclavicular sprain classification

Grade	Acromioclavicular ligament	Coracoclavicular ligament	Acromioclavicular instability
1	Stretched	Intact	None
2	Torn	Stretched	Moderate in anteroposterior plane; mild to moderate in vertical plane
3	Torn	Torn	Marked in anteroposterior plane; marked in vertical plane

are injured. This injury may be due to a direct blow to the lateral aspect of the shoulder or a fall on an outstretched arm. AC separations are classified as grades 1, 2, and 3, depending on which ligaments are torn (Table 25.2).

Diagnosis

Following an AC separation, the athlete complains of immediate pain near the AC joint that is made worse with arm movement, especially abduction. On examination, the athlete is tender over the AC joint and the clavicle may be riding above the level of the acromion. Pulling down on the arm elicits more pain. The athlete may feel more pain and a popping sensation when the arm is abducted beyond 90 degrees. Marked swelling and ecchymosis are present in severe cases.

Performing the *crossover test* can help distinguish the three grades of AC separation. Have the athlete touch the top of the uninjured shoulder with the hand of the injured one. Push down on the elbow while the athlete resists the movement. With grade 1 injuries, the athlete can still resist movement, although it is painful. With grade 2 injuries, the athlete is unable to resist downward pressure on the elbow. With grade 3 injuries, the athlete is unable to touch the top of the uninjured shoulder. If a grade 2 or 3 injury is suspected, an AP roentgenographic view of both shoulders should be obtained to compare the AC spacing of the injured and uninjured shoulder. Fracture of the clavicle, acromion, coracoid, or humerus must be ruled out. If plain films are normal, stress radiographs done with 5 to 10 pounds of weight strapped to both arms may show elevation of the distal clavicle compared to the opposite side. With grade 2 injuries, the clavicle is elevated by one-half the width of the AC joint. With grade 3 injuries, the distal clavicle is movable and rides above the acromion (Fig. 25.2).

Management

All AC separations should be treated acutely with ice and a sling applied for immobilization. Further treatment is based on the severity of the injury.

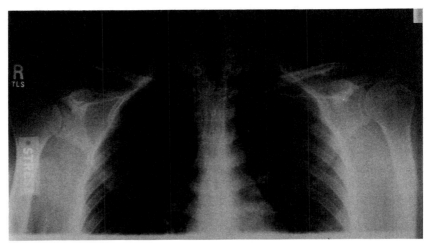

FIGURE 25.2. Stress roentgenogram showing a markedly displaced right distal clavicle indicative of a grade 3 acromioclavicular separation.

Athletes with grade 1 injuries begin shoulder strengthening when they are pain-free at rest, which is usually 2 to 7 days after injury. They may return to their sport when they have normal, pain-free range of motion. A grade 2 injury requires a somewhat longer period of immobilization, usually 10 to 14 days, before beginning strengthening exercises. Recovery usually takes 2 to 3 weeks. Considerable disagreement exists regarding operative versus nonoperative treatment of grade 3 AC separations.[10] Factors to consider include concomitant injuries, cosmetic result, and anticipated future use. An orthopedic surgeon should be involved in the care of any athlete with a grade 3 AC separation.

Knee Ligament Injuries: Anterior Cruciate Ligament

The anterior cruciate ligament (ACL) is the main AP stabilizer of the knee joint. Partial or complete tears of this ligament may be associated with tears of the lateral capsular ligament as well as avulsion fractures of the tibial plateau. The most common mechanism of injury for an ACL injury is a hyperextension deceleration force on the knee with or without rotation. This injury occurs during change of direction on an athletic field or landing after a rebound on the basketball court. A direct blow to the front of the knee or a lateral blow with rotation may also tear the ACL.

Diagnosis

The athlete may feel something snap or hear a loud "pop" following an ACL injury, and there is immediate pain and moderate-to-severe swelling within the first 2 hours after injury. The early onset of joint effusion, indicating a hemarthrosis, is highly suggestive of an ACL injury and is present 60% to 70% of the time.[11,12] Range of motion of the knee is markedly reduced, and there is generalized tenderness about the entire knee joint.

The best way to detect an ACL injury is the *Lachman test*[12]: With the hamstring muscles relaxed, the knee is placed in 15 degrees of flexion. With one hand on the femur just above the knee to stabilize it, the tibia is pulled forward with the opposite hand placed over the tibial tuberosity. If the ACL is intact, the tibia comes to a firm stop. If the ligament is torn, the tibia continues forward sluggishly as if attached to a rubber band. The *anterior drawer test* is similar to the Lachman test but is less reliable. If ligament testing is difficult because of a large joint effusion or the athlete's pain level, reexamination 7 to 10 days after injury is more reliable. A radiograph of the knee is necessary to rule out a tibial plateau fracture.

Management

Acute management of an ACL tear includes ice, elevating the knee to reduce swelling, and use of a knee immobilizer and crutches. Athletes with only mild laxity and a firm endpoint on ligament testing can usually be managed with a functional rehabilitation program. The rehabilitation program for ACL injuries emphasizes early return of motion and quadriceps and hamstring muscle strengthening and stretching.[13] Protective bracing during those activities that put high demands on knee stability may be appropriate for certain athletes. Athletes with marked joint laxity or complaints of giving away on twisting or pivoting motions should be referred to an orthopedic surgeon for possible arthroscopic repair.

Knee Ligament Injuries—Collateral Ligament Tear

The usual mechanism of injury of a collateral ligament tear of the knee is a valgus or varus stress applied to the knee with the foot planted. The injury usually occurs as a result of a direct blow to either the medial or lateral side of the joint, but it can also occur from a noncontact, twisting motion. Medical collateral ligament sprains are the most common knee injuries in downhill skiing.[14] The medial collateral ligament has two major components: the tibial collateral ligament and the medial capsular ligament. The medial capsular ligament is the deeper of the two, and injuries to it are associated with tears of the medial meniscus and the anterior cruciate ligament.

Diagnosis

Symptoms and physical examination findings for collateral ligament tears depend on the severity of the injury, as listed in Table 25.3. Physical

TABLE 25.3. Collateral ligament tear classification

Grade	Symptom	Examination
1	Pain on running, cutting Knee stable	Pain with stressing No instability
2	Immediate pain, swelling Knee feels unstable	Increased pain Unstable at 30 degrees Stable at 0 degrees
3	Severe pain, unable to walk Gross instability	Unstable at 0 degrees

examination tests for stability of the collateral ligaments are best performed on the uninjured knee first to establish what is "normal" for the athlete. To test the stability of the medial collateral ligament, with one hand above and one hand below the knee, apply a valgus stress to the knee in 30 degrees of flexion as well as maximal extension. Opening of the joint relative to the uninjured knee indicates at least partial instability. Instability at full extension is indicative of an associated anterior or posterior cruciate ligament tear. The stability test for the lateral collateral ligament is performed in a similar manner except that hand position is reversed and a varus stress is applied. In skeletally immature athletes with a suspected medial collateral ligament tear, stress films are necessary to rule out a femoral epiphyseal rupture.

Management

After an acute collateral ligament injury, the athlete should apply ice and elevate the knee to reduce swelling. A knee immobilizer and crutches are helpful until the patient can bear weight without pain. Early functional knee rehabilitation has been shown to be an effective treatment for grades 1 and 2 and some grade 3 collateral ligament sprains.[15] However, all grade 3 sprains should be referred to an orthopedist for consideration of surgery, especially if there are associated meniscal or cruciate ligament injuries. The rehabilitation program for collateral ligament injuries emphasizes quadriceps muscle strengthening and hamstring stretching. Varus and valgus stresses on the knee are best avoided until complete recovery has been achieved, usually within 4 to 6 weeks.

Meniscal Injuries

The medial or lateral meniscus of the knee can tear during a single traumatic event, or a more minor injury may occur after a degenerative process from overuse activities. Acute meniscal tears most often follow a twisting motion of the knee, usually when the athlete is running or cutting. Tears of the medial meniscus are twice as common as lateral tears and are one of the most common acute knee injuries.[12]

Diagnosis

The athlete with a meniscal tear complains of immediate knee pain. Joint line swelling often occurs within 12 to 24 hours after the injury. If the meniscal tear has displaced a fragment of cartilage into the joint, the athlete may complain of the knee locking in a flexed position or getting "stuck" during motion. On examination, a mild effusion may be present, and there is often joint line tenderness. The *McMurray test* is used to detect a meniscal tear. Begin with the knee in maximum flexion and the foot externally rotated (or internally rotated to detect a medial meniscus tear). While maintaining the rotation, bring the knee into full extension. A *painful* pop or click felt over the joint line indicates a positive test. This test has limited diagnostic sensitivity but may be an indication for further evaluation. Plain films are usually nondiagnostic during the evaluation of meniscal tears, but magnetic resonance imaging is helpful for delineating the location and extent of a meniscal tear.

Management

Ice, elevation, and knee immobilization are important during the first 24 to 48 hours after the acute injury. Weight-bearing should be avoided for the first few days or until pain and swelling are decreased. A suspected meniscal injury without an associated ligamentous injury causing instability can be managed initially with symptomatic treatment and knee rehabilitation. If there is no improvement with this regimen or it is crucial to get the athlete back to participation, arthroscopy should be considered for diagnosis and treatment. In the active athlete, most meniscal tears require arthroscopic repair. Partial meniscectomy, if possible, is preferable to complete meniscectomy because of the risk of degenerative changes.[16]

Patellar Dislocation and Subluxation

Complete, usually lateral displacement of the patella from the femoral groove constitutes a patellar dislocation. The dislocation results from a valgus or twisting force on the knee with contraction of the quadriceps muscles as occurs in a baseball swing or a sidestep cut. Subluxation (partial or transient displacement) of the patella may occur during everyday activities or as a result of much less force than is the case for a dislocation. Patellofemoral malalignment and imbalance in the medial and lateral quadriceps muscles are predisposing factors for patellar dislocation and subluxation.

Diagnosis

The athlete experiences immediate pain and a sensation of obvious malalignment of his or her knee after a dislocation. Usually the patella "goes out" with the knee in flexion and may "go back into place" when the knee is extended. Swelling usually occurs within the first 2 hours. Athletes with patellar subluxation may only feel a sensation of slipping or instability when twisting or pivoting on the knee. With chronic subluxation, mild recurrent swelling is often present. If the patella has already been reduced, a large effusion with hypermobility and marked apprehension on movement of the patella laterally is present. In athletes with subluxation, the apprehension test is positive in two-thirds of cases.[17] The uninjured knee should be examined carefully for any signs of predisposing conditions. With first-time dislocations especially, radiographs should be obtained, including an infrapatellar view to rule out an avulsion fracture of the medial patellar facet or the lateral femoral condyle.

Management

To reduce a dislocated patella, the hip is first flexed to relax the quadriceps muscles, and then the knee is gently extended while applying pressure along the lateral patellar edge. Reduction is usually accomplished without anesthesia, but if the patella has been dislocated for a long time with subsequent marked muscle spasm, local anesthesia around the patella or sedation of the athlete may be required. For first-time dislocations, improved healing occurs with immobilization for 4 to 6 weeks in full extension, followed by functional rehabilitation. Functional patellar braces may help alleviate knee pain secondary to patellar malalignment and instability, but controlled studies are needed to more specifically define indications for their use.[18] With recurrent dislocations or subluxations, a shorter period of immobilization can be used with even more emphasis placed on functional rehabilitation. Athletes with recurrent disabling subluxation should be referred to an orthopedic surgeon for possible extensor mechanism reconstructive surgery to improve patellofemoral biomechanics.

Ankle Sprains

Ankle sprains are one of the most common athletic injuries in any sport or athletic activity.[19] Eighty-five percent of all ankle sprains involve the lateral ligaments (anterior and posterior talofibular and calcaneofibular). Lateral sprains occur after an inversion injury often with the foot in some degree of plantar flexion. Medial ankle sprains or injury to the deltoid ligament result from eversion injuries, such as when a basketball player comes down from a rebound and steps on another player's foot.

Diagnosis

After a twisting injury of the ankle, the athlete experiences immediate pain, a sensation of a "pop," and decreased weight-bearing ability. The onset and degree of swelling present is related to the severity of the injury as well as how active the athlete is after the injury. The range of motion limitation and the athlete's weight-bearing ability after injury are useful guides to the severity of the injury. Weight-bearing can be tested simply by asking the athlete to stand on both feet, then stand on the injured foot alone, and finally raise up on the toes of the injured foot. Marked difficulty with these maneuvers indicates a more severe injury.

The degree of ligament laxity after an ankle sprain is tested using the anterior drawer and inversion stress tests. The *anterior drawer test* is performed by stabilizing the distal tibia and grasping the heel with the other hand and pulling forward. The ankle should be in a neutral position and the calf muscles relaxed to perform this test optimally. Significant forward translation of the ankle during this maneuver indicates laxity of the anterior talofibular ligament. The *inversion stress test* is performed by stabilizing the tibia with one hand, grasping the heel with the other hand, and inverting the foot. Excessive motion of the ankle with this maneuver indicates laxity of the calcaneofibular ligament. With any ankle sprain, it is important to palpate along the length of the tibia and fibula to detect associated fractures or disruption of the interosseous membrane. After ankle inversion, point tenderness at the base of the fifth metatarsal may indicate an avulsion fracture that results from disruption of the peroneus brevis muscle.

Ankle roentgenograms need not be obtained from all athletes with ankle sprains. Mild ankle sprains with only minimal swelling and pain and good weight-bearing ability do not require radiographic evaluation. AP, lateral, and mortise views of the ankle should be obtained for moderate-to-severe ankle sprains to rule out associated fractures or ankle instability as evidenced by widening of the ankle mortise.

Management

Early mobilization of ankle sprains has been shown to be an effective treatment for all injuries regardless of the severity.[20,21] A 24- to 48-hour period of ice, elevation, and rest followed by early weight-bearing and functional rehabilitation returns the athlete to his or her activity sooner and prevents loss of mobility or strength in the ankle. Ankle rehabilitation is essential for the prevention of chronic ankle instability after an acute sprain. An effective ankle rehabilitation program emphasizes range of motion, exercises to improve plantar flexion and dorsiflexion, and exercises to stretch and strengthen calf muscles. For the motivated or especially active athlete, a wobble board can be used for proprioception training.

Use of functional bracing such as a lace-up support or an Aircast brace may help athletes resume their usual activities sooner by preventing reinjury and providing increased stability of the ankle during the rehabilitation phase. Unless gross instability is present, immobilization of the ankle for longer than 7 to 10 days should be avoided to prevent muscle atrophy and loss of ankle motion.

Gamekeeper's (Skier's) Thumb

Gamekeeper's thumb or skier's thumb involves a sprain of the ulnar collateral ligament of the metacarpophalangeal (MCP) joint of the thumb. The mechanism of injury is a fall on an outstretched hand, causing forced abduction of the thumb such as occurs from a fall during skiing while holding a ski pole. This injury is also common in football, wrestling, and baseball.

Diagnosis

After this injury, pain is felt primarily over the MCP joint and is made worse by abducting or extending the thumb. Mild-to-moderate swelling and ecchymosis may be present; and pinch strength may be decreased, especially with grade 3 injuries. Point tenderness is noted over the ulnar aspect of the MCP joint. Radial stress applied to the MCP joint with the joint at 0 and 30 degrees of flexion tests the integrity of the ulnar collateral ligament. This examination may be difficult in the acute setting because of pain and swelling, and a digital block may be necessary to define the extent of the injury. A roentgenogram of the thumb is indicated in all patients with a significant thumb sprain before stressing the joint, since an associated avulsion fracture at the base of the proximal phalanx occurs in 20% of cases.

Management

Detecting the presence of a complete tear is essential to adequately treat thumb sprains. Complete tears of the ulnar collateral ligament, as demonstrated by marked laxity in full extension, require surgical repair in most cases.[22] Grade 1 and 2 thumb sprains are best treated with a thumb spica cast or splint protection for 4 to 6 weeks. Rehabilitation exercises are started at 3 to 4 weeks and consist of strengthening exercises of the forearm flexors, extensors, and the intrinsic muscles of the hand used for pinch and handgrip. A shorter period of immobilization may be used in athletes with only partial tears and no instability. During activity, the thumb can be protected by taping it to the index finger to prevent excessive abduction.

Overuse Syndromes

Most athletic injuries seen by family physicians are overuse injuries.[23] Overuse syndromes result from microtrauma to soft tissues secondary to repetitive motion or activity. Over time, this repetitive microtrauma causes a local inflammatory process, leading to pain and loss of function. Biomechanical factors such as malalignment or muscle imbalance, poor training techniques, and faulty equipment predispose the athlete to overuse injuries. Overuse syndromes most commonly involve the musculotendinous unit, resulting in tendinitis or tenosynovitis. Repetitive mechanical trauma to a joint may result in synovitis or arthritis, and repetitive overuse stress on bones results in periostitis or stress fractures. Overuse injuries are classified according to grades as listed in Table 25.4. Treatment plans for overuse injuries attempt to control inflammation and restore normal function and mobility. Complete rest from activity is rarely necessary. Modification of activity and an appropriate rehabilitation program are the hallmarks of successful treatment.

Shoulder Impingement Syndrome

Shoulder impingement syndrome, also known as swimmer's shoulder or rotator cuff tendinitis, is a painful arc syndrome caused by impingement of the supraspinatus and biceps tendon by the overlying coracoacromial ligament or anterior border of the acromium. After repetitive overhand

TABLE 25.4. Guide to overuse injuries

Grade	History	Physical examination	Treatment
1	Pain, usually hours after activity "Soreness"	Generalized tenderness	Ice
2	Pain late in activity or just after activity	Localized pain	Ice Decrease activity 25%
3	Pain early or in middle of activity	Point tenderness Erythema Swelling	Ice Decrease activity 50% NSAID
4	Pain at rest	Grade 3 signs plus decreased range of motion Impaired function	Ice Rest NSAID

NSAID = nonsteroidal antiinflammatory drug.

motion, the bursa interposed between the coracoacromial ligament and the underlying supraspinatus tendon wears out. The supraspinatus and biceps tendons are subjected to constant pressure from the head of the humerus, leading to degenerative changes and repeated microtrauma causing inflammation. It is most frequently seen in swimmers using freestyle, backstroke, or butterfly strokes but is also a common cause of shoulder pain in other athletes participating in overhead-use sports.

Diagnosis

The athlete with shoulder impingement complains of anterior shoulder pain radiating to the deltoid area. As many as 80% of swimmers experience significant shoulder pain at some time.[24] A "snapping" sensation at the overhand phase of the swimming stroke is also characteristic of impingement syndrome. Examination of the shoulder reveals point tenderness over the coracoacromial ligament. Pain elicited with either of the following maneuvers suggests shoulder impingement. With the arm at 90 degrees of forward flexion and the elbow at 90 degrees, internally rotate the shoulder to elicit pain. Forward flexion past 180 degrees with the forearm pronated causes pain at the anterior acromion if impingement is present.

Management

Control of inflammation with ice massage and nonsteroidal antiinflammatory drugs (NSAIDs) are useful when symptoms of impingement are most prominent. Modification of the swimmer's workout to include varying strokes, decreasing total yardage, or use of a kickboard helps decrease the stress placed on the shoulder. Rehabilitation exercises that emphasize stretching of the rotator cuff muscles and strengthening of internal and external rotators as well as weighted shoulder flexibility exercises to increase clearance under the coracoacromial arch help speed recovery.

Tennis Elbow

Lateral epicondylitis, better known as tennis elbow, is periostitis at the attachment of the extensor carpi radialis brevis tendon to the lateral epicondyle. Although fewer than 5% of patients with lateral epicondylitis actually play tennis, it is the most common overuse problem of tennis players. In addition to tennis, lateral epicondylitis is a common overuse syndrome with any activity that requires gripping. It is common in athletes with poor tennis stroke technique or who use a small grip size.

Diagnosis

Dull, aching lateral elbow pain, often more pronounced with the backhand stroke, is characteristic of tennis elbow. Swelling is uncommon, and rest from the offending activity usually relieves the symptoms. On examination, there is point tenderness over the lateral epicondyle, and pain is reproduced by shaking hands or extending the middle finger against resistance.

Management

Ice massage alternated with cross-fiber friction massage helps control inflammation. The ice reduces local edema, and the friction massage then promotes blood flow to the area, which helps wash out inflammatory cells. NSAIDs help control the pain and reduce the inflammation. Because the risk of tendon rupture after steroid injection in the lateral epicondyle area is low, this modality should be considered as a first-line treatment to control inflammation. Use of a counterforce brace placed just distal to the lateral epicondyle reduces the amount of friction over the epicondyle and diminishes pain.[25] Modification of the athlete's tennis game to include improved backhand technique and a slightly larger grip size are also useful for treating tennis elbow. After the athlete is pain-free, a rehabilitation program emphasizing stretching and strengthening of the forearm extensors and flexors can help prevent this problem from recurring.

Patellofemoral Pain Syndrome

Patellofemoral pain syndrome describes several conditions characterized by peripatellar pain. Patellofemoral pain is the most frequent knee problem seen in most running clinics and typically occurs in the recreational runner who is progressing (i.e., increasing mileage or speed in his or her training program).[26] The risk factors associated with running include excessive mileage, rapid change in the training routine, and improper running shoes. Patellofemoral pain may also be due to a biomechanical abnormality of the hips, knees, ankles, or feet. Leg length discrepancies, femoral anteversion, an increased Q angle (the angle formed by the intersection of the line of pull of the quadriceps and the patellar tendon), external tibial torsion, patella alta (high-riding patella), tight hamstring muscles, a poorly developed vastus medialis obliquus, and excessive pronation of the feet are conditions that may lead to patellofemoral pain syndrome.

Diagnosis

Athletes with patellofemoral pain syndrome complain of peripatellar aching soreness that is often worse when descending stairs, squatting, or kneeling. The pain may be aggravated after prolonged sitting with the knee in a flexed position, also known as the "movie sign." Depending on the severity of the condition, the pain may occur at any time during physical activity but typically comes on a few hours after activity and is relieved with rest. Examination of the athlete with patellofemoral pain syndrome begins with a search for factors that may predispose to this condition. With the athlete standing, inspect for an increased Q angle, patellar alignment, foot malalignment, or leg length discrepancy, each of which may aggravate symptoms. Examination of the knee joint may reveal tenderness of the medial or lateral patella with motion. Crepitus may be felt during flexion and extension of the knee but is a nonspecific finding. The athlete may experience pain with the *patellofemoral grinding test,* which is performed by displacing the patella distally with the hand and then asking the athlete to contract the quadriceps.[27] Effusion is not typical of patellofemoral pain syndrome, and in fact, examination of the knee can be normal despite the presence of continued symptoms. The tangential or "sunrise" radiographic view of the knee can confirm the presence of patellofemoral malalignment, if suspected clinically, but films of the knee are most often normal.

Management

Treatment of patellofemoral pain syndrome focuses on correction of any biomechanical abnormality combined with a functional rehabilitation program. Orthotics for foot malalignment and functional bracing for patellar malalignment help alleviate symptoms. Modification of activity to include decreased mileage or pace for the runner or avoidance of activities requiring excessive flexion are often useful therapies. The rehabilitation program for patellofemoral pain syndrome emphasizes hamstring stretching and quadriceps muscle strengthening.[28] Icing the knee before and after exercise and using NSAIDs allow a quicker return to activity.

Shin Splints

Shin splints is a commonly used but imprecise term to describe musculotendinous inflammation of the lower extremity related to myositis, periostitis, or fasciitis. It is a common overuse syndrome of runners, aerobic dance enthusiasts, and track and field athletes. Risk factors for the development of shin splints include a rapid increase in activity or running mileage, running on hard surfaces, excessive use of foot dorsiflexors, and faulty shoe wear.

Diagnosis

Athletes with shin splints complain of aching pain or discomfort in the leg during exercise or immediately after exercise depending on the severity. Anteromedial pain is common, and on examination there is often tenderness along the tibia that is made worse with active dorsiflexion. During examination of the athlete with shin splints, it is important to look for signs of lower extremity compartment syndrome, such as muscle weakness, paresthesias, decreased skin temperature, or slow capillary refill. The presence of point or percussion tenderness on the tibial shaft or localized swelling may indicate a more serious problem, such as a stress fracture.

Management

Treatment goals for shin splints focus on symptomatic relief and correction of the cause of the shin splints. Pre- and postactivity stretching of the lower extremity muscles, a decrease in intensity or duration of the activity, postactivity icing, and use of NSAIDs are helpful modalities for relieving symptoms. Use of proper foot wear, a change to a softer running surface, and modification of training schedule or switching to low-impact aerobics help the athlete to prevent recurrent problems with shin splints.

Plantar Fasciitis

Plantar fasciitis is inflammation of the plantar fascia at its insertion on the base of the calcaneus. It is the most common cause of heel pain in runners.[29] Predisposing factors for this condition are usually biomechanical, including flat feet, hyperpronation, and tight calf muscles. Athletes who resume a training program after time off from running or overweight athletes are at risk for developing plantar fasciitis.

Diagnosis

The pain associated with plantar fasciitis is usually localized to the base of the heel at the point of the insertion of the fascia into the calcaneus. The pain is worse in the morning and is sometimes relieved with activity. On examination, there is point tenderness just anterior to the calcaneus, and swelling and pain may extend along the medial arch in severe cases. Runners with plantar fasciitis often continue running until the condition progresses from an acute state to a chronic state, which is much more difficult to treat. The presence of a heel spur, seen on the foot roentgenogram, is indicative of a more chronic problem and is not a useful clue to the diagnosis or management of this condition.

Management

The goals of therapy for plantar fasciitis are to decrease acute inflammation and correct the underlying biomechanical problem. Ice massage, NSAIDs and decreased activity help alleviate inflammatory symptoms. Orthotics such as a heel pad or a plantar arch support may help athletes with hyperpronation or flat feet.[30] Proper shoe wear with excellent heel and arch support are necessary if this condition is to be prevented. Rehabilitation exercises for plantar fasciitis emphasize heel cord and calf muscle stretching and strengthening exercises for the soleus (heel lifts) and intrinsic muscles of the foot (lifting objects with the toes). It is useful to counsel the athlete to be patient with the rehabilitation program, as successful treatment of plantar fasciitis often takes up to 8 weeks.

References

1. McKeag DB, Hough DO, Berglund TB, Davenport MP. The role of the family physician in sports medicine. Phys Sports Med 1983;11:101–13.
2. Bailes JE, Maroon JC. Management of cervical spine injuries in athletes. Clin Sports Med 1989;8:43–58.
3. Vegso TT, Lehman RC. Field evaluation and management of head and neck injuries. Clin Sports Med 1987;6:1–15.
4. Cantu RC. When to return to contact sports after a cerebral concussion. Sports Med Dig 1988;10:1–2.
5. Kelly JP, Nichols JS, Filley CM, et al. Concussion in sports—guidelines for the prevention of catastrophic outcome. JAMA 1991;266:2867–9.
6. Mohtadi NG. Advances in the understanding of anterior instability of the shoulder. Clin Sports Med 1991;10:863–70.
7. Kulund DN. The injured athlete, 2nd ed. Philadelphia: Lippincott, 1988:331–2.
8. Aronen JC, Regan K. Decreasing the incidence of recurrence of first time anterior shoulder dislocations with rehabilitation. Am J Sports Med 1984;12:283–91.
9. Rowe CR, Zarins B. Recurrent transient subluxation of the shoulder. J Bone Joint Surg [Am] 1981;63:863–72.
10. Taft TN, Wilsen FC, Oglesby JW. Dislocation of the acromioclavicular joint. J Bone Joint Surg [Am] 1987;69:1045–51.
11. Noyes FR, Bassett RW, Grood ES, Butler DL. Arthroscopy in acute traumatic hemarthrosis of the knee: incidence of anterior cruciate tears and other injuries. J Bone Joint Surg [Am] 1980;62:687–95.
12. Jensen JE, Conn RR, Hazelrigg G, Hewett JE. Systematic evaluation of acute knee injuries. Clin Sports Med 1985;4:295–312.
13. Montgomery JB, Steadman JR. Rehabilitation of the injured knee. Clin Sports Med 1985;4:333–43.
14. Marshall JL, Johnson RJ. Mechanisms of the most common ski injuries. Phys Sports Med 1977;5:49–54.
15. Hastings DE. The non-operative management of collateral ligament injuries of the knee joint. Clin Orthop 1980;147:22–28.
16. Northmove-Ball MD, Dandy DJ, Jackson RW. Arthroscopic, open partial, and total meniscectomy: a comparative study. J Bone Joint Surg [Am] 1983;65:400–4.
17. Henry JH. Conservative treatment of patellofemoral subluxation. Clin Sports Med 1989;8:261–78.
18. Cherf J, Paulos LE. Bracing for patellar instability. Clin Sports Med 1990;9:813–21.
19. Mack RP. Ankle injuries in athletics. Clin Sports Med 1982;1:71–84.
20. Konradsen L, Holmer P, Sandergaard L. Early mobilizing treatment for grade III ankle ligament injuries. Foot Ankle 1992;12:69–73.

21. Linde F, Huass I, Furgensen V, Madsen F. Early mobilizing treatment in lateral ankle sprains. Scand J Rehabil Med 1986;18:17–21.
22. Kahler DM, McLue FC. Metacarpophalangeal and proximal interphalangeal joint injuries of the hand, including the thumb. Clin Sports Med 1992;11: 57–76.
23. McKeag DB. The concept of overuse—the primary care aspects of overuse syndromes in sports. Prim Care 1984;11:43–59.
24. Johnson JE, Sim FH, Scott SG. Musculoskeletal injuries in competitive swimmers. Mayo Clin Proc 1987;62:289–304.
25. Nirschl RP. Soft-tissue injuries about the elbow. Clin Sports Med 1986;5: 637–52.
26. Clement DB, Taunton JE, Smart GM, McNicol KL. A survey of overuse running injuries. Phys Sports Med 1981;9:47–58.
27. Hoppenfeld S. Physical examination of the knee joint by complaint. Orthop Clin North Am 1979;10:3–20.
28. Brunet ME, Stewart GW. Patellofemoral rehabilitation. Clin Sports Med 1989;8:319–29.
29. Bazzoli AS, Pollina FS. Heel pain in recreational runners. Phys Sports Med 1989;17:55–61.
30. Newell SG, Miller SJ. Conservative treatment of plantar fascial strain. Phys Sports Med 1977;5:68–73.

CASE PRESENTATION

Subjective

PATIENT PROFILE

Kendra Nelson is a 16-year-old white female high school sophomore.

PRESENTING PROBLEM

"Ankle injury."

PRESENT ILLNESS

Three hours ago, Kendra twisted her left ankle while playing basketball in the high school gym. She noted immediate pain and swelling, and she can bear almost no weight on the ankle.

PAST MEDICAL HISTORY

Kendra had a similar ankle sprain about 4 months ago.

SOCIAL HISTORY, HABITS, FAMILY HISTORY

These are unchanged since her last office visit for viral influenza 7 months ago (see Chapter 10).

- What additional history regarding the injury might be helpful?
- How might today's problem relate to the injury 4 months ago?
- What might be significant regarding the immediate care provided at the school?
- What might be the meaning of this injury to Kendra? How would you inquire about this?

Objective

GENERAL

The patient hops, rather than walks, to the examination room using the left lower extremity only for balance.

VITAL SIGNS

Blood pressure, 102/64; pulse, 74.

EXAMINATION

The left ankle is swollen and ecchymotic. It is tender laterally, and there is limited range of motion. The dorsalis pedis pulse is normal.

LABORATORY

An office x-ray with routine views of the ankle reveals soft tissue injury with swelling most prominent laterally. There are no bony abnormalities, and the ankle mortise is intact.

- What more would you include in the physical examination?
- What would be evidence on physical examination to help differentiate between soft tissue injury and fracture?
- Have you seen other patients with similar findings? If so, what was the diagnostic assessment and outcome of therapy?
- What are possible complications of this injury, and how would you examine for these?

Assessment

- Based on the findings described above, what is your diagnosis? How would you explain this to Kendra?
- Describe the tissue and pathologic changes involved in this injury.
- What are the implications of this injury for the family and the school?
- If the ankle mortise seemed unstable, what would you do differently?

Plan

- What would be your therapy of this injury? How would you explain your plan to Kendra and her parents?
- Kendra asks about weight-bearing, return to school, and participation in sports. What would you advise?
- What should you tell the school about the injury? How will you communicate this information?
- What follow-up would you advise?

26

Occupational Hazards

GEOFFREY GOLDSMITH, SANDRA B. NICHOLS, AND
HENRY F. SIMMONS

Unraveling the nature of occupational exposures requires a collaborative undertaking that involves the physician, patient, and often the employer. At times, regulatory agencies such as the Occupational Safety and Health Administration (OSHA) are involved in determining the offending occupational agent and preventing future exposures.

Clinical Approach to Patients Exposed to Occupational Hazards

Patient History

A sample occupational history appears in Figure 26.1. A 2-week symptom diary is recommended to correlate workplace exposures and the onset, duration, intensity, aggravation, and alleviation of the patient's signs and symptoms.

Clues to the work relatedness of the illness may be that the symptoms become worse during or at the end of the day and are better on the weekend. Symptoms may clear during holidays only to return by the first or second day of work. Several months of exposure may occur before a patient is sensitized to a chemical at work, although irritants can generate symptoms within minutes of exposure. Furthermore, the work conditions change periodically at the workplace. Ventilation systems may fail and periodically expose employees to higher levels of irritants or toxins. Cold weather may necessitate shutting a window, which can lead to a significant increase in airborne levels of chemicals resulting in respiratory complaints. Thus the clinician should ask the patient about specific patterns to the symptoms that parallel changes in the workplace environment.

Some patients provide the physician an exact name of the suspected offending chemical and even an information sheet (material safety data sheet, or MSDS) that describes the toxicology of a particular chemical.

Even when the type of chemical exposure is clear, the physician must determine the severity of exposure, which is a function of the chemical's toxicity, the amount of time the worker is in contact with the chemical agent, the dose of exposure and the time exposed. The patient should be asked about the use of protective equipment at work (gloves, aprons, masks, hearing protectors) that would lessen the effective "dose" of chemical that enters the body.

The patient's past medical problems, medications, habits, and hobbies are critical elements of the occupational history. Each of these factors may point to the patient's increased susceptibility to workplace irritants or allergens, or they may point to preexisting medical conditions that may mimic workplace-related disorders. For example, asthma symptoms could be due to occupational asthma or a flare-up of intrinsic asthma. It is well known that cigarette smoking adds to the risk of respiratory disease; therefore, a smoking history is important to determine in patients suspected of occupationally induced lung disease.

Workplace Database

After a thorough medical history, the nature of the occupational environment is quantified. The "workplace history" involves an intensive review of the industrial processes and procedures to which the patient is exposed.

Most employers are required to maintain a log (OSHA Form 200) of work time lost to injuries and illnesses. These data can assist the clinician to identify whether the patient is suffering from a disorder similar to that experienced by coworkers. Occupational diseases sometimes become obvious only when viewing the signs and symptoms in terms of the larger group of coworkers rather than on an individual patient basis. If coworkers are similarly affected, the possibility is increased that the patient's complaints are work-related.

The physician should request a copy of the log. The employer may be hesitant to provide it; but if the clinician believes that it contains essential information he or she may wish to contact the union or the plant manager to explain the rationale for reviewing these records (Table 26.1).

Physicians may demand access to the names of the chemicals at the patient's workplace. Federal law requires that the employer who uses, produces, or distributes hazardous chemicals must maintain information sheets (MSDS) on all the workplace chemicals to which employees are exposed and make this information available to the treating physician.

The patient's complaints may relate to nonchemical exposures, for example, excessive noising, radiation, repetitive motion, heat, or cold. The physician should review the worker's job activities with both the patient and the patient's supervisor.

PATIENT I.D.

Age:

Sex:

Race:

I. Patient symptoms: Note changes in patient symptoms over time

1. Diagram: onset (x), severity (0–5), and duration (2-week symptom log).

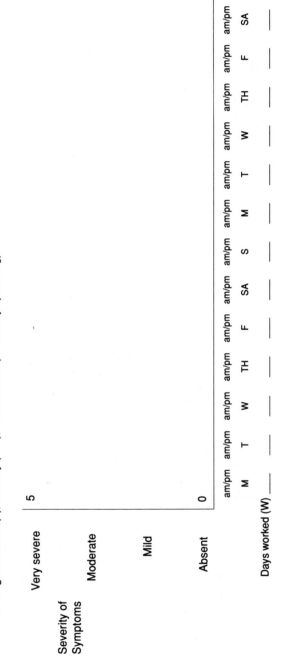

RECORD

Note changes at work (new
responsibilities, processes, A-C/heat protection). _____

_____

_____

2. Current work duties (describe day-to-day duties). _____

_____

3. Work history.

	Years worked	Description of job	Exposures, illness, injury
This position			
Prior position			
Prior position			
Prior position			

Figure 26.1. Occupational history record.

4. Current workplace exposures (biologic, noise, chemicals, radiation, psychological, heat/cold, repetitive movement). _____

5. Personal protection used on job. _____

6. How often is protective equipment used? _____

7. Other workers affected with similar complaints? _____

8. Family members with similar complaints? _____

9. Past medical history (especially systems review related to current complaints). _____

10. Past sensitivities to workplace processes. _____

11. Exposed to "spill" at work? _____

12. Family member(s) being exposed to chemicals? _____

13. Neighborhood exposures? _____

14. Hobbies and habits (avocational exposures)? _____
    a. Cigarettes? _____
    b. Alcohol? _____
    c. Painting, woodworking, other hobbies? _____

15. Allergies. _____

16. Medications. _____

II. Workplace factors

A. Identifying data
   1. Company name _____
   2. Supervisor name _____
     Telephone no. _____
   3. Company industrial hygienist _____
     Telephone no. _____
   4. Company nurse _____
     Telephone no. _____
   5. Union _____
     Telephone no. _____
   6. Company safety representative _____
     Telephone no. _____

B. Products, processes, and exposures
   7. Company products and processes _____
   8. Potential exposures (quantify) _____
   9. Health records/safety data _____

TABLE 26.1. Sources of information to assist in
clinical exposure cases

Employer
　Safety committee
　Plant manager
　Toxicologist or industrial hygienist

Union
　Union safety committee
　National urban office

State
　State OSHA office
　Department of Labor
　Department of Agriculture

Medical library
　Reference librarian assistance for Toxline, Chemline, Cancer
　　and Occupational Hazard Databases

Hospital
　Poison control center

Federal agencies
　National Institute for Occupational Safety and Health (NIOSH)
　Federal OSHA office—Technical Data Center
　　Office of Toxic Substances

Private agencies
　American Industrial Hygiene Association
　National Safety Council

Requesting Assistance from OSHA

Physicians can request a worksite visit by the local OSHA office to assist in analyzing potential exposures. Such requests are not taken lightly by OSHA or the employer. Many employment sites, however, do not have the resources to maintain an industrial hygienist or safety staff and welcome an OSHA visit. There may be delays between the physician's request and the time that an OSHA workplace visit is conducted because of the heavy workload of the OSHA inspectors. Some employers may not accept the physician's recommendations or be unable to do so because of financial or business reasons. The clinician is not empowered to force the employer to make specific changes to remedy the situation. The local OSHA office is valuable when the employer disagrees with the physician about the need for workplace changes. The OSHA staff can visit employers on an "invited"-by-employer basis without giving citations, although OSHA does have the authority to visit and cite employers for violations of the OSHA law.

Laboratory Assessment

There are no standard laboratory profiles for a patient who has been exposed to industrial chemicals. The laboratory evaluation is related to the toxicology of the specific chemical agent. Often the services of a regional toxicology laboratory is required to perform the specialized tests that relate to the chemical exposure. It is important that the clinician fastidiously follow the recommendations for specimen collection and shipping. This point is critical given the low levels of toxins one is trying to detect in some occupation-related exposures. For example, use of a standard specimen bottle may introduce an unacceptable level of contaminants when attempting to measure trace levels of pesticide in a fat sample.

Prevention

Prevention is the principal goal of occupational medicine. The clinician may request that the workplace change its manufacturing process, consider substituting other chemicals, improve ventilation, or have a stronger compliance program for employees using protective equipment. The physician's duty to the patient includes more than diagnosis and treatment. The physician advises the patient on personal hygiene, health surveillance, and legal rights under OSHA or Worker's Compensation laws.

Solvents

By definition, a solvent is a substance that dissolves another material. A diverse array of chemicals, ranging from water to complex organic molecules, serve as solvents. Accordingly, there are few workplaces involved in industrial processes that are entirely free of these agents. However, solvents find their widest application as cleaners, degreasers, paint bases, and adhesive components. As the quantities and types of solvents vary from site to site, so does the opportunity for exposure, absorption, and intoxication. When one considers that about 9.8 million workers are exposed annually to solvents in the United States, the health consequences are obvious.[1]

Widely used solvents include aromatic and aliphatic hydrocarbons, ketones, and various halocarbons. The hydrocarbons and ketones include such entities as *n*-hexane, methyl-*n*-butyl ketone, benzene, toluene, and xylenes; the halocarbons encompass such chlorocarbons as methylene chloride, trichloroethane, trichlorethylene, and perchlorethylene.

Many of these chemicals are readily volatile at atmospheric pressure and ambient temperatures, which makes them an inhalation risk. Furthermore, many penetrate the intact skin, providing additional opportunities for intoxication. After absorption, some are excreted unchanged, whereas others are metabolized to reactive intermediates that have special toxicities, such as that of benzene on bone marrow.[2]

Diagnosis and Treatment

The various kinds of toxicity fall into broad categories, which include possible damage to the kidneys, liver, skin, mucous membranes, lungs, and nervous system. For example, the halocarbons share the capacity to injure both the liver and the kidneys. They also have the potential to sensitize the myocardium to circulating catecholamines and may therefore be arrhythmogenic in the setting of acute intoxication. Also, all the agents can cause defatting dermatitis, a mild inflammatory process arising from the leaching of fat from the skin after prolonged contact. Most of them can also irritate the eye and upper airway mucosa. Although ingestions pose an additional aspiration risk, which varies with the viscosity of the involved chemical, they do not commonly occur in the industrial setting. Finally, all the solvents are potentially neurotoxic.[3]

Three basic categories of solvent neurotoxicity occur. The first is central nervous system (CNS) depression, which is identical to that associated with the lipophilic general anesthetics. It is a property of most of the hydrocarbon and halocarbon solvents. The second category is a complex of poorly defined neuropsychiatric complaints that have been associated with prolonged exposures to solvents. Typical examples include claims of impaired mentation and depression. The third is a peripheral neuropathy that is unique to solvents such as n-hexane and methyl-n-butyl ketone. The injury is likely attributable to the generation of metabolites that directly damage peripheral neurons by reacting with their chemical components.

Workers who experience brief exposures to large concentrations of airborne solvents may complain of nothing more than nonspecific headache and dizziness. However, frank inebriation manifested as ataxia, slurred speech, and poor judgment resembling ethanol intoxication may ensue. If sufficient amounts of the substances have been absorbed, profound coma with respiratory suppression and hypotension appears.

A diagnosis of acute solvent intoxication should be considered in patients with either nonspecific complaints (e.g., dizziness) or altered mental status after work in a contaminated atmosphere. If an individual requires stabilization of vital signs after removal from the contaminated area, standard Advanced Cardiac Life Support (ACLS) techniques are appropriate. Epinephrine should be avoided whenever possible owing to the propensity of some solvents to enhance development of catecholamine-induced arrhythmias. Once life-threatening problems have been resolved, hepatic and renal function should be assessed. Determining serum levels of solvents or their metabolites is of no value in the management of acute intoxication. The consequences of secondary hypoxic encephalopathy and protracted hypotension that may accompany severe intoxication are complex management problems. Supportive care remains the mainstay of therapy.[4]

Prolonged contact with lesser concentrations of many solvents has been suggested to be the cause of assorted neuropsychiatric dysfunctions.[5] Typical complaints include fatigue, memory disturbance, irritability, and depression. A conclusive causal relation is difficult to demonstrate, as the signs and symptoms are not specific. Furthermore, even when neuropsychiatric testing is abnormal, comparable preexposure data are seldom available. When evaluating such patients, it is important to assess the premorbid psychiatric status and to search for other causes of the symptoms, such as substance abuse or functional illness.

Solvent-associated peripheral neuropathy has been observed after chemical abuse (e.g., glue sniffing) and as a consequence of industrial exposure. When *n*-hexane is involved, the polyneuropathy may partially or totally disappear within months to years after exposure.[6] Another solvent that has been implicated is methyl-*n*-butyl ketone, which shares the metabolite, 2,5-hexanedione, a classic neurotoxicant, with hexane. Methylethyl ketone (which is not itself a cause of peripheral neuropathy) apparently potentiates the effects of methyl-*n*-butyl ketone and *n*-hexane.[7] There is no specific therapy for these syndromes. Affected workers simply must avoid ongoing exposure.

Prevention

The prevention of solvent-associated diseases is best accomplished by strict industrial monitoring of workplace concentrations, ensuring adequate ventilation, and where high-level exposure is unavoidable through the use of an appropriate respirator. An additional option includes the episodic measurement of urinary metabolites, which are associated with some of the solvents as indexes of exposure. Finally, periodic physical examinations should include questionnaires to elicit neuropsychiatric complaints and blood work to assess liver and kidney function.

Regulation

The use of solvents in the workplace is closely regulated by various federal agencies, such as OSHA. Limitations have been placed on the concentrations that are acceptable for both short exposures and for a 40-hour, 5-day work week. Although the levels do offer protection to most workers exposed, there are individuals with hypersensitivity to the toxic effects of the solvents who may not tolerate these levels.

Organophosphates

The organophosphates (insecticides) are readily absorbed after gastrointestinal, conjunctival, dermal, or inhalational exposure. The interval between exposure and onset of symptoms varies with the chemical route of entry and degree of exposure. Symptoms almost always occur within 24 hours. Onset of symptoms is most rapid after inhalational exposure and slowest with dermal contact, although a skin lesion may accelerate dermal absorption.

The organophosphate insecticides are highly toxic chemicals. They act by covalently binding to cholinesterases. Acetylcholine is the most important chemical transmitter at synaptic junctions. Acetylcholinesterase breaks down acetylcholine. The toxicologic effects of the organophosphates are due to the inhibition of acetylcholinesterase in the nervous system, resulting in the accumulation of acetylcholine at synapses and myoneural junctions. The overabundance of acetylcholine initially excites and/or paralyzes transmission in cholinergic synapses, which include (1) the CNS; (2) the parasympathetic nerve endings, such as in sweat glands (muscarinic effect); and (3) the motor nerves and ganglionic fibers of autonomic ganglia (variable effect). The signs and symptoms of organophosphate poisoning are thus expressions of these three effects caused by excess acetylcholine.[8]

Signs and Symptoms of Poisoning

Diagnosis is based on a history of acute exposure and the presence of CNS nicotinic and muscarinic manifestations. The breath often has a garlic-like odor. The most commonly reported early symptoms are headache, nausea, and dizziness. Anxiety and restlessness are prominent. As the poisoned state worsens, it manifests as muscle twitching, weakness, tremors, excessive salivation, miosis, lacrimation, and weakness. The development of ataxia, confusion psychosis, convulsion, paralysis, pulmonary edema, bradycardia, or cardiac arrhythmia indicates severe poisoning, and aggressive emergency management must be initiated.

Laboratory Assessment

Laboratory data may be used to confirm the diagnosis. If there are strong clinical indications of acute organophosphate poisoning, treat patient immediately—do not wait for laboratory confirmation. Laboratory confirmation may be obtained by measuring decreases in the plasma pseudocholinesterases (PChE) and red blood cell acetycholinesterase (AChE) activities.

The PChE activity is a sensitive indicator of exposure but is not as reliable as AChE activity. PChE can be depressed secondary to medical illness or chronic organophosphate exposure. The AChE activity provides a more reliable measure of the acute toxic effect of organophosphate. A 25% or greater depression in activity from baseline generally indicates true exposure. Other useful laboratory tests are electrolytes; complete blood count; glucose, creatinine, and liver enzyme levels; arterial blood gases; electrocardiogram; and chest roentgenogram.[9]

Emergency Treatment

The emergency team should avoid direct contact with the heavily contaminated clothing and vomitus; they should always wear gloves and remove all the patient's clothing as rapidly as possible. The following steps are then followed.

1. Initiate acute life support.
2. Evaluate the airway, breathing, and circulatory status, and stabilize.
3. Clear and maintain the airway; assist ventilation if necessary.
4. Pay careful attention to respiratory muscle weakness and observe for sudden respiratory arrest.
5. Document level of consciousness and determine if the patient needs glucose, thiamine, and naloxone because of the possibility of other reasons for altered consciousness.
6. Observe the patient 6 to 8 hours to rule out delayed-onset symptoms resulting from skin absorption or fat storage.
7. Contact the regional poison control center for more specifics.

Specific Drugs and Antidotes

Specific treatment includes the antimuscarinic agent atropine and the enzyme reactivator pralidoxime. Atropine is a physiologic antidote for organophosphate poisoning. It should be initiated immediately on clinical suspension of organophosphate poisoning.

When treating *adults,* give atropine 0.5 to 2.0 mg IV. Repeat every 5 to 15 minutes until there is satisfactory drying of bronchial secretions and decreased wheezing. For severe poisonings, several grams of atropine may be required. If patients do not respond after 3 to 4 mg of atropine, they probably will not benefit from higher doses unless bradycardia is caused by excessive cholinergic input. Atropinization is maintained by repeated doses for 2 to 12 hours or longer depending on the severity of the poisoning.

When treating *children,* give atropine 0.02 to 0.05 mg/kg IV. Repeat every 5 to 10 minutes until satisfactory atropinization is achieved or until a maximum dose of 0.5 mg has been given.

Pralidoxime (2-PAM) acts to regenerate the enzyme activity. It displaces the covalently bonded organophosphate. The drug should be given as soon as the patient has been stabilized with acute life support and atropine and after blood has been obtained for the red blood cell AChE assay. Administer 2-PAM AChE reactivator in cases of severe poisoning by organophosphate pesticides in which respiratory depression, muscle weakness, and twitching are severe. When administered early (usually 48 hours after poisoning), pralidoxime relieves the nicotinic, muscarinic, and CNS effects of organophosphate poisoning. It should be given immediately. Adults are given 1 to 2 g IV slowly. Children are given 25 to 50 mg/kg IV slowly (maximum, 1 g). The dose may be repeated every 6 to 8 hours to control muscular weakness and fasciculation. 2-PAM is most effective if started within the first 24 hours after the exposure.

To decontaminate a patient, remove all contaminated clothing and wash the exposed area, including hair and nails, with copious amounts of soap and water. Take extreme care not to contaminate yourself. Contaminated clothing should be discarded. Do not induce emesis because of the danger of respiratory arrest or seizures. Perform gastric lavage, protecting the airway with a cuffed endotracheal tube if the patient is obtunded. Instill activated charcoal and sorbitol in an aqueous slurry. Monitor the cardiac and pulmonary status closely. The patient may require 5 to 14 days of hospitalization. Continued monitoring of glucose and cholinesterase is essential.

Carbamate

Carbamate insecticides are less toxic than the organophosphates. They have a broad spectrum of uses as agricultural and household garden insecticides. Like organophosphates, carbamates inhibit AChE enzyme, which allows excessive accumulation of acetylcholine at muscarinic, nicotinic, and CNS receptors. The carbamates are absorbed by all routes, including inhalation, ingestion, and dermal absorption.[10]

Carbamates are not highly lipophilic and do not cause delayed or persistent toxicity. The 1990 Annual Report of the American Association of Poison Control Centers (AAPCC) National Data Collection System noted 5263 exposures to carbamate insecticides with 1084 patients treated at a health care facility; there was one death. Although the carbamate insecticide is a cholinesterase inhibitor, it is considered reversible. The clinical syndrome is more benign and of much shorter duration than that caused by the organophosphates. The carbamates penetrate the CNS poorly, and so convulsions are uncommon.

Signs and Symptoms of Poisoning

The signs and symptoms of cholinergic excess usually occur within 30 minutes but may not develop until 1 to 2 hours after exposure. Malaise, muscle weakness, dizziness, and sweating are commonly reported as early symptoms of poisoning. Miosis, dyspnea, bronchospasm, headache, and salivation have also been reported. Severe neurologic sequelae including convulsion are less common than with organophosphate poisoning.

Laboratory Findings

Serum and red blood cell cholinesterase values are not reliable unless a substantial amount of N-methylcarbamate has been absorbed. Absorption of some N-methylcarbamates can be confirmed by analysis of urine for their unique metabolites. Use clinical judgment to diagnose and treat this poisoning.

Emergency Treatment

Initiate ACLS by maintaining the airway and assist ventilation if necessary. Observe the patient for 4 to 6 hours after exposure. A few patients require prolonged observation. Administer atropine 0.5 to 2.0 mg IV. Repeat every 5 to 10 minutes until manifestations of cholinergic input are reversed (i.e., decreased bradycardia, bronchorrhea, and wheezing). 2-PAM is not recommended; it is thought to be contraindicated for carbaryl poisonings, as it may reduce the antidotal effect of atropine. When a physician is faced with a critically ill patient exhibiting signs and symptoms of cholinesterase inhibition, either from an unknown insecticide or a combination organophosphate and carbamate exposure, several authors have noted that a trial with 2-PAM is clearly indicated.[8–10]

Pyrethrum and Pyrethrins

Pyrethrum and pyrethin products are widely used insecticides of biologic origin. They incite dermal and respiratory allergies, which are thought to be exacerbated by the noninsecticidal ingredients. Acute human poisoning is rare. The 1990 Annual Report of the AAPCC National Data Collection System reported 4354 exposures to pyrethrins alone, with 1314 patients treated at a health care facility and no deaths. About 50% of the patients who are sensitive to ragweed exhibit a cross reaction to pyrethrum. The refined pyrethrins are probably less allergenic but appear to retain some sensitized properties.[11,12]

There are more than 2000 products containing pyrethrum and its related compounds. Pyrethrums are derived from flowers of the chrysanthemum. The six active chemicals in pyrethrum are known collectively as the pyrethrins. Synthetic derivatives of the pyrethrins are known as the pyrethroids.

Signs and Symptoms of Poisoning

Toxicity to humans is primarily associated with hypersensitivity reactions and direct irritant effect. Anaphylaxis has occurred, as has asthma, acute rhinitis, dermatitis, pneumonitis, and shock. Pyrethrums are absorbed by inhalation or ingestion. Inhalation of these compounds may precipitate wheezing in asthmatics. Inhalation or pulmonary aspiration may also cause a hypersensitivity pneumonitis. Ingestion by massive oral doses may affect the CNS, resulting in seizures, coma, or respiratory arrest. Anaphylactic reactions including bronchospasm, oropharyngeal edema, and shock may occur in hypersensitive individuals.

Laboratory Assessment

There are no laboratory tests that are specific for identifying these compounds. Other useful laboratory studies are arterial blood gases, chest roentgenograms, and pulmonary function tests.

Emergency Treatment

ACLS is initiated if indicated. In most cases, antihistamines effectively control most hypersensitivity reactions. If severe asthma, oropharyngeal edema, or shock occurs, the patient may require epinephrine, theophylline, bronchodilators, or corticosteroids. If the patient has ingested a large amount of pyrethrin substance, it may be necessary to empty the stomach by intubation and perform lavage with activated charcoal and a cathartic. Aggressive decontamination of skin and eyes with soap and water (skin) is suggested.

References

1. Organic solvents in the workplace. MMWR 1987;36:282–3.
2. Barceloux, DG. Halogenated solvents. In: Sullivan JB, Krieger GR, editors. Hazardous materials toxicology: clinical principles of environmental health. Baltimore: Williams & Wilkins, 1992:732–47.
3. Gerarde HW. Toxicological studies on hydrocarbons. IX. The aspiration hazard and toxicity of hydrocarbons and hydrocarbon mixtures. Arch Environ Health 1963;6:35–47.
4. Goldfrank LR, Kulberg AG, Bresnitz EA. Hydrocarbons. In: Goldfrank LR, Flomenbaum NE, Lewin NA, et al., editors. Goldfrank's toxicologic emergencies. Norwalk, CT: Appleton & Lange, 1990:759–68.
5. Spencer PS, Schaumburg HH. Organic solvent neurotoxicity—facts and research needs. Scand J Work Environ Health 1985;1(Suppl 11):53–60.
6. Arlien-Sorborg P. n-Hexane. In: Solvent neurotoxicity. Boca Raton, FL: CRC Press, 1992:178.

7. Ralston WH, Hilderbrand RL, Uddi DE, et al. Potentiation of 2,5-hexane-dione neurotoxicity by methyl ethyl ketone. Toxicol Appl Pharmacol 1985;81:319–27.
8. Haddad L, Winchester J. Clinical management of poisoning and drug overdose, 2nd ed. Philadelphia: Saunders, 1990:1076–103.
9. Olson K. Poisoning and drug overdose. Norwalk, CT: Appleton & Lange, 1990.
10. Zwiener RJ, Ginsburg CM. Organophosphate and carbamate poisoning in infants and children. Pediatrics 1988;81:121–6.
11. Recognition and management of pesticide poisons, 4th ed. Washington, DC: Environmental Protection Agency, 1989.
12. Litovitz TL, Schmitz BF, Holm KC, Klein-Schwantz W. 1990 Annual Report of the American Association of Poison Control Data Centers National Data Collection System. Am J Emerg Med 1991;9:461–509.

CASE PRESENTATION

Subjective

PATIENT PROFILE

Samuel Nelson is a 48-year-old single white male farm worker.

PRESENTING PROBLEM

"Weak and shaky."

PRESENT ILLNESS

Samuel Nelson is brought to the office by his employer who owns a local orchard and who reports that Samuel had spent the morning driving a sprayer through the orchard rows. Toward the end of the morning—a half-hour ago—Samuel was noted to be weak, restless, and slightly confused. He was brought immediately to the physician's office.

PAST MEDICAL HISTORY

A record review reveals that Mr. Nelson is a heavy smoker and has had chronic obstructive pulmonary disease for more than 5 years. He had pneumonia treated as an outpatient 3 years ago.

SOCIAL HISTORY, HABITS, FAMILY HISTORY

These were recorded at his last visit about 7 months ago (see Chapter 13), and no additional information is available at this time.

- What additional data might help clarify what has happened to this patient?
- What are some common chemicals to which farm workers are exposed, and how would you inquire about these?
- How could you help clarify the patient's mental status?
- What are diagnostic possibilities, other than occupational exposure to chemicals, that might explain these symptoms? How might you elicit information about these possibilities?

Objective

VITAL SIGNS

Blood pressure, 150/100; pulse, 82; respirations, 26; temperature, 37.2°C.

EXAMINATION

The patient is lying on the examination table, apparently restless and tremulous. There is a faint garlic-like odor to the breath. The pupils of both eyes appear constricted. There is copious lacrimation and salivation. The neck is supple and the skin is moist. The chest shows an increased AP diameter with distant breath sounds and scattered bronchi at both bases. The heart has a regular sinus rhythm without murmurs. The abdominal muscles appear somewhat tight.

- What more—if anything—would you include in the physical examination? Why?
- What is the significance of the physical findings described?
- What—if any—laboratory tests should be obtained at this time?
- What are the possible risks to health care providers? Describe precautions that should be taken by the physician and staff when examining and treating this patient.

Assessment

- What is the apparent cause of the patient's acute problem? Describe the pathophysiology.
- What are the possible implications of this preexisting chronic obstructive pulmonary disease?
- What are the immediate risks to the patient?
- Describe the workplace implications of this problem. What is the personal physician's role?

Plan

- What should be your immediate therapy?
- What would you do next? Office observation? Consultation? Hospitalization? Describe your role if the patient is hospitalized.
- What are the workers' compensation implications of this event?
- What follow-up would you advise?

Index